STUDY GUIDE FOR
Lewis's

Medical-Surgical Nursing

Assessment and Management
of Clinical Problems

STUDY GUIDE FOR
Lewis's
Medical-Surgical Nursing
Assessment and Management of Clinical Problems

Twelfth Edition

Mariann M. Harding, PhD, RN, CNE, FAADN
Professor of Nursing
Kent State University Tuscarawas
New Philadelphia, Ohio

Jeffrey Kwong, RN, DNP, MPH, ANP-BC, FAANP, FAAN
Professor
Division of Advanced Nursing Practice, School of Nursing
Rutgers University
Newark, New Jersey

Debra Hagler, PhD, RN, ACNS-BC, CNE, CHSE,
    ANEF, FAAN
Clinical Professor
Edson College of Nursing and Health Innovation
Arizona State University
Phoenix, Arizona

Courtney Reinisch, RN, DNP, FNP-BC
Associate Professor
School of Nursing
Montclair State University
Montclair, New Jersey

Prepared By

Collin Bowman-Woodall, MSN, RN
Assistant Clinical Professor
UCSF School of Nursing
San Francisco, California

ELSEVIER

Elsevier
3251 Riverport Lane
St. Louis, Missouri 63043

STUDY GUIDE FOR LEWIS'S MEDICAL-SURGICAL NURSING, TWELFTH EDITION   ISBN: 978-0323792387

Notice

Practitioners and researchers must always rely on their own experience and knowledge in evaluating and using any information, methods, compounds or experiments described herein. Because of rapid advances in the medical sciences, in particular, independent verification of diagnoses and drug dosages should be made. To the fullest extent of the law, no responsibility is assumed by Elsevier, authors, editors or contributors for any injury and/or damage to persons or property as a matter of products liability, negligence or otherwise, or from any use or operation of any methods, products, instructions, or ideas contained in the material herein.

Previous editions copyrighted 2020, 2017, 2014, 2011, 2007, 2004, 2000, 1996, 1992, 1987, and 1983 by Mosby, Inc., an affiliate of Elsevier Inc.

Executive Content Strategist: Henderson Lee
Content Development Specialist: Rebecca Leenhouts
Publishing Services Manager: Deepthi Unni
Project Manager: Sindhuraj Thulasingam
Design Direction: Gopalakrishnan Venkataraman

Printed in Canada

Last digit is the print number: 9   8   7   6   5   4   3   2   1

Working together
to grow libraries in
developing countries

www.elsevier.com • www.bookaid.org

CONTENTS

Professional Nursing

1. Using the American Nurses Association's definition of nursing, which activities are within the domain of nursing? **Select all that apply**.
   _____ a. Implementing intake and output for a patient who is vomiting
   _____ b. Establishing and implementing a stress management program for family caregivers of patients with Alzheimer's disease
   _____ c. Explaining the risks associated with the planned surgical procedure when a preoperative patient asks about risks
   _____ d. Developing and performing a study to compare the health status of older patients who live alone with the status of older patients who live with family members
   _____ e. Identifying the effect of an investigational drug on patients' hemoglobin levels
   _____ f. Using a biofeedback machine to teach a patient with cancer how to manage chronic pain
   _____ g. Preventing pneumonia in an immobile patient by implementing frequent turning, coughing, and deep breathing
   _____ h. Determining and giving fluid replacement therapy needed for a patient with serious burns
   _____ i. Testifying to legislative bodies about the effect of health policies on culturally, socially, and economically diverse populations

2. A nurse who has worked on an orthopedic unit for several years is encouraged by the nurse manager to become certified in orthopedic nursing. What will certification in nursing require and/or provide? **Select all that apply.**
   a. A certain amount of clinical experience
   b. Successful completion of an examination
   c. Membership in specialty nursing organizations
   d. Professional recognition of expertise in a specialty area
   e. An advanced practice role that requires graduate education

3. When guiding nurses in how to perform professionally, which describes a competent level of nursing care based on the nursing process?
   a. Standards of Professional Performance
   b. Standards of Practice
   c. Quality and Safety Education for Nurses
   d. State Nurse Practice Act

4. What are the 6 competencies from Quality and Safety Education for Nurses (QSEN) that are expected of new nursing graduates?
   a.
   b.
   c.
   d.
   e.
   f.

5. Place the steps of the evidence-based practice (EBP) process in order, using 1 as the first step and 6 as the last step.
   _____ Share the results of the EBP change
   _____ Ask a clinical question
   _____ Critically analyze the evidence
   _____ Find and collect the evidence
   _____ Evaluate patient outcomes
   _____ Implementing the evidence in practice

6. The following is an example of an evidence-based practice (EBP) clinical question. "In adult seizure patients, is restraint or medication more effective in protecting them from injury during a seizure?" Which word(s) in the question identify(ies) the *C* part of the PICOT format?
   a. Restraint
   b. Or medication
   c. During a seizure
   d. Adult seizure patients
   e. Protecting them from injury

7. Two nurses are establishing a smoking cessation program to assist patients with chronic lung disease to stop smoking. What would the nurses do to offer the most effective program with the best outcomes?
   a. Search for an article that describes nursing interventions that are effective for smoking cessation.
   b. Develop a clinical question that will allow patients to compare different cessation methods during the program.
   c. Keep comprehensive records that detail each patient's progress and ultimate outcomes from participation in the program.
   d. Use evidence-based clinical practice guidelines developed from randomized controlled trials of smoking cessation methods.

8. The nurse is working in a health care facility where uniform electronic health records are used. What is the primary purpose of such a record?
   a. To reduce the cost of health care by eliminating paper records.
   b. To keep the patient's medical information more private than handwritten records.
   c. To provide a single place for health care members to review, update, document, and order patient care.
   d. To provide a single record, making the patient's medical information accessible to any care givers in any health system.

9. Match the phases of the nursing process with the descriptions (phases may be used more than once).

   Descriptions
   _____ a. Analysis of data
   _____ b. Priority setting
   _____ c. Nursing interventions
   _____ d. Data collection
   _____ e. Identifying patient strengths
   _____ f. Measuring patient achievement of goals
   _____ g. Setting goals
   _____ h. Identifying health problems
   _____ i. Modifying the plan of care
   _____ j. Documenting care provided

   Nursing Process Phases
   1. Assessment
   2. Diagnosis
   3. Planning
   4. Implementation
   5. Evaluation

10. During the diagnosis phase of the nursing process, assessment data is analyzed to make conclusions, referred to as clinical problems. Clinical problems are not the same as medical diagnoses. Which statements are examples of clinical problems? **Select all that apply.**
    a. Fatigue due to sleep deprivation
    b. Sepsis due to gram negative infection
    c. Hypervolemia due to increased sodium intake
    d. Constipation due to irregular defecation habits
    e. Chronic obstructive pulmonary disease due to history of smoking
    f. Myocardial infarction due to coronary artery occlusion

11. For the clinical problems and patient outcomes listed below, identify a specific nursing intervention to help the patient reach the outcome.
    a. Clinical problem: impaired tissue integrity due to immobility.
       Patient outcome: patient will have skin integrity free of pressure injuries.

    b. Clinical problem: constipation due to inadequate fluid and fiber intake.
       Patient outcome: patient will have daily soft bowel movements in 1 week.

12. A patient with a seizure disorder is admitted to the hospital after a sustained seizure. When she tells the nurse that she has not taken her medication regularly, the nurse identifies that there is a lack of knowledge regarding her medication regimen. Using the Nursing Outcomes Classification (NOC), the nurse identifies an outcome of *Compliance behavior: prescribed medications,* with the indicator *Takes medication at intervals prescribed, at a target rate of 3 (sometimes demonstrated).* When the nurse tries to teach the patient about the medication regimen, the patient tells the nurse that she knows about the medication but does not always have the money to refill the prescription. Where was the mistake made in the nursing process with this patient?
    a. Planning
    b. Diagnosis
    c. Evaluation
    d. Assessment
    e. Implementation

13. What are the 5 rights of delegating nursing care? **Select all that apply**.
    a. Right time
    b. Right task
    c. Right patient
    d. Right person
    e. Right dosage
    f. Right circumstance
    g. Right supervision and evaluation
    h. Right directions and communication

14. Delegation is a process used by the RN to provide safe and effective care in an efficient manner. What nursing interventions would not be delegated to assistive personnel (AP) but would be performed by the RN? **Select all that apply.**
    a. Administering patient medications
    b. Ambulating stable patients
    c. Performing patient assessment
    d. Evaluating the effectiveness of patient care
    e. Feeding patients at mealtime
    f. Performing sterile procedures
    g. Providing patient teaching
    h. Obtaining vital signs on a stable patient
    i. Helping with patient bathing

15. Match the following care planning tools to the description statement(s). There may be more than 1 tool per statement, and the tools will be used more than once.

   Tools
   1. Nursing Care Plan
   2. Concept Maps
   3. Clinical Pathway

   Description Statements
   _____ A plan that directs an entire health care team
   _____ Used as guides for routine nursing care
   _____ Used in nursing education to teach the nursing process and care planning
   _____ A description of patient care needed at specific times during treatment
   _____ Should be personalized and specific to each patient
   _____ A visual diagram representing relationships among patient problems, interventions, and data
   _____ Used for high-volume or high-risk and predictable case types

16. Which nursing actions are in response to the National Patient Safety Goals? **Select all that apply.**
   a. Use restraints to prevent patient falls.
   b. Administer all medications ordered by physicians.
   c. Wash hands before and after every patient contact.
   d. Conduct a "time-out" when too tired to provide care.
   e. Quickly communicate test results to the right staff person.
   f. Evaluate the initial existence of pressure ulcers before patient dismissal.

17. Which quality-of-care measures influence the payment for healthcare services by third-party payers? **Select all that apply.**
   a. Clinical outcomes
   b. Patient satisfaction
   c. Use of evidence-based practice
   d. Adoption of information technology
   e. Occurrence of a serious reportable event

18. The Affordable Care Act (ACA) encourages groups of doctors, hospitals, and other health care providers to unite to coordinate care for Medicare patients. What are these groups called?
   a. National Quality Forum (NQF)
   b. Preferred Provider Organization (PPO)
   c. Accountable Care Organization (ACO)
   d. Health Maintenance Organization (HMO)

Social Determinants of Health

1. A 62-year-old black man has been diagnosed with lung cancer and is scheduled for surgery. What would the nurse recognize as the most likely major determinant of this patient's health?
   a. He is a black man.
   b. He chose to smoke all his adult life.
   c. His father died of lung cancer at about the same age.
   d. His lack of experience limits his ability to understand and act on health information.

2. A 73-year-old white woman is brought to the emergency department by a neighbor who found the woman experiencing severe abdominal and lower back pain for 2 days associated with nausea and vomiting for the last 24 hours. She has always refused medical care of any kind and lives by herself "up the mountain" off a dirt road in rural West Virginia. She gave birth to 2 children with the help of a midwife. Both of her children left for the West Coast years ago and she rarely sees them. She was not married to the father of her children, and she has not seen him in years. She has barely made a living by sewing for a doll company and receives a small amount of public assistance. As ill as she is, she is insisting that she will return home after she sees the doctor. List at least 4 factors in this situation that contribute to health disparities.
   a.
   b.
   c.
   d.

3. Which individual conditions may be associated with limited health literacy which lead to health disparities? **Select all that apply.**
   a. Age
   b. Place
   c. Gender
   d. Race/ethnicity
   e. Language barrier
   f. Income/education

4. Cultural safety describes care that prevents cultural imposition. The nurse must be aware of and include the knowledge of which factors to provide culturally safe patient care? **Select all that apply.**
   a. Values
   b. Culture
   c. Ethnicity
   d. Stereotyping
   e. Acculturation
   f. Ethnocentrism

5. What are 4 basic characteristics of culture?
   a. Ever present, shared by all members, expected by all members, adapted to individuals
   b. Dynamic, shared values, provides a baseline for judging other cultures, learned from parents
   c. Ever present, not always shared by all members, not accepted by the group, learned at school
   d. Dynamic, not always shared by all members, adapted to specific conditions, learned by communication and imitation

6. What specific component of acquiring cultural competence is reflected in creating a safe environment for collection of relevant cultural data during the health history and physical examination?
   a. Cultural skill
   b. Cultural encounter
   c. Cultural awareness
   d. Cultural knowledge

7. Identify 1 example of how each of the following cultural factors may affect the nursing care of a patient of a different culture and 1 example of the functioning of a health care team made up of individuals from different cultures.

Cultural Factor	Effect on Nursing Care	Health Care Team
Time orientation		
Economic factors		
Nutrition		
Personal space		
Beliefs and practices		

8. When ordering a food tray for a patient who identifies as Islamic, what would the nurse consider about this patient's diet?
   a. They do not eat pork.
   b. They do not eat shellfish.
   c. They are likely vegetarian.
   d. They do not eat any type of meat.

9. There are 5 groups that comprise social determinants of health (SDH). In the table below, enter each SDH group in the left column. In the right column, provide a description about how each group affects a person's health.

Social Determinant of Health	Health Disparity

10. What would the nurse expect when a Mexican woman requests a *curandero*?
    a. She is requesting a folk healer.
    b. She is requesting a religious leader.
    c. She is requesting a female health care provider.
    d. She is requesting a midwife.

11. When the nurse takes a surgical consent form to an Asian woman for a signature after the surgeon has provided the information about the recommended surgery, the patient refuses to sign the consent form. What is the *best* response by the nurse?
    a. "Didn't you understand what the doctor told you about the surgery?"
    b. "Are there others with whom you want to talk before making this decision?"
    c. "Why won't you sign this form? Do you want to do what the doctor recommended?"
    d. "I'll have to call the surgeon and have your surgery cancelled until you can make a decision."

12. Match each patient statement to its social determinant of health group.
    a. "I have a very supportive spouse."   1. Economic stability
    b. "I don't have the money to pay for medications."   2. Education
    c. "I live in a high-crime area."   3. Health care
    d. "I lost my job and have no insurance."   4. Community context
    e. "I quit high-school and earned a GED."   5. Neighborhood

13. What drug class has a different response in blacks when compared with the usual response in European Americans?
    a. Analgesics
    b. Anticoagulants
    c. Benzodiazepines
    d. Antihypertensive agents

14. Some cultures avoid direct eye contact while others observe silence. Which cultural groups may not return a direct gaze or are comfortable with silence? **Select all that apply.**
    a. Arab
    b. Asian
    c. Blacks
    d. Hispanic
    e. Native American

15. What would the nurse do to communicate with a patient who does not speak the predominant language? **Select all that apply.**
    a. Pantomime words while verbalizing the specific words.
    b. Speak slowly and enunciate clearly in a slightly louder voice.
    c. Use family members rather than strangers as interpreters to increase the patient's feeling of comfort.
    d. Use a website or phrase books that translate from both the nurse's language and the patient's language.
    e. Avoid the use of any words known in the patient's language because the grammar and pronunciation may be incorrect.

16. What measures would the nurse use to reduce health care disparities? **Select all that apply.**
    a. Use cultural competency guidelines.
    b. Use a family member as the interpreter.
    c. Use standardized, evidence-based care guidelines.
    d. Complete the health history as rapidly as possible.
    e. Consider racial and cultural differences in planning care.

Health History and Physical Examination

1. During the day, while being admitted to the nursing unit from the emergency department, a patient tells the nurse that she is short of breath and has pain in her chest when she breathes. Her respiratory rate is 28 breaths/min, and she is coughing up yellow sputum. Her skin is hot and moist, and her temperature is 102.2°F (39°C). The laboratory results show white blood cell count elevation and the sputum result is pending. The patient says that coughing makes her head hurt and that she aches all over. Identify the subjective and objective assessment data for this patient.

Subjective	Objective

2. For the patient described in Question 1, the data will lead the night shift nurse to complete a focused nursing assessment of which body part(s)?
   a. Abdomen
   b. Arms and legs
   c. Head and neck
   d. Anterior and posterior chest

3. Give an example of a sensitive way to ask a patient each of the following questions.
   a. Is the patient on antihypertensive medication having a side effect of impotence?
   b. Has the patient with a history of alcohol use disorder had recent alcohol intake?
   c. Who are the sexual contacts of the patient with gonorrhea?
   d. Does the patient skip taking medications because they cost too much?

4. The nurse prepares to interview a patient for a nursing history but finds the patient in obvious pain. What is the nurse's best action at this time?
   a. Delay the interview until the patient is free of pain.
   b. Administer pain medication before initiating the interview.
   c. Gather as much information as quickly as possible by using closed-ended questions that require brief answers.
   d. Ask only those questions pertinent to the specific problem and complete the interview when the patient is more comfortable.

5. While the nurse is obtaining a health history, the patient tells the nurse, "I am so tired, I can hardly function." What is the nurse's best action at this time?
   a. Stop the interview and leave the patient alone to be able to rest.
   b. Arrange another time with the patient to complete the interview.
   c. Question the patient further about the characteristics of the symptoms.
   d. Reassure the patient that the symptoms will improve when treatment has had time to be effective.

6. Rewrite each of the following questions asked by the nurse so that it is an open-ended question designed to gather information about the patient's functional health patterns.
   a. Are you having any pain?
   b. Do you have good relationship with your spouse?
   c. How long have you been ill?
   d. Do you exercise regularly?

7. A patient has come to the health clinic and reports having diarrhea for 3 days. He says the stools occur 5 or 6 times per day and are very watery. Every time he eats or drinks something, he has an urgent diarrhea stool. He denies being out of the country, but did attend a large family reunion held at a campground in the mountains about a week ago. Using PQRST, what areas of symptom investigation still need to be addressed to provide additional important information? **Select all that apply.**
   a. Timing
   b. Quality
   c. Severity
   d. Palliative
   e. Radiation
   f. Precipitating factors

8. The following data are obtained from a patient during a nursing history. Organize these data according to Gordon's functional health patterns. Patterns may be used more than once, and some data may apply to more than 1 pattern.

   Data

   _____ a. 78-year-old woman
   _____ b. Married, 3 grown children who all live out of town
   _____ c. Cares for an invalid husband at home daily with the help of homemaker
   _____ d. Vision corrected with glasses; hearing normal
   _____ e. Height 5 ft, 8 in; weight 170 lb
   _____ f. Considers herself a stress eater; eats when stressed
   _____ g. 5-year history of adult-onset asthma; smokes 2 or 3 cigarettes a day
   _____ h. Coughing, wheezing, with stated shortness of breath
   _____ i. Moderate light-yellow sputum
   _____ j. Says she now has no energy to care for husband
   _____ k. Awakens 3 or 4 times per night to use a bronchodilator inhaler
   _____ l. Uses a laxative twice a week for bowel function; no urinary problems
   _____ m. Feels her health is good for her age
   _____ n. Allergic to codeine and aspirin
   _____ o. Has esophageal reflux and eats bland food
   _____ p. Can usually handle the stress of caring for her husband but if she becomes overwhelmed, asthma worsens
   _____ q. Has been menopausal for 26 years; no sexual activity
   _____ r. Takes medications for asthma, hypertension, and hypothyroidism and uses diazepam PRN for anxiety
   _____ s. Goes out for lunch with friends weekly
   _____ t. Says she misses going to church with her husband but watches religious services with him on TV

   Pattern

   1. Demographic data
   2. Important health information
   3. Health-perception/health-management pattern
   4. Nutrition-metabolic pattern
   5. Elimination pattern
   6. Activity-exercise pattern
   7. Sleep-rest pattern
   8. Cognitive-perceptual pattern
   9. Self-perception/self-concept pattern
   10. Role-relationship pattern
   11. Sexuality-reproductive pattern
   12. Coping–stress tolerance pattern
   13. Value-belief pattern

9. What is an example of a pertinent negative finding during a physical assessment?
   a. Chest pain that does not radiate to the arm
   b. Elevated blood pressure in a patient with hypertension
   c. Pupils that are equal and react to light and accommodation
   d. Clear lung sounds in a patient with chronic bronchitis

10. Match the following data with the assessment technique used to obtain the information.

   Data
   a. Normal blood flow through arteries
   b. Abnormal blood flow in carotid artery
   c. Tympany of the abdomen
   d. Pitting edema
   e. Cyanosis of the lips
   f. Hyperactive peristalsis
   g. Bruising of the lateral left thigh
   h. Cool, clammy skin

   Assessment Technique
   1. Inspection
   2. Palpation
   3. Percussion
   4. Auscultation

11. What is the correct sequence of examination techniques that should be used when assessing the patient's abdomen?
   a. Inspection, palpation, auscultation, percussion
   b. Palpation, percussion, auscultation, inspection
   c. Auscultation, inspection, percussion, palpation
   d. Inspection, auscultation, percussion, palpation

12. When performing a physical assessment, what approach is most important for the nurse to use?
   a. A head-to-toe approach to avoid missing an important area
   b. The same systematic, efficient sequence for all assessments
   c. A sequence that is least revealing and embarrassing for the patient
   d. An approach that allows time to collect the nursing history data while performing the assessment

13. The nurse is performing a physical assessment on a 90-year-old male patient who has been bedridden for the past year. Which adaptations would be appropriate when assessing the patient? **Select all that apply.**
   a. Make sure that a family member is with him.
   b. Handle the skin with care because of potential fragility.
   c. Keep the patient warm and comfortable during the assessment.
   d. Allow the patient to watch TV to distract him from any painful assessments.
   e. Place the patient in a position of comfort and avoid unnecessary changes in position.

14. In what patient situations would a comprehensive assessment be performed? **Select all that apply.**
   a. Reports of chest pain
   b. On initial admission to the telemetry unit
   c. On initial evaluation by the home health nurse
   d. Found lying on the floor, unresponsive, with moist skin
   e. On arrival in the surgery holding area of the operating room

15. Which assessment tools can be used to assess the cardiac system? **Select all that apply.**
   a. Watch
   b. Stethoscope
   c. Reflex hammer
   d. Ophthalmoscope
   e. Blood pressure cuff

16. What is the term used for assessment data that the patient reports?
   a. Focused
   b. Objective
   c. Subjective
   d. Comprehensive

17. On the first encounter with the patient, the nurse will complete a general survey. Which features are included? **Select all that apply.**
   a. Mental state and behavior
   b. Lung sounds and bowel tones
   c. Body temperature and pulses
   d. Speech and body movements
   e. Body features and obvious physical signs
   f. Abnormal heart murmur and limited mobility

Patient and Caregiver Teaching

1. In each of these nursing situations, identify the *general goal* of the patient and caregiver teaching.

Nursing Situation	Goal
Teaching a new mother about the recommended infant immunization schedule	
Discussing recommended lifestyle changes with a patient who has a newly diagnosed heart disease	
Counseling a patient with a breast biopsy that is positive for cancer	
Demonstrating the proper condom application to sexually active teenagers	

2. What is meant by this statement: "Every interaction with a patient or caregiver is potentially a teachable moment"?

3. Which statements describe the teaching-learning process? **Select all that apply.**
   a. Learning can occur without teaching.
   b. Teaching may make learning more efficient.
   c. Teaching must be well planned to be effective.
   d. Learning has not occurred when there is no change in behavior.
   e. Teaching uses a variety of methods to influence knowledge and behavior.

4. From the list of adult learning principles, identify which one(s) is (are) used in these examples of patient teaching. A principle may be used more than once, and more than 1 principle may be used for each example of patient teaching.

Examples of Patient Teaching	Principles
_____ a. The nurse explains why it is important for a patient who has Parkinson's disease to walk with wide placement of the feet.	1. Learner's need to know
_____ b. The nurse asks a patient what is most important to her to learn about managing a new colostomy.	2. Learner's readiness to learn
_____ c. The nurse teaches a patient how to reduce the risks for stroke after the patient has had a transient ischemic attack.	3. Learner's prior experiences 4. Learner's motivation to learn
_____ d. The nurse provides a variety of printed materials and Internet resources for a patient to use to learn about impaired kidney function.	5. Learner's orientation to learning 6. Learner's self-concept
_____ e. When caring for a patient with newly diagnosed asthma, the nurse explains that asthma is a disorder the patient can control and allows the patient to decide when teaching should be done and who else should be included.	
_____ f. The patient diagnosed with diabetes requests to perform blood glucose monitoring and insulin administration while being taught by the nurse.	
_____ g. During preoperative teaching of a patient scheduled for a total hip replacement, the nurse compares the postoperative care with that of the patient's prior back surgery.	

5. A patient with diabetes tells the nurse that he cannot see any reason to change his eating habits because he is not overweight. What action does the nurse determine as the most appropriate for a patient at this stage of the Transtheoretical Model of Health Behavior Change?
   a. Help the patient set priorities for managing his diabetes.
   b. Arrange for the dietitian to describe what dietary changes are needed.
   c. Explain that dietary changes can help prevent long-term complications of diabetes.
   d. Emphasize that he must change behaviors if he is going to control his blood glucose levels.

6. Revise the following medical terms into phrases that a patient with limited health literacy would be able to understand.
   a. Acute myocardial infarction
   b. Intravenous pyelogram
   c. Diabetic retinopathy

7. Which action by a nurse demonstrates an empathetic approach to patient teaching?
   a. Assesses the patient's needs before developing the teaching plan
   b. Provides positive nonverbal messages that promote communication
   c. Reads and reviews educational materials before distributing them to patients and families
   d. Overcomes personal frustration when patients are discharged before teaching is complete

8. Describe 1 strategy that could be used to overcome these common barriers to teaching patients and caregivers.

Barrier	Strategy
Lack of time	
Your feeling as a teacher	
Nurse–patient differences	

9. The nurse assesses a 48-year-old male patient and his family for learning needs related to the myocardial infarction the patient had 2 days ago. While doing an assessment, the nurse finds out that the patient's father died at age 52 years from a myocardial infarction. Which assessment area will influence the teaching plan for this patient and family?
   a. Learner characteristics
   b. Physical characteristics
   c. Psychologic characteristics
   d. Sociocultural characteristics

10. Which strategy should the nurse use to promote a patient's self-efficacy during the teaching-learning process?
    a. Emphasize the relevancy of the teaching to the patient's life.
    b. Begin with concepts and tasks that are easily learned to promote success.
    c. Provide stimulating learning activities that encourage motivation to learn.
    d. Encourage the patient to learn independently without instruction from others.

11. Identify the teaching interventions that are indicated for the following patient characteristics:

Patient Characteristic	Teaching Intervention
Impaired hearing	
Patient sees no need for a change in health behaviors	
Drowsiness caused by use of sedatives	
Presence of pain	
Uncertain reading ability	
Visual learning style	
Primary language is not English	

12. A 68-year-old female patient admitted due to a stroke 3 days ago has weakness on her right side. She states, "I will never be able to take care of myself. I don't want to go to therapy this afternoon." After listening to her, which statement would be included as part of a motivational interview?
    a. "Why not?"
    b. "If you go to therapy, I'll give you a back rub when you get back."
    c. "I know you are tired but look how much easier walking was today than it was last week."
    d. "Well, with that attitude, you will have trouble. The doctor ordered therapy because he thought it would help."

13. Write a learning goal for the patient taking potassium-wasting diuretics who does not know what foods are high in potassium.

14. Which teaching strategies should be used when it is difficult to reach the desired goals of the session? **Select all that apply.**
    a. DVD
    b. Role play
    c. Discussion
    d. Printed material
    e. Lecture-discussion
    f. Web-based programs

15. When selecting audiovisual and written materials as teaching strategies, what is important for the nurse to do?
    a. Provide the patient with these materials before the planned learning experience.
    b. Ensure that the materials include all the information the patient will need to learn.
    c. Review the materials before use for accuracy and appropriateness to learning needs and goals.
    d. Assess the patient's auditory and visual ability because these functions are necessary for these strategies to be effective.

16. A patient with a breast biopsy positive for cancer tells the nurse that she has been using information from the Internet to try to make a decision about her treatment choices. When counseling the patient, what should the nurse consider? **Select all that apply.**
    a. The patient should be taught how to identify reliable and accurate information available online.
    b. All sites used by the patient should be evaluated by the nurse for accuracy and appropriateness of the information.
    c. Most information from the Internet is incomplete and inaccurate and should not be used to make important decisions about treatment.
    d. The Internet is an excellent source of health information, and online education programs can provide patients with better instruction than is available at clinics.
    e. The patient should be encouraged to use sites established by universities, the government, or reputable health organizations, such as the American Cancer Society, to access reliable information.

17. Identify what short-term evaluation technique is appropriate to assess whether the patient has met the following learning goals.

Learning Goal	Evaluation Technique
The patient will demonstrate to the nurse the preparation and administration of a subcutaneous insulin injection to himself with correct technique before discharge.	
Before discharge, the patient will identify 5 serious side effects of Coumadin that should be reported to the health care provider.	
The patient's spouse will select the foods highest in potassium for each meal from the hospital menu with 80% accuracy.	
The patient will state "no shortness of breath" when ambulating unassisted with the walker each of 3 times a day.	
The patient's caregiver will state that they are ready to change the patient's dressing today.	

18. What is the best example of documentation regarding patient teaching about wound care?
    a. "The patient was taught care of wound and dressing changes."
    b. "The patient demonstrated correct technique of wound care following instruction."
    c. "The patient and caregiver state that they understand the purposes of wound care."
    d. "Written instructions about wound care and dressing changes were given to the patient."

19. Which teaching strategies should the nurse plan to use for a patient from the Baby Boomer generation? **Select all that apply.**
    a. Podcast
    b. Role playing
    c. Group teaching
    d. Lecture-discussion
    e. A game or game system
    f. Patient education TV channels

20. An 88-year-old male patient with dementia and a fractured hip is admitted to the clinical unit accompanied by his daughter who is his caregiver. The daughter looks tired and disheveled. About 6 months ago she moved in with her father to keep him safe when he started wandering away from his home. She has no money because of her inability to work. She has inadequate information and is concerned about what will happen to her father after this hospitalization. Her brother calls on the phone to tell her what to do but does not come to visit or help out. There is conflict in the family related to decisions about caregiving. She has no respite from caregiving responsibilities and is socially isolated with loss of friends from an inability to have time for herself. What are the best coping strategies to teach this patient's daughter? **Select all that apply.**
    a. Keep a journal.
    b. Get regular exercise.
    c. Join a support group.
    d. Go on a weight-loss diet.
    e. Use humor to relieve stress.
    f. Take time to read more books.

Chronic Illness and Older Adults

1. A 78-year-old female patient is admitted with nausea, vomiting, anorexia, diarrhea, and dehydration. She has a history of diabetes and, 2 years ago, had a stroke with residual right-sided weakness. Which characteristics of chronic illness would the nurse identify in this patient? **Select all that apply.**
   a. Self-limiting
   b. Residual disability
   c. Permanent impairments
   d. Infrequent complications
   e. Need for long-term management
   f. Nonreversible pathologic changes

2. Seven tasks required for daily living with chronic illness have been identified. From Table 5.4, select at least 1 of these tasks that would specifically apply to the following common chronic conditions in older adults.

Chronic Condition	Task
Diabetes	
Visual impairment	
Heart disease	
Hearing impairment	
Alzheimer disease	
Arthritis	
Orthopedic impairment	

3. Consider the differences between primary and secondary prevention. Fill in the blanks.
   a. Actions aimed at early detection of disease and interventions to prevent progression of disease are considered _____ prevention.
   b. Following a proper diet, getting appropriate exercise, and receiving immunizations against specific diseases are considered _____ prevention.

4. What is the leading cause of death in the United States?
   a. Cancer
   b. Diabetes
   c. Heart disease
   d. Stroke
   e. Chronic obstructive pulmonary disease

5. According to the Corbin and Strauss chronic illness trajectory, which statement describes a patient with an unstable condition?
   a. Life-threatening situation
   b. Increasing disability and symptoms
   c. Gradual return to acceptable way of life
   d. Loss of control over symptoms and disease course

6. Which statement(s) about older people are myths and illustrate the concept of ageism? **Select all that apply.**
   a. You can't teach an old dog new tricks.
   b. Old people are not sexually active.
   c. Most old people live independently.
   d. Most older adults can no longer learn new information.
   e. Most older people lose interest in life and wish they would die.

7. For each of the clinical problems listed, identify at least 2 normal expected physiologic changes related to aging that could be etiologic factors of the diagnosis. Changes related to aging are found in the chapters identified in Table 5.5.
   a. Nutritionally compromised (see Table 44.5)
      Change:
      Change:
   b. Activity intolerance (see Table 66.1)
      Change:
      Change:
   c. Risk for injury (see Table 60.2; Table 22.1)
      Change:
      Change:
   d. Impaired urinary elimination (see Table 49.2)
      Change:
      Change:
   e. Impaired respiratory function (see Table 27.1)
      Change:
      Change:
   f. Risk for impaired skin integrity (see Table 24.1)
      Change:
      Change:
   g. Inadequate tissue perfusion (see Table 35.1)
      Change:
      Change:
   h. Impaired bowel elimination (see Table 43.5)
      Change:
      Change:

8. Which statement made by the older adult would the nurse identify as the presence of age-associated memory impairment?
   a. "I just can't seem to remember the name of my granddaughter."
   b. "I make out lists to help me remember what I need to do, but I can't seem to use them."
   c. "I forgot that I went to the grocery store this morning and didn't realize it until I went again this afternoon."
   d. "I forget movie stars' names more often now, but I can remember them later after the conversation is over."

9. Indicate what the acronym *SCALES* stands for in assessment of nutrition indicators in frail older adults.

S	
C	
A	
L	
E	
S	

10. When working with older patients who identify with a specific ethnic group, which factor would the nurse identify as increasing the risk for health care problems?
    a. Living with extended families who isolate the patient.
    b. Living in rural areas where services are not readily available.
    c. Eating ethnic foods that do not provide all the essential nutrients.
    d. Having less income to spend for medications and health care services.

11. An 83-year-old woman is being discharged from the hospital following stabilization of her international normalized ratio (INR) levels (used to assess effectiveness of warfarin therapy). She has chronic atrial fibrillation and has been on warfarin (Coumadin) for several years. Discharge instructions include returning to the clinic weekly for INR testing. Which patient statement indicates that she may be unable to have the testing done?
    a. "When I have the energy, I have taken the bus to get this test done."
    b. "I will need to ask my son to bring me into town every week for the test."
    c. "Should I just keep taking the same pill every day until I can get a ride to town?"
    d. "It is important to have this test every week. I have several church friends who can bring me."

12. The old-old population (85 years and older) has an increased risk for frailty. However, old age is just one element of frailty. Identify at least 3 other assessment findings that are considered criteria for frailty.
    a.
    b.
    c.

13. An 80-year-old woman is brought to the emergency department by her daughter, who says her mother has refused to eat for 6 days. The mother says she stays in her room all the time because the family is mean to her when she eats or watches TV with them. She says her daughter brings her only 1 meal a day, and that meal is cold leftovers from the family's meals days before.
    a. What types of elder mistreatment may be present in this situation?
    b. How would the nurse assess the situation to determine whether abuse is present?
       The daughter says her mother is too demanding and she just cannot cope with caring for her mother 24 hours a day.
    c. What may be an appropriate clinical problem for the daughter?
    d. What resources can the nurse suggest to the daughter?

14. What are 3 common factors known to precipitate placement in a long-term care facility?
    a.
    b.
    c.

15. An 88-year-old woman is brought to the health clinic for the first time by her 64-year-old daughter. During the initial comprehensive nursing assessment of the patient, what would the nurse do?
    a. Ask the daughter whether the patient has any urgent needs or problems.
    b. Interview the patient and daughter together so that pertinent information can be confirmed.
    c. Refer the patient for an interprofessional comprehensive geriatric assessment because at her age she will have multiple needs.
    d. Obtain a comprehensive health history using physical, psychologic, functional, developmental, socioeconomic, and cultural assessments.

16. What is a mental status assessment of the older adult especially important in determining?
    a. Potential for independent living
    b. Eligibility for federal health programs
    c. Service and placement needs of the person
    d. Whether the person should be classified as frail

17. What is the most important nursing measure in the rehabilitation of an older adult to prevent loss of function from inactivity and immobility?
    a. Using assistive devices, such as walkers and canes
    b. Teaching good nutrition to prevent loss of muscle mass
    c. Performance of active and passive range-of-motion (ROM) exercises
    d. Performance of risk appraisals and assessments related to immobility

18. Since most older adults take at least 6 prescription drugs, what are 4 nursing interventions that can specifically help prevent problems caused by multiple drug use in older patients?
    a.
    b.
    c.
    d.

19. Which nursing actions would show the nurse's understanding of the concept of providing safe care without using restraints? **Select all that apply.**
    a. Placing patients with fall risk in low beds
    b. Asking simple yes-or-no questions to clarify patient needs
    c. Making hourly rounds on patients to assess for pain and toileting needs
    d. Placing a disruptive patient near the nurses' station in a chair with a seat belt
    e. Applying a jacket vest loosely so that the patient can turn but cannot climb out of bed

20. When teaching a 69-year-old patient about self-care, what will promote health? **Select all that apply.**
    a. Proper diet
    b. Immunizations
    c. Teaching chair yoga
    d. Demonstrating balancing techniques
    e. Participation in health promotion activities

21. The 58-year-old male patient will be transferred from the acute care clinical unit of the hospital to another care area. The patient needs complicated dressing changes for several months. To which practice setting(s) could the patient be transitioned? **Select all that apply.**
    a. Acute rehabilitation
    b. Long-term acute care
    c. Intermediate care facility
    d. Transitional subacute care
    e. Programs for All-Inclusive Care for the Elderly (PACE)

Caring for Lesbian, Gay, Bisexual, Transgender, Queer or Questioning, and Gender Diverse Patients

1. What term is sometimes used if genitalia or chromosomal make up cannot be categorized?
   a. Biologic sex
   b. Intersex
   c. Transgender
   d. Gender dysphoria

2. Match the culture to its reference which describes gender beyond binary (male/female) constructs or those who identify as the opposite gender than their biologic sex.
   _____ a. Indigenous American   1. Hijras
   _____ b. India   2. Two-spirit
   _____ c. Albanian   3. Burrnesha

3. The nurse is caring for a patient classified as having gender dysphoria. Which statement best describes gender dysphoria?
   a. There is a conflict between a person's gender identity and their biologic sex.
   b. The person's gender identity, role, or expression differs from cultural norms.
   c. The person does not define themselves as one gender or the other.
   d. The person identifies their gender based on their romantic attraction to others.

4. Match each term describing gender and sexual identity to its meaning or significance.
   _____ a. Straight (heterosexual)   1. No sexual attraction for partnered sexuality
   _____ b. Gay or lesbian (homosexual)   2. Attracted to more than 1 gender
   _____ c. Bisexual   3. Gender identity matches biologic sex
   _____ d. Cisgender   4. Attracted to same biologic sex
   _____ e. Gender non-conforming   5. Biologic or sex traits not clearly categorized
   _____ f. Intersex   6. Gender identity differs from binary norms
   _____ g. Asexual   7. Attracted to opposite gender

5. Which statements about health disparities and inequities among LGBTQ+ populations are true? Select all that apply.
   a. Cisgender people have a higher rate of poverty than do LGBTQ+ persons.
   b. LGBTQ+ persons have higher rates of substance use compared to the non-LGBTQ+ persons.
   c. Depression is not a significant issue for LGBTQ+ persons.
   d. Mental health disorders are more prevalent among transgender persons compared to heterosexuals.
   e. LGBTQ+ youth have considered attempting suicide at a higher rate than transgender and non-binary youth.
   f. Gay and bisexual men have higher rates of obesity than heterosexual men.
   g. Black men having sex with men (MSM) have higher rates of HIV infection than Hispanic/Latino (MSM) men.
   h. Lesbian and bisexual women have a higher incidence of human papilloma virus (HPV) infections than do gay and bisexual men.
   i. Lung cancer rates are higher in men who have sex with men (MSM).
   j. LGBTQ+ populations have a higher victimization rate compared to heterosexual populations.

6. After introducing yourself as the nurse, what is the best way to determine how to address the patient who identifies as transgender?
   a. Use *he/she* for the pronoun based on their first name.
   b. Ask the patient their preferred name.
   c. Use the name listed on their legal identification.
   d. Refer to the patient using a neutral pronoun like *they*.

7. A patient who is assigned as male at birth is transitioning to become female. Which hormone would the nurse expect to be prescribed to help the patient grow breasts?
   a. Testosterone
   b. Oxytocin
   c. Estradiol
   d. Progesterone

8. A patient assigned as female at birth wants a prescription for testosterone to develop male characteristics. Which health condition may contraindicate its use?
   a. History of deep vein thrombosis
   b. History of migraines
   c. History of renal disease
   d. History of cardiovascular disease

9. The nurse is asking a patient about who to contact in case of an emergency. The patient states that he is in a polyamorous relationship. How would the nurse interpret this?
   a. The patient has 1 partner of the opposite sex.
   b. The patient has 1 partner of the same sex.
   c. The patient has more than 1 partner of either sex.
   d. The patient doesn't have a partner to list as a contact.

10. Match the gender affirming surgical procedures to their correct descriptions.
    _____ a. Phalloplasty   1. Removal of the uterus
    _____ b. Mastectomy   2. Creating a penis from existing genital tissue
    _____ c. Orchiectomy   3. Removal of breast tissue
    _____ d. Hysterectomy   4. Creating a penis using various body tissues
    _____ e. Metoidioplasty   5. Removal of the testicles

11. A patient transitioning from male to female undergoes facial feminization surgery. Which intervention should the nurse prioritize postoperatively?
    a. Applying ice packs to reduce facial swelling
    b. Monitoring the patient's airway
    c. Administering opioids to decrease pain
    d. Encouraging the patient to use the incentive spirometer

CASE STUDY Gender Affirming Surgery

Patient Profile

A.J. is a 32-year-old biologic male who has identified as a female for the last 5 years. A.J. is being admitted for gender affirming surgery beginning with facial feminization.

©Valeria Blanc/iStock.com

Subjective Data
- Diagnosed with gender dysphoria
- History of hypertension, takes enalapril
- History of type I diabetes, takes insulin
- In a monogamous relationship with a male partner
- Prescribed gender affirming hormone therapy, estrogen and an anti-androgen

Postoperative Objective Data
- Vital signs: BP 145/85 mm Hg, HR 120 beats/min, RR 28 breaths/min, temperature 99.7°F (37.6°C), oxygen saturation 93% on room air
- Lethargic, arousable to name, oriented to person and place
- Inspiratory stridor
- Coarse bilateral breath sounds
- Facial edema
- Head wrap dressing clean, dry, and intact
- Bilateral peri-orbital bruising
- Small amount of sanguineous oral drainage
- Reports 7 out of 10 incisional pain
- FSBS 205 mg/dL

Questions

1. The patient has the following medications ordered. **Choose the most likely options for the information missing from the table below by selecting from the lists of options provided.**

Medication	Dose, Route, Frequency	Drug Class	Indication
Enalapril	5 mg PO once daily	1	Hypertension
Hydromorphone	2	Opioid	Acute pain
3	4 mg IV every 6 hours PRN	Antiemetic	Nausea/vomiting
Spironolactone	50 mg PO twice daily	Potassium-sparing diuretic	4
Ketorolac	5	Non-steroidal antiinflammatory	Acute Pain
6	25 mg IV every 6 hours PRN	Antiemetic	Nausea/vomiting

Options for 1	Options for 2 and 5	Options for 3 and 6	Options for 4
Angiotensin II receptor blocker	650 mg PO every 6 hr PRN	Promethazine	Hypertension
Thiazide diuretic	400 mg PO every 6 hr PRN	Prochlorperazine	Androgen inhibitor
Alpha-adrenergic blocker	15 mg IV every 6 hr	Ondansetron	Hypokalemia
Beta blocker	0.5 mg IV every 1 hr PRN	Hydroxyzine	Heart failure
Angiotensin-converting enzyme inhibitor	25 mcg IV every 30 min PRN	Haloperidol	Diabetes

2. **Choose the most likely options for the information missing from the statements below by selecting from the lists of options provided.**

_____1_____ is classified as a female sex hormone that is used to promote feminine characteristics during gender transition. The nurse should teach the client about anticipated effects which include _____2_____, _____2_____, and decreased testicular size. The nurse should also discuss potential risks which include _____3_____, _____3_____, and prolactinomas. Persons who want to transition should consider the benefits versus the risks to make an informed decision about gender affirming hormone therapy.

Options for 1	Options for 2	Options for 3
Oxytocin	Increased libido	Breast cancer
Progesterone	Breast growth	Polycythemia
Estradiol	Skin softening	Venous thromboembolic event

Options for 1	Options for 2	Options for 3
Testosterone	Facial hair growth	Prostate cancer
Calcitonin	Amenorrhea	Hyperkalemia
Estriol	Increased abdominal fat	Anemia
Prolactin	Increased muscle mass	Renal disease

3. Use an X to indicate whether the nursing actions below are <u>Indicated</u> (appropriate or necessary), <u>Contraindicated</u> (could be harmful), or <u>Non-Essential</u> (makes no difference or is unnecessary).

Nursing Action	Indicated	Contraindicated	Non-Essential
Administer 10 units NPH insulin, IV			
Administer 2 mg morphine sulfate IV			
Administer 500 mL 0.9% normal saline bolus			
Elevate the HOB to a minimum of 30 degrees			
Insert an oral pharyngeal airway			
Insert an additional peripheral IV			
Apply ice packs to eyes and cheeks			
Administer O_2 6 L/min using simple face mask			
Teach the patient how to perform pursed-lip breathing			

4. For each assessment finding, use an X to indicate whether the <u>intervention</u> was Effective (helped to meet expected outcomes), <u>Ineffective</u> (did not help to meet expected outcomes), or <u>Unrelated</u> (not related to the expected outcomes).

Assessment Finding	Effective	Ineffective	Unrelated
Reports 3 out of 10 incisional pain			
Temperature 99°F (37.2°C)			
O_2 saturation 94%			
Heart rate 100 beats/min			
FSBS 220 mg/dL			
Awake, oriented to person, place and time			
Breath sounds clear			

5. The nurse begins to develop a plan of care identifying postoperative interventions and teaching needs prior to discharge. What would the nurse include in this patient's plan of care? Select all that apply.
   _____ A.   Teach the patient to continue using ice packs to eyes and cheeks for the next 7 days.
   _____ B.   Help the patient out of bed to sit in a chair on postoperative day 0.
   _____ C.   Keep the HOB less than 30 degrees while the patient is in bed.
   _____ D.   Administer oxycodone PO every 4-6 hours as needed for pain.
   _____ E.   Teach the patient to increase dietary intake of green leafy vegetables, such as spinach.
   _____ F.   Inform the patient to contact their health care provider if they experience palpitations.
   _____ G.   Encourage the patient to use the incentive spirometer 10 times/hour while awake.

Stress Management

1. When a patient at the clinic is informed that testing indicates the presence of gonorrhea, the patient sighs and says, "That, I can handle." What does the nurse understand about the patient in this situation?
   a. The patient is in denial about the possible complications of gonorrhea.
   b. The patient does not perceive the gonorrhea infection as a threatening stressor.
   c. The patient does not have other current stressors that require adaptation or coping mechanisms.
   d. The patient knows how to cope with gonorrhea from dealing with previous gonorrhea infections.

2. The student nurse is depressed. He is trying to study for an important examination but cannot focus. Yesterday he received news that his mother was diagnosed with metastatic breast cancer. What effect could the stress on the student's mind and spirit *most likely* have on the student's body?
   a. The student's stress will cause failure of the examination.
   b. The student's stress will contribute to physical illness.
   c. The student's worry will affect his driving to see his mother.
   d. The student's emotional stress will cause bad feelings about the examination.

3. Identify 4 key personal characteristics that promote adaptation to stressors.
   a.
   b.
   c.
   d.

4. Using the word and phrase list below, fill in the boxes with the numbers of the words or phrases that illustrate the physiologic responses to stress.

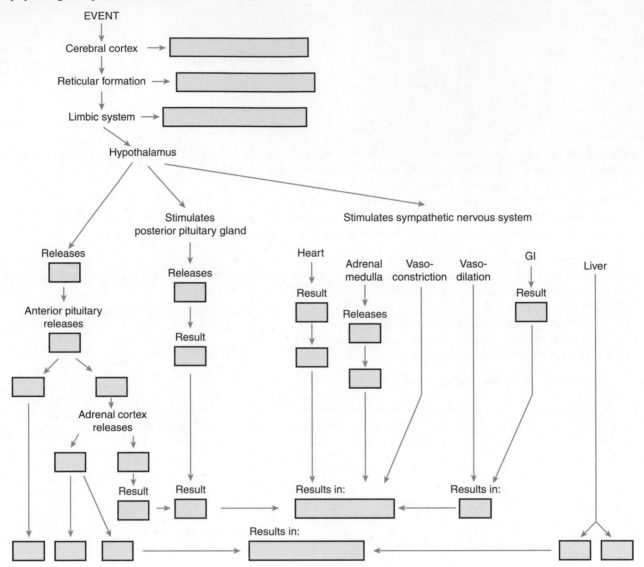

Word and Phrase List

1. Interpretation of event
2. ↑ ADH (antidiuretic hormone)
3. Cortisol
4. ↑ Blood volume
5. ↑ HR and stroke volume
6. ↑ Water retention
7. Wakefulness and alertness
8. ↑ Sympathetic response
9. β-Endorphin
10. Self-preservation behaviors
11. ↑ Cardiac output
12. Corticotropin-releasing hormone
13. Aldosterone
14. ACTH (adrenocorticotropic hormone)
15. Blunted pain perception
16. ↑ Gluconeogenesis
17. ↑ Epinephrine and norepinephrine
18. ↓ Digestion
19. ↑ Proopiomelanocortin (POMC)
20. ↑ Systolic blood pressure
21. ↓ Inflammatory response
22. Glycogenolysis
23. ↑ Blood to vital organs and large muscles
24. ↑ Blood glucose
25. ↑ Na and H_2O reabsorption

5. Using the diagram in Question 4 and the physiologic responses that are noted, identify 8 objective clinical or laboratory manifestations and 4 subjective findings that the nurse may expect.

Objective Manifestations	**Subjective Findings**
a.	a.
b.	b.
c.	c.
d.	d.
e.	
f.	
g.	
h.	

6. While caring for a female patient with Alzheimer's disease and her caregiver husband, the nurse finds that the patient's husband is experiencing increased asthma problems. What is a possible explanation for this finding?
   a. Progressive worsening of asthma occurs in people as they age.
   b. Chronic and intense stress can cause exacerbation of immune-based diseases.
   c. The husband is probably smoking more to help him cope with needing to care continually for his wife.
   d. The husband inadequately copes with his wife's condition by unconsciously forgetting to take his medications.

7. Identify the behaviors listed as either positive coping (P) or negative coping (N) strategies.
   _____ a. Smoking cigarettes
   _____ b. Ignoring a situation
   _____ c. Joining a support group
   _____ d. Starting an exercise program
   _____ e. Increasing time spent with friends

8. A patient has recently had a myocardial infarction. What emotion-focused coping strategies would the nurse encourage him to use to adapt to the physical and emotional stress of his illness? **Select all that apply.**
   a. Use meditation.
   b. Plan dietary changes.
   c. Start an exercise program.
   d. Do favorite escape activities (e.g., playing cards).
   e. Share feelings with spouse or other family members.

9. While teaching relaxation therapy to a patient with fibromyalgia, what does the nurse recognize as being most important to incorporate?
   a. Exercise
   b. Relaxation breathing
   c. Soft background music
   d. Progressive muscle relaxation

10. After receiving the assigned patients for the day, the nurse determines that stress-relieving interventions are a priority for which patient?
   a. The man with peptic ulcer disease
   b. The newly admitted woman with cholecystitis
   c. The man with a bacterial exacerbation of chronic bronchitis
   d. The woman who is 1 day postoperative for knee replacement

11. A 32-year-old man is admitted to the hospital with an acute exacerbation of Crohn's disease. What coping strategies may be suggested by the nurse during his hospitalization? **Select all that apply.**
   a. Humor
   b. Exercise
   c. Journaling
   d. A cleansing diet
   e. Relaxation therapy

CASE STUDY Stress

Patient Profile
M.J., a 26-year-old single female, is admitted to the hospital with right lower quadrant pain rated as 8 on a scale of 0 to 10; 10 to 12 watery, blood-streaked stools in the past 24 hours; and a low-grade fever. She has a 7-year history of inflammatory bowel disease.

(©azndc/iStock/Thinkstock)

Subjective Data
Patient relates the following:
- Has been hospitalized 4 times in the past year.
- Is not currently working because of the illness and has no income.
- Has no health insurance.
- Her boyfriend has lived with her for 2 years.
- Does not want her boyfriend to visit because she thinks he has enough problems of his own.
- Has been in bed for the past week because of pain, weakness, nausea, and malaise and has been crying and is depressed.
- Talks weekly with her sister.
- Has 2 dogs at home.

Objective Data
- Height: 5 ft, 6 in (168 cm)
- Weight: 104 lb (47.3 kg)
- Hemoglobin: 10.5 g/dL (105 g/L)
- Hematocrit: 30%
- Temp: 100°F (37.8°C)

Questions
1. What physiologic and psychologic stressors can be identified or anticipated in M.J.'s situation? What is the effect of these stressors? **Use an X to identify if the stressor is <u>Physiologic</u> or <u>Psychologic</u>, and the <u>Effect</u> (result of a stressor).**

Assessment Finding	Physiologic	Psychologic	Effect
Weight 47.3 kg			
Pain 8 out of 10			
No health insurance			
Inflammatory bowel disease			
Hematocrit 30%			
Hospitalized 4 times during the last year			
Chronic disease			
Depression			

2. What factors, identified in the nursing assessment, could negatively impact M.J.'s adaptation to stress? **Select all that apply.**
_____A. Her refusal to seek support from her boyfriend
_____B. Multiple hospitalizations
_____C. Has a live-in boyfriend
_____D. 7-year history of IBD
_____E. Lack of employment
_____F. Weakness
_____G. Talks with her sister weekly
_____H. Has pets

3. **What nursing actions would the nurse implement to enhance M.J.'s adaptation to stress? Use an X to identify if the intervention is <u>Indicated</u> (will help), <u>Contraindicated</u> (will not help or could be harmful), or is <u>Non-Essential</u> (makes no difference).**

Nursing Action	Indicated	Contraindicated	Non-Essential
Avoid meditation			
Administer pain medication			
Obtain a physical therapy consult			
Promote restful sleep			

Nursing Action	Indicated	Contraindicated	Non-Essential
Teach relaxation breathing			
Restrict visitors			
Consult with a social worker			

4. Which assessment findings indicate that M.J. is responding to therapies?
   Use an X to identify if the interventions were <u>Effective</u> (helped to meet expected outcomes), <u>Ineffective</u> (did not help to meet expected outcomes), or <u>Unrelated</u> (not related to the expected outcomes).

Assessment Finding	Effective	Ineffective	Unrelated
Gains 2 pounds in 2 weeks			
Walks the dogs twice daily			
Refuses to tell her sister about her recent hospitalization			
Has 3 stools per day			
Cries twice a week about her disease			
Platelet count 128,000/mm^3			

5. **Choose the most likely options for the information missing from the statements below by selecting from the lists of options provided.**

   M.J. expresses to the nurse how concerned she is about the future. The nurse assigns _____**1**_____ as the priority clinical problem. The nurse considers several coping strategies when making recommendations to M.J. One coping strategy is for M.J. to participate in _____**2**_____ by coloring in a coloring book. Another recommendation is to write down her thoughts, which is a form of _____**2**_____. M.J. says she is going to find a support group, which the nurse recognizes as an example of _____**3**_____. Other relaxation strategies the nurse would recommend are _____**4**_____, _____**4**_____, and _____**4**_____.

Options for 1	Options for 2	Options for 3	Options for 4
Acute pain	Humor	Stressors	Yoga
Nutritionally compromised	Exercise	Problem-focused coping	Qigong
Fatigue	Journaling	Relaxation	Working
Difficulty coping	Pet therapy	Emotion-focused coping	Tai Chi
Decisional conflict	Art therapy	Mind-body-spirit connection	Traveling
Health Maintenance Alteration	Biofeedback	Reticular formation	Problem-solving

Sleep and Sleep Disorders

1. Which statement about sleep is accurate?
   a. Lack of sleep causes medical and psychiatric disorders.
   b. Adults generally need at least 5 hours of sleep every 24 hours.
   c. During sleep an individual is not consciously aware of his or her environment.
   d. Less than 10% of adults report at least 1 sleep problem, such as difficulty falling asleep.

2. What are clinical manifestations of insomnia? **Select all that apply.**
   a. Narcolepsy
   b. Fragmented sleep
   c. Long sleep latency
   d. Morning headache
   e. Daytime sleepiness
   f. Difficulty concentrating

3. What is a typical parasomnia?
   a. Cataplexy
   b. Hypopnea
   c. Sleep apnea
   d. Sleep terrors

4. What regulates the cyclic changes between waking and sleep?
   a. Fluctuating levels of melatonin
   b. The environmental light-dark cycles
   c. Suprachiasmatic nucleus in hypothalamus
   d. A variety of neurotransmitters released from the nervous system

5. Match the descriptions to the stages of sleep. Some descriptions may have more than 1 stage, and some stages may be used more than once.

   Description
   _____ a. Brain waves resemble wakefulness
   _____ b. Deepest sleep
   _____ c. Associated with specific electroencephalogram (EEG) waveforms
   _____ d. Most vivid dreaming occurs
   _____ e. 20% to 25% of sleep
   _____ f. Person easily awakened
   _____ g. Most of the night of sleep
   _____ h. Slow eye movements
   _____ i. Slowed heart rate, decreased body temperature
   _____ j. Decreased occurrence in older adults

   Sleep Stage
   1. N1
   2. N2
   3. N3
   4. Rapid eye movement (REM)

6. List at least 3 behaviors or practices that can contribute to insomnia.
   a.
   b.
   c.

7. A polysomnography (PSG) may be done on a patient with signs and symptoms of a sleep disorder. What measures and observations does this study include? **Select all that apply.**
   a. Heart rate monitoring
   b. Noninvasive oxygen saturation (SpO$_2$)
   c. Surface body temperature fluctuations
   d. Blood pressure monitoring (noninvasive)
   e. Airflow measured at the nose and mouth
   f. Muscle tone measured by electromyogram (EMG)
   g. Respiratory effort around the chest and abdomen
   h. Eye movements recorded by electrooculogram (EOG)
   i. Brain activity recorded by EEG
   j. Actigraph watch worn on the wrist to monitor motor activity
   k. Gross body movements monitored via cameras and microphones

8. What is the best therapy to try first for insomnia?
   a. Complementary therapies, such as melatonin
   b. Over-the-counter medications, such as diphenhydramine
   c. Benzodiazepine-receptor agents (e.g., zolpidem [Ambien])
   d. Cognitive-behavioral therapies, such as relaxation therapy

9. Which statement indicates to the nurse that a patient taught sleep hygiene practices needs further instruction?
   a. "Once I go to bed, I should get up if I am not asleep after 20 minutes."
   b. "It's okay to have my usual 2 glasses of wine in the evening before bed."
   c. "A couple of crackers with cheese and a glass of milk may help to relax before bed."
   d. "I should go to the gym earlier in the day so that I'm done at least 6 hours before bedtime."

10. The patient is reporting insomnia and daytime fatigue. Which beverage would be the best option for this patient with an afternoon snack?
    a. Cola
    b. Green tea
    c. A&W root beer
    d. Decaffeinated coffee

11. A nurse caring for a patient in the intensive care unit (ICU) implements strategies to create an environment conducive to sleep. Which strategy would be most effective?
    a. Turning off the lights in the room during the night
    b. Having the television on at all times for background noise
    c. Silencing the alarms on the bedside monitor and infusion pumps
    d. Administering ordered analgesics around the clock, even if the patient denies pain

12. Which medication is a first-line nonamphetamine wake-promotion drug that is used to treat narcolepsy?
    a. Pitolisant (Wakix)
    b. Modafinil (Provigil)
    c. Amitriptyline (Elavil)
    d. Solriamfetol (Sunosi)

13. The nurse in a clinic is talking with a patient who will be traveling from the Midwest time zone to Moscow to attend a 4-day conference. The patient asks the nurse how he can minimize the effects of jet lag. What are at least 2 recommendations that the nurse could give to the patient?

14. Place the events below in the order they occur in the patient with obstructive sleep apnea (beginning with 1).
    _____ a. Apnea lasting 10 to 90 seconds
    _____ b. Brief arousal and airway opened
    _____ c. Generalized startle response, snorting, or gasping
    _____ d. Hypoxemia and hypercapnia
    _____ e. Narrowing of air passages with muscle relaxation and/or partial or complete obstruction of the pharynx caused by the tongue and soft palate falling backward
    _____ f. Risk factors: obesity, neck circumference 16 inches or larger, age older than 65 years
    _____ g. Occurs 180 to 400 times during 6 to 8 hours of sleep

15. The health care provider (HCP) has ordered continuous positive airway pressure (CPAP) for a patient with severe obstructive sleep apnea. How will CPAP help the patient?
    a. Prevent airway occlusion by bringing the tongue forward
    b. Be easily tolerated by both the patient and patient's bed partner
    c. Provide enough positive pressure in the airway to prevent airway collapse
    d. Deliver a high inspiratory pressure and a low expiratory pressure to prevent airway collapse

16. While caring for a patient following an uvulopalatopharyngoplasty (UPPP), the nurse monitors the patient for which complications during the immediate postoperative period?
    a. Snoring and foul-smelling breath
    b. Infection and electrolyte imbalance
    c. Loss of voice and severe sore throat
    d. Airway obstruction and hemorrhage

17. An older patient asks the nurse why she has so much trouble sleeping. What is the most appropriate response by the nurse?
    a. "Disturbed sleep is a normal result of aging."
    b. "Have you tried any over-the-counter medications to help you sleep?"
    c. "Don't worry. You don't need as much sleep as you did when you were younger."
    d. "Tell me more about the trouble you are having. There may be some things we can do to help."

18. Nurses who rotate shifts or work nights are at risk for developing shift work sleep disorder characterized by insomnia, sleepiness, and fatigue. Identify at least 3 negative implications for the nurse.

19. What strategies could decrease the distress of rotating shifts for nurses? **Select all that apply.**
    a. Take a brief onsite nap.
    b. Use sleep hygiene practices.
    c. Sleep just before going to work.
    d. Maintain consistent sleep/wake schedules even on days off (if possible).
    e. Negotiate to control work schedule rather than having someone else impose the schedule.

CASE STUDY   Sleep Disorder

Patient Profile

W.D., a 75-year-old man with Parkinson's disease, was admitted to the hospital for surgical repair of a right fractured hip. He fell when he slipped on a bathroom rug.

(Rauluminate/iStock/Thinkstock)

Subjective Data
- Has a history of chronic insomnia and uses various over-the-counter sleep aids without relief
- Usually drinks a few glasses of wine at night while watching TV in his bed
- Lives alone and is very anxious about who will take care of him after surgery
- History of osteoarthritis, reports the pain is worse in the morning; takes over-the-counter NSAIDs a few times per week
- History of hypertension, takes atenolol
- History of heart failure, takes furosemide before bed, captopril, and digoxin; denies shortness of breath
- History of type 2 diabetes, takes glipizide
- States he has a persistent cough that wakes him up at night

Objective Data
- Total hip arthroplasty postoperative day 0
- Estimated blood loss during surgery was 75 mL
- Reports 3 out of 10 incisional pain
- Dorsalis pedis pulses: left foot 3+, right foot 2+
- Capillary refill < 3 seconds in all 4 extremities
- Right foot cooler than left foot
- Alert and oriented x4
- Vital signs: HR 86 beats/min, BP 150/80 mm Hg, RR 14 breaths/min, oxygen saturation 95% on room air, temperature 96.6°F (35.9°C)
- Right hip dressing 50% saturated with serosanguineous drainage

Questions

1. Which factors may be contributing to his history of chronic insomnia? **Select all that apply.**

_____a. Alcohol consumption
_____b. Parkinson's disease
_____c. Use of over-the-counter sleep aids
_____d. Age
_____e. Diuretic medication
_____f. Heart failure
_____g. Type 2 diabetes
_____h. Osteoarthritis
_____i. ACE inhibitor medication

2. **Referring to the information in the Patient Profile above, highlight or place a check mark next to the assessment findings that require follow-up by the nurse.**

3. Based on the patient information above, use an X to indicate whether the nursing actions listed below are <u>Indicated</u> (appropriate or necessary), <u>Contraindicated</u> (not appropriate or could be harmful), or <u>Non-Essential</u> (makes no difference or is unnecessary) for the client's care at this time.

Nursing Action	Indicated	Contraindicated	Non-Essential
Initiate O_2 therapy			
Administer opioid pain medication			
Position the patient onto his right side			
Prepare to administer a blood transfusion			
Administer the ordered antihypertensive medication			
Turn the TV off prior to patient's bedtime			
Allow the patient to nap during the day			
Place patient in a private room			
Schedule physical therapy in the early afternoon			
Administer the furosemide at 9 PM			

4. The nurse is creating a discharge teaching plan for when W.D. is discharged home. **For each patient statement, use an X to indicate which statement indicates that teaching is Effective (the patient understands) and which statement indicates that teaching is Ineffective (the patient needs additional teaching).**

Health Teaching	Effective	Ineffective
"I will continue to take furosemide at bedtime."		
"I will contact my primary HCP to ask about changing captopril to a different medication."		
"I will avoid drinking a cup of coffee in the morning."		
"I will stop using the Internet several hours before bedtime."		
"I can drink 7-Up with dinner."		
"I will get up and read a book if I cannot fall asleep within 20 minutes after going to bed."		

5. The patient is prescribed the following medications. **Choose the most likely options for the information missing from the table below by selecting from the lists of options provided.**

Medication	Dose, Route, Frequency	Drug Class	Indication
1	25 mg PO twice daily	ACE inhibitor	HTN & heart failure
Oxycodone	**2**	Opioid	Acute pain
3	25-100 mg PO three times/day	Decarboxylase inhibitor	Parkinson's disease
Furosemide	20 mg PO once daily	Loop diuretic	**4**
Atenolol	50 mg once daily	**5**	Hypertension
Glipizide	**6**	Sulfonylurea	Type 2 diabetes
Digoxin	0.125 mg once daily	**7**	**8**

Options for 1 and 3	Options for 2 and 6	Options for 5 and 7	Options for 4 and 8
Captopril	200 mg PO every 6 hr PRN	Alpha-adrenergic blocker	Hypertension
Metoprolol	5-10 mg PO every 4 hr PRN	ACE inhibitor	Heart failure
Digoxin	15 mg IV every 6 hr PRN	Angiotensin II receptor blocker	Hyperkalemia
Carbidopa-levodopa	5 mg PO twice daily	Loop diuretic	Parkinson's disease
Zolpidem	50 mg PO twice daily	Cardiac glycoside	Diabetes
Trazodone	100 mg PO once daily	Beta blocker	Sleep aid

Pain

1. Pain has been defined as "whatever the person experiencing the pain says it is, existing whenever the patient says it does." This definition is problematic for the nurse when caring for which type of patient?
   a. A patient placed on a ventilator
   b. A patient with a history of opioid addiction
   c. A patient with decreased cognitive function
   d. A patient with pain resulting from severe trauma

2. On the first postoperative day following a bowel resection, the patient reports abdominal and incisional pain rated 9 on a scale of 0 to 10. Postoperative orders include morphine (4 mg IV q4hr) for pain and may repeat morphine (4 mg IV) for breakthrough pain. The nurse determines that it has been only 1¾ hours since the last dose of morphine and wants to wait a little longer. What effect does the nurse's action have on the patient?
   a. Protects the patient from addiction and toxic effects of the drug
   b. Prevents hastening or causing a patient's death from respiratory dysfunction
   c. Contributes to unnecessary suffering and physical and psychosocial dysfunction
   d. Shows the nurse understands the adage of "start low and go slow" in giving analgesics

3. List and briefly describe the 5 dimensions of pain.
   a.
   b.
   c.
   d.
   e.

4. Once generated, what may block the transmission of an action potential along a peripheral nerve fiber to the dorsal root of the spinal cord?
   a. Nothing can stop the action potential along an intact nerve until it reaches the spinal cord.
   b. The action potential must cross several synapses, points at which the impulse may be blocked by drugs.
   c. Transmission may be interrupted by drugs (e.g., local anesthetics) that act on peripheral sodium channels.
   d. The nerve fiber produces neurotransmitters that may activate nearby nerve fibers to transmit pain impulses.

5. A patient comes to the clinic reporting a dull pain in the anterior and posterior neck. On examination, the nurse notes that the patient has full range of motion (ROM) of the neck and no throat redness or enlarged head or neck lymph nodes. What will be the nurse's next appropriate assessment indicated by these findings?
   a. Palpating the liver
   b. Auscultating bowel sounds
   c. Inspecting the patient's ears
   d. Palpating for the presence of hip pain

6. While caring for an unconscious patient, the nurse discovers a stage 2 pressure injury on the patient's heel. During care of the wound, what is the nurse's understanding of the patient's perception of pain?
   a. The patient will have a behavioral response if pain is perceived.
   b. The area should be treated as a painful lesion, using gentle cleansing and dressing.
   c. The area can be thoroughly scrubbed because the patient is not able to perceive pain.
   d. All nociceptive stimuli that are transmitted to the brain result in the perception of pain.

7. Using number 1 as the first process and number 4 as the last process, number in order the nociceptive processes that occur to communicate tissue damage to the central nervous system (CNS).

    _____ a. Perception

    _____ b. Modulation

    _____ c. Transmission

    _____ d. Transduction

8. Match the following types of pain in the left column with a category of pain from the upper right column and an example of the source of the pain from the lower right column.

    Types of Pain

    _____ a. Pain from loss of afferent input

    _____ b. Pain persisting from sympathetic nervous system (SNS) activity

    _____ c. Pain caused by dysfunction in the CNS

    _____ d. Pain arising from skin and subcutaneous tissue; well localized

    _____ e. Pain arising from muscles and bones; localized or diffuse and radiating

    _____ f. Pain felt along the distribution of peripheral nerve(s) from nerve damage

    _____ g. Pain arising from visceral organs; well or poorly localized; referred cutaneously

    Categories of Pain
    1. Nociceptive pain
    2. Neuropathic pain

    Sources of Pain
    3. Sunburn
    4. Pancreatitis
    5. Osteoarthritis
    6. Poststroke pain
    8. Trigeminal neuralgia
    9. Postmastectomy pain

9. Amitriptyline is prescribed for a patient with chronic pain from fibromyalgia. When the nurse explains that this drug is an antidepressant, the patient states that she is in pain, not depressed. What is the nurse's best response to the patient?
    a. Antidepressants will improve the patient's attitude and prevent a negative emotional response to the pain.
    b. Chronic pain almost always leads to depression, and the use of this drug will prevent depression from occurring.
    c. Some antidepressant drugs relieve pain by releasing neurotransmitters that prevent pain impulses from reaching the brain.
    d. Certain antidepressant drugs are metabolized in the liver to substances that numb the ends of nerve fibers, preventing the onset of pain.

10. A patient with trigeminal neuralgia has moderate to severe burning and shooting pain. In helping the patient manage the pain, what does the nurse recognize about this type of pain?
    a. Includes treatment with adjuvant analgesics
    b. Will be chronic and require long-term treatment
    c. Responds to small to moderate round-the-clock doses of oral opioids
    d. Can be well controlled with salicylates or nonsteroidal antiinflammatory drugs (NSAIDs)

11. In the following scenario, identify the assessment finding that corresponds to the elements of a pain assessment. A 62-year-old male patient is admitted to the medical unit from the emergency department. On arrival, he is trembling and nearly doubled over with severe, cramping abdominal pain. He indicates that he has severe right upper quadrant pain that radiates to his back and he is more comfortable walking bent forward than lying in bed. He notes that he has had several similar bouts of abdominal pain in the last month but "not as bad as this. This is the worst pain I can imagine." The other episodes lasted only about 2 hours. Today he had an acute onset of pain and nausea after eating fish and chips at a fast-food restaurant about 4 hours ago.

Element of Pain Assessment	Assessment Finding
Onset	
Duration and pattern of pain	
Location	
Intensity	
Quality	
Associated symptoms	
Management strategies	

12. List the 10 basic principles that should guide the treatment of all pain.
    a.
    b.
    c.
    d.
    e.
    f.
    g.
    h.
    i.
    j.

13. A patient with advanced colorectal cancer has continuous, poorly localized abdominal pain at an intensity of 5 on a scale of 0 to 10. How would the nurse teach the patient to use pain medications?
    a. On an around-the-clock schedule
    b. As often as necessary to keep the pain controlled
    c. By alternating 2 different types of drugs to prevent tolerance
    d. When the pain cannot be controlled with distraction or relaxation

14. A patient who has been taking ibuprofen and imipramine (Tofranil) for control of cancer pain is having increased pain. What would the nurse recommend to the health care provider (HCP) as an appropriate change in the medication plan?
    a. Add PO oxycodone to the other medications.
    b. Substitute PO ketorolac, an NSAID, for imipramine.
    c. Add transdermal fentanyl (Duragesic) to the use of the other medications.
    d. Substitute PO hydrocodone with acetaminophen for the other medications.

15. A patient with chronic cancer-related pain has started using MS Contin for pain control and has developed common side effects of the drug. The nurse reassures the patient that tolerance will develop to most of these side effects but that continued treatment will most likely be required for what?
    a. Pruritus
    b. Dizziness
    c. Constipation
    d. Nausea and vomiting

16. A postoperative 68-year-old opioid-naive patient is receiving morphine by patient-controlled analgesia (PCA) for postoperative pain. What is the reason for not starting the PCA analgesic with a basal dose of analgesic?
    a. Opioid overdose
    b. Nausea and itching
    c. Lack of pain control
    d. Adverse respiratory outcomes

17. Which measures or drugs may be effective in controlling pain in the physiologic pain process stage of transduction? **Select all that apply.**
    a. Distraction
    b. Corticosteroids
    c. Epidural opioids
    d. Local anesthetics
    e. Antiseizure medications
    f. Nonsteroidal antiinflammatory drugs (NSAIDs)

18. A patient is receiving a continuous infusion of morphine via an epidural catheter after major abdominal surgery. Which actions would the nurse include in the plan of care? **Select all that apply.**
    a. Label the catheter as an epidural access.
    b. Assess the patient's pain relief frequently.
    c. Use sterile technique when caring for the catheter.
    d. Monitor the patient's level of consciousness (LOC).
    e. Monitor patient vital signs (BP, heart rate, respirations).
    f. Assess the motor and sensory function of the patient's lower extremities.

19. A patient with multiple injuries following an automobile accident tells the nurse that he has "bad" pain but that he can "tough it out" and does not need pain medication. To gain the patient's participation in pain management, what is most important for the nurse to explain to the patient?
    a. Patients have a responsibility to keep the nurse informed about their pain.
    b. Unrelieved pain has many harmful effects on the body that can impair recovery.
    c. Using pain medications rarely leads to addiction when they are used for actual pain.
    d. Nonpharmacologic therapies can be used to relieve his pain if he is afraid to use pain medications.

20. The patient has chronic pain that is no longer relieved with oral morphine. Which medication would the nurse expect to be ordered to provide better pain relief for this patient?
    a. Fentanyl
    b. Hydrocodone
    c. Intranasal butorphanol
    d. Morphine sustained-release

21. After the family members of a postoperative patient leave, the patient tells the nurse that his family gave him a headache by fussing over him so much. What is an appropriate intervention by the nurse?
    a. Administer the PRN analgesic prescribed for his postoperative pain.
    b. Ask the patient's permission to use acupressure to ease his headache.
    c. Reassure the patient that his headache will subside now that his family has gone.
    d. Teach the patient biofeedback methods to relieve his headaches by controlling cerebral blood flow.

CASE STUDY   Pain

Patient Profile

R.D. is a 62-year-old man, with chronic pain from metastatic cancer, is being evaluated for a change in his pain therapy.

(BananaStock/Thinkstock)

Subjective Data
- Desires 0 pain but will accept pain level of 3 to 4 on a scale of 0 to 10.
- He has been taking 2 Percocet tablets every 4 hrs while awake, but his pain is usually a 4 to a 5 with the medication.
- Patient reports that pain varies over 24 hours from 5 to 10.
- Always awakens in the morning with pain at 10 with nervousness, nausea, and a runny nose.
- When pain becomes severe, he stays in bed and concentrates on blocking the pain by emptying his mind.
- Is worried that increased pain means his disease is worsening.
- Is afraid to take additional doses or other opioids because he fears addiction.

Objective Data
- Height: 6 ft 0 in (183 cm)
- Weight: 150 lbs (68 kg)
- Rigid posturing, slow gait

Questions

1. Use an X to indicate which data from the nursing assessment are characteristic of the affective, behavioral, and cognitive dimensions of the pain experience.

Assessment Finding	Affective	Behavioral	Cognitive
Worried about worsening disease			
Stays in bed with severe pain			
Empties his mind to block pain			
Afraid of addiction			
Rigid posture with slow gait			

2. The nurse performs a physical assessment on R.D. and documents the following nurse's note. **Highlight the findings in the note below that indicate this patient's pain is not well managed.**

NURSE'S NOTE:

The patient reports his current pain is 5 out of 10 and describes it as constant. He seems preoccupied as I have to repeat questions. He is fidgety and grimaces when he moves. Vital signs: HR 98 beats/min, RR 20 breaths/min, BP 155/82 mm Hg, SpO$_2$ 96% on room air, Temp. 37.1°C. He requests the urinal to void. He reports feeling rested over the past 3 days. Had his neighbor drive him to the appointment because he cannot concentrate.

3. Patients can become physically dependent on opioids placing them at risk of withdrawal when the drug is abruptly stopped or decreased. **For each assessment finding use an X to indicate if the finding is <u>Associated</u> (is a manifestation) with withdrawal or is <u>Unrelated</u> (is not a manifestation) to the withdrawal syndrome.**

Assessment finding	Associated	Unrelated
Oliguria		
Diaphoresis		
Chills		
Bradycardia		
Rhinorrhea		
Constipation		
Hypoxemia		
Insomnia		

4. Choose the most likely options for the information missing from the table below by selecting from the lists of options provided.

Medication	Drug Class	Nursing Consideration
Gabapentin	Antiseizure	1
2	Mu agonist	QT prolongation
Duloxetine	3	Decreased libido
4	NSAID	GI bleeding
Celecoxib	5	6
7	Corticosteroid	8

Options for 2, 4, and 7	Options for 3 and 5	Options for 1, 6, and 8
Dexamethasone	Cox-II inhibitor	Drowsiness
Gabapentin	Mu agonist	Hyperglycemia
Duloxetine	NSAID	QT prolongation
Diclofenac	SNRI	Cardiovascular thrombotic events
Celecoxib	Antiseizure	GI bleeding
Methadone	Corticosteroid	Decreased libido

5. Which statements indicate to the nurse that therapy and teaching are effective? **Select all that apply.**
_____ A. "The goal is to be able to perform ADLs."
_____ B. "I will double the amount of Percocet medication when my pain is severe."
_____ C. "I will use heat and cold occasionally to manage pain."
_____ D. "I will keep a journal about my pain."
_____ E. "I will learn to tolerate 10 out of 10 pain as the disease progresses."
_____ F. "If the pain therapies are effective, I will be pain free."
_____ G. "I will take additional acetaminophen for breakthrough pain."
_____ H. "I will incorporate meditation."
_____ I. "I will be able to drive when the pain is tolerable."

Palliative and End-of-Life Care

1. Palliative care is any form of care or treatment that focuses on reducing the severity of disease symptoms to prevent and relieve suffering and improve quality of life for patients with serious life-threatening illnesses. What are the specific goals of palliative care? **Select 6 that apply.**
   a. Regard dying as a normal process.
   b. Minimize the financial burden on the family.
   c. Provide relief from symptoms, including pain.
   d. Affirm life and neither hasten nor postpone death.
   e. Prolong the patient's life with aggressive new therapies.
   f. Support holistic patient care and enhance quality of life.
   g. Offer support to patients to live as actively as possible until death.
   h. Help the patient and family identify and access pastoral care services.
   i. Offer support to the family during the patient's illness and their own bereavement.

2. The husband and daughter of a Hispanic woman dying from pancreatic cancer refuse to consider using hospice care. What would the nurse do first?
   a. Assess their understanding of what hospice care services are.
   b. Ask them how they will care for the patient without hospice care.
   c. Talk directly to the patient and family to see if the nurse can change their minds.
   d. Accept their decision because they are Hispanic and prefer to care for their own family members.

3. List the 2 criteria for admission to a hospice program.
   a.
   b.

4. For each of the following body systems, identify 3 physical manifestations that the nurse would expect to see in a patient approaching death.

   Respiratory
   a.
   b.
   c.

   Skin
   a.
   b.
   c.

   Gastrointestinal
   a.
   b.
   c.

   Musculoskeletal
   a.
   b.
   c.

5. A terminally ill patient is unresponsive and has cold, clammy skin with mottling on the extremities. The patient's husband and 2 grown children are arguing at the bedside about where the patient's funeral should be held. What would the nurse do first?
   a. Ask the family members to leave the room if they are going to argue.
   b. Take the family members aside and explain that the patient may be able to hear them.
   c. Tell the family members that this decision is premature because the patient has not yet died.
   d. If the patient regains consciousness, the patient should be asked because it is their decision.

6. A 20-year-old patient with a massive head injury is on life support, including a ventilator to maintain respirations. What 3 criteria for brain death are necessary to discontinue life support?
   a.
   b.
   c.

7. A patient with end-stage liver failure tells the nurse, "If I can just live to see my first grandchild who is expected in 5 months, then I can die happy." The nurse recognizes that the patient is showing which stage of grieving?
   a. Prolonged grief disorder
   b. Kübler-Ross's stage of bargaining
   c. Kübler-Ross's stage of depression
   d. The new normal stage of the Grief Wheel

8. A terminally ill man tells the nurse, "I have never believed there is a God or an afterlife, but now it is too terrible to imagine that I will not exist. Why was I here in the first place?" What does this statement help the nurse recognize about the patient's needs?
   a. He is experiencing spiritual distress.
   b. This man will not have a peaceful death.
   c. He needs to be reassured that his feelings are normal.
   d. There should be a referral to a clergyman to discuss his beliefs.

9. In most states, which legal documents include directives to physicians, durable power of attorney for health care, and medical power of attorney?
   a. Natural death acts
   b. Allow natural death
   c. Advance care planning
   d. Do-not-resuscitate order

10. A patient is receiving care to manage symptoms of a terminal illness when the disease no longer responds to treatment. What is this type of care?
    a. Terminal care
    b. Palliative care
    c. Supportive care
    d. Maintenance care

11. A patient in the last stages of life is experiencing shortness of breath and air hunger. Based on practice guidelines, what is the most appropriate action by the nurse?
    a. Apply oxygen.
    b. Give bronchodilators.
    c. Administer antianxiety agents.
    d. Use any methods that make the patient more comfortable.

12. What does end-of-life care involve?
    a. Constant assessment for changes in physiologic functioning.
    b. Administering large doses of analgesics to keep the patient sedated.
    c. Providing as little physical care as possible to prevent disturbing the patient.
    d. Encouraging the patient and family members to verbalize their feelings of sadness, loss, and forgiveness.

13. The dying patient and family have many interrelated psychosocial and physical care needs. Which ones can the nurse manage with the patient and family? **Select all that apply.**
    a. Anxiety
    b. Fear of pain
    c. The dying process
    d. Care being provided
    e. Anger toward the nurse
    f. Feeling powerless and hopeless

14. A deathly ill patient from a culture different than the nurse's is admitted. Which question is appropriate to help the nurse provide culturally competent care?
    a. "If you die, will you want an autopsy?"
    b. "Are you interested in learning about palliative or hospice care?"
    c. "Do you have any preferences for what happens if you are dying?"
    d. "Tell me about your expectations of care during this hospitalization."

CASE STUDY   End-of-Life Palliative Care

(SylvieBouchard/
iStock/Thinkstock)

Patient Profile

S.J., a 42-year-old woman, had unsuccessful treatment for breast cancer 1 year ago and now has metastasis to the lung and vertebrae. She lives at home with her husband, 15-year-old daughter, and 12-year-old son. She has been referred to hospice because of her deteriorating condition and increasing pain. Her husband is an accountant and tries to do as much of his work at home as possible so that he can help care for his wife. Their children have become withdrawn, choosing to spend as much time as possible at their friends' homes and doing outside activities.

Subjective Data

- S.J. reports that she stays in bed most of the time because it is too painful to stand and sit.
- She reports her pain as an 8 on a scale of 0 to 10 while taking oral MS Contin every 12 hours.
- She reports shortness of breath with almost any activity, such as getting up to go to the bathroom.
- S.J. says she knows she is dying, but her greatest suffering results from her children not caring about her.
- She and her husband have not talked with the children about her dying.
- Her husband reports that he does not know how to help his wife anymore and that he feels guilty sometimes when he just wishes it were all over.

Objective Data

- Height: 5 ft 2 in (157 cm)
- Weight: 97 lbs (44 kg)
- Skin intact
- Vital signs: Temp 99°F (37.2°C), HR 92 beats/min, RR 30, breaths/min 102/60 mm Hg

Questions

1. Indicate which assessment finding listed in the far-left column is applicable to the clinical problem. Note that some assessment findings may be applied to more than one clinical problem or may not be used at all.

Assessment Finding	Clinical Problem	Appropriate Assessment Finding for Clinical Problem
Stays in bed due to pain	Difficulty coping	
Her children don't care about her	Caregiver Role Strain	
Shortness of breath with activity	Grief	
S.J. and her husband haven't talked to their children about her dying		
Husband feels guilty because he wishes it was all over		
Husband tries to do as much work at home to help care for S.J.		
Husband doesn't know how to help S.J. anymore		
Children are withdrawn spending most of their time out of the house		

2. What other assessment data should the nurse obtain from S.J. and her husband before making any decisions about care of the family?

   Use an X to indicate if the assessment data is Essential (is necessary or appropriate) or Non-essential (is unnecessary or is inappropriate) for the care of S.J. and her husband at this time.

Assessment Data	Essential	Non-Essential
Reasons for not discussing her impending death with their children		
Funeral plans		
Assessment of spiritual needs		
S.J.'s dying preferences		
Assessment of S.J.'s functional status		
Determine if S.J. is competent to make decisions		
Assessment of how S.J. and her husband are coping		

3. What nursing actions would the nurse include when planning care for S.J.?

   Use an X to indicate if the nursing action is Indicated (is necessary or appropriate), Contraindicated (could be harmful), or Non-essential (is unnecessary or makes no difference) for the care of S.J. at this time.

Nursing Action	Indicated	Contraindicated	Non-Essential
Avoid the use of opioids			
Insert a nasogastric feeding tube			
Place S.J. on neutropenic precautions			
Auscultate lung sounds			
Apply sequential compression stockings			
Obtain an arterial blood gas (ABG)			
Implement every 2-hour turning schedule			
Consult the palliative care team			
Recommend a chiropractor			

4. What would the nurse tell S.J. and her family regarding what to expect as S.J. approaches the end of life? **Select all that apply**.

   _____A. She may report seeing or talks to deceased loved ones.
   _____B. She may seem withdrawn and won't respond because she cannot hear.
   _____C. She may become hungry and thirsty in the last days of life.
   _____D. She may experience delirium and restlessness in the last days of life.
   _____E. Her skin color may become mottled or cyanotic in the last days of life.
   _____F. The children should be encouraged to say goodbye.
   _____G. She may sleep more often.
   _____H. She may have difficulty swallowing.
   _____I. Opioids will be withheld if she experiences respiratory difficulty.

5. **Choose the most likely options for the information missing from the statements below by selecting from the options provided.**

   There are _____**1**_____ domains of palliative care. Domain 3 is _____**2**_____. An example of domain 2, physical aspects of care, is _____**3**_____. Caregivers should have specific roles along with resources, which is part of domain _____**4**_____. A hospice program has 2 criteria. They are _____**5**_____ and _____**5**_____.

Options for 1 and 4	Options for 2
1	Care structure and processes
2	Ethical and legal aspects
3	Social aspects of care
4	Physical aspects of care
5	Spiritual, religious, and existential aspects of care
6	Culture care
7	Care of the patient nearing end of life
8	Psychologic and psychiatric aspects

Options for 3	Options for 5
Beliefs of a higher power	Patient has less than 3 months to live
Access to transportation	One physician determines the patient is terminal
Symptom management	Patient must agree in writing
Establishing a plan of care	Two physicians determine the patient is terminal
Accepting cultural variations	Death is guaranteed in 6 months
Obtaining an advance directive	Patient cannot be discharged from hospice care
Involving hospice services	Patient must have Medicare
Mental health treatment	Includes curative care

Substance Use Disorders

1. What is the definition of substance use disorder (SUD)?
   a. A compulsive need to experience pleasure
   b. Behavior associated with maintaining an addiction
   c. Absence of a substance will cause withdrawal symptoms
   d. Overuse and dependence on a substance that negatively affects functioning

2. What term is used to describe a decreased effect of a substance following repeated exposure?
   a. Relapse
   b. Tolerance
   c. Abstinence
   d. Withdrawal

3. As health care professionals, nurses have a responsibility to help reduce the use of tobacco. List the recommended "5 *A's*" as brief clinical interventions.
   a.
   b.
   c.
   d.
   e.

4. On admission to the hospital for a knee replacement, a patient who has smoked for 20 years expresses an interest in quitting. What is the best response by the nurse?
   a. "Good for you! You should talk to your doctor about that."
   b. "Why did you ever start in the first place? It's so hard to quit."
   c. "Since you will not be able to smoke while you are in the hospital, just don't start again when you are discharged."
   d. "Great! While you are here, I'll help you make a plan and work with your doctor to get you what you need to quit smoking."

5. List 2 major health problems commonly seen in the acute care setting related to the use of the following substances.

   Nicotine
   a.
   b.

   Alcohol
   a.
   b.

   Cocaine and amphetamines
   a.
   b.

   Opioids
   a.
   b.

   Cannabis
   a.
   b.

6. What are the physiologic effects associated with cocaine and amphetamines? **Select all that apply.**
   a. Drowsiness
   b. Nasal damage
   c. Constricted pupils
   d. Sexual dysfunction
   e. Increase in appetite
   f. Tachycardia with hypertension

7. Which substance, when used by the patient with SUD, can cause euphoria, drowsiness, decreased respiratory rate, and slurred speech?
   a. Opioids
   b. Alcohol
   c. Cannabis
   d. Depressants

8. Which manifestations are experienced by a patient when withdrawing from sedative-hypnotic addiction? **Select all that apply.**
   a. Seizures
   b. Violence
   c. Suicidal thoughts
   d. Tremors and anxiety
   e. Sweating, nausea, and cramps

9. The nurse is encouraging a woman who smokes 1½ packs of cigarettes per day to quit with the use of nicotine replacement therapy. The woman asks how the nicotine in a patch or gum differs from the nicotine she gets from cigarettes. What would the nurse explain about nicotine replacement?
   a. It includes a substance that eventually creates an aversion to nicotine.
   b. It provides a noncarcinogenic nicotine, unlike the nicotine in cigarettes.
   c. It prevents the weight gain that is a concern to women who stop smoking.
   d. It eliminates the thousands of toxic chemicals that are inhaled with smoking.

10. Match the following drugs used for treatment of cocaine toxicity with their specific uses. Answers may be used more than once.

Drug	Uses
_____ a. haloperidol (Haldol)	1. Tachycardia
_____ b. IV lidocaine	2. Hallucinations
_____ c. IV diazepam (Valium)	3. Dysrhythmias
_____ d. propranolol (Inderal)	4. Seizures
_____ e. risperidone (Risperdal)	
_____ f. IV lorazepam (Ativan)	
_____ g. procainamide	

11. A patient who is a heavy caffeine user has been NPO all day in preparation for a late afternoon surgery. What assessment findings may indicate the patient is experiencing caffeine withdrawal?
    a. A headache
    b. Nervousness
    c. Mild tremors
    d. Shortness of breath

12. The third day after a patient with alcohol use disorder was admitted for acute pancreatitis, the nurse finds that the patient is experiencing alcohol withdrawal delirium. What are the signs of withdrawal delirium on which the nurse based this judgment? **Select all that apply.**
    a. Apathy
    b. Seizures
    c. Disorientation
    d. Severe depression
    e. Cardiovascular collapse
    f. Visual and auditory hallucinations

13. Which question is the best approach to use to assess a newly admitted patient's use of addictive drugs?
    a. "How do you relieve your stress?"
    b. "You don't use any illegal drugs, do you?"
    c. "Which alcohol or recreational drugs do you use?"
    d. "Do you have any addictions we should know about to prevent complications?"

14. Which program would the nurse recognize will stop the behavior that leads to the most preventable cause of death in the United States?
    a. Prohibit alcohol use in public places.
    b. Prevent tobacco use in children and adolescents.
    c. Motivate individuals to enter addiction treatment.
    d. Recognize addictions as illnesses rather than crimes.

15. A young woman is brought to the emergency department by police who found her lying on a downtown sidewalk. The initial nursing assessment finds that she is unresponsive and has a weak pulse of 112 beats/minute; shallow respirations of 8 breaths/minute; and cold, clammy skin. Identify the 2 medications that would most likely be administered immediately and explain why they would be given to this patient.
    a.
    b.

16. A patient with a history of alcohol use disorder (AUD) is admitted to the hospital following an automobile accident. What assessment information is most important for the nurse to obtain to plan care for the patient?
    a. When the patient last had alcohol intake
    b. How much alcohol has recently been used
    c. What type of alcohol has recently been ingested
    d. The patient's current blood alcohol concentration

17. A patient in alcohol withdrawal is at risk for injury due to sensorimotor deficits, seizure activity, and confusion. Which nursing intervention is most important?
    a. Provide a darkened, quiet environment free from external stimuli.
    b. Force fluids to help in diluting the alcohol concentration in the blood.
    c. Monitor vital signs often to detect an extreme autonomic nervous system response.
    d. Use restraints as necessary to prevent the patient from reacting violently to hallucinations.

18. What is an important postoperative intervention indicated for the patient with AUD who is alcohol intoxicated and undergoing emergency surgery?
    a. Monitor weight because of malnutrition.
    b. Give an emergency dose of IV magnesium.
    c. Decrease pain medication to prevent cross-tolerance to opiates.
    d. Closely monitor for signs of withdrawal and respiratory and cardiac problems.

19. During admission to the emergency department, a patient with chronic alcoholism is intoxicated and very disoriented and confused. Which drug will the nurse administer first?
    a. IV thiamine
    b. IV benzodiazepines
    c. IV haloperidol (Haldol)
    d. IV naloxone in normal saline

20. The nurse is working with a patient at the clinic who does not want to quit smoking even though he is having trouble breathing at times and has a frequent cough. Which clinical practice guideline strategies would the nurse use with this patient?
    a. Cost, cough, cleanliness, Chantix
    b. Ask, advise, assess, assist, arrange
    c. Deduce, describe, decide, deadline
    d. Relevance, risks, rewards, roadblocks, repetition

21. When assessing an older patient for substance use, the nurse specifically asks the patient about the use of alcohol and which other types of medications?
    a. Opioids
    b. Sedative-hypnotics
    c. Central nervous system stimulants
    d. Prescription and over-the-counter medications

CASE STUDY Cocaine Toxicity

Patient Profile

N.C. is a 28-year-old man who was admitted to the emergency department with chest pain, tachycardia, dizziness, nausea, and severe migraine-like headache.

(monkeybusinessimages/
iStock/Thinkstock)

Subjective Data
- Thinks he is having a heart attack
- Admits he was at a party earlier in the evening drinking alcohol, smoking pot, and snorting cocaine
- Reports he became irritable and restless
- Reports having an increased need for cocaine in the past few months

Objective Data
- Appears extremely nervous and irritable
- Appears pale and diaphoretic
- Has tremors
- BP 210/110 mm Hg, HR 100 beats/min, RR 30 breaths/min

Questions

1. Indicate which assessment finding listed in the far-left column is a sign or symptom of the potential complication. Note that some assessment findings will be used more than once.

Assessment Finding	Potential Complication	Appropriate Assessment Finding for Complication
Nervous and irritable	Myocardial Infarction	
Chest pain	Stroke	
BP 210/110 mm Hg	Psychosis	
Paranoia		
Pale and diaphoretic		
Dizziness		
Migraine-like headache		
Nausea		

2. What interventions would the nurse implement to treat N.C.?

   Use an X to indicate if the nursing intervention is <u>Indicated</u> (appropriate or necessary), <u>Contraindicated</u> (could be harmful), or <u>Non-Essential</u> (unnecessary).

Nursing Intervention	Indicated	Contraindicated	Non-Essential
Obtain a 12-lead ECG			
Obtain a blood alcohol level			
Administer acetaminophen 650 mg PO			
Institute seizure precautions			
Administer 500 mL D_5W bolus IV			
Administer 0.4 mg SL nitroglycerin			
Insert an oropharyngeal airway to keep airway patent			
Apply sequential compression devices			

3. When performing the *Drug Abuse Screening Test (DAST-10)*, which questions would the nurse ask N.C.? *Select all that apply.*

   _____A. Have you ever been arrested for drug possession or use?

   _____B. Have you engaged in illegal activities in order to obtain drugs?

   _____C. Have you had "blackouts" or "flashbacks" as a result of drug use?

   _____D. Have you ever coerced someone else to do drugs with you?

_____E. Do you use more than 1 drug at a time?

_____F. Have you neglected your family because of your use of drugs?

_____G. Do you ever feel bad or guilty about your drug use?

_____H. Have you or someone else been injured as a result of your drug use?

4. Use an X in the right column to indicate which teaching about withdrawal from cocaine and alcohol, listed in the left column, is appropriate for the nurse to provide N.C.

Potential Teaching	Appropriate Teaching
"You may experience severe mood swings."	
"You can drink one alcoholic beverage each day to avoid severe withdrawal symptoms."	
"You shouldn't crave cocaine, but you may crave alcohol during the first few days."	
"You should sleep when you desire."	
"You should take a multivitamin daily."	
"There is an antidote to treat cocaine withdrawal, but not alcohol withdrawal."	
"You may need to be hospitalized if your withdrawal symptoms are severe."	

Inflammation and Healing

1. A patient with an inflammatory disease has the following clinical manifestations. Identify the primary chemical mediators involved in producing the manifestation and the physiologic change that causes the manifestation.

Clinical Manifestation	Chemical Mediators	Physiologic Change
Fever		
Redness		
Edema		
Leukocytosis		

2. In a patient with leukocytosis with a shift to the left, what would the nurse recognize as the cause?
   a. The complement system has been activated to enhance phagocytosis.
   b. Monocytes are released into the blood in larger-than-normal amounts.
   c. The response to cellular injury is not adequate to remove damaged tissue and promote healing.
   d. The demand for neutrophils causes the release of immature neutrophils from the bone marrow.

3. What does the mechanism of chemotaxis accomplish?
   a. Causes the transformation of monocytes into macrophages
   b. Involves a pathway of chemical processes resulting in cellular lysis
   c. Attracts the accumulation of neutrophils and monocytes to an area of injury
   d. Slows the blood flow in a damaged area, allowing migration of leukocytes into tissue

4. What effect does the action of the complement system have on inflammation?
   a. Modifies the inflammatory response to prevent stimulation of pain
   b. Increases body temperature, resulting in destruction of microorganisms
   c. Produces prostaglandins and leukotrienes that increase blood flow, edema, and pain
   d. Increases inflammatory responses of vascular permeability, chemotaxis, and phagocytosis

5. Key interventions for treating initial soft tissue injury and resulting inflammation are remembered using the acronym *RICE*. What are the most important actions for the emergency department nurse to do for the patient with an ankle injury?
   a. Reduce swelling, shine light on wound, control mobility, and get the history of the injury.
   b. Rub the wound clean, immobilize the area, cover the area protectively, and exercise the leg.
   c. Rest with immobility, apply a cold compress and/or a compression bandage, and elevate the ankle.
   d. Rinse the wounded ankle, get x-rays of the ankle, carry the patient, and extend the ankle with a splint.

6. What is characteristic of chronic inflammation?
   a. It may last 2 to 3 weeks.
   b. The injurious agent persists or repeatedly injures tissue.
   c. Infective endocarditis is an example of chronic inflammation.
   d. Neutrophils are the predominant cell type at the site of inflammation.

7. During the healing phase of inflammation, which cells would be most likely to regenerate?
   a. Skin
   b. Neurons
   c. Cardiac muscle
   d. Skeletal muscle

8. Place the following events that occur during healing by primary intention in sequential order from 1 (first) to 10 (last).
   a. _____ Blood clots form
   b. _____ Approximation of wound edges
   c. _____ Avascular, pale, mature scar present
   d. _____ Enzymes from neutrophils digest fibrin
   e. _____ Epithelial cells migrate across wound surface
   f. _____ Fibroblasts migrate to site and secrete collagen
   g. _____ Budding capillaries result in pink, vascular friable wound
   h. _____ Healing area contracts by movement of myofibroblasts
   i. _____ Macrophages ingest and digest cellular debris and red blood cells
   j. _____ Fibrin clot serves as meshwork for capillary growth and epithelial cell migration

9. What is the main difference between healing by primary intention and healing by secondary intention?
   a. Primary healing requires surgical debridement for healing to occur.
   b. Primary healing involves suturing 2 layers of granulation tissue together.
   c. Presence of more granulation tissue in secondary healing results in a larger scar.
   d. Healing by secondary intention takes longer because more steps in the healing process are necessary.

10. A patient who had abdominal surgery 3 months ago calls the clinic reporting severe abdominal pain and cramping, vomiting, and bloating. What would the nurse suspect is the most likely cause?
    a. Infection
    b. Adhesion
    c. Contracture
    d. Evisceration

11. A patient had a complicated vaginal hysterectomy. The student nurse provided perineal care after the patient had a bowel movement. The student nurse tells the nurse there was a lot of light-brown, smelly drainage seeping from the vaginal area. What complication would the nurse suspect?
    a. Dehiscence
    b. Hemorrhage
    c. Keloid formation
    d. Fistula formation

12. Which nutrients aid in capillary synthesis and collagen production by the fibroblasts in wound healing?
    a. Fats
    b. Proteins
    c. Vitamin C
    d. Vitamin A

13. What role do B-complex vitamins play in wound healing?
    a. Decrease metabolism
    b. Protect protein from being used for energy
    c. Provide metabolic energy for the inflammatory process
    d. Coenzymes for fat, protein, and carbohydrate metabolism

14. The patient is admitted from home with a clean stage 2 pressure injury. What would the nurse expect to observe when doing a wound assessment?
    a. Adherent gray necrotic tissue
    b. Clean, moist granulating tissue
    c. Red-pink wound bed, without slough
    d. Creamy ivory to yellow-green exudate

15. What type of dressing will the nurse most likely use for the patient in Question 14?
    a. Hydrocolloid
    b. Transparent film
    c. Absorptive dressing
    d. Negative pressure wound therapy

16. The patient's wound is not healing, so the health care provider (HCP) is going to send the patient home with negative pressure wound therapy. What will the caregiver need to understand about the use of this device?
    a. The wound must be cleaned daily.
    b. The patient will be placed in a hyperbaric chamber.
    c. The occlusive dressing must be sealed tightly to the skin.
    d. The diet will not be as important with this sort of treatment.

17. When caring for patients, what is the most important precaution for preventing transmission of infections?
    a. Wearing face and eye protection during routine daily care of the patient
    b. Wearing nonsterile gloves when in contact with body fluids, excretions, and contaminated items
    c. Wearing a gown to protect the skin and clothing during patient care activities likely to soil clothing
    d. Hand washing after touching fluids and secretions, removing gloves, and between patient contacts

18. Which patient is at the greatest risk for developing a pressure injury?
    a. A 42-year-old obese woman with type 2 diabetes
    b. A 78-year-old man who is confused and malnourished
    c. A 30-year-old man who is comatose after a head injury
    d. A 65-year-old woman who has urge and stress incontinence

19. What is the most important nursing intervention for the prevention and treatment of pressure injuries?
    a. Using pressure-reduction devices
    b. Repositioning the patient frequently
    c. Massaging pressure areas with lotion
    d. Using lift sheets and trapeze bars to facilitate patient movement

20. The patient is transferring from another facility with the description of a sore on her sacrum that is deep enough to see the muscle. What stage of pressure injury would the nurse expect to see on admission?
    a. Stage 1
    b. Stage 2
    c. Stage 3
    d. Stage 4

21. Documentation indicates a patient has a stage 3 pressure injury on their right hip. What would the nurse expect to observe when assessing the patient's right hip?
    a. Exposed bone, tendon, or muscle
    b. An abrasion, blister, or shallow crater
    c. Deep crater through subcutaneous tissue to fascia
    d. Persistent redness (or bluish color in darker skin tones)

22. Which nursing interventions for a patient with a stage 4 sacral pressure injury are *most* appropriate to assign or delegate to a licensed practical/vocational nurse (LPN/VN)? **Select all that apply.**
    a. Assess and document wound appearance.
    b. Teach the patient pressure injury risk factors.
    c. Assist the patient to change positions at frequent intervals.
    d. Choose the type of dressing to apply to the pressure injury.
    e. Measure the size (width, length, depth) of the pressure injury.

CASE STUDY   Inflammation

Patient Profile

G.K., a 28-year-old female patient who has type 1 diabetes, is admitted to the hospital with cellulitis of her left lower leg. She had been applying heating pads to the leg for the last 48 hours, but the leg has become more painful and she has developed chills.

(Ivan_Kochergin/
iStock/Thinkstock)

Subjective Data
- Reports severe pain and heaviness in her leg
- Reports that she cannot bear weight on her leg and has been in bed for 3 days
- Lives alone and has not had anyone to help her with meals

Objective Data

Physical Examination
- Irregular shape, 2-cm diameter, 1-cm deep, open wound above the left medial malleolus with moderate amount of thick, yellow drainage
- Left leg red and edematous from ankle to knee
- Left calf measurement is 3 inches larger than the right calf
- Temp: 102°F (38.9°C)

Laboratory Tests
- White blood cell (WBC) count: 18,300/μL (18.3 × 10^3/L; 80% neutrophils, 12% bands)
- Wound culture: *Staphylococcus aureus*
- Blood glucose: 204 mg/dL

Questions

1. **Choose the most likely options for the information missing from the statements below by selecting from the lists of options provided.**

   As a result of her cellulitis and open wound, the patient is at risk of developing _____**1**_____ and _____**1**_____. The nurse would monitor for the following assessment findings: _____**2**_____, ____**2**_____, and _____**2**_____. The nurse informs the other health care team members that _____**3**_____, _____**3**_____, and _____**3**_____ are indicated.

Options for 1	Options for 2	Options for 3
Diabetic ketoacidosis	Kussmaul breathing	Cleansing the wound with alcohol
Neurovascular complications	Dyspnea	Irrigating the wound using 0.9% NSS
Hyperosmolar Hyperglycemic Syndrome	Leukocytosis	Elevating LLE above the level of the heart
Sepsis	Diminished left dorsalis pedis pulse	Increasing oral fluid intake
Hypoglycemia	Fever	Applying ice packs to LLE
Dysrhythmias	Chest pain	Applying SCDs bilaterally

2. The wound care nurse has been consulted about the management of G.K.'s wound above the left medial malleolus. **Match each of the wound care options (Column A) with its uses (Column C) using the choices provided in Column B.**

A. Wound Care Dressings	B. Choices for Use	C. Correct Wound Care Dressing for Its Use
1. Alginates	Prophylactic in non-healing wounds	
2. Hydrocolloids	Used to prevent pressure injuries	
3. Antimicrobials	Used on almost any wound	
4. Hydrogels	Used for minor wounds	
5. Transparent films	Necrotic wounds	
6. Nonadherent	Wounds with light drainage	
7. Foams	Wounds with heavy exudate	
8. Gauze	Dry, uninfected wounds	

3. **Highlight the findings in the nurse's notes below that are indicative of sepsis.**

NURSE'S NOTES

4. Patient reports 3/10 pain in LLE on a 0 to 10 pain intensity scale. Pulse 110 beats/min, increased since admission, BP 90/55 mm Hg decreased since admission. Temp:102.2°F (39°C). Capillary refill is > 3 sec in all extremities. Patient is lethargic, oriented x4. Skin is hot & dry. Poor appetite, bowel sounds hypoactive. FSBG 152 mg/dL. Breath sounds CTA. - B. Gibbs, RN **Based on the clinical data above, use an X to indicate whether the nursing actions below are <u>Indicated</u> (appropriate or necessary), <u>Contraindicated</u> (could be harmful), or <u>Non-essential</u> (makes no difference or are unnecessary) for the client's care at this time.**

Nursing Action	Indicated	Contraindicated	Non-Essential
Administer acetaminophen 650 mg PO			
Teach the patient to use an incentive spirometer			
Check FSBG before meals and at bedtime			
Cleanse the ankle wound with hydrogen peroxide			
Assess the patient's hemoglobin A1C			
Administer D_5W at 125 mL/hr			
Weigh the client daily			

5. G. K. is being discharged home. What health teaching will the nurse include as part of the discharge instructions? **Select all that apply**.

_____ A. "Stop taking the antibiotics when the pain in your left leg subsides."

_____ B. "Notify your health care provider if you continue to have fevers."

_____ C. "Elevate your left leg above the level of your heart as much as possible."

_____ D. "You can use crutches until it is comfortable to put full weight on your left leg."

_____ E. "Avoid strenuous activity until your health care provider tells you otherwise."

_____ F. "You can alternate between acetaminophen and ibuprofen as needed for pain."

_____ G. "You may soak in hot tubs to promote wound healing."

Genetics

1. Which term is the definition for physical traits expressed by an individual?
   a. Allele
   b. Genomics
   c. Phenotype
   d. Chromosomes

2. Which definition is the best description of the term *genotype*?
   a. Genetic identity of an individual
   b. Transmission of a disease from parent to child
   c. Basic unit of heredity; arranged on chromosome
   d. Family tree containing genetic characteristics and disorders of that family

3. A 26-year-old man was adopted. What health information related to his biologic parents and family will be most useful to him when he gets married? **Select all that apply.**
   a. Cholecystitis occurring in family members
   b. Occurrence of prostate cancer in 1 uncle
   c. Ages of family members diagnosed with diseases
   d. Kidney stones present in extended family members
   e. Age and cause of death of deceased family members

4. The new parents of an infant born with Down syndrome ask the nurse what happened to cause the chromosomal abnormality. What is the best response by the nurse?
   a. "During cell division of the reproductive cells there is an error causing an abnormal number of chromosomes."
   b. "A mutation in 1 of the chromosomes created an autosomal recessive gene that is expressed as Down syndrome."
   c. "An abnormal gene on 1 of the 2 chromosomes was transferred to the fetus, causing an abnormal chromosome."
   d. "A process of translocation caused the exchange of genetic material between the 2 chromosomes in the cell, resulting in abnormal chromosomes."

5. When a father has Huntington's disease with a heterozygous genotype, the nurse uses the Punnett square to illustrate the inheritance patterns and the probability of transmission of the autosomal dominant disease. The mother does not carry the Huntington's disease gene. Complete the subsequent Punnett square to illustrate this inheritance pattern, using "H" as the normal gene and "h" as the gene for Huntington's disease.

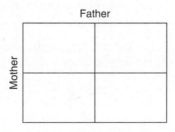

There is a _____ % chance that offspring will be unaffected.

There is a _____ % chance that offspring will be affected.

6. Which statements accurately describe(s) genetic testing? **Select all that apply.**
   a. Results of genetic testing may raise psychologic and emotional issues.
   b. An ethical issue that is raised with genetic testing is protection of privacy to prevent discrimination.
   c. Genetic testing of the mother can be used to determine an unborn child's risk of having genetic conditions.
   d. An example of genetic testing that is required by all states is premarital testing of women for the hemophilia gene.
   e. Genetic testing for *BRCA1* and *BRCA2* mutations can identify women who may choose to have mastectomies to prevent breast cancer.

7. Tay-Sachs disease is an autosomal recessive disease. Both parents have been identified as heterozygous. There is a _____ % chance that their offspring will be affected.

8. A couple lost a second baby to miscarriage. They are both considering having genetic testing done before trying to get pregnant again. What would the nurse include when teaching about genetic testing?
   a. A particular genetic test will tell them if there is a specific genetic change that could cause a genetic condition to the child.
   b. The test results will identify the diseases their children will inherit from them.
   c. Genetic testing will determine if they are predisposed to developing a genetic disease.
   d. Genetic testing kits that are available on the Internet are just as good as and less costly than going to a genetic counselor.

9. The daughter of a man with Huntington's disease is having presymptomatic genetic testing done. What does a positive result mean for her?
   a. She will get the disease.
   b. She is a carrier of Huntington's disease.
   c. She will be at increased risk for developing the disease.
   d. She must change her diet, exercise, and environment to prevent the disease.

10. A 21-year-old patient says no one in his family has type 1 diabetes, but he has had it since childhood. He asks how diabetes was transmitted to him. How would the nurse explain this disease?
    a. It is a single gene disorder.
    b. It is a chromosome disorder.
    c. It is an acquired genetic disorder.
    d. It is a multifactorial genetic disorder.

11. The health care provider (HCP) plans to prescribe trastuzumab (Herceptin) for the patient with breast cancer. What testing will the HCP order before prescribing this medication?
    a. HER-2 protein levels
    b. *BRCA2* gene mutation
    c. *BRCA1* gene mutation
    d. Stage II cancer identification

12. The HCP is having difficulty finding the appropriate dose for the patient taking warfarin (Coumadin). What can the nurse suggest that may solve this problem?
    a. Pharmacogenomic testing
    b. Start bivalirudin (Angiomax) IV
    c. Change from warfarin (Coumadin) to clopidogrel (Plavix) and aspirin
    d. Change from warfarin (Coumadin) to enoxaparin (Lovenox) injections

13. A 20-year-old patient has a family history of colon cancer. Genetic testing shows he has the gene for familial adenomatous polyposis (FAP). What would the nurse include when teaching the patient?
    a. How to change his diet
    b. Reason for annual colonoscopies
    c. Need for a referral for gene therapy
    d. Not to have children so that they will not be affected

14. Which statement accurately describes gene therapy?
    a. May activate a mutated gene that is functioning improperly
    b. Is often done by replacing a healthy gene with a mutated gene
    c. Is an investigational technique used to treat genetic diseases with no cure
    d. Introduces a new gene into reproductive cells to help fight a genetic disease

15. The National Marrow Donor Program obtains hematopoietic stem cells from donors for recipients in need. When discussing this donation with the donor, what would the nurse share about these stem cells?
    a. They must come from an embryo or umbilical cord.
    b. These cells will form new blood cells for the recipient.
    c. Taking these cells will cause the donor to become anemic.
    d. These cells must be removed with a bone marrow aspiration.

CASE STUDY Genetics

Patient Profile
D.L., a 26-year-old woman, is concerned about having children because her younger brother has Duchenne muscular dystrophy (MD). She is seeking genetic testing.

(thoth11/iStock/ Thinkstock)

Subjective Data
* She is engaged to be married.
* She has many questions about her risks.

Objective Data
* Her eyes are darting around the room.
* Her hands and feet are trembling.
* She is chewing her fingernails.

Questions
1. **Choose the most likely options for the information missing from the statements below by selecting from the lists of options provided.**

   Duchenne muscular dystrophy is a _____**1**_____ disorder which affects _____**2**_____. Other disorders that share this category are _____**3**_____ and _____**3**_____. Carriers are_____**4**_____.

Options for 1	Options for 2	Options for 3	Options for 4
Autosomal recessive	Males and females equally	Thalassemia	Sons of affected females
Autosomal dominant	Usually males	Hemophilia	Daughters of affected females
X-linked recessive	Usually females	Huntington's disease	Sons of affected males
Heterozygous	Daughters of affected males	Cystic fibrosis	Daughters of affected males
Multifactorial inherited	Sons of affected males	Wiskott-Aldrich syndrome	Affected parents

2. During genetic testing, D.L. learns that she has the BRCA gene. What is true about the BRCA gene? **Select all that apply**.
    _____A. She has a higher risk of developing colon cancer.
    _____B. She has a higher risk of developing ovarian cancer.
    _____C. BRCA is a protective gene.
    _____D. If she has a daughter, her daughter will inherit the BRCA gene.
    _____E. It is an x-linked recessive genetic disorder.
    _____F. It is an autosomal dominant genetic disorder.
    _____G. BRCA is an inherited mutation.
    _____H. She has a higher risk of developing breast cancer.

3. What statements made by D.L. indicate genetic counseling was successful?

For each client response, use an X to indicate whether the nurse's teaching was <u>Effective</u> (response indicates that the client understands), <u>Ineffective</u> (response indicates that the client does not understand), or <u>Unrelated</u> (response is not related to the nurse's health teaching).

Client's Response	Effective	Ineffective	Unrelated
"I will not have any children since they will develop Duchenne muscular dystrophy."			
"I will have bilateral mastectomies since I will develop breast cancer."			
"I will consult an oncologist about the chances of developing ovarian cancer."			
"I will have my eggs harvested and consider preimplantation genetic diagnosis before getting pregnant."			
"I will eat healthy and exercise to reduce my risks of developing cancer."			

4. Choose the most likely options for the information missing from the table by selecting from the lists of options provided.

Medication	Drug Class	Pharmacogenetic Role	Indication
abacavir	2	HLA-B*5701	HIV/AIDS
crizotinib	Kinase inhibitor	ALK	4
vemurafenib	6	BRAF V600E	melanoma
1	anticoagulant	VKORC1	Deep vein thrombosis
5	Monoclonal antibody	3	Breast cancer
clopidogrel	antiplatelet	7	8

Options for 1 and 5	Options for 2 and 6	Options for 3 and 7	Options for 4 and 8
Abacavir	Kinase inhibitor	HER-2	Deep vein thrombosis
Warfarin	Nucleoside reverse transcriptase inhibitor	ALK	Breast cancer
Vemurafenib	Anticoagulant	CYP2C19	Coronary artery disease
Trastuzumab	Antiplatelet	HLA-B*5701	Non-small cell lung cancer
Clopidogrel	Monoclonal antibody	BRAF V600E	HIV/AIDS
Crizotinib	Antiviral	VKORC1	Melanoma

Immune Responses and Transplantation

1. Which type of immunity is the result of contact with the antigen through infection and is the longest lasting type of immunity?
   a. Innate immunity
   b. Natural active acquired immunity
   c. Artificial active acquired immunity
   d. Artificial passive acquired immunity

2. What accurately describes artificial passive acquired immunity? **Select all that apply.**
   a. Gamma globulin injection
   b. Immunization with antigen
   c. Immediate effect, lasting a short time
   d. Maternal immunoglobulins in neonate
   e. Boosters may be needed for extended protection

3. How does an antigen stimulate an immune response?
   a. It circulates in the blood, where it comes in contact with circulating macrophages.
   b. It is captured and processed by a macrophage and then presented to lymphocytes.
   c. It is a foreign protein that has antigenic determinants different from those of the body.
   d. It combines with larger molecules that are capable of stimulating production of antibodies.

4. Which T lymphocytes are involved in direct attack and destruction of foreign pathogens?
   a. Dendritic cells
   b. Natural killer cells
   c. T helper (CD4) cells
   d. T cytotoxic (CD8) cells

5. How does interferon help the body's natural defenses?
   a. Directly attacks and destroys virus-infected cells
   b. Augments the immune response by activating phagocytes
   c. Induces production of antiviral proteins in cells that prevent viral replication
   d. Is produced by viral infected cells and prevents the transmission of the virus to adjacent cells

6. What is included in the humoral immune response?
   a. Surveillance for malignant cell changes
   b. Production of antigen-specific immunoglobulins
   c. Direct attack of antigens by activated B lymphocytes
   d. Releasing cytokines responsible for destruction of antigens

7. Where and into what do activated B lymphocytes differentiate?
   a. Spleen; natural killer cells that destroy infected cells
   b. Bone marrow; plasma cells that secrete immunoglobulins
   c. Thymus; memory B cells that retain a memory of the antigen
   d. Bursa of Fabricius; helper cells that in turn activate additional B lymphocytes

8. Which immunoglobulin is responsible for the primary immune response and forms antibodies to ABO blood antigens?
   a. IgA
   b. IgD
   c. IgG
   d. IgM

9. Which immunoglobulins will initially protect a newborn baby who is being exclusively breastfed? **Select all that apply.**
   a. IgA
   b. IgD
   c. IgE
   d. IgG
   e. IgM

10. Which characteristic describes IgE? **Select all that apply.**
    a. Assists in parasitic infections
    b. Responsible for allergic reactions
    c. Present on the lymphocyte surface
    d. Assists in B-lymphocyte differentiation
    e. Predominant in secondary immune response
    f. Protects body surfaces and mucous membranes

11. What are the important functions of cell-mediated immunity? **Select all that apply.**
    a. Fungal infections
    b. Transfusion reactions
    c. Rejection of transplanted tissues
    d. Contact hypersensitivity reactions
    e. Immunity against pathogens that survive inside cells

12. A 69-year-old woman asks the nurse whether it is possible to "catch" cancer because many of her friends of the same age have been diagnosed with different kinds of cancer. In responding to the woman, the nurse understands that which factor increases the incidence of tumors in older adults?
    a. An increase in autoantibodies
    b. Decreased activity of the bone marrow
    c. Decreased differentiation of T lymphocytes
    d. Decreased size and activity of the thymus gland

13. What describes the occurrence of a type IV or delayed hypersensitivity reaction?
    a. Antigen links with specific IgE antibodies bound to mast cells or basophils releasing chemical mediators
    b. Cellular lysis or phagocytosis through complement activation following antigen-antibody binding on cell surfaces
    c. Sensitized T lymphocytes attack antigens or release cytokines that attract macrophages that cause tissue damage
    d. Antigens combined with IgG and IgM too small to be removed by mononuclear phagocytic system deposit in tissue and cause fixation of complement

14. What are examples of type I or IgE-mediated hypersensitivity reactions? **Select all that apply.**
    a. Asthma
    b. Urticaria
    c. Angioedema
    d. Allergic rhinitis
    e. Atopic dermatitis
    f. Contact dermatitis
    g. Anaphylactic shock
    h. Transfusion reactions
    i. Goodpasture syndrome

15. Which type of hypersensitivity reaction occurs with rheumatoid arthritis and acute glomerulonephritis?
    a. Type I or IgE-mediated hypersensitivity reaction
    b. Type II or cytotoxic hypersensitivity reaction
    c. Type III or immune-complex–mediated hypersensitivity reaction
    d. Type IV or delayed hypersensitivity reaction

16. For the patient with allergic rhinitis, which therapy should the nurse expect to be ordered first?
    a. Corticosteroids
    b. Immunotherapy
    c. Antipruritic drugs
    d. Sympathomimetic/decongestant drugs

17. A patient was given an IM injection of penicillin in the gluteus maximus and developed dyspnea and weakness within minutes following the injection. Which additional assessment findings indicate that the patient is having an anaphylactic reaction? **Select all that apply.**
    a. Wheezing
    b. Hypertension
    c. Rash on arms
    d. Constricted pupils
    e. Slowed strong pulse
    f. Feeling of impending doom

18. The patient is admitted from a nearby park with an apparent anaphylactic reaction to a bee sting. He is experiencing dyspnea and hypotension with swelling at the site. Beginning with number 1 as the top priority, number the following actions the nurse should implement in the order of priority for this patient.
    a. _____ Remove the stinger
    b. _____ Ensure a patent airway
    c. _____ Prepare to administer epinephrine
    d. _____ Start IV for fluid and medication access
    e. _____ Anticipate intubation with severe respiratory distress
    f. _____ Have diphenhydramine and nebulized albuterol available

19. Which rationale describes treatment of atopic allergies with immunotherapy?
    a. It decreases the levels of allergen-specific T helper cells.
    b. It decreases the level of IgE so that it does not react as readily with an allergen.
    c. It stimulates increased IgG to bind with allergen-reactive sites, preventing mast cell–bound IgE reactions.
    d. It gradually increases the amount of allergen in the body until it is no longer recognized as foreign and does not elicit an antibody reaction.

20. A nurse develops contact dermatitis after wearing latex gloves. What accurately describes this?
    a. This demonstrates a type I allergic reaction to natural latex proteins.
    b. Use of powder-free latex gloves prevents the development of symptoms.
    c. Use of oil-based hand cream when wearing gloves prevents latex allergy.
    d. This demonstrates a type IV allergic reaction to chemicals used in the manufacture of latex gloves.

21. A 32-year-old male veteran tells the nurse he gets a headache, sore throat, shortness of breath, and nausea when his girlfriend wears perfume and when he was painting her apartment. He is afraid he has cancer. What does the nurse suspect may be the patient's problem?
    a. He has posttraumatic stress disorder.
    b. He has multiple chemical sensitivities.
    c. He needs to wear a mask when he paints.
    d. He is looking for an excuse to break up with his girlfriend.

22. Although the cause of autoimmune disorders is unknown, which factors are believed to be present in most conditions? **Select all that apply.**
    a. Younger age
    b. Male gender
    c. Inheritance of susceptibility genes
    d. Initiation of autoreactivity by triggers
    e. Frequent viruses throughout the lifetime

23. Why is plasmapheresis indicated in the treatment of autoimmune disorders?
    a. To obtain plasma for analysis and evaluation of specific autoantibodies
    b. To decrease high lymphocyte levels in the blood to prevent immune responses
    c. To remove autoantibodies, antigen-antibody complexes, and inflammatory mediators of immune reactions
    d. To add monocytes to the blood to promote removal of immune complexes by the mononuclear phagocyte system

24. Before the patient receives a kidney transplant, a crossmatch test is ordered. What does a positive crossmatch indicate?
    a. Paternity and predicts risk for certain diseases
    b. Tissue type match for a successful transplantation
    c. Racial background and predicts risk for certain diseases
    d. Cytotoxic antibodies to the donor, which contraindicate transplanting this donor's organ

25. What is the most common cause of secondary immunodeficiency disorders?
    a. Chronic stress
    b. T-cell deficiency from HIV
    c. Drug-induced immunosuppression
    d. Common variable hypogammaglobulinemia

26. Which characteristics are seen with acute transplant rejection? **Select all that apply.**
    a. Treatment is supportive
    b. Only occurs with transplanted kidneys
    c. Organ must be removed when it occurs
    d. The recipient's T cytotoxic lymphocytes attack the foreign organ
    e. Long-term use of immunosuppressants necessary to combat the rejection
    f. Usually reversible with additional or increased immunosuppressant therapy

27. The patient is experiencing fibrosis and glomerulopathy a year after a kidney transplant. Which type of rejection is occurring?
    a. Acute
    b. Chronic
    c. Delayed
    d. Hyperacute

28. What are the most common immunosuppressive agents initially used to prevent rejection of transplanted organs?
    a. Cyclosporine, sirolimus, and muromonab-CD3
    b. Prednisone, polyclonal antibodies, and cyclosporine
    c. Azathioprine, mycophenolate mofetil, and sirolimus
    d. Tacrolimus, prednisone, and mycophenolate mofetil

29. The patient has received a bone marrow transplant. Soon after the transplant, there is a rash on the patient's skin. She says her skin is itchy and she has severe abdominal pain. What best summarizes what is happening to the patient and how she will be treated?
    a. Graft rejection occurring; treat with different immunosuppressive agents
    b. Dry skin and nausea are side effects of immunosuppressants; decrease the dose
    c. Transplanted bone marrow is attacking her tissue; prevent with immunosuppressive agents
    d. Dry skin from the dry air and nausea from the food in the hospital; treat with humidifier and home food

CASE STUDY Allergy

(deepblue/iStock/
Thinkstock)

Patient Profile
M.W., a 70-year-old male patient, has been diagnosed with chronic allergic rhinitis. His health care provider prescribed oral antihistamines for control of his symptoms, which have not been completely effective. He is to undergo skin testing to identify specific allergens.

Subjective Data
- Itching of eyes, nose, and throat
- Stuffy nose, head congestion

Objective Data
- Clear nasal drainage; reddened eyes and lacrimation

Questions
1. What assessments of M.W. should the nurse include? **Use an X to indicate if the assessment is __Essential__ (necessary or appropriate) or __Unrelated__ (not relevant or unnecessary).**

Assessment	Essential	Unrelated
History of past and present allergies		
Auscultate lung sounds		
History of genitourinary problems		
Family history of allergies		
History of neurologic problems		
Presence of pets in the home		
Assess for presence of peripheral edema		

2. M.W. wants to proceed with allergy testing, which can cause an anaphylactic reaction that can be life-threatening. Indicate which nursing action listed in the far-left column is appropriate for the potential complication. Note that not all nursing actions will be used.

Nursing Action	Potential Complication	Appropriate Nursing Action for Complication
Normal saline 1 L bolus	Bronchospasm	
Epinephrine 0.5 mg IM	Hypotension	
Incentive spirometer	Hypoxemia	
Supine with raised legs		
Nebulized albuterol		
High-flow oxygen via face mask		
IV diphenhydramine		

3. Which of the following are applicable when performing intradermal skin testing? **Select all that apply.**
_____A. Apply a tourniquet below the site if the patient has a severe allergic reaction.
_____B. Have intubation equipment at the bedside.
_____C. Administer epinephrine IM or IV if the patient has an anaphylactic reaction.
_____D. Skin testing cannot be performed if the patient has food allergies.
_____E. Skin testing should be performed to confirm allergic rhinitis.
_____F. If the patient is allergic to an allergen, reactions will occur within 72 hours when using scratch or intradermal methods.
_____G. There are 3 different methods of skin testing.
_____H. Negative results means the patient does not have an allergic disorder.

4. M.W. has been diagnosed with an allergy to household dust. What methods would the nurse recommend to manage this type of allergy? **Use an X to indicate if the recommendation will be <u>Effective</u> (helps manage the allergy), <u>Ineffective</u> (doesn't help manage the allergy), or <u>Unrelated</u> (is not related to the management of this allergy).**

Recommendation	Effective	Ineffective	Unrelated
Use a duster wand to dust furniture			
Use a steam vacuum to clean floors			
Wear hypoallergenic jewelry			
Change air filters in furnaces and AC units			
Use a HEPA-filter air purifier			
Open windows to improve airflow			

5. Choose the most likely options for the information missing from the table below by selecting from the lists of options provided.

Medication	Drug Class	Nursing Consideration
Fluticasone	1	Adherence is important
2	Decongestant	3
Montelukast	LTRA	4
5	Anticholinergic	May cause nosebleeds
Cetirizine	6	Minimal sedation
7	Antihistamine (1st generation)	8

Options for 2, 5, and 7	Options for 1 and 6	Options for 3, 4, and 8
Diphenhydramine	Anticholinergic	Adherence is important
Fluticasone	Antihistamine (2nd generation)	May cause nosebleeds
Pseudoephedrine	LTRA	Monitor LFTs
Montelukast	Decongestant	Minimal sedation
Cetirizine	Antihistamine (1st generation)	Use with caution in HTN
Ipratropium bromide	Corticosteroid	Report palpitations

15

Infection

1. To what is the increase in emerging and untreatable infections attributed? **Select all that apply.**
   a. Global travel and bioterrorism
   b. The evolution of infectious agents
   c. Use of antibiotics to treat viral infections
   d. Transmission of infectious agents from humans to animals
   e. An increased number of immunosuppressed and chronically ill people

2. Name 4 common antibiotic-resistant organisms: _____, _____, _____, and _____.

3. What are the recommended measures to prevent the transmission of health care–associated infections (HAIs)? **Select all that apply.**
   a. Empty bedpans as soon as possible.
   b. Limit fresh flowers in patient rooms.
   c. Remove urinals from bedside tables.
   d. Use of personal protective equipment.
   e. Wash hands or use alcohol-based sanitizer.
   f. Make sure patients wear sandals in the shower.

4. A patient with diarrhea has been diagnosed with *Clostridium difficile*. Along with standard precautions, which kind of transmission-based precautions will be used when the nurse is caring for this patient?
   a. Droplet precautions
   b. Contact precautions
   c. Isolation precautions
   d. Airborne precautions

5. A 78-year-old patient has developed an infection caused by *Haemophilus influenzae*. In addition to standard precautions, what would the nurse use for protection when working within 3 feet of the patient?
   a. Mask
   b. Gown
   c. Shoe covers
   d. Particulate respirator

6. An 82-year-old male patient with cardiac disease who is in the intensive care unit (ICU) is beginning to have decreased cognitive function. What would the nurse initially suspect as a potential cause of this change?
   a. Fatigue
   b. Infection
   c. ICU psychosis
   d. Medication allergy

7. The nurse determines that the patient understands the teaching about decreasing the risk for antibiotic-resistant infection when the patient makes which statement?
   a. "I know I should take the antibiotic for 1 day after I feel better."
   b. "I want an antibiotic ordered for my cold so that I can feel better sooner."
   c. "I always save some pills because I get the illness again after I first feel better."
   d. "I will follow the directions for taking the antibiotic so that I will get over this infection."

8. SARS-CoV-2 is an RNA virus that is thought to primarily enter the host through cells found in which body system?
   a. Eyes
   b. Skin
   c. Respiratory tract
   d. Gastrointestinal tract

9. What personal protective equipment would the nurse don before caring for a patient with COVID-19? **Select all that apply.**
   a. Goggles
   b. Surgical mask
   c. N95 mask or PAPR
   d. Gown
   e. Gloves
   f. Hair cover

10. Antibiotics are either bacteriocidal or bacteriostatic. Which class of antibiotics would the nurse recognize as having both properties?
    a. Tetracyclines
    b. Sulfonamides
    c. Cephalosporins
    d. Macrolides

11. What would the nurse do prior to initiating antibiotic therapy?
    a. Obtain the patient's temperature
    b. Ask the patient about antibiotic resistance
    c. Collect any ordered blood or specimen cultures
    d. Administer probiotics to reduce the risk of diarrhea

12. When teaching a patient about proper use of antibiotics, which patient statements indicate additional teaching is necessary? **Select all that apply.**
    a. "I will not share my antibiotics."
    b. "Washing my hands frequently is important."
    c. "I will ask for antibiotics to treat any sore throats."
    d. "I will stop taking the antibiotics once my fever goes away."
    e. "I will take the antibiotics at the same time each day until they are gone."
    f. "I will save any unused antibiotics for future use."

13. Antiviral therapy is only available to treat a small number of viruses. Which antiviral drug has been approved to treat COVID-19?
    a. Acyclovir
    b. Remdesivir
    c. Oseltamivir
    d. Valacyclovir

14. In each of the following situations, identify which option has the highest risk for human immunodeficiency virus (HIV) transmission?
    a. Transmission to women or to men during heterosexual intercourse
    b. Hollow-bore needle used for vascular access or used for IM injection
    c. First 2 to 4 weeks of infection or 1 year after infection
    d. Perinatal transmission from HIV-infected mothers taking antiretroviral therapy (ART) or HIV-infected mothers using no therapy
    e. A splash exposure of HIV-infected blood on skin with an open lesion or a needle-stick exposure to HIV-infected blood

15. Using number 1 as the first event and number 7 as the last event, place in order the following events of HIV infection of a cell.

_____ a. The release of reverse transcriptase converts HIV ribonucleic acid (RNA) into a single strand of DNA.

_____ b. Viral DNA is spliced into cell genome using the enzyme integrase.

_____ c. HIV binds with CD4$^+$ T cell protein receptors on the outside of the cell (fusion).

_____ d. Viral DNA directs the cell to replicate infected daughter cells and makes more HIV.

_____ e. Viral RNA enters the host CD4$^+$ T cell.

_____ f. Long strands of viral RNA are cut in the presence of protease and released before CD4$^+$ T cell destruction.

_____ g. Single-stranded viral DNA replicates into double-stranded DNA.

16. In the table below, indicate which event of HIV infection of a cell is controlled by each drug. Refer to Question 9 for the events which will also be the mechanism of action of the drug.

Drug	Mechanism of Action
Attachment inhibitors	
Entry inhibitors	
Reverse transcriptase inhibitors	
Integrase inhibitors	
Protease inhibitors	

17. What is the main reason that the normal immune response does not contain HIV infection?
    a. CD4$^+$ T cells become infected with HIV and are destroyed.
    b. The virus inactivates B cells, preventing the production of HIV antibodies.
    c. Natural killer cells are destroyed by the virus before the immune system can be activated.
    d. Monocytes ingest infected cells, differentiate into macrophages, and shed viruses in body tissues.

18. Which characteristic corresponds with the acute stage of HIV infection?
    a. Burkitt's lymphoma
    b. Temporary fall of CD4$^+$ T cells
    c. *Pneumocystis jiroveci* pneumonia
    d. Fever, sore throat, and lymphadenopathy

19. Which finding supports the diagnosis of acquired immunodeficiency syndrome (AIDS) in the person with HIV?
    a. Flu-like symptoms
    b. Oral hairy leukoplakia
    c. CD4$^+$ T cells 200–500/µL
    d. Cytomegalovirus retinitis

20. Why do opportunistic diseases develop in a person with AIDS?
    a. They are side effects of drug treatment of AIDS.
    b. They are sexually transmitted to people during exposure to HIV.
    c. They are characteristic in people with stimulated B and T lymphocytes.
    d. These infections or tumors occur in a person with an incompetent immune system.

21. Which characteristics describe *Pneumocystis jiroveci* infection, an opportunistic disease that can be associated with HIV?
    a. May cause fungal meningitis
    b. Diagnosed by lymph node biopsy
    c. Pneumonia with dry, nonproductive cough
    d. Viral retinitis, stomatitis, esophagitis, gastritis, or colitis

22. Which opportunistic disease associated with AIDS is characterized by vascular lesions of the skin, mucous membranes, and viscera?
    a. Kaposi sarcoma
    b. *Candida albicans*
    c. Herpes simplex type 1 infection
    d. Varicella-zoster virus infection

23. A patient comes to the clinic and requests testing for HIV infection. Before the testing, what is most important for the nurse to do?
    a. Ask the patient to identify all sexual partners.
    b. Determine when the patient thinks exposure to HIV occurred.
    c. Explain that all test results must be repeated at least twice to be valid.
    d. Discuss prevention practices to prevent transmission of the HIV to others.

24. The "rapid" HIV antibody testing is performed on a patient at high risk for HIV infection. What would the nurse explain about this test?
    a. The test measures the activity of the HIV and reports viral loads as real numbers.
    b. This test is highly reliable, and in 5 minutes the patient will know if HIV infection is present.
    c. If the results are positive, another blood test and a return appointment for results will be necessary.
    d. This test detects drug-resistant viral mutations that are present in viral genes to evaluate resistance to antiretroviral drugs.

25. Treatment with 2 nucleoside reverse transcriptase inhibitors (NRTIs) and an integrase inhibitor is prescribed for a patient with HIV infection. The patient asks why so many drugs are necessary for treatment. What would the nurse explain is the main reason for combination therapy?
    a. Cross-resistance between specific antiretroviral drugs is reduced when drugs are given in combination.
    b. Combinations of antiretroviral drugs decrease the potential for developing antiretroviral-resistant HIV variants.
    c. Side effects of the drugs are reduced when smaller doses of 3 different drugs are used rather than large doses of 1 drug.
    d. When CD4$^+$ T-cell counts are < 500/μL, a combination of drugs that have different actions is more effective in slowing HIV growth.

26. What is one of the most significant factors in determining when to start ART in a patient with HIV infection?
    a. Whether the patient has high levels of HIV antibodies
    b. Confirmation that the patient has contracted HIV infection
    c. The patient's readiness to commit to a complex, lifelong, uncomfortable drug regimen
    d. Whether the patient has a support system to help manage the treatment regimen and costs

27. After teaching a patient with HIV infection about using antiretroviral drugs, which statement by the patient indicates to the nurse that further teaching is needed?
    a. "I should never skip doses of my medication, even if I develop side effects."
    b. "By taking my HIV medications I will be able to lower by CD4$^+$ cell count."
    c. "I should not use any over-the-counter drugs without checking with my health care provider (HCP)."
    d. "If I develop a headache with nausea and vomiting, I should report it to my HCP."

28. What prophylactic measures are routinely used as early as possible in HIV infection to prevent opportunistic and debilitating secondary problems?
    a. Isoniazid to prevent tuberculosis
    b. Zoster virus vaccination to prevent shingles
    c. Trimethoprim/sulfamethoxazole for toxoplasmosis
    d. Vaccines for pneumococcal pneumonia, influenza, and hepatitis A and B

29. A patient diagnosed with HIV 1 year ago has no symptoms of HIV-related illness and does not want to start ART at this time. What is the best nursing intervention for the patient at this stage of illness?
    a. Assist with end-of-life issues
    b. Provide care during acute exacerbations
    c. Provide physical care for chronic diseases
    d. Teach the patient about immune enhancement

30. Identify at least 3 ways to eliminate or reduce the risk for HIV transmission related to sexual intercourse and drug use and 2 ways to reduce the risk for perinatal transmission.

Sexual Intercourse	Drug Use	Perinatal Transmission
a.	a.	a.
b.	b.	b.
c.	c.	

31. A patient with advanced AIDS has confusion because of neurologic changes. When planning care for the patient, what would the nurse consider as the highest priority?
    a. Maintain a safe patient environment
    b. Provide a quiet, nonstressful environment to avoid overstimulation
    c. Use memory cues, such as calendars and clocks, to promote orientation
    d. Provide written instructions of directions to promote understanding and orientation

CASE STUDY   HIV Infection

Patient Profile
A.K., a 28-year-old single man, is seen at a health clinic for flu-like symptoms. He is worried that he may have HIV.

(Image Source Pink/
Image Source/Thinkstock)

Subjective Data
- Says he has a history of multiple sex partners
- Reports vague symptoms of fatigue and headache
- Reports occasional night sweats

Objective Data
- Tests positive for HIV antibody
- Temp: 100°F (37.8°C)
- Enlarged cervical and femoral lymph nodes

Questions

1. What additional tests may be performed for this patient? **Use an X to indicate if the tests below are Anticipated (appropriate or necessary) or Non-essential (makes no difference or is unnecessary).**

Diagnostic Test	Anticipated	Non-Essential
CBC with differential		
CD4$^+$ T cell count		
Echocardiogram		
Viral load count		
Arterial blood gas		
Hepatitis B and C serology		
Spiral CT scan		

2. What counseling activities would the nurse prioritize and perform during A.K.'s visit? **Use an X to indicate if the counseling activities below are Indicated (appropriate or necessary), Contraindicated (could be harmful), or Non-essential (makes no difference or is unnecessary).**

Counseling Activity	Indicated	Contraindicated	Non-Essential
Provide resources for emotional support			
Evaluate suicide risk			
Discuss completing an Advance Directive			
Discuss clinical manifestations of AIDS			
Discuss end-of-life planning			
Contact tracing			
Treatment options			
Provide ideas about how to tell his coworkers			

3. **Complete the following sentences by choosing the most likely option for the missing information from the lists of options provided.**

To help prevent developing opportunistic infections, A.K. should get the following vaccines: _____**1**_____, _____**1**_____, and _____**1**_____. The nurse discusses risk reduction methods with A.K. which include _____**2**_____ and _____**2**_____. Combination ART is recommended for A.K. The nurse explains that ART _____**3**_____. If A.K. doesn't respond to treatment, tests can be performed to identify if he has developed a resistance to the ART medications. These tests are the _____**4**_____ assay and the _____**4**_____ assay.

Options for 1	Options for 2	Options for 3	Options for 4
Gardasil	using PrEP	is curative	HIV antigen
Pneumococcal	abstaining from sex	is palliative	Phenotype
Rabies	using a condom	is painful	HLA-B*5701
Hepatitis B	adhering to ART	reduces viral load	CCR5
Influenza	avoiding kissing	doesn't have side effects	Genotype
Tetanus	self-isolation	is not expensive	CXCR4

4. What information would the nurse include when teaching A.K. about taking ART medications? **Select all that apply.**
   _____A. Adherence is a key component of ART.
   _____B. Notify your HCP before taking herbals or OTC medications.
   _____C. ART medications cannot be changed.
   _____D. Take the medications at different times each day.
   _____E. Combination therapy reduces the risk of drug resistance.
   _____F. If the viral load becomes undetectable, you may stop taking these medications.
   _____G. Use pillboxes to help you remember to take the medications.
   _____H. Involve family or friends to help you remember to take these medications.

5. There is a potential for A.K. to develop opportunistic infections due to HIV infection. **Indicate which assessment finding listed in the far-left column is applicable to the opportunistic infection. Note that some assessment findings may apply to more than one opportunistic infection.**

Assessment Finding	Opportunistic Infection	Appropriate Assessment Finding for Opportunistic Infection
Use of accessory muscles	*Pneumocystis jiroveci*	
Night sweats	Kaposi sarcoma	
Fever	*Cryptococcus neoformans*	
Swollen lymph nodes		
Impaired memory		
Hyperpigmented lesions		
Seizures		

16

Cancer

1. The nurse is presenting a community education program related to cancer prevention. Based on current cancer death rates, what would the nurse emphasize as the most important preventive action for both women and men?
   a. Smoking cessation
   b. Routine colonoscopies
   c. Frequent imaging tests
   d. Regular examination of reproductive organs

2. What defect in cellular proliferation is involved in the development of cancer?
   a. A rate of cell proliferation that is more rapid than that of normal body cells
   b. Shortened phases of cell life cycles with occasional skipping of G1 or S phases
   c. Rearrangement of stem cell RNA that causes abnormal cellular protein synthesis
   d. Indiscriminate and continuous proliferation of cells with loss of contact inhibition

3. What does the presence of carcinoembryonic antigens (CEAs) and α-fetoprotein (AFP) on cell membranes show has happened to the cells?
   a. They have shifted to more immature metabolic pathways and functions.
   b. They have spread from areas of original development to different body tissues.
   c. They produce abnormal toxins or chemicals that show abnormal cellular function.
   d. They have become more differentiated because of repression of embryonic functions.

4. What factor differentiates a malignant tumor from a benign tumor?
   a. It causes death.
   b. It grows at a faster rate.
   c. It is often encapsulated.
   d. It invades and metastasizes.

5. A patient is admitted with acute myelogenous leukemia and a history of Hodgkin's lymphoma. What is the nurse most likely to find in the patient's history?
   a. Work as a radiation chemist
   b. Epstein-Barr virus diagnosed in vitro
   c. Intense tanning throughout the lifetime
   d. Alkylating agents for treating the Hodgkin's lymphoma

6. Which mutated tumor suppressor gene is most likely to contribute to many types of cancer, including bladder, breast, colorectal, and lung?
   a. *p53*
   b. *APC*
   c. *BRCA1*
   d. *BRCA2*

7. Cancer cells go through stages of development. What accurately describes the stage of promotion? **Select all that apply.**
   a. Obesity is an example of a promoting factor.
   b. The stage is characterized by increased growth rate and metastasis.
   c. Withdrawal of promoting factors will reduce the risk of cancer development.
   d. Tobacco smoke is a complete carcinogen that is capable of both initiation and promotion.
   e. Promotion is the stage of cancer development in which there is an irreversible alteration in the cell's DNA.

8. A patient was told about having carcinoma in situ, and the student nurse wonders what this is. How would the nurse explain this to the student nurse?
   a. Evasion of the immune system by cancer cells
   b. Lesion with histologic features of cancer except invasion
   c. Capable of causing cellular alterations associated with cancer
   d. Tumor cell surface antigens that stimulate an immune response

9. Which word identifies a mutation of protooncogenes?
   a. Oncogenes
   b. Retrogenes
   c. Oncofetal antigens
   d. Tumor angiogenesis factor

10. What is the name of a tumor from the embryonal mesoderm tissue of origin found in the anatomic site of the meninges that has malignant behavior?
    a. Meningitis
    b. Meningioma
    c. Meningocele
    d. Meningeal sarcoma

11. A patient's breast tumor originates from embryonal ectoderm. It has moderate dysplasia and moderately differentiated cells. It is a small tumor with minimal lymph node involvement and no metastases. What is the best description of this tumor?
    a. Sarcoma, grade II, $T_3N_4M_0$
    b. Leukemia, grade I, $T_1N_2M_1$
    c. Carcinoma, grade II, $T_1N_1M_0$
    d. Lymphoma, grade III, $T_1N_0M_0$

12. The nurse is counseling a group of people over the age of 50 years with average risk for cancer about screening tests for cancer. Which is recommended to screen for colorectal cancer?
    a. Barium enema every year
    b. Colonoscopy every 10 years
    c. Fecal occult blood every 5 years
    d. Annual prostate-specific antigen (PSA) and digital rectal examination

13. A small lesion is found in a patient's lung when an x-ray is done for cervical spine pain. What is the definitive method of determining if the lesion is malignant?
    a. Lung scan
    b. Tissue biopsy
    c. Oncofetal antigens in the blood
    d. CT or positron emission tomography (PET) scan

14. A patient with a genetic mutation of *BRCA1* and a family history of breast cancer is admitted to the surgical unit where she is scheduled for a bilateral simple mastectomy. What is the reason for this procedure?
    a. Prevent breast cancer
    b. Diagnose breast cancer
    c. Cure or control breast cancer
    d. Provide palliative care for untreated breast cancer

15. Match the surgical procedures with their primary purposes in cancer treatment *(answers may be used more than once)*.

Surgical Procedure	**Primary Purpose**
_____ a. Mammoplasty	1. Cure, control, or both
_____ b. Bowel resection	2. Supportive care
_____ c. Laminectomy to relieve spinal cord compression	3. Palliation
_____ d. Insertion of feeding tube into stomach	4. Rehabilitation
_____ e. Colostomy to bypass bowel obstruction	
_____ f. Placement of a central venous catheter	
_____ g. Debulking procedure to enhance radiation therapy	
_____ h. Surgical fixation of bones at risk for pathologic fracture	

16. Which condition would most likely be cured with chemotherapy as a treatment measure?
    a. Neuroblastoma
    b. Small cell lung cancer
    c. Small tumor of the bone
    d. Large hepatocellular carcinoma

17. Which classification of chemotherapy drugs is cell cycle phase–nonspecific, breaks the DNA helix that interferes with DNA replication, and crosses the blood–brain barrier?
    a. Nitrosoureas
    b. Antimetabolites
    c. Mitotic inhibitors
    d. Antitumor antibiotics

18. What is the nurse trying to prevent when using many precautions during IV administration of vesicant chemotherapy agents?
    a. Septicemia
    b. Extravasation
    c. Catheter occlusion
    d. Anaphylactic shock

19. For which type of cancer would the nurse expect the use of the intravesical route of regional chemotherapy delivery?
    a. Bladder
    b. Leukemia
    c. Osteogenic sarcoma
    d. Metastasis to the brain

20. Which delivery system would be used to deliver regional chemotherapy for metastasis from a primary colorectal cancer?
    a. Intrathecal
    b. Intraarterial
    c. Intravenous
    d. Intraperitoneal

21. When teaching the patient with cancer about chemotherapy, which approach should the nurse take?
    a. Avoid telling the patient about side effects of the drugs to prevent anticipatory anxiety.
    b. Assure the patient that side effects from chemotherapy are uncomfortable but not life threatening.
    c. Explain that antiemetics, antidiarrheals, and analgesics will be given as needed to control side effects.
    d. Tell the patient that chemotherapy-related alopecia is usually permanent but can be managed with lifelong use of wigs.

22. Which normal tissues manifest early, acute responses to pelvic radiation therapy?
    a. Spleen and liver
    b. Kidney and nervous tissue
    c. Bone marrow and gastrointestinal (GI) mucosa
    d. Hollow organs, such as the stomach and bladder

23. Which instructions would the nurse include when teaching a patient about skin care related to external radiation?
    a. Keep the area shaved of hair.
    b. Keep the area covered if it is sore.
    c. Dry the skin thoroughly after cleansing.
    d. Avoid extreme temperatures to the area.

24. What is important for the nurse to be aware of when caring for a patient undergoing brachytherapy?
    a. The patient will undergo simulation to identify and mark the field of treatment.
    b. The patient is a source of radiation, and personnel must wear film badges during care.
    c. The goal of this treatment is only palliative, and the patient should be aware of the expected outcome.
    d. Computerized dosimetry is used to determine the maximum dose of radiation to the tumor within an acceptable dose to normal tissue.

25. To prevent the debilitating cycle of fatigue-depression-fatigue in patients receiving radiation therapy, what would the nurse encourage the patient to do?
    a. Implement a walking program.
    b. Ignore the fatigue as much as possible.
    c. Do the most stressful activities when fatigue is tolerable.
    d. Schedule rest periods throughout the day whether fatigue is present or not.

26. When the patient asks about the late effects of chemotherapy and high-dose radiation, what would the nurse plan to include when describing these effects?
    a. Third space syndrome
    b. Secondary malignancies
    c. Chronic nausea and vomiting
    d. Persistent myelosuppression

27. What describes a primary use of immunotherapy in cancer treatment?
    a. Protects normal, rapidly reproducing cells of the GI system from damage during chemotherapy
    b. Prevents the fatigue associated with chemotherapy and high-dose radiation as seen with bone marrow depression
    c. Enhances or supplement the effects of the host's immune responses to tumor cells that produce flu-like symptoms
    d. Depresses the immune system and circulating lymphocytes as well as increase a sense of well-being by replacing central nervous system deficits

28. While caring for a patient who is at the nadir of chemotherapy, what is the nurse's top priority?
    a. Diarrhea
    b. Grieving
    c. Risk for infection
    d. Nutritional intake

29. An allogeneic hematopoietic stem cell transplant is planned for a patient with acute myelogenous leukemia. What information would the nurse include when teaching the patient about this procedure?
    a. There is no risk for graft-versus-host disease because the donated marrow is treated to remove cancer cells.
    b. The patient's bone marrow will be removed, treated, stored, and then reinfused after intensive chemotherapy.
    c. There is no need for post transplant protective isolation because the stem cells are infused directly into the blood.
    d. Peripheral stem cells are obtained from a donor who has a human leukocyte antigen (HLA) match with the patient.

30. During initial chemotherapy, a patient with leukemia develops hyperkalemia and hyperuricemia which the nurse recognizes as an oncologic emergency. What treatment would the nurse anticipate as the priority?
    a. Increase urine output with hydration therapy
    b. Establish electrocardiographic (ECG) monitoring
    c. Administer a bisphosphonate, such as pamidronate (Aredia)
    d. Restrict fluids and administer hypertonic sodium chloride solution

31. The patient with advanced cancer is having difficulty with pain control and expresses fear about becoming addicted to the opioids. What would the nurse do first?
    a. Administer a nonsteroidal antiinflammatory drug.
    b. Assess the patient's vital signs and behavior to determine the medication to use.
    c. Have the patient keep a pain diary to better assess the patient's potential addiction.
    d. Obtain a detailed pain history including quality, location, intensity, duration, and type of pain.

32. Which factors will help a patient in coping positively with having cancer? **Select all that apply.**
    a. Feeling of control
    b. Strong support system
    c. Internalization of feelings
    d. Possibility of cure or control
    e. Easier adaptability of a young person
    f. Not having had to cope with previous stressful events

CASE STUDY Cancer

(pixelheadphoto/
iStock/Thinkstock)

Patient Profile

R.M. is a 58-year-old man who was recently diagnosed with metastatic lung cancer. He began treatment with chemotherapy through a peripherally inserted central catheter (PICC) 5 days ago.

Subjective Data
- Reports almost continuous nausea, which becomes severe and causes vomiting following chemotherapy
- Reports no appetite and feels hot
- Expresses no hope that the chemotherapy will lead to a positive outcome

Objective Data
- Temp: 99.7°F (37.4°C)
- WBC count: 3200/μL (3.2 × 10^9/L)
- Neutrophils: 500/μL (0.5 × 10^9/L)
- Skin warm with decreased turgor

Questions

1. What assessment data indicate that R.M. may have an infection? **Use an X to indicate if the assessment finding is <u>Significant</u> (indicates an infection) or <u>Unrelated</u> (does not indicate an infection).**

Assessment Finding	Significant	Unrelated
Reports no appetite		
WBC count: 3200/μL		
Decreased skin turgor		
Temp: 99.7°F (37.4°C)		
Nausea and vomiting		
Neutrophils: 500/μL		
Expresses no hope		

2. What factors may be contributing to his negative attitude towards chemotherapy? **Select all that apply**.
   _____A. He experiences side effects from chemotherapy.
   _____B. He feels that he lacks control over his body.
   _____C. His daughter is providing emotional support.
   _____D. Other people he knows have died from cancer.
   _____E. He openly expresses his concerns and feelings.
   _____ F. Friends and family members are unable to visit him
   _____G. Mediation has been useful in managing his stress.
   _____H. He is on a medical leave of absence from his job.

3. What nursing interventions are appropriate to treat the following clinical problems? **Indicate which nursing intervention in the left column is appropriate for the clinical problem. Note some interventions may be used more than once.**

Nursing Intervention	Clinical Problem	Appropriate Nursing Intervention for Clinical Problem
Encourage small frequent meals	Hyperthermia	
Administer antiemetics as needed	Impaired Immunity	
Monitor temperature every 4 hours	Impaired Gastrointestinal Function	
Administer acetaminophen 650 mg PR q. 8 hours PRN	Nutritionally Compromised	
Keep a food diary to track daily calories and fluids		
Monitor weight frequently		
Institute neutropenic precautions		
Administer 500 mL 0.9% normal saline bolus		
Perform frequent oral care		

4. Choose the most likely options for the information missing from the text below by selecting from the lists of options provided. There are many hematopoietic growth factors used in cancer treatment. _____1_____ treats anemia related to chemotherapy, but side effects include _____2_____ and _____2____. _____3_____ can treat neutropenia caused by chemotherapy. Side effects include _____4_____ and ____4_____. Oprelvekin is a drug that can be used to treat _____5_____. If the patient experiences _____6_____ and _____6_____ as side effects from this drug, the nurse should notify the health care provider.

Options for 1 and 3	Options for 2, 4 and 6	Options for 5
Oprelvekin	Hypertension	Anemia
Sargramostim	Bone pain	Leukocytosis
Pegfilgrastim	Shortness of breath	Thrombocytopenia
Epoetin alfa	Thrombosis	Polycythemia
Ondansetron	Tachycardia	Neutropenia
Sandostatin	Nausea and vomiting	Myeloid cell recovery

5. When teaching R.M. and his family about how to prevent infection, which statements indicate teaching has been effective?
Use an X to indicate if the teaching has been Effective (helps prevent infection), Ineffective (does not help to prevent an infection) or is Unrelated (isn't related to helping prevent infection).

Teaching	Effective	Ineffective	Unrelated
"I will perform frequent hand washing with anti-bacterial soap."			
"I can walk barefoot around the house, as long as I wear shoes outside."			
"I will use a clean technique when changing the PICC dressing."			
"I need to report fevers to my HCP."			
"I will use an electric razor to shave."			
"I will refer to online cancer resources to learn coping strategies."			

Fluid, Electrolyte, and Acid-Base Imbalances

1. A patient with consistent dietary intake who loses 1 kg of weight in 1 day has lost _____ mL of fluid.

2. A man who weighs 90 kg has a total body water content of approximately _____ L.

3. Which statements about fluid in the human body are true? **Select all that apply.**
   a. The primary hypothalamic mechanism of water intake is thirst.
   b. Third spacing refers to the abnormal movement of fluid into interstitial spaces.
   c. A cell surrounded by hypoosmolar fluid will shrink and die as water moves out of the cell.
   d. A cell surrounded by hyperosmolar fluid will shrink and die as water moves out of the cell.
   e. Concentrations of Na^+ and K^+ in interstitial and intracellular fluids are maintained by the sodium-potassium pump.

4. Match the following descriptions with the mechanisms of fluid and electrolyte movement.

   Description
   _____ a. Force exerted by a fluid
   _____ b. Uses a protein carrier molecule
   _____ c. Pressure exerted by plasma proteins
   _____ d. Adenosine triphosphate (ATP) required
   _____ e. Force determined by osmolality of a fluid
   _____ f. Flow of water from low-solute concentration to high-solute
          concentration
   _____ g. Passive movement of molecules from a high concentration to lower
          concentration

   Mechanisms
   1. Osmosis
   2. Diffusion
   3. Active transport
   4. Oncotic pressure
   5. Osmotic pressure
   6. Facilitated diffusion
   7. Hydrostatic pressure

5. A patient has a serum Na^+ of 147 mEq/L (147 mmol/L), blood urea nitrogen (BUN) of 6 mg/dL (2.1 mmol/L), and a blood glucose level of 126 mg/dL (7.0 mmol/L).

$$\text{Plasma osmolality} = (2 \times Na) + \left(\frac{BUN}{2.8}\right) + \left(\frac{Glucose}{18}\right)$$

The patient's effective serum osmolality is _____ mOsm/kg. Is the patient's plasma osmolality normal, increased, or decreased?

6. As fluid circulates through the capillaries, there is movement of fluid between the capillaries and interstitium. What describes the fluid movement that would cause edema? **Select all that apply.**
   a. Plasma hydrostatic pressure is less than plasma oncotic pressure.
   b. Plasma oncotic pressure is higher than interstitial oncotic pressure.
   c. Plasma hydrostatic pressure is higher than plasma oncotic pressure.
   d. Plasma hydrostatic pressure is less than interstitial hydrostatic pressure.
   e. Interstitial hydrostatic pressure is lower than plasma hydrostatic pressure.

7. Using the options in the 2nd table below, fill in the blanks in the table below to indicate the direction of fluid shift and the mechanism of fluid movement that is involved. **Answers may be used more than once.**

Event or Factor	Direction of Fluid Shift	Mechanism of Fluid Movement Involved
Burns		
Dehydration		
Fluid overload		
Hyponatremia		
Low serum albumin		
Administration of 10% glucose		
Application of elastic bandages		

Options:

Direction of Fluid Shifts	Mechanism of Fluid Movement Involved
1. From blood vessels to interstitium 2. From extracellular compartment to the cell 3. From cell to extracellular compartment 4. From interstitium to vessels	a. Osmosis b. Plasma hydrostatic pressure c. Interstitial hydrostatic pressure d. Tissue oncotic pressure e. Oncotic pressure

8. A woman has ham with gravy and green beans cooked with salt pork for dinner.
   a. How could this meal affect the woman's serum osmolality?
   b. What fluid regulation mechanisms are stimulated by the intake of these foods?

9. What stimulates aldosterone secretion from the adrenal cortex?
   a. Excessive water intake
   b. Increased serum osmolality
   c. Decreased serum potassium
   d. Decreased sodium and water

10. While caring for an 84-year-old patient, the nurse monitors the patient's fluid and electrolyte balance recognizing what as a normal change of aging?
    a. Hyperkalemia
    b. Hyponatremia
    c. Decreased insensible fluid loss
    d. Increased plasma oncotic pressures

11. The nurse is admitting a patient to the clinical unit from surgery. Being alert to potential fluid volume alterations, what assessment data will be important for the nurse to monitor to identify early changes in the patient's postoperative fluid volume? **Select all that apply.**
    a. Intake and output
    b. Skin turgor
    c. Lung sounds
    d. Respiratory rate
    e. Level of consciousness

12. Which patient is at risk for hypernatremia?
    a. Has an aldosterone deficiency
    b. Has prolonged vomiting and diarrhea
    c. Receives excessive IV 5% dextrose solution
    d. Has impaired consciousness and decreased thirst sensitivity

13. In a patient with sodium imbalances, the primary clinical manifestations are related to alterations in what body system?
    a. Kidneys
    b. Cardiovascular system
    c. Musculoskeletal system
    d. Central nervous system

14. Match the electrolyte imbalances with their associated causes. **Answers may be used more than once and imbalances may have more than 1 associated cause.**

Electrolyte Imbalance	Cause
a. Metabolic alkalosis	1. Hypernatremia
b. Parathyroidectomy	2. Hyponatremia
c. Diabetes insipidus	3. Hyperkalemia
d. Fleet enemas	4. Hypokalemia
e. Primary polydipsia	5. Hypercalcemia
f. Excess milk of magnesia use	6. Hypocalcemia
g. Early burn stage	7. Hyperphosphatemia
h. Chronic alcoholism	8. Hypophosphatemia
i. Vitamin D deficiency	9. Hypermagnesemia
j. Osmotic diuresis	10. Hypomagnesemia
k. Prolonged immobilization	
l. Hyperaldosteronism	
m. Chronic kidney disease	
n. Loop and thiazide diuretics	

15. A patient is taking diuretic drugs. Which fluid or electrolyte imbalance can occur in this patient? **Select all that apply.**
    a. Hyperkalemia
    b. Hyponatremia
    c. Hypocalcemia
    d. Hypotonic fluid loss
    e. Hypertonic fluid loss

16. Which potential complication is related to both hyperkalemia and hypokalemia?
    a. Seizures
    b. Paralysis
    c. Dysrhythmias
    d. Acute kidney injury

17. Which disorder is hyperkalemia often associated?
    a. Hypoglycemia
    b. Metabolic acidosis
    c. Respiratory alkalosis
    d. Decreased urine potassium levels

18. In a patient with a positive Chvostek's sign, the nurse would expect the IV administration of which medication?
    a. Calcitonin
    b. Vitamin D
    c. Loop diuretics
    d. Calcium gluconate

19. A patient with chronic kidney disease has hyperphosphatemia. What is a commonly associated electrolyte imbalance?
    a. Hypokalemia
    b. Hyponatremia
    c. Hypocalcemia
    d. Hypomagnesemia

20. What is the normal pH range of the blood and what ratio of base to acid does this reflect?
    a. 7.32 to 7.42; 25 to 2
    b. 7.32 to 7.42; 28 to 2
    c. 7.35 to 7.45; 20 to 1
    d. 7.35 to 7.45; 30 to 1

21. What are the characteristics of the carbonic acid–bicarbonate buffer system? **Select all that apply.**
    a. The lungs eliminate CO_2
    b. Neutralizes HCl acid to yield carbonic acid and salt
    c. H_2CO_3 formed by neutralization dissociates into H_2O and CO_2
    d. Shifts H^+ in and out of cell in exchange for other cations, such as potassium and sodium
    e. Free basic radicals dissociate into ammonia and OH^-, which combines with H^+ to form water

22. What are characteristics of the phosphate buffer system? **Select all that apply.**
    a. Neutralizes a strong base to a weak base and water
    b. Resultant sodium biphosphate is eliminated by kidneys
    c. Free acid radicals dissociate into H^+ and CO_2, buffering excess base
    d. Neutralizes a strong acid to yield sodium biphosphate, a weak acid, and salt
    e. Shifts chloride in and out of red blood cells in exchange for sodium bicarbonate, buffering both acids and bases

23. A patient who has a large amount of carbon dioxide in the blood also has what in the blood?
    a. Large amount of carbonic acid and low hydrogen ion concentration
    b. Small amount of carbonic acid and low hydrogen ion concentration
    c. Large amount of carbonic acid and high hydrogen ion concentration
    d. Small amount of carbonic acid and high hydrogen ion concentration

24. Match the acid–base imbalances with their mechanisms.

Acid–Base Imbalance	Mechanism
_____ a. Increased carbonic acid (H_2CO_3)	1. Metabolic acidosis
_____ b. Decreased carbonic acid (H_2CO_3)	2. Metabolic alkalosis
_____ c. Increased base bicarbonate (HCO_3^-)	3. Respiratory acidosis
_____ d. Decreased base bicarbonate (HCO_3^-)	4. Respiratory alkalosis

25. What is a compensatory mechanism for metabolic alkalosis?
    a. Shifting of bicarbonate into cells in exchange for chloride
    b. Kidney conservation of bicarbonate and excretion of hydrogen ions
    c. Deep, rapid respirations (Kussmaul respirations) to increase CO_2 excretion
    d. Decreased respiratory rate and depth to retain CO_2 and kidney excretion of bicarbonate

26. Match the acid–base imbalances with their common causes. **Answers may be used more than once.**

Cause	Acid–Base Imbalance
_____ a. Renal failure	1. Metabolic acidosis
_____ b. Severe shock	2. Metabolic alkalosis
_____ c. Diabetic ketosis	3. Respiratory acidosis
_____ d. Respiratory failure	4. Respiratory alkalosis
_____ e. Prolonged vomiting	
_____ f. Baking soda used as antacid	
_____ g. Mechanical over ventilation	
_____ h. Sedative or opioid overdose	
_____ i. Response to anxiety, fear, and pain	

27. A patient with a pH of 7.29 has metabolic acidosis. Which value is useful in determining whether the cause of the acidosis is an acid gain or a bicarbonate loss?
    a. $PaCO_2$
    b. Anion gap
    c. Serum Na^+ level
    d. Bicarbonate level

28. Identify the acid–base imbalances represented by the following laboratory values.

    a. pH 7.50
       PaCO₂ 30 mm Hg
       HCO₃⁻ 24 mEq/L
       PaO₂ 79 mm Hg
       Interpretation:

       _____

       _____

    b. pH 7.20
       PaCO₂ 25 mm Hg
       HCO₃⁻ 15 mEq/L
       PaO₂ 96 mm Hg
       Interpretation:

       _____

       _____

    c. pH 7.26
       PaCO₂ 56 mm Hg
       HCO₃⁻ 24 mEq/L
       PaO₂ 68 mm Hg
       Interpretation:

       _____

       _____

    d. pH 7.62
       PaCO₂ 48 mm Hg
       HCO₃⁻ 45 mEq/L
       PaO₂ 98 mm Hg
       Interpretation:

       _____

       _____

    e. pH 7.44
       PaCO₂ 54 mm Hg
       HCO₃⁻ 36 mEq/L
       PaO₂ 90 mm Hg
       Interpretation:

       _____

       _____

    f. pH 7.35
       PaCO₂ 60 mm Hg
       HCO₃⁻ 40 mEq/L
       PaO₂ 84 mm Hg
       Interpretation:

       _____

       _____

29. To provide free water and intracellular fluid hydration for a patient with acute gastroenteritis who is NPO, which IV fluid would the nurse expect to administer?
    a. Dextrose 5% in water
    b. Dextrose 10% in water
    c. Lactated Ringer's solution
    d. Dextrose 5% in normal saline (0.9%)

30. What is an example of an appropriate IV solution to treat an extracellular fluid volume deficit?
    a. D₅W
    b. 3% saline
    c. Lactated Ringer's solution
    d. Dextrose 5% in 0.45% saline

31. On assessment of a central venous access device (CVAD) site, the nurse notes that the transparent dressing is loose along 2 sides. What should the nurse do immediately?
    a. Wait and change the dressing when it is due.
    b. Tape the 2 loose sides down and document.
    c. Apply a gauze dressing over the transparent dressing and tape securely.
    d. Remove the dressing and apply a new transparent dressing using sterile technique.

32. A patient just had a CVAD inserted. Using number 1 as the first action and number 8 as the last action, number the following nursing actions related to care of the CVAD.
    _____ a. Perform hand hygiene.
    _____ b. Flush each line with 10 mL of normal saline.
    _____ c. Use strict sterile technique to change the dressing.
    _____ d. Clamp unused lines after flushing if not using positive pressure valve caps.
    _____ e. Assess the CVAD insertion site for redness, edema, warmth, drainage, and pain.
    _____ f. Use friction to cleanse the CVAD insertion site with chlorhexidine-based preparation.
    _____ g. Turn the patient's head to the side away from the CVAD insertion site when changing the caps.
    _____ h. Obtain chest x-ray results to verify placement of the catheter in the distal end of the superior vena cava.

33. A patient is scheduled to have a tunneled catheter placed for administration of chemotherapy for breast cancer. When preparing the patient for the catheter insertion, what does the nurse explain about this method of chemotherapy administration?
    a. Decreases the risk for extravasation at the infusion site
    b. Reduces the incidence of systemic side effects of the drug
    c. Does not become occluded as peripherally inserted catheters can
    d. Allows continuous infusion of the drug directly to the area of the tumor

34. The nurse is reviewing a patient's morning laboratory results. Which result would most concern the nurse?
    a. Serum Na^+ of 150 mEq/L
    b. Serum Mg^{2+} of 1.1 mEq/L
    c. Serum PO_4^{3-} of 4.5 mg/dL
    d. Serum Ca^{2+} (total) of 8.6 mg/dL

CASE STUDY   Fluid and Electrolyte Imbalance

Patient Profile
P.B., a 69-year-old woman who lives alone, is admitted to the hospital because of weakness and confusion. She has a history of chronic heart failure and chronic diuretic use.

(© Thinkstock)

Objective Data
Physical Examination
- Neurologic: Confusion, slow to respond to questioning, generalized weakness
- Cardiovascular: BP 90/62 mm Hg, HR 112 beats/min, peripheral pulses weak; ECG shows sinus tachycardia
- Pulmonary: RR 12 and shallow
- Other findings: Decreased skin turgor, dry mucous membranes

Laboratory Results
- Serum electrolytes
  - Na^+: 141 mEq/L (141 mmol/L)
  - K^+: 2.5 mEq/L (2.5 mmol/L)
  - Cl^-: 85 mEq/L (85 mmol/L)
  - HCO_3^-: 40 mEq/L (40 mmol/L)
- BUN: 42 mg/dL (15 mmol/L)
- Hct: 52%
- Arterial blood gases
  - pH: 7.52
  - $PaCO_2$: 55 mm Hg
  - PaO_2: 88 mm Hg
  - HCO_3^-: 34 mEq/L (34 mmol/L)

Questions
1. Highlight or place a check mark next to the laboratory results that are abnormal.
2. Indicate which assessment finding listed in the far-left column is applicable to the clinical problem. Note that some assessment findings may be applied to more than one clinical problem.

Assessment Finding	Clinical Problem	
Confusion	Electrolyte imbalance	
Sinus tachycardia	Metabolic Alkalosis	
Generalized weakness	Fluid imbalance	
Decreased skin turgor		
Dry mucous membranes		
Hct 52%		
pH 7.52		
HCO_3^- 34 mEq/L		
Weak peripheral pulses		
Shallow respirations		
BP 90/62 mm Hg		

3. What nursing actions would be included in this patient's plan of care? **Use an X to indicate if the nursing action is Indicated (is appropriate or necessary), Contraindicated (is not appropriate or could be harmful), or Non-essential (is unnecessary or irrelevant).**

Nursing Action	Indicated	Contraindicated	Non-Essential
Continuous cardiac monitoring			
3% saline infusion			
Auscultate breath sounds			
Monitor urine output			
Apply oxygen 4 L/min via nasal cannula			
Place patient on falls precautions			
Perform passive range of motion exercises			

4. What would the nurse teach P.B. before she is discharged? **Select all that apply**.
   _____A. Drink at least 1500 mL per day, even if she isn't thirsty
   _____B. Increase sodium intake to conserve water
   _____C. Report any signs of edema to your HCP
   _____D. Avoid cola beverages
   _____E. Feeling palpitations is expected
   _____F. Report diuresis to your HCP
   _____G. Monitor your weight monthly
   _____H. Eat green leafy vegetables, like spinach

5. **Choose the most likely options for the information missing from the statements below by selecting from the lists of options provided.**

   _____1_____ solutions are known as volume or plasma expanders. They have large molecules that increase _____2_____. _____3_____ is a colloid that is available in 2 concentrations. The __4__ solution is similar to plasma while the __4__ solution is hypertonic. All colloids affect blood coagulation by interfering with _____5_____.

Options for 1	Options for 2	Options for 3
Crystalloid	Diffusion	Albumin
Hypertonic	Hydrostatic pressure	Whole blood
Hypotonic	Oncotic pressure	Saline
Colloid	Osmosis	Lactated Ringer's
Isotonic	Active transport	Dextrose

Options for 4	Options for 5
3%	Factor II
5%	Factor III
10%	Factor X
25%	Factor VIII
50%	Factor IX

Preoperative Care

1. Which procedures are done for curative purposes? **Select all that apply.**
   a. Gastroscopy
   b. Rhinoplasty
   c. Tracheotomy
   d. Hysterectomy
   e. Herniorrhaphy

2. A patient is scheduled for a hemorrhoidectomy at an ambulatory surgery center. What is an advantage of performing surgery at an ambulatory center?
   a. Fewer diagnostic studies and perioperative medications are necessary.
   b. Preoperative and postoperative teaching by the nurse isn't necessary.
   c. There isn't a need to provide psychologic support to alleviate fears of pain and discomfort.
   d. A preoperative nursing assessment related to possible risks and complications is not performed.

3. A patient, who is being admitted to the surgical unit for a hysterectomy, paces the floor repeatedly saying, "I just want this over." What would the nurse do to promote a positive surgical outcome?
   a. Ask the patient what her specific concerns are about the surgery.
   b. Redirect the patient's attention to the necessary preoperative preparations.
   c. Reassure the patient that the surgery will be over soon and she will be fine.
   d. Tell the patient she should not be so anxious because she is having a common, safe surgery.

4. Many common herbal products can cause surgical complications. Which herbs would the nurse teach the patient to avoid before surgery to prevent an increased risk for bleeding? **Select all that apply.**
   a. Garlic
   b. Fish oil
   c. Valerian
   d. Vitamin E
   e. Astragalus
   f. Ginkgo biloba

5. When the nurse asks a preoperative patient about allergies, the patient reports a history of seasonal environmental allergies and allergies to a variety of fruits. What would the nurse do next?
   a. Note this information in the patient's record as hay fever and food allergies.
   b. Place an allergy alert wristband that identifies the specific allergies on the patient.
   c. Ask the patient to describe the nature and severity of any allergic responses experienced from these agents.
   d. Notify the anesthesia care provider (ACP) because the patient may have an increased risk for allergies to anesthetics.

6. During a preoperative review of systems, the patient reveals a history of renal disease. Which preoperative diagnostic studies should be performed?
   a. Electrocardiogram (ECG) and chest x-ray
   b. Serum glucose and complete blood count (CBC)
   c. Arterial blood gases (ABGs) and coagulation tests
   d. Blood urea nitrogen (BUN), serum creatinine, and electrolytes

7. During a preoperative physical examination, which problem would the nurse consider as causing an increased risk of compromised respiratory function during or after surgery?
   a. Obesity
   b. Dehydration
   c. Enlarged liver
   d. Decreased peripheral pulses

8. What type of procedural information should be given to a patient in preparation for ambulatory surgery? **Select all that apply.**
   a. How pain will be controlled
   b. Any fluid and food restrictions
   c. Characteristics of monitoring equipment
   d. What odors and sensations may be experienced
   e. Technique and practice of coughing and deep breathing, if appropriate

9. The nurse asks a preoperative patient to sign a surgical consent form as specified by the surgeon and then signs the form after the patient signs. What is the nurse doing by this action?
   a. Witnessing the patient's signature
   b. Obtaining informed consent from the patient for the surgery
   c. Verifying that the consent for surgery is truly voluntary and informed
   d. Ensuring that the patient is mentally competent to sign the consent form

10. When the nurse prepares to administer a preoperative medication to a patient, the patient tells the nurse that they really do not understand what the surgeon plans to do.
    a. What action would the nurse take?
    b. What condition of informed consent has not been met?

11. A patient scheduled for hip replacement surgery in the early afternoon is NPO but receives and ingests a breakfast tray with clear liquids on the morning of surgery. What would the nurse expect when the ACP is notified?
    a. Surgery will be performed as scheduled.
    b. Surgery will be rescheduled for the following day.
    c. Surgery will be postponed for 8 hours after the fluid intake.
    d. A nasogastric tube will be inserted to remove the fluids from the stomach.

12. What is the reason for using preoperative checklists on the day of surgery?
    a. The patient is correctly identified and preoperative medications administered.
    b. All preoperative orders and procedures have been carried out and documented.
    c. Voiding is the last procedure before the patient is transported to the operating room.
    d. Patients' families have been informed as to where they can accompany and wait for patients.

13. What is a common reason that a nurse may need extra time when preparing older adults for surgery?
    a. Difficulty coping
    b. Limited adaptation to stress
    c. Diminished vision and hearing
    d. Need to include caregivers in activities

14. The nurse is reviewing the laboratory results for a preoperative patient. Which result would be immediately reported to the surgeon?
    a. Serum K^+ of 3.8 mEq/L
    b. Hemoglobin of 15 g/dL
    c. Blood glucose of 100 mg/dL
    d. White blood cell (WBC) count of 18,500/μL

15. The nurse is preparing a patient for transport to the operating room for a right knee arthroscopy. What actions would the nurse take at this time? **Select all that apply.**
    a. Ensure that the patient has voided.
    b. Verify that the informed consent is signed.
    c. Complete preoperative nursing documentation.
    d. Verify that the right knee is marked with indelible marker.
    e. Ensure that the history and physical examination (H&P), diagnostic reports, and vital signs are on the chart.

CASE STUDY Preoperative Patient

Patient Profile

C.J., a 44-year-old male construction worker, is scheduled for a bronchoscopy for a biopsy of a right lung lesion. He initially sought medical care for hemoptysis and increasing fatigue. When the nurse asked him to sign the operative permit, he stated that he was not certain if he should go ahead with the procedure because he fears a diagnosis of cancer.

(Thinkstock)

Subjective Data
- Never been hospitalized
- No medical problems except mild obesity
- Has a history of cigarette smoking 28 pack-years
- Is married with 2 children, ages 6 and 8 years; both children have cystic fibrosis
- Is fearful that his wife will not be able to manage without him

Objective Data
- Diagnostic studies: chest x-ray revealed mass in upper lobe of right lung
- Hematocrit 31%

Questions

1. C.J. will be an outpatient for the bronchoscopy. What preoperative teaching would the nurse provide? **Select all that apply.**
   _____A. He may eat toast on the morning of surgery.
   _____B. He may drive himself home the same day after recovering from surgery.
   _____C. All valuables should be left at home.
   _____D. Do not have anything by mouth after midnight.
   _____E. Bring a photo ID and health insurance information.
   _____F. He can use a ride share service to take him home after the procedure.
   _____G. He will need to be discharged with a responsible adult.
   _____H. He can take ibuprofen for pain the night before surgery.
   _____I. It is fine to drink black coffee without sugar or milk 3 hours before surgery.

2. Indicate which assessment finding listed in the far-left column is applicable to the clinical problem. Note that some assessment findings may be applied to more than one clinical problem.

Assessment Finding	Clinical Problem	Appropriate Assessment Finding for Clinical Problem
28 pack-years smoker	Anxiety	
"Wife will not be able to manage without him."	Risk for impaired respiratory function	
Never been hospitalized	Substance Use	
Mild obesity		
Mass in upper lobe of right lung		
Hematocrit 31%		
Fears diagnosis		
Has 2 children with cystic fibrosis		

3. Complete the following sentences by choosing the most likely option for the missing information from the lists of options provided. C.J. isn't sure if he should proceed with the procedure. The nurse must confirm _____**1**_____consent has occurred before the procedure can proceed. This type of consent is the responsibility of the _____**2**_____. Topics that need to be discussed are _____**3**_____, _____**3**_____, and _____**3**_____. If the patient still has questions about the procedure, the nurse would _____**4**_____.

Options for 1	Options for 2	Options for 3	Options for 4
Surgical	Anesthesiologist	Risks	Get consent from his wife
Procedural	Circulator	Surgical techniques	Notify the anesthesia provider
Informed	CRNA	Benefits	Document in the nurse's notes
Pathology	Surgeon	Options	Notify the surgeon
Implied	Scrub technician	Alternatives	Cancel the procedure

4. What would the nurse teach C.J. preoperatively?

Use an X to indicate if the teaching is <u>Indicated</u> (is appropriate or necessary), <u>Contraindicated</u> (is not appropriate or could be harmful), or <u>Non-essential</u> (is unnecessary or irrelevant).

Teaching	Indicated	Contraindicated	Non-Essential
"You will need to take deep breaths and cough."			
"You will need a blood transfusion after this type of procedure."			
"You will be monitored for at least an hour after the procedure."			
"You will need to eat and drink before you will be discharged home."			
"You will not have any pain after the procedure."			
"You may have shortness of breath immediately after the procedure."			

5. Several medications may be administered preoperatively.

Choose the most likely options for the information missing from the table by selecting from the lists of options provided.

Medication	Dose, Route	Drug Class	Indication
4	1 g IV	Antibiotic	Infection prophylaxis
Glycopyrrolate	1	Anticholinergic	3
Midazolam	2 mg IV	2	7
Scopolamine	1 mg transdermal	5	Prevent N/V
Fentanyl	8	Opioid	Relieve pain
6	4 mg IV	Antiemetic	Prevent N/V

Options for 1 and 8	Options for 2 and 5	Options for 3 and 7	Options for 4 and 6
1 g IV	Anticholinergic	Procedural sedation	Midazolam
2 mg IV	Antiemetic	Decrease respiratory secretions	Scopolamine
50 mcg IV	Benzodiazepine	Infection prophylaxis	Ondansetron
0.2 mg IV	Opioid	Prevent N/V	Cefazolin
4 mg IV	Antibiotic	Decrease heart rate	Fentanyl
1 mg transdermal	Beta-blocker	Treat hypertension	Glycopyrrolate

Intraoperative Care

1. What is the physical environment of a surgery suite primarily designed to promote?
   a. Electrical safety
   b. Medical and surgical asepsis
   c. Comfort and privacy of the patient
   d. Communication among the surgical team

2. When transporting an inpatient from another area in the hospital to the surgical department, which area is this nurse able to access?
   a. Sterile core
   b. Holding area
   c. Corridors of surgical suite
   d. Unprepared operating room

3. Which nursing actions are performed by the scrub nurse? **Select all that apply.**
   a. Prepares instrument table
   b. Documents intraoperative care
   c. Remains in the sterile area of the operating room (OR)
   d. Checks mechanical and electrical equipment
   e. Passes instruments to surgeon and assistants
   f. Monitors blood and other fluid loss and urine output

4. What is the main goal of the circulating nurse during preparation of the OR, transferring and positioning the patient, and assisting the anesthesia team?
   a. Avoiding any type of injury to the patient
   b. Maintaining a clean environment for the patient
   c. Providing for patient comfort and sense of well-being
   d. Preventing breaks in aseptic technique by the sterile members of the team

5. Goals for patient safety in the OR include the Universal Protocol. What is included in this protocol?
   a. All surgical centers of any type must submit reports on patient safety infractions to the accreditation agencies.
   b. Members of the surgical team stop whatever they are doing to check that all sterile items have been prepared properly.
   c. Members of the surgical team pause right before surgery to meditate for 1 minute to decrease stress and possible errors.
   d. A surgical timeout is performed just before the procedure is started to verify patient identity, surgical procedure, and surgical site.

6. What action by the scrub nurse is considered a break in sterile technique?
   a. Touches the mask with sterile gloved hands.
   b. Touches sterile gloved hands to the gown at chest level.
   c. Touches the drape at the incision site with sterile gloved hands.
   d. Touches the lower arm to the instruments on the instrument tray.

7. During surgery, a patient is at risk of perioperative positioning injury. What is a common risk factor for this type of injury?
   a. Skin lesions
   b. Break in sterile technique
   c. Musculoskeletal deformities
   d. Electrical or mechanical equipment failure

8. Which short-acting barbiturate is most often used for induction of general anesthesia?
   a. Nitrous oxide
   b. Propofol (Diprivan)
   c. Isoflurane (Forane)
   d. Methohexital (Brevital)

9. Because of the rapid elimination of volatile liquids used for general anesthesia, what would the nurse anticipate the patient will need early in the recovery period from anesthesia?
   a. Warm blankets
   b. Analgesic medication
   c. Observation for respiratory depression
   d. Airway protection in anticipation of vomiting

10. What is the main advantage of using midazolam as an adjunct to general anesthesia?
    a. Amnestic effect
    b. Analgesic effect
    c. Prolonged action
    d. Antiemetic effect

11. Identify the rationale for the use of each of the following drugs during surgery and list 1 nursing intervention indicated in the care of the patient postoperatively which is related to the drug.

Drug	Use	Nursing Intervention
ketamine (Ketalar)		
fentanyl (Sublimaze)		
desflurane (Suprane)		
succinylcholine (Anectine)		
dexmedetomidine (Precedex)		

12. Monitored anesthesia care (MAC) is being considered for a patient undergoing a cervical dilation and endometrial biopsy in the clinic. The patient asks the nurse, "What is MAC?" How would the nurse respond?
    a. It can be administered only by anesthesiologists or nurse anesthetists.
    b. It would never be used outside of the OR because of the risk of serious complications.
    c. It is so safe that it can be administered by nurses with direction from health care providers.
    d. It provides maximum flexibility to match the sedation level with the patient and procedure needs.

13. Match the methods of local and regional anesthetic administration with their descriptions.

Description	Method of Anesthesia
a. Injection of agent into subarachnoid space	1. Nerve block
b. Injection of anesthetic agent directly into tissues	2. IV nerve block
c. Injection of a specific nerve with an anesthetic agent	3. Spinal block
d. Injection of anesthetic agent into space around the vertebrae	4. Epidural block
e. Injection of agent into veins of extremity after limb is exsanguinated	5. Local infiltration

14. The patient will be placed under moderate sedation to allow realignment of a fracture in the emergency department. When the family asks about this type of sedation, what would the nurse tell them?
    a. Inhalation agents will be used
    b. High levels of sedation are required
    c. Is frequently used for traumatic injuries
    d. Patients remain responsive and breathe without assistance

15. What condition would the nurse anticipate may occur during epidural and spinal anesthesia?
    a. Spinal headache
    b. Hypotension and bradycardia
    c. Loss of consciousness and seizures
    d. Downward extension of nerve block

16. A patient scheduled for a procedure is expected to receive ketamine (Ketalar). What would the nurse include in patient teaching?
    a. Hallucinations may occur, so the patient will receive midazolam.
    b. An indwelling catheter may be needed if urinary retention occurs.
    c. Antiemetics will be given beforehand to reduce nausea and vomiting.
    d. Using ketamine will allow the patient to be fully awake during the procedure.

17. A preoperative patient reports that an uncle died during surgery because of a fever and cardiac arrest. Knowing the patient is at risk for malignant hyperthermia, the preoperative nurse alerts the surgical team. How would the operative team proceed?
    a. The surgery will be canceled.
    b. Specific precautions will be taken to safely anesthetize the patient.
    c. Dantrolene will be given to prevent hyperthermia during surgery.
    d. The patient will be placed on a cooling blanket during the surgical procedure.

18. Which anesthetic agent is it most important to monitor the patient for malignant hyperthermia?
    a. Ketamine
    b. Pancuronium
    c. Succinylcholine
    d. Dexmedetomidine

CASE STUDY   Intraoperative Patient

Patient Profile

T.M., a 76-year-old male retired police officer, is admitted to the OR for an inguinal hernia repair. He has a history of severe chronic obstructive pulmonary disease (COPD) and heart failure; therefore, the anesthesia care provider (ACP) has decided to use spinal anesthesia. The preoperative nurse has verified the baseline data, which includes vital signs, height, weight, age, allergies, level of consciousness, NPO status, and comfort level. A signed informed consent is on the chart. T.M. has no allergies.

(Anita_Bonita/
iStock/Thinkstock)

Questions

1. When transferring the patient from the preoperative department to the operating room, what information would the preoperative nurse include in the hand-off communication to the circulating nurse?

Use an X to indicate if the information shared during the hand-off is <u>Essential</u> (necessary or important information to include) or <u>Non-Essential</u> (unnecessary or unimportant information to include).

Information to Report	Essential	Non-Essential
Height		
Vital signs		
History of COPD		
Type of surgery		
Plans for discharge home		
Allergies		
NPO status		
Baseline comfort level		
History of heart failure		
Retired police officer		

2. T.M. has been given midazolam 1 mg in the preoperative department. What nursing actions would be taken when T.M. arrives in the OR?

Use an X to indicate if the nursing action is <u>Indicated</u> (appropriate or necessary), Contraindicated (could be harmful), or <u>Non-Essential</u> (makes no difference or is unnecessary).

Nursing Action	Indicated	Contraindicated	Non-Essential
Have the patient stand to transfer from the gurney to the OR table.			
Perform a *Time Out*			

Nursing Action	Indicated	Contraindicated	Non-Essential
Position the patient			
Update the family upon arrival			
Attaches monitoring equipment (BP cuff, ECG leads, etc.)			
Cut off the patient's ID bracelet to make room for an additional IV			
Have the patient sign the surgical consent form			

3. How should the incisional site be prepped for surgery? **Select all that apply.**
   _____A. The groin is cleansed with alcohol.
   _____B. The lower abdomen is cleansed with an antimicrobial agent.
   _____C. The groin is shaved with a blade razor.
   _____D. Allow the prep solution to pool under the patient to keep the area clean.
   _____E. The groin is cleansed with an antimicrobial agent.
   _____F. The surgical area should be prepped from distal toward the incision site.
   _____G. The prep agent should be allowed to fully dry.
   _____H. The surgical area should be prepped from the clean area to the dirty area.
   _____I. Drape the area before prepping the surgical site.
   _____J. Use clippers to remove hair near the surgical site.

4. Indicate which nursing action listed in the far-left column is applicable to the clinical problem. Note that some nursing actions may be applied to more than one clinical problem.

Nursing Action	Clinical Problem	Appropriate Nursing Action for Clinical Problem
Allows skin prep fumes to dispel	Risk for injury	
Antibiotic is administered minutes before incision is made	Hypothermia	
Uses Bair hugger	Risk for infection	
Confirms patient has had CHG bath		
Only exposes surgical site		
Checks electrical equipment		
The circulating nurse monitors aseptic technique for self and others		
Correctly places the grounding pad		

5. T.M. has spinal anesthesia to repair an inguinal hernia. What complications of spinal anesthesia would the CRNA monitor T.M. for during surgery?

   For each assessment finding, use an X to indicate if the assessment finding is <u>Expected</u> (no follow-up is required) or <u>Requires Nursing Follow-Up</u> (could be harmful to the patient).

Assessment Finding	Expected	Requires Nursing Follow-Up
Temperature 36.4°C		
BP 90/42 mm Hg		
HR 52 beats/min		
RR 18 breaths/min		
Cannot feel or move his legs		
Tingling in arms and hands		
SpO$_2$ 97% on 4 L/min nasal cannula		
Feels like he cannot take a deep a breath		

Postoperative Care

1. What does progression of patients through various phases of care in a postanesthesia care unit (PACU) primarily depend on?
   a. Condition of patient
   b. Type of anesthesia used
   c. Preference of surgeon
   d. Type of surgical procedure

2. Upon admission of a patient to the PACU, what is the nurse's priority assessment?
   a. Vital signs
   b. Surgical site
   c. Respiratory adequacy
   d. Level of consciousness

3. How is the surgical information about the patient relayed to the PACU nurse?
   a. A copy of the written operative report
   b. A verbal report from the circulating nurse
   c. A verbal report from the anesthesia care provider (ACP)
   d. An explanation of the surgical procedure from the surgeon

4. To prevent agitation during the patient's recovery from anesthesia, when would the nurse begin orientation to the environment?
   a. When the patient is awake
   b. When the patient first arrives in the PACU
   c. When the patient becomes agitated or frightened
   d. When the patient can be aroused and recognize where they are

5. On admission to the PACU, what is included in the routine assessment of the patient's cardiovascular function?
   a. Monitoring arterial blood gases
   b. Electrocardiographic (ECG) monitoring
   c. Determining fluid and electrolyte status
   d. Direct arterial blood pressure monitoring

6. Postoperative atelectasis or aspiration of gastric contents will cause what respiratory complication?
   a. Hypoxemia
   b. Hypercapnia
   c. Hypoventilation
   d. Airway obstruction

7. What would the nurse do to prevent airway obstruction in the postoperative patient who is unconscious or semiconscious?
   a. Encourage deep breathing
   b. Elevate the head of the bed
   c. Administer oxygen per mask
   d. Position the patient in a side-lying position

8. What is most important for the nurse to do to promote effective coughing, deep breathing, and ambulation in the postoperative patient?
   a. Teach the patient controlled breathing.
   b. Explain the rationale for these activities.
   c. Provide adequate and regular pain medication.
   d. Use an incentive spirometer to motivate the patient.

9. While assessing a patient in the PACU, the nurse finds that the patient's blood pressure (BP) is below the preoperative baseline. What assessment finding indicates that the patient has residual vasodilating effects of anesthesia?
   a. A urinary output > 30 mL/hr
   b. An oxygen saturation of 88%
   c. A normal pulse with warm, dry, pink skin
   d. A narrowing pulse pressure with normal pulse

10. A patient in the PACU has emergence delirium manifested by agitation and thrashing. What would the nurse assess for first?
    a. Hypoxemia
    b. Neurologic injury
    c. Distended bladder
    d. Cardiac dysrhythmias

11. The PACU nurse applies warm blankets to a postoperative patient who is shivering and has a body temperature of 96.0°F (35.6°C). What treatment may also be necessary to treat the patient?
    a. Oxygen therapy
    b. Vasodilating drugs
    c. Antidysrhythmic drugs
    d. Analgesics or sedatives

12. Which patient is ready for discharge from Phase I PACU care to the clinical unit?
    a. Arouses easily, pulse is 112 beats/min, respiratory rate is 24 breaths/min, dressing is saturated, arterial oxygen saturation by pulse oximetry (SpO_2) is 88%
    b. Awake, vital signs stable, dressing is dry and intact, no respiratory depression, SpO_2 is 92%
    c. Difficult to arouse, pulse is 52 beats/min, respiratory rate is 22 breaths/min, dressing is dry and intact, SpO_2 is 91%
    d. Arouses, BP higher than preoperative and respiratory rate is 10 breaths/min, no excess bleeding, SpO_2 is 92%

13. Which clinical problems common in postoperative patients has ambulation been found to be an appropriate intervention? **Select all that apply.**
    a. Surgical wound healing
    b. Risk for aspiration from decreased level of consciousness
    c. Impaired physical mobility due to decreased muscle strength
    d. Impaired airway clearance from decreased respiratory excursion
    e. Constipation from decreased physical activity and impaired GI motility
    f. Risk for inadequate tissue perfusion caused by a potential venous thromboembolism

14. A patient who had major surgery is experiencing emotional stress as well as physiologic stress from the effects of surgery. What can this stress cause?
    a. Diuresis
    b. Hyperkalemia
    c. Fluid retention
    d. Impaired blood coagulation

15. In addition to ambulation, which nursing intervention could be implemented to prevent or treat the postoperative complication of syncope?
    a. Monitor vital signs after ambulation.
    b. Do not allow the patient to eat before ambulation.
    c. Slowly progress to ambulation with slow changes in position.
    d. Have the patient deep breathe and cough before getting out of bed.

16. Which tubes drain gastric contents? **Select all that apply.**
    a. T-tube
    b. Penrose
    c. Nasogastric tube
    d. Indwelling catheter
    e. GI tube

17. What drainage is drained using a Hemovac drain?
    a. Bile
    b. Urine
    c. Gastric contents
    d. Wound drainage

18. The nurse observes drainage on the surgical dressing when the patient is transferred from the PACU to the clinical unit. In what order of priority would the nurse perform the following actions? **Number the options using 1 for the first action and 5 for the last action.**
    _____ a. Reinforce the surgical dressing.
    _____ b. Change the dressing and assess the wound as ordered.
    _____ c. Notify the surgeon of excessive drainage type and amount.
    _____ d. Recall the report from PACU for the number and type of drains in use.
    _____ e. Note and record the type, amount, and color and odor of the drainage.

19. Thirty-six hours postoperatively, a patient has a temperature of 100°F (37.8°C). What is the most likely cause for this elevated temperature?
    a. Dehydration
    b. Wound infection
    c. Lung congestion and atelectasis
    d. Normal surgical stress response

20. The health care provider has ordered IV morphine every 2-4 hrs PRN for a patient following major abdominal surgery. When would the nurse plan to administer the morphine?
    a. Before all planned painful activities
    b. Every 2 to 4 hours during the first 48 hours
    c. Every 4 hours as the patient requests the medication
    d. After assessing the nature and intensity of the patient's pain

21. What would the nurse include in postoperative discharge instructions?
    a. Need for follow-up care with home care nurses
    b. Directions for maintaining routine postoperative diet
    c. Written information about self-care during recuperation
    d. Need to restrict all activity until surgical healing is complete

---

CASE STUDY Postoperative Patient

(© szefei/iStock/ Thinkstock)

Patient Profile
S.B., a 63-year-old alert and oriented woman, is admitted to the PACU following a cystoscopy for recurrent bladder infections and recent hematuria. The procedure was scheduled as outpatient surgery and performed under IV sedation.

Postoperative Orders
- Vital signs per routine
- Remove IV before discharge
- Patient to void before discharge
- Ciprofloxacin (Cipro) 500 mg PO every 6 hrs for 10 days
- Acetaminophen 300 mg/codeine 30 mg 1 or 2 tabs every 3 hrs PRN pain
- Patient to call HCP office to schedule follow-up appointment

Questions
1. What nursing actions would be implemented postoperatively to help S.B. meet discharge criteria?

Use an X to indicate whether the nursing actions below are Indicated (appropriate or necessary), Contraindicated (could be harmful), or Non-Essential (unnecessary or makes no difference) for this patient's care.

Nursing Action	Indicated	Contraindicated	Non-Essential
Administer 0.4 mg naloxone IV to reverse sedation			

Nursing Action	Indicated	Contraindicated	Non-Essential
Administer B&O suppository for bladder spasms			
Offer oral fluids			
Contact ride-share for transport home			
Report gross hematuria to the HCP			
Apply sequential compression device			
Observe dressing for drainage			
Use bladder scan if patient is unable to void			

2. The nurse is assisting S.B. out of bed to ambulate to the bathroom.

For each assessment finding, use an X to indicate if the finding is <u>Expected</u> (finding is expected for this patient), <u>Unexpected</u> (finding could indicate a problem that needs follow-up) or <u>Unrelated</u> (isn't useful or isn't relevant data).

Assessment Finding	Expected	Unexpected	Unrelated
Temperature 37.9°C			
Patient reports burning during urination			
BP 95/45 mm Hg			
HR 110 beats/min			
SpO2 96% on room air			
Patient reports feeling sleepy			
Patient reports being thirsty			
Needs assistance during ambulation			
Reports nausea with movement			

3. What discharge instructions would the nurse include when teaching S.B. about self-care? **Select all that apply.**
   _____A. Don't drive until your HCP says it's okay
   _____B. You may resume normal activity as tolerated in 24 hours
   _____C. You may take a bath or shower starting tomorrow
   _____D. Change your dressing every day until the wound heals
   _____E. Strain your urine and collect any sediment in a specimen container
   _____F. Notify your HCP if you have a fever > 101°F
   _____G. Drink lots of fluid, especially water
   _____H. Advance your diet as tolerated, starting with mild bland foods
   _____I. You may take acetaminophen for pain, but don't exceed 3000 mg per day

4. Discharging a patient from PACU to home versus to the clinical unit may have different criteria.

Use an X to indicate if the nursing action is applicable to <u>Discharge Home</u> or <u>Discharge to the Clinical Unit</u>. Note some nursing actions may apply to both.

Nursing Action	Discharge Home	Discharge to Clinical Unit
PO opioid administered 15 minutes before discharge		
SBAR Hand-off		
Must be accompanied by an adult		
Pain is controlled or tolerable to the patient		
Patient is able to ambulate		
Is able to eat and drink without nausea or vomiting		
Vital signs are at baseline or stable for the patient		

Nursing Action	Discharge Home	Discharge to Clinical Unit
Understands postoperative self-care		
IV is removed		
Patient is arousable, but goes to sleep easily		

5. There are potential respiratory complications that can affect postoperative patients. Nurses in the PACU must continually assess for the presence of these complications and know how to intervene.

For each <u>Potential Complication</u> indicate which nursing action listed in the far-left column is an appropriate intervention for these potential complications postoperatively. Note that some nursing actions may not be used or used more than once.

Nursing Action	Potential Complication	Appropriate Nursing Action for Each Complication
Head tilt or jaw thrust	Laryngospasm	
Use incentive spirometry	Airway obstruction caused by tongue	
Administer furosemide 20 mg IV	Atelectasis	
Stimulate patient as needed		
Ambulate patient		
Use ambu bag to apply positive pressure ventilation		
Insert an artificial airway		
Have patient cough and deep breathe		
Perform chest physiotherapy		
Administer oxygen per protocol		

Emergency and Disaster Nursing

1. Using the Emergency Severity Index (ESI), triage the following patient situations present in an emergency department (ED) as ESI level 1, 2, 3, 4, or 5.

_____a. A 6-year-old child with a temperature of 103.2°F (39.6°C)

_____b. A 22-year-old woman with asthma in acute respiratory distress

_____c. An infant who has been vomiting for 2 days

_____d. A 50-year-old man with low back pain and spasms

_____e. A 32-year-old woman who is unconscious following an automobile accident

_____f. A 40-year-old woman with rhinitis and a cough

_____g. A 58-year-old man with midsternal chest pain

_____h. A 16-year-old teenager with an angulated forearm following a sports injury

2. When a nurse is performing a primary survey in the ED, what is being assessed?
   a. Whether the personnel of the ED are adequate to treat the patient
   b. The acuity of the patient's condition to determine priority of care
   c. Whether the patient is responsive enough to provide needed information
   d. The status of airway, breathing, circulation, disability, and exposure/environmental control

3. During the primary survey, the nurse observes asymmetric chest wall movement. What intervention would the nurse do first?
   a. Check a central pulse.
   b. Stabilize the cervical spine.
   c. Apply direct pressure to the wound.
   d. Start bag-mask ventilation with 100% oxygen.

4. During the secondary survey of a trauma patient in the ED, why is it important that the nurse obtain details of the incident?
   a. The mechanism of injury can predict specific injuries.
   b. Key facts may be forgotten when needed later for legal actions.
   c. Alcohol use associated with many accidents can affect treatment of injuries.
   d. Many types of accidents or trauma must be reported to government agencies.

5. What nursing intervention is done during the "E" step of the primary survey?
   a. Obtain full set of vital signs.
   b. Remove the patient's clothing and assess.
   c. Elicit history and head-to-toe assessment.
   d. Assess mental status and capillary refill for signs of shock.

6. When is the placement of a nasogastric tube contraindicated during emergency care?
   a. Inhalation injury
   b. Head or facial trauma
   c. Intraabdominal bleed
   d. Cervical spine fracture

7. In assessing the emergency patient's health history, what information is obtained using the mnemonic SAMPLE?
   a. Skin, anatomy of injuries, mucous membranes, peripheral edema, leukocytosis, eczema location
   b. Stiffness, approximate weight, motor function, palpable swelling, labored breathing, edema severity
   c. Symptoms, allergies, medications, past health history, last meal, and events/environment leading to the illness or injury
   d. Sentience, abdominal sounds, memory loss, people exposed to, last medication, earliest availability of past medical records

8. A 63-year-old trauma patient has open wounds, and the nurse asks the patient about her tetanus immunization status. Which situation would tetanus and diphtheria toxoids with acellular pertussis (Tdap) vaccine be given to the patient?
   a. Had 3 doses of tetanus toxoid as a child
   b. Has had a dose of tetanus toxoid in the past 10 years
   c. Is unsure of the history of tetanus toxoid vaccinations
   d. Has not had a dose of tetanus toxoid in the past 3 years

9. In which patient situation would therapeutic hypothermia be started in the ED?
   a. 48-year-old male found unconscious by neighbors; on ED arrival, he is moaning and moving all extremities
   b. 62-year-old man defibrillated by emergency medical technicians (EMTs); on ED arrival, he is not responsive, his heart rhythm and BP are stable
   c. 30-year-old female who has heat exhaustion after a marathon; on ED arrival, she is hypotensive and extremely diaphoretic with a temperature of 102.6°F (39.2°C)
   d. 38-year-old female found face down in her bathtub; she has a history of seizures; on ED arrival, she is responsive to pain only and she was intubated by paramedics with evidence of pulmonary edema; her pulse oximetry is 91%

10. After the death of a 36-year-old man from a massive head injury, what would be appropriate for the ED nurse to do?
    a. Ask the family members to consider donating their loved one's organs.
    b. Notify an organ procurement agency that a death has occurred that could result in organ donation.
    c. Explain to the family what a generous act it would be to donate the patient's organs to another patient who needs them.
    d. Ask the family to check the patient's driver's license to determine whether he had designated approval of donation of his organs in case of death.

11. What heat-related emergency would the healthy athlete with inadequate fluid intake be most likely to experience after exercise?
    a. Heatstroke
    b. Heat attack
    c. Heat cramps
    d. Heat exhaustion

12. Which statements describe heat exhaustion? **Select all that apply.**
    a. Volume and electrolyte depletion
    b. Treated with rapid cooling methods
    c. High risk of mortality and morbidity
    d. Rectal temperature of 99.6°F to 104°F (37.5°C to 40°C)
    e. Causes mild confusion, diaphoresis, and dilation of pupils

13. What intervention would the nurse perform during rewarming of a patient's toes with deep frostbite?
    a. Apply sterile dressings to blisters.
    b. Place the feet in a cool water bath.
    c. Massage the digits to increase circulation.
    d. Ensure that IV analgesics are administered.

14. A patient is brought to the ED following a skiing accident after which he was not found for several hours. He is rigid and has slowed respiratory and heart rates. What would the nurse do first during the primary assessment?
    a. Start active core rewarming interventions.
    b. Monitor the core temperature by the axillary route.
    c. Manage and maintain ABCs (airway, breathing, circulation).
    d. Expose the patient to check for areas of frostbite and other injuries.

15. A homeless man is brought to the ED in severe hypothermia with a temperature of 85°F (29.4°C). What would the nurse expect to find on initial assessment?
    a. Shivering and lethargy
    b. Fixed and dilated pupils
    c. BP not obtainable by Doppler
    d. Respirations of 6 to 8 per minute

16. What condition occurs with saltwater drowning but not with freshwater drowning?
    a. Destruction of surfactant
    b. Noncardiogenic pulmonary edema
    c. Water moves from alveoli to capillary bed and circulation
    d. Fluid is drawn into the alveoli from the pulmonary capillaries

17. What is the first priority in managing the patient after drowning?
    a. Reversing acidosis
    b. Correcting hypoxia
    c. Maintaining fluid balance
    d. Preventing cerebral edema

18. The ascending paralysis caused by the bite of a wood or dog tick may cause respiratory arrest unless what happens?
    a. The tick is removed.
    b. Antibiotics are administered.
    c. An antidote for the neurotoxin is given.
    d. Hemodialysis is started to remove the neurotoxin.

19. A patient was bitten by the neighbor's dog 8 hours ago. What treatment would the nurse plan to provide?
    a. Report the bite to the police.
    b. Give rabies prophylaxis.
    c. Start prophylactic IV antibiotics.
    d. Dress the wound to prevent exposure to neurotoxins.

20. The patient is admitted with severe acidosis after trying to commit suicide by ingesting aspirin. What would be used to treat this patient?
    a. Milk
    b. Cathartics
    c. Hemodialysis
    d. Whole bowel irrigation

21. For which ingested poisons may gastric lavage be considered? **Select all that apply.**
    a. Bleach
    b. Aspirin
    c. Drain cleaner
    d. Iron supplements
    e. Amitriptyline (Elavil)

22. An unresponsive patient is admitted to the ED with nausea, vomiting, and diaphoresis. The patient's family brought an empty container of acetaminophen that was found nearby. A large oral gastric tube is inserted. What does the nurse prepare to give first?
    a. GoLYTELY
    b. Ipecac syrup
    c. Gastric lavage
    d. Activated charcoal

23. Which biologic agent of terrorism is a bacterial neurotoxin that causes paralysis and respiratory failure with death occurring without treatment?
    a. Botulism
    b. Smallpox
    c. Tularemia
    d. Mustard gas

24. Which agent of terrorism does not have an established treatment for those exposed to it?
    a. Plague
    b. Anthrax
    c. Tularemia
    d. Hemorrhagic fever

25. Which biologic agents of terrorism can currently be protected against with a vaccine? **Select all that apply.**
    a. Plague
    b. Anthrax
    c. Botulism
    d. Smallpox
    e. Tularemia
    f. Hemorrhagic fever

26. When a patient is admitted with hemorrhagic fever, what treatment would the nurse provide?
    a. Parenteral analgesics
    b. Supportive treatment
    c. Warfarin administration
    d. Care of the rodent or mosquito bite

27. As a member of a volunteer disaster medical assistance team, what would the nurse be expected to do?
    a. Triage casualties of a tornado that hit the local community.
    b. Assist with implementing the hospital's emergency response plan.
    c. Train citizens of communities how to respond to mass casualty incidents.
    d. Deploy to local or other communities with disasters to provide medical assistance.

CASE STUDY   Heatstroke

Patient Profile

M.M., age 72 years, was taking a short break from nailing new shingles on his roof during the summer when he lost consciousness, collapsed, and fell off the roof onto his yard. His wife called 911 and he is brought to the ED accompanied by his wife.

(NADOFOTOS/ iStock/ Thinkstock)

Subjective Data
• Wife states that M.M. has been working all week on the roof even though he has not felt well for the last day or two.

Objective Data
• Vital signs: Temp 106.6°F (41.4°C), HR 124 beats/min weak and thready, RR 36 breaths/min and shallow, BP 82/40 mm Hg
• Skin hot, dry, and ashen

Questions
1. What interventions would the nurse expect to implement upon admission to the ED?

Use an X to indicate if the nursing action is <u>Indicated</u> (appropriate or necessary), <u>Contraindicated</u> (could be harmful), or <u>Non-essential</u> (makes no difference or is unnecessary).

Nursing Action	Indicated	Contraindicated	Non-Essential
C-spine precautions			
Oxygen via 6 L/min nasal cannula			
Establish IV access using 16G catheters			
Infuse normal saline 0.9% at 30 mL/hr			
Remove patient's clothing			
Insert an indwelling urinary catheter			
Clean and dress abrasions and cuts			
Assess pupils			
Auscultate bowel sounds			

2. What diagnostic test results would the nurse expect when caring for M.M.?

Use an X to indicate if the diagnostic test result is <u>Expected</u> (a finding consistent with the patient's admission data) or <u>Unexpected</u> (a finding inconsistent with the patient's admission data).

Diagnostic Test Result	Expected	Unexpected
CT scan shows cerebral contusion		
Na 120 mEq/L		
K 2.9 mEq/L		
Hct 22%		
12-lead ECG shows sinus tachycardia with PVCs		
Creatinine 0.8 mg/dL		
PaO$_2$ 85 mm Hg		

3. How would the nurse treat this patient's hyperthermia? **Select all that apply.**
_____A. Place wet sheets over patient's bare body.
_____B. Use an air conditioning unit to blow on patient.
_____C. Administer cool IV fluids.
_____D. Insert an NG tube and lavage using lukewarm fluid.
_____E. Use fans to blow on patient.
_____F. Place ice packs in armpits and groins.
_____G. Use Bair hugger machine to blow cool air.
_____H. Use drugs to prevent shivering.

4. For each clinical problem, indicate which nursing action is appropriate to improve or resolve the problem. Note that not all nursing actions may be used.

Nursing Action	Clinical Problem	Appropriate Nursing Action for Clinical Problem
Passive ROM every 4 hours	Fluid imbalance	
1000 mL bolus of normal saline 0.9%	Electrolyte imbalance	
Maintain urine output 1 mL/kg/hr	Impaired mobility	
Place patient on kinetic bed		
Administer KCL 10 mEq IVPB over 1 hour		
Administer oxygen to keep SpO$_2$ > 94%		
Apply sequential compression devices		
Continuous cardiac monitoring		
Administer 3% saline as ordered		
Maintain CVP ≥ 8 mm Hg		

5. Upon M.M.'s discharge home, what discharge instructions would the nurse include to prevent future episodes of heatstroke? **Select all that apply.**
_____A. Limit your exposure outside on hot days.
_____B. Drink lots of water to stay hydrated.
_____C. If you experience muscle cramps, wait 2 hours before resuming strenuous activities.
_____D. You can drink beer after working all day in the hot sun.
_____E. If you feel lightheaded, seek a cooler environment.
_____F. Wear loose breathable clothing on hot, humid days.
_____G. Your wife should check on you periodically throughout the day.

Assessment and Management: Visual Problems

1. Use the following terms to fill in the labels in the illustration below.

Terms

anterior chamber	optic nerve
choroid	posterior
ciliary body	chamber
cornea	pupil
iris	retina
lens	sclera
optic disc	vitreous humor

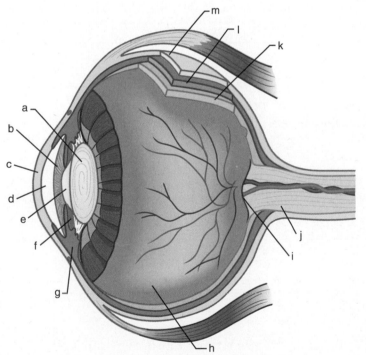

a. _____

b. _____

c. _____

d. _____

e. _____

f. _____

g. _____

h. _____

i. _____

j. _____

k. _____

l. _____

m. _____

2. What is in the posterior cavity of the eye?
   a. Zonules
   b. Cornea
   c. Aqueous humor
   d. Vitreous humor

3. What is the function of the sclera?
   a. Secrete aqueous humor
   b. Focus light rays on the retina
   c. Protective outer layer of the eyeball
   d. Photoreceptor cells stimulated in dim environments

4. What accurately describes the conjunctiva?
   a. Junction of the upper and lower eyelids
   b. Point where the optic nerve exits the eyeball
   c. Transparent mucous membrane lining the eyelids
   d. Drains tears from the surface of the eye into the lacrimal canals

5. Which tissue nourishes the ciliary body, iris, and part of the retina?
   a. Pupil
   b. Cones
   c. Choroid
   d. Canal of Schlemm

6. Identify the cranial nerves that are responsible for the following eye functions.

Eye Function	Cranial Nerve
Elevating eyelids	
Closing eyelids	
Visual acuity	

7. Identify the causes of the following assessment findings of the eye that are associated with aging.

Assessment Finding	Cause
Floaters	
Ectropion	
Pinguecula	
Arcus senilis	
Yellowish sclera	
Dry, irritated eyes	
Decreased pupil size	
Changes in color perception	

8. When obtaining a health history from a patient with cataracts, it is most important for the nurse to ask about the use of which drug?
   a. Corticosteroids
   b. Oral hypoglycemic agents
   c. β-Adrenergic blocking agents
   d. Antihistamines and decongestants

9. Identify a specific finding identified by the nurse during assessment of each of the patient's functional health patterns that indicates either a risk factor for visual problems or the response of the patient to an eye problem.

Functional Health Pattern	Risk Factor or Response to Visual Problem
Health perception–health management	
Nutritional-metabolic	
Elimination	
Activity-exercise	
Sleep-rest	
Cognitive-perceptual	
Self-perception–self-concept	
Role-relationship	
Sexuality-reproductive	
Coping–stress tolerance	
Value-belief	

10. Describe what is meant by the finding that the patient has a visual acuity of right eye: 20/40; left eye: 20/50.

11. The nurse documents PERRLA following assessment of a patient's eyes. What assessment finding supports this statement?
    a. A slightly oval shape of the pupils
    b. The presence of nystagmus on far lateral gaze
    c. Dilation of the pupil when a light is shined in the opposite eye
    d. Constriction of the pupils when an object is brought closer to the eyes

12. Identify the assessment techniques used to obtain the following assessment data.

Assessment Data	Assessment Technique
Peripheral vision field	
Extraocular muscle functions	
Near visual acuity	
Visual acuity	
Intraocular pressure	

13. In which group of patients would the nurse expect to find a yellow cast to the sclera?
    a. Infants
    b. Older persons
    c. Persons with brown irises
    d. Patients with eye infections

14. What would the nurse use to determine the presence of corneal abrasions or defects in a patient with an eye injury?
    a. A tonometer
    b. Fluorescein dye
    c. Pocket penlight
    d. An ophthalmoscope

15. What are possible abnormal assessment findings when assessing the eyelid? **Select all that apply.**
    a. Ptosis
    b. Strabismus
    c. Blepharitis
    d. Anisocoria
    e. Swollen pinna

16. When the patient has a diagnosis of hyperthyroidism, which abnormal eye assessment may be present?
    a. Light intolerance
    b. Unequal pupil size
    c. Protrusion of eyeball
    d. Deviation of eye position

17. When examining the patient's eye with an ophthalmoscope, which finding would most concern the nurse?
    a. No blood vessels in the macula
    b. Depression at the center of the optic disc
    c. A break in the retina at the site of the macula
    d. Pieces of liquefied vitreous in the vitreous chamber

18. To prepare a patient for a fluorescein angiography, what would the nurse explain about the test?
    a. Measures curvature of the cornea
    b. Involves IV dye injection to evaluate blood flow through retinal blood vessels
    c. Includes application of eyedrops containing a dye that will localize arterial abnormalities in the retina
    d. Anesthetizes the eye so that probes can be inserted into the anterior chamber to measure intraocular pressure

19. Myopia is present in 30% of Americans. Which characteristics are associated with myopia? **Select all that apply.**
    a. Excessive light refraction
    b. Abnormally short eyeball
    c. Unequal corneal curvature
    d. Corrected with concave lens
    e. Image focused in front of retina

20. The patient is diagnosed with presbyopia. What explanation of this condition would the nurse give the patient?
    a. Absence of the lens
    b. Abnormally long eyeballs
    c. Correctable with cylinder lens
    d. Loss of accommodation associated with age

21. What would the nurse do to determine if an unconscious patient has contact lenses in their eyes?
    a. Use a penlight to shine a light obliquely over the eyeball.
    b. Apply drops of fluorescein dye to the eye to stain the lenses yellow.
    c. Touch the cornea lightly with a dry cotton ball to see if the patient reacts.
    d. Tense the lateral canthus to cause a lens to be ejected if it is present in the eye.

22. What surgical choices are available for correction of a refractive error? **Select all that apply .**
    a. LASIK
    b. Contact lenses
    c. Corrective lenses
    d. Intraocular lens implantation
    e. Photorefractive keratectomy (PRK)

23. A patient tells the nurse on admission that he is legally blind. What does the nurse understand about the patient's vision?
    a. Has lost usable vision but has some light perception
    b. Will need time for grieving and adjusting to living with total blindness
    c. Will be dependent on others to ensure a safe environment for functioning
    d. May be able to perform many tasks and activities with vision enhancement techniques

24. Identify 5 nursing measures that would be implemented to increase a visually impaired patient's safety and comfort.
    a.
    b.
    c.
    d.
    e.

25. A patient is admitted to the emergency department with a wood splinter embedded in the right eye. Which intervention by the nurse is most appropriate?
    a. Irrigate the eye with a large amount of sterile saline.
    b. Carefully remove the splinter with a pair of sterile forceps.
    c. Cover the eye with a dry sterile patch and a protective shield.
    d. Apply light pressure on the closed eye to prevent bleeding or loss of aqueous humor.

26. What best describes pink eye?
    a. Blindness
    b. Acute bacterial conjunctivitis
    c. Epidemic keratoconjunctivitis
    d. Chronic inflammation of sebaceous glands

27. When the patient describes inflammation of the cornea, what would the nurse document?
    a. Keratitis
    b. Blepharitis
    c. Hordeolum
    d. Conjunctivitis

28. What would the nurse teach all patients with conjunctival infections to use?
    a. Artificial tears to moisten and soothe the eyes
    b. Dark glasses to prevent the discomfort of photophobia
    c. Iced moist compresses to the eyes to promote comfort and healing
    d. Frequent and thorough hand washing to avoid spreading the infection

29. Endophthalmitis can be a complication of intraocular surgery or penetrating ocular injury. What manifestations are expected when the nurse assesses a patient with this disorder? **Select all that apply.**
    a. Ocular pain
    b. Photophobia
    c. Eyelid edema
    d. Reddened sclera
    e. Bleeding conjunctiva
    f. Decreased visual acuity

30. A patient with early cataracts tells the nurse that he is afraid cataract surgery may cause permanent visual damage. What would the nurse teach the patient?
    a. The cataracts will only worsen with time and should be removed as early as possible to prevent blindness.
    b. Cataract surgery is very safe, and with the implantation of an intraocular lens, the need for glasses will be eliminated.
    c. Progression of the cataracts can be prevented by avoidance of ultraviolet (UV) light and good dietary management.
    d. Vision enhancement techniques may improve vision until surgery becomes an acceptable way to maintain desired activities.

31. A 60-year-old patient is being prepared for outpatient cataract surgery. When obtaining admission data from the patient, what would the nurse expect to find in the patient's history?
    a. A painless, sudden, severe loss of vision
    b. Blurred vision, colored halos around lights, and eye pain
    c. A gradual loss of vision with abnormal color perception and glare
    d. Light flashes, floaters, and a "cobweb" in the field of vision with loss of central or peripheral vision

32. A patient with bilateral cataracts is scheduled for an extracapsular cataract extraction with an intraocular lens implantation of 1 eye. What would the nurse do preoperatively?
    a. Assess the visual acuity in the unoperated eye to plan the need for postoperative assistance.
    b. Inform the patient that the operative eye will need to be patched for 3 to 4 days postoperatively.
    c. Assure the patient that vision in the operative eye will be improved to near normal on the first postoperative day.
    d. Teach the patient routine coughing and deep-breathing techniques to use postoperatively to prevent respiratory complications.

33. For the patient with a retinal break, what extraocular techniques may be used with sclera buckling to seal the break by creating an inflammatory reaction that causes a chorioretinal adhesion or scar? **Select all that apply.**
    a. Cryopexy
    b. Vitrectomy
    c. Pneumatic retinopexy
    d. Laser photocoagulation
    e. Penetrating keratoplasty

34. Following a pneumatic retinopexy, what does the nurse need to know about the postoperative care for the patient?
    a. Specific positioning and activity restrictions are likely to be required for days or weeks.
    b. The patient is frequently hospitalized for 7 to 10 days on bed rest until healing is complete.
    c. Patients experience little or no pain, and development of pain indicates hemorrhage or infection.
    d. Reattachment of the retina commonly fails, and patients can be expected to grieve for loss of vision.

35. What nursing action is most important for the patient with age-related dry macular degeneration (AMD)?
    a. Teach the patient how to use topical eyedrops for treatment of AMD.
    b. Emphasize the use of vision enhancement techniques to improve what vision is present.
    c. Encourage the patient to undergo laser treatment to slow the deposit of extracellular debris.
    d. Explain that nothing can be done to save the patient's vision because there is no treatment for AMD.

36. A patient with wet AMD is treated with photodynamic therapy. What would the nurse instruct the patient to do after the procedure?
    a. Maintain the head in an upright position for 24 hours.
    b. Avoid blowing the nose or causing jerking movements of the head.
    c. Completely cover all the skin to avoid a thermal burn from sunlight.
    d. Expect to experience blind spots where the laser has caused retinal damage.

37. What is an important health promotion nursing intervention for a middle-aged adult related to glaucoma?
    a. Teach people at risk for glaucoma about early signs and symptoms of the disease.
    b. Prepare patients with glaucoma for lifestyle changes necessary to adapt to eventual blindness.
    c. Promote measurements of intraocular pressure every 2 to 4 years for early detection and treatment of glaucoma.
    d. Inform patients that glaucoma is curable if eye medications are administered before visual impairment has occurred.

38. When teaching the patient about the new diagnosis of glaucoma, which characteristics relate only to primary open-angle glaucoma (POAG)? **Select all that apply.**
    a. Gradual loss of peripheral vision
    b. Treated with iridotomy or iridectomy
    c. Causes loss of central vision with corneal edema
    d. May be caused by increased production of aqueous humor
    e. Treated with cholinergic agents, such as pilocarpine (Pilocar)
    f. Resistance to aqueous outflow through trabecular meshwork

39. Which characteristics of glaucoma are associated with only acute primary angle-closure glaucoma (PACG)? **Select all that apply.**
    a. Caused by lens blocking papillary opening
    b. Treated with trabeculoplasty or trabeculectomy
    c. Causes loss of central vision with corneal edema
    d. Treated with β-adrenergic blockers, such as betaxolol (Betoptic)
    e. Causes sudden, severe eye pain associated with nausea and vomiting
    f. Treated with hyperosmotic oral and IV fluids to lower intraocular pressure

40. The health care provider (HCP) has prescribed optic drops of betaxolol (Betoptic), latanoprost, and pilocarpine (Pilocar) in addition to oral acetazolamide (Diamox) for treatment of a patient with chronic open-angle glaucoma. What is the rationale for the use of each of these drugs in the treatment of glaucoma?

Drug	Rationale for Use
Betaxolol	
Latanoprost	
Pilocarpine	
Acetazolamide	

CASE STUDY Chronic Open-Angle Glaucoma

Patient Profile
A.G., a 52-year-old woman, is being seen in her ophthalmologist's office for a routine eye examination. Her last examination was 5 years ago.

(XiXinXing/iStock/ Thinkstock)

Subjective Data
- Reports no current ocular problems
- Has not kept annually scheduled examinations because her eyes have not bothered her
- Takes metoprolol tartrate (Lopressor) for hypertension
- Has a family history of glaucoma
- Uses over-the-counter diphenhydramine for seasonal allergies

Objective Data
- BP 130/78 mm Hg
- HR 72 beats/min

Ophthalmic Examination
- Visual acuity: Right eye 20/20, Left eye 20/20
- Intraocular pressure: Right eye 25 mm Hg, Left eye 28 mm Hg; by Tono-Pen tonometry
- Direct and indirect ophthalmoscopy: small, scattered retinal hemorrhages; optic discs appear normal with no cupping
- Perimetry (visual field) testing: loss of lateral 80-95° peripheral vision in both eyes

Interprofessional Care
The HCP prescribes betaxolol (Betoptic) 1 drop both eyes. The nurse instructs A.G. on the reasons for the drug and how to do punctal occlusion.

Questions

1. What assessment findings are relevant to diagnose acute primary open-angle glaucoma (POAG)?

   For each assessment finding, use an X to indicate if the finding is <u>Expected</u> (occurs in POAG), is <u>Unexpected</u> (doesn't occur in POAG), or is <u>Unrelated</u> (is not related to POAG).

Assessment Finding	Expected	Unexpected	Unrelated
Severe eye pain			
Opacity of the lens			
Loss of peripheral vision			
Blurred vision			
Left eye IOP 28 mm Hg			
Eyelid ptosis			
Light gray optic disc			

2. **Highlight the abnormal findings in the ophthalmic exam.**
   Patient denies pain or pressure
   Visual acuity: Right eye 20/20, Left eye 20/20
   Intraocular pressure by Tono-Pen tonometry: Right eye 25 mm Hg, Left eye 28 mm Hg
   Direct and indirect ophthalmoscopy: small, scattered retinal hemorrhages; optic discs appear normal with no cupping
   Perimetry (visual field) testing: loss of lateral 80-95° peripheral vision in both eyes

3. The nurse is teaching A.G. about how to correctly administer the eyedrops. What statements by the patient indicate the teaching is effective?

   For each statement, use an X to indicate if teaching is <u>Effective</u> (the patient understands how to correctly administer the eyedrop) or is <u>Ineffective</u> (the patient needs more education).

Patient Statement	Effective	Ineffective
"I will wash my hands before administering the eyedrop."		
"I will touch the tip of the eyedrop bottle to my lower eyelid to make sure the medicine goes in."		
"If more than one medication is prescribed, I will wait several minutes between eyedrops."		
"I will use punctal occlusion to prevent systemic absorption."		
"I need to lay down to administer the eyedrops."		
"I should keep my eyes closed for approximately 10 minutes after the eyedrop has been instilled."		

4. What discharge teaching would the nurse provide A.G.? **Select all that apply.**
   _____A. If she experiences increased fatigue, report it to the HCP.
   _____B. The medication may increase her heart rate.
   _____C. Call 911 if she experiences any respiratory distress.
   _____D. Keep all eye appointments to monitor the POAG.
   _____E. It is normal to have loss of vision.
   _____F. Report moderate to severe eye pain to the HCP.
   _____G. You will have to sleep at a 30-degree angle.
   _____H. Report dizziness or lightheadedness to the HCP.
   _____I. You can stop your eyedrops once your glaucoma is cured.

Assessment and Management: Auditory Problems

1. What organ maintains balance and equilibrium?
   a. Cochlea
   b. Organ of Corti
   c. Ossicular chain
   d. Semicircular canals

2. How does the eustachian tube assist the auditory system?
   a. Transmits sound stimuli to the brain
   b. Sets bones of the middle ear in motion
   c. Allows for equalization of pressure in the middle ear
   d. Transmits stimuli from the semicircular canals to the brain

3. Which changes of aging can impair hearing in the older adult? **Select all that apply.**
   a. Atrophy of eardrum (middle ear)
   b. Increased hair growth (external ear)
   c. Increased production and dryness of cerumen (external ear)
   d. Increased vestibular apparatus in semicircular canals (inner ear)
   e. Decreased cochlear efficiency from increased blood supply (inner ear)
   f. Neuron degeneration in auditory nerve and central pathways (inner ear)

4. What report by the patient would cause the nurse to suspect presbycusis?
   a. Ringing in the ears
   b. A sensation of fullness in the ears
   c. Difficulty understanding the meaning of words
   d. A decrease in the ability to hear high-pitched sounds

5. Describe the significance of the following questions when obtaining subjective data during assessment of the auditory system.

Question	Significance
Do you have a history of childhood ear infections or ruptured eardrums?	
Do you use any over-the-counter or prescription medications on a regular basis?	
Have you ever been treated for a head injury?	
Is there a history of hearing loss in your parents?	
Have you been exposed to excessive noise levels in your work or recreational activities?	
Has the amount of social activities you are involved in changed?	

6. What accurately describes an assessment of the ear?
   a. Major landmarks of the tympanic membrane include the umbo, handle of malleus, and cone of light.
   b. The presence of a retracted eardrum on otoscopic examination is indicative of positive pressure in the middle ear.
   c. In chronic otitis media, the nurse would expect to find a lack of landmarks and a bulging eardrum on otoscopic examination.
   d. To straighten the ear canal in an adult before insertion of the otoscope, the nurse grasps the auricle and pulls downward and backward.

7. What findings indicats sensorineural hearing loss? **Select all that apply.**
   a. Positive Rinne test
   b. Negative Rinne test
   c. Weber lateralization to impaired ear
   d. Weber lateralization to good ear
   e. External or middle ear pathology
   f. Inner ear or nerve pathway pathology

8. Results of an audiometry indicate that a patient has a 10-dB hearing loss at 8000 Hz. What is the most appropriate action by the nurse?
   a. Encourage the patient to start learning to lip-read
   b. Speak at a normal speed and volume with the patient
   c. Avoid words in conversation that have many high-pitched consonants
   d. Discuss the advantages and disadvantages of various hearing aids with the patient

9. When does caloric testing indicate disease of the vestibular system of the ear?
   a. Hearing is improved with irrigation of the external ear canal
   b. No nystagmus is elicited with application of water in the external ear
   c. The patient experiences intolerable pain with irrigation of the external ear
   d. With cool water irrigation, nystagmus is produced opposite the side of instillation

10. Identify a specific finding identified by the nurse during assessment of each of the patient's functional health patterns that indicates either a risk factor for hearing problems or the response of the patient to an ear problem.

Functional Health Pattern	Risk Factor for or Response to Hearing Problem
Health perception–health management	
Nutritional-metabolic	
Elimination	
Activity-exercise	
Sleep-rest	
Cognitive-perceptual	
Self-perception–self-concept	
Role-relationship	
Sexuality-reproductive	
Coping–stress tolerance	
Value-belief	

11. What is the role of the nurse in hearing preservation?
    a. Advise patients to keep the ears clear of wax with cotton-tipped applicators.
    b. Monitor patients at risk for drug-induced ototoxicity for tinnitus and vertigo.
    c. Promote the use of ear protection in work and recreational activity with noise levels above 75 dB.
    d. Advocate for MMR (measles, mumps, rubella) immunization in susceptible women as soon as pregnancy is confirmed.

12. Number the following high-noise environments from 1 indicating the highest risk for ear injury to 6 indicating the lowest risk for ear injury.

_____ a. Gas lawn mower for 10 hours

_____ b. Heavy factory noise for 8 hours

_____ c. Using a chainsaw continuously for 2 hours

_____ d. Working in a quiet home office for 8 hours

_____ e. Guiding jet planes to and from airport gates

_____ f. Sitting in front of amplifiers at a rock concert

13. A 74-year-old man has moderate presbycusis and heart disease. He takes 1 aspirin a day, as an antiplatelet agent, and uses quinidine, furosemide (Lasix), and enalapril (Vasotec) for his heart condition. What risk factors does he have for hearing loss and ototoxicity?

14. Which nursing action would be included in the management of the patient with external otitis?
    a. Irrigate the ear canal with body temperature saline several hours after instilling lubricating eardrops.
    b. Insert an ear wick deep into the ear before each application of eardrops to disperse the medication.
    c. Teach the patient to prevent further infections by instilling antibiotic drops into the ear canal before swimming.
    d. Administer eardrops without touching the dropper to the auricle and position the ear upward for 2 minutes afterward.

15. What knowledge is needed by the nurse to best care for a patient with chronic otitis media? **Select all that apply.**
    a. A culture and sensitivity of drainage determines treatment.
    b. It is an infection in the inner ear that may lead to headaches.
    c. Full feeling in the ear, popping, and decreased hearing indicate effusion.
    d. Formation of an acoustic neuroma may destroy the structures of the middle ear or invade the dura of the brain.
    e. The patient who has had a tympanoplasty should protect the ear from infection and sudden pressure changes in the ear.

16. While caring for a patient with otosclerosis, which finding would the nurse expect in the patient's history and physical assessment?
    a. Strong family history of the disease
    b. Symptoms of sensorineural hearing loss
    c. Positive Rinne test and lateralization to the better ear on Weber testing
    d. Immediate and consistent improvement in hearing at the time of surgical treatment

17. The nurse identifies a patient is at risk for injury following a stapedectomy based on what knowledge about this surgery?
    a. Nystagmus may result from perilymph disturbances caused by surgery.
    b. Stimulation of the labyrinth during surgery may cause vertigo and loss of balance.
    c. Blowing the nose or coughing may precipitate dislodgement of the tympanic graft.
    d. Postoperative tinnitus may decrease the patient's awareness of environmental hazards.

18. What makes up the triad of symptoms that occur with inner ear problems? **Select all that apply.**
    a. Vertigo
    b. Nausea
    c. Tinnitus
    d. Sensorineural hearing loss
    e. Inflammation of the ear canal

19. What is an appropriate nursing intervention for the patient during an acute attack of Ménière's disease?
    a. Frequent repositioning
    b. A quiet, darkened room
    c. A television for diversion
    d. Padded side rails on the bed

20. What knowledge guides the nurse when providing care for a patient with an acoustic neuroma?
    a. Widespread metastasis usually occurs before symptoms of the tumor are noticed.
    b. Facial nerve function will be sacrificed during surgical treatment to preserve hearing.
    c. Early diagnosis and treatment of the tumor can preserve hearing and vestibular function.
    d. Treatment is usually delayed until hearing loss is significant because a neuroma is a benign tumor.

21. What characteristics are associated with conductive hearing loss? **Select all that apply.**
    a. Presbycusis
    b. Speaks softly
    c. Related to otitis media
    d. Result of ototoxic drugs
    e. Hears best in noisy environment
    f. May be caused by impacted cerumen

22. What factors may be associated with sensorineural loss? **Select all that apply.**
    a. Head trauma
    b. Otitis media
    c. Exposed to noise trauma
    d. Otosclerosis
    e. Patient's mother has hearing loss
    f. Ménière's disease

23. When teaching a patient to use a hearing aid, where does the nurse encourage the patient to initially use the aid?
    a. Outdoors, where sounds are distinct
    b. At social functions, where simultaneous conversations take place
    c. In a quiet, controlled environment to experiment with tone and volume
    d. In public areas such as malls or stores, where others will not notice its use

CASE STUDY Ménière's Disease

Patient Profile
B.C., a 41-year-old woman, is seen in the urgent care clinic with reports of dizziness and ringing in her right ear.

Subjective Data
- No medical history
- Reports pressure in her right ear
- Reports episodic dizziness lasting several days with nausea
- No history of falls but needs to lie down during dizziness episodes
- Denies using any medication

Objective Data
- BP 125/70 mm Hg
- HR 102 beats/min
- Temperature 100.2°F (37.9°C)

Interprofessional Care
The HCP prescribes meclizine 25 mg once daily and bed rest during episodes of vertigo. The nurse also instructs B.C. to change her diet and address stress management.

Questions
1. Which assessment findings would the nurse expect in this patient with Ménière's disease?

   Use an X to indicate whether the assessment finding is <u>Expected</u> (is an expected finding in this disease), Un<u>expected</u> (is not an expected finding in this disease), or <u>Unrelated</u> (isn't related to this disease).

Assessment Finding	Expected	Unexpected	Unrelated
Symptoms began at 25 years of age			
Sensorineural hearing loss			
Visual floaters			
Ear congestion			
"Drop attacks"			
Conductive hearing loss			
Nystagmus			
Headaches			

2. What lifestyle changes would the nurse recommend to B.C.?

Use an X to indicate whether the lifestyle change is <u>Indicated</u> (appropriate), <u>Contraindicated</u> (is inappropriate or could be harmful), or <u>Non-Essential</u> (makes no difference or is unnecessary).

Lifestyle Change	Indicated	Contraindicated	Non-Essential
"You should restrict eating canned foods."			
"You can drink tea, coffee, or cola."			
"You need to avoid chocolate."			
"You must avoid all alcoholic beverages."			
"Take prescribed antibiotics as directed."			
"Work with audiology to learn vestibular exercises."			
"Take acetaminophen or ibuprofen for headaches."			
"Avoid riding as a passenger in cars."			

3. **Choose the most likely options for the information missing from the statements below by selecting from the lists of options provided.**
   _____1_____ is an over-the-counter medication that is recommended to treat acute _____2_____. When teaching B.C. about this medication, the nurse recommends taking it _____3_____ because this medication can cause _____4_____. If the medication is taken during the day, it is recommended that the patient does not _____5_____ until she knows how the medication will affect her. Other common side effects include _____6_____, _____6_____, and _____6_____.

Options for 1	Options for 2	Options for 3	Options for 4
Meclizine	Nausea	In the morning	Headaches
Diphenhydramine	Headaches	Before meals	Dry mouth
Scopolamine	Vertigo	After meals	Fatigue
Lorazepam	Ear pressure	Before bed	Insomnia
Ondansetron	Anxiety	Midday	Drowsiness
Sumatriptan	Pain	With water	Nausea

Options for 5	Options for 6
Exercise	Dry mouth
Weigh herself	Nausea
Eat	Fatigue
Get out of bed	Headaches
Drive	Vertigo
Watch TV	Nystagmus

4. What would the nurse include when doing discharge teaching with B.C.? **Select all that apply.**
   _____A. Protect yourself from sun exposure.
   _____B. Find a dark quiet room during episodes of vertigo.
   _____C. Avoid heights, like climbing ladders, if experiencing dizziness.
   _____D. Engage in stress relieving activities like yoga.
   _____E. Don't watch TV when experiencing symptoms.
   _____F. It is unsafe to work so you may need to apply for disability.
   _____G. Don't go to movie theaters, even if you are asymptomatic.

5. How would the nurse communicate with B.C. and other patients with hearing impairments?

Use an X to indicate whether the technique is <u>Indicated</u> (is appropriate), <u>Contraindicated</u> (is inappropriate), or <u>Unrelated</u> (makes no difference or is unnecessary).

Communication Technique	Indicated	Contraindicated	Unrelated
Maintain eye contact			
Exaggerate facial expressions			
Speak loudly in impaired ear			
Use simple sentences			
Keep patient in upright position			
Write if necessary			
Have patient avoid sudden position changes			

Assessment: Integumentary System

1. Use the following terms to fill in the labels in the illustration below.

Terms

adipose tissue	connective tissue	hair shaft	stratum germinativum
apocrine sweat gland	hair follicle	stratum corneum	epidermis
arrector pili muscle	sebaceous gland	eccrine sweat gland	nerves
blood vessels	dermis	melanocyte	subcutaneous tissue

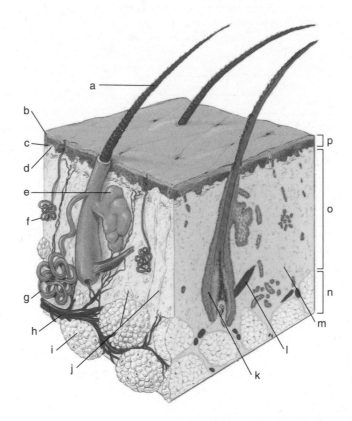

a. _____   g. _____   m. _____

b. _____   h. _____   n. _____

c. _____   i. _____   o. _____

d. _____   j. _____   p. _____

e. _____   k. _____

f. _____   l. _____

2. When the nurse is assessing the skin of an older adult, which factor is likely to contribute to dry skin?
   a. Increased bruising
   b. Excess perspiration
   c. Decreased extracellular fluid
   d. Chronic ultraviolet light exposure

3. When obtaining important health information from a patient during assessment of the skin, what is most important for the nurse to ask about?
   a. A history of freckles as a child.
   b. Patterns of weight gain and loss.
   c. Communicable childhood illnesses.
   d. Skin problems related to the use of medications.

4. Identify 1 specific finding identified by the nurse during assessment for each of the patient's functional health patterns that would indicate a risk factor for skin problems or a patient response to a skin problem.

Functional Health Pattern	Risk Factor for or Response to Skin Problem
Health perception–health management	
Nutritional-metabolic	
Elimination	
Activity-exercise	
Sleep-rest	
Cognitive-perceptual	
Self-perception–self-concept	
Role-relationship	
Sexuality-reproductive	
Coping–stress tolerance	
Value-belief	

5. When performing a physical assessment of the skin, what would the nurse do first?
   a. Palpate the temperature of the skin with the fingertips.
   b. Assess the degree of turgor by pinching the skin on the forearm.
   c. Inspect specific lesions before performing a general examination of the skin.
   d. Ask the patient to undress completely so that all areas of the skin can be inspected.

6. Which statements are true about skin and skin care? **Select all that apply.**
   a. One of the detrimental effects of obesity on the skin is increased sweating.
   b. Ultraviolet (UV) exposure from tanning beds is safer and causes less damage than UV from the sun.
   c. The nutrient that is critical in maintaining and repairing the structure of epithelial cells is vitamin C.
   d. Exposure to UV rays is believed to be the most important factor in the development of skin cancer.
   e. The photosensitivity caused by various drugs can be blocked using topical hydrocortisone.
   f. Photosensitivity results when certain chemicals in body cells and tissues absorb light from the sun and release energy that harms the tissues and cells.

7. The nurse sees that redness remains after palpation of a discolored lesion on the patient's leg. Which problem does this describe?
   a. Varicosities
   b. Intradermal bleeding
   c. Dilated blood vessels
   d. Erythematous lesions

8. A woman calls the health clinic and describes a rash that she has over the abdomen and chest. She tells the nurse that the rashes are raised, fluid-filled, like small blisters that are distinct.
   a. Identify the type of primary skin lesion described by this patient.
   b. What is the distribution terminology for these lesions?
   c. What other information does the nurse have to document the critical components of these lesions?

9. What is the main difference between an excoriation and an ulcer?
   a. Ulcers do not penetrate below the epidermal junction.
   b. Excoriations involve only thinning of the epidermis and dermis.
   c. Excoriations will form crusts or scabs, while ulcers remain open.
   d. An excoriation heals without scarring because the dermis is not involved.

10. A patient has a plaque lesion on the dorsal forearm. Which type of biopsy is most likely to be used for diagnosis of the lesion?
    a. Punch biopsy
    b. Shave biopsy
    c. Incisional biopsy
    d. Excisional biopsy

11. What is the most common diagnostic test used to determine a causative agent of skin infections?
    a. Culture
    b. Tzanck test
    c. Immunofluorescent studies
    d. Potassium hydroxide (KOH) slides

12. The patient asks the nurse what telangiectasia looks like. Which is the best description for the nurse to give the patient?
    a. A circumscribed, flat discoloration
    b. Small, superficial, dilated blood vessels
    c. Benign tumor of blood or lymph vessels
    d. Tiny purple spots resulting from tiny hemorrhages

13. An active athletic person calls the clinic and describes her feet as having a linear break-throughs in the skin. What is the best documentation of this problem?
    a. Scales
    b. Fissure
    c. Pustule
    d. Comedo

14. A home health nurse is visiting an older obese woman who has recently had hip surgery. She tells the patient's caregiver that the patient has intertrigo. How would the nurse explain this to the caregiver?
    a. It is thickening of the skin.
    b. It is dermatitis in the folds of her skin.
    c. It is a loss of color in diffuse areas of her skin.
    d. It is a firm plaque caused by fluid in the dermis.

15. When assessing a black patient, the nurse notes ashen color of the nail beds. What would the nurse do next?
    a. Palpate for rashes on the legs.
    b. Assess for jaundice in the sclera of the eye.
    c. Assess the mucous membranes for cyanosis.
    d. Assess for pallor of the skin on the buttocks.

16. The patient is visiting the free clinic to refill her medications. During the generalized assessment, the nurse documents alopecia; an increased heart rate; warm, moist, flushed skin; and thin nails. The patient also says she is anxious and has lost weight lately. Which systemic problem will the nurse suspect and communicate to the health care provider?
    a. Hyperthyroidism
    b. Systemic lupus erythematosus
    c. Vitamin B_1 (thiamine) deficiency
    d. Human immunodeficiency virus (HIV) infection

Integumentary Problems

1. Which statements describe malignant melanoma? **Select all that apply.**
   a. Related to chemical exposure
   b. Neoplastic growth of melanocytes
   c. Skin cancer with highest mortality rate
   d. Irregular color and asymmetric shape
   e. Frequently occurs on previously damaged skin

2. What is the most common type of skin cancer which has pearly borders?
   a. Actinic keratosis
   b. Basal cell carcinoma
   c. Malignant melanoma
   d. Squamous cell carcinoma

3. What skin condition has hyperkeratotic scaly lesions, is a precursor of squamous cell carcinoma, and may be treated with topical fluorouracil (5-FU)?
   a. Actinic keratosis
   b. Basal cell carcinoma
   c. Malignant melanoma
   d. Squamous cell carcinoma

4. What characteristic is commonly seen with dysplastic nevus syndrome?
   a. Associated with sun exposure
   b. Precursor of squamous cell carcinoma
   c. Slow-growing tumor with rare metastasis
   d. Lesion has irregular color and asymmetric shape

5. Describe what is indicated by the *ABCDEs* of malignant melanoma.
   A.
   B.
   C.
   D.
   E.

6. A 66-year-old patient is scheduled to have a basal cell carcinoma on the cheek excised in the health care providers office. What discharge teaching is most important for the nurse to include?
   a. You will probably need radiation as well after the excision.
   b. It is good you are having it removed to avoid massive tissue destruction.
   c. It is too bad you can't have this done by laser because it leaves less scarring.
   d. Using the prescribed ointment and an adhesive bandage will promote the healing with less scarring.

7. When considering the initial treatment for newly diagnosed malignant melanoma, what would the nurse expect? **Select all that apply.**
   a. Shave biopsy
   b. Mohs surgery
   c. Surgical excision
   d. Localized radiation
   e. 5-FU
   f. Topical nitrogen mustard

8. A 78-year-old woman who has had chronic respiratory disease for 30 years weighs 212 lb (96.4 kg) and is 5 ft 1 in (152.5 cm) tall. She has recently completed corticosteroid and antibiotic treatment for an exacerbation of her respiratory disease. Identify 4 specific predisposing factors for bacterial skin infection in this patient.
   a.
   b.
   c.
   d.

9. What is the name for papillomavirus infection seen on the skin?
   a. Furuncle
   b. Carbuncle
   c. Erysipelas
   d. Plantar wart

10. Which description characterizes seborrheic keratosis?
    a. White, patchy yeast infection
    b. Warty, irregular papules or plaques
    c. Excessive turnover of epithelial cells
    d. Deep inflammation of subcutaneous tissue

11. Which skin condition occurs as an allergic reaction to mite eggs?
    a. Scabies
    b. Impetigo
    c. Folliculitis
    d. Pediculosis

12. Which skin conditions are more common in immunosuppressed patients? **Select all that apply.**
    a. Acne
    b. Lentigo
    c. Candidiasis
    d. Herpes zoster
    e. Herpes simplex 1
    f. Kaposi sarcoma

13. What instructions would the nurse include when teaching a patient with hives?
    a. Apply topical benzene hexachloride.
    b. Avoid contact with the causative agent.
    c. Gradually expose the area to increasing amounts of sunlight.
    d. Use over-the-counter antihistamines routinely to prevent the condition.

14. A nurse caring for a disheveled patient with poor hygiene observes that the patient has small red lesions flush with the skin on the head and body. The patient reports severe itching at the sites. What would the nurse look for when assessing the patient?
    a. Nits on the shafts of head hair
    b. The presence of ticks attached to the scalp
    c. A history of sexually transmitted infections
    d. The presence of burrows in the interdigital webs

15. A patient with a contact dermatitis is treated with calamine lotion. What is the reason for using this base for a topical preparation?
    a. A suspension of oil and water to lubricate and prevent drying
    b. An emulsion of oil and water used for lubrication and protection
    c. Insoluble powders suspended in water that leave a residual powder on the skin
    d. A mixture of a powder and ointment that causes drying when moisture is absorbed

16. A patient with psoriasis is being treated with psoralen plus ultraviolet A light (PUVA) phototherapy. The nurse would teach the patient to wear protective eyewear that blocks all UV rays for how long?
    a. Continuously for 6 hours after taking the medication
    b. Until the pupils are able to constrict on exposure to light
    c. For 12 hours following treatment to prevent retinal damage
    d. For 24 hours following treatment when outdoors or when indoors near a bright window

17. Identify 1 instruction the nurse would provide to a patient receiving the following medications for skin problems.

Medication	Nursing Instruction
Topical antibiotics	
Topical corticosteroids	
Systemic antihistamines	
Topical fluorouracil	
Topical immunomodulators	

18. Match the invasive interventions with conditions that they are used to treat *(interventions may be used for more than 1 condition)*.

    Interventions
    _____ a. Electrodessication or electrocoagulation
    _____ b. Excision
    _____ c. Mohs surgery
    _____ d. Curettage
    _____ e. Cryosurgery

    Conditions
    1. Malignant melanoma
    2. Common and genital warts
    3. Basal and squamous cell carcinomas
    4. Telangiectasia
    5. Lesions involving the dermis
    6. Seborrheic keratoses

19. What are the most appropriate compresses to use to promote comfort for a patient with inflamed, pruritic dermatitis?
    a. Cool tap water compresses
    b. Cool acetic acid compresses
    c. Warm sterile saline compresses
    d. Warm potassium permanganate compresses

20. What is an appropriate intervention to promote debridement and removal of scales and crusts of skin lesions?
    a. Warm oatmeal baths
    b. Warm saline compresses
    c. Cool sodium bicarbonate baths
    d. Cool magnesium sulfate compresses

21. Identify the reason for using the following interventions to control pruritus.

Intervention	Rationale
Cool environment	
Topical menthol, camphor, or phenol	
Soaks and baths	

22. A female patient with chronic skin lesions of the face and arms tells the nurse that she cannot stand to look at herself in the mirror anymore because of her appearance. Based on this information, which clinical problem would the nurse prioritize?
    a. Anxiety as a result of personal appearance
    b. Disturbed body image from her perception of unsightly lesions
    c. Lack of knowledge about how to use cover-up makeup techniques
    d. Social isolation and decreased activities as a result of poor self-image

23. To prevent lichenification related to chronic skin problems, what does the nurse encourage the patient to do?
    a. Use measures to control itching.
    b. Wear sterile gloves when touching the lesions.
    c. Use careful hand washing and safe disposal of soiled dressings.
    d. Use topical antibiotics with wet-to-dry dressings over the lesions.

24. What is the most common reason patients request elective cosmetic surgery?
    a. Improve self-image
    b. Remove deep acne scars
    c. Lighten the skin in pigmentation problems
    d. Prevent skin changes associated with aging

25. Which skin condition would be treated with laser surgery?
    a. Preauricular lesion
    b. Redundant soft tissue conditions
    c. Obesity with subcutaneous fat accumulation
    d. Fine wrinkle reduction or facial lesion removal

26. What type of skin graft is used to transfer skin and subcutaneous tissue to large areas of deep tissue destruction?
    a. Skin flap
    b. Free graft
    c. Soft tissue extension
    d. Free graft with vascular anastomoses

27. A patient who is receiving chemotherapy calls the HCP's office and reports itching in her groin and under her breasts. What would the nurse ask about before making an appointment for the patient to see the HCP?
    a. Her height and weight
    b. What the areas look like
    c. If chemotherapy was completed
    d. What medications she is taking

28. A patient with diabetes and chronic obstructive pulmonary disease has been treated with high-dose corticosteroids for the past several years. Which skin manifestations could be related to these comorbidities? **Select all that apply.**
    a. Acne
    b. Increased sweating
    c. Dry, coarse, brittle hair
    d. Impaired wound healing
    e. Erythematous plaques of the shins
    f. Decreased subcutaneous fat over extremities

CASE STUDY   Cellulitis

Patient Profile
W.B., a 72-year-old man, cut his left lower arm with a kitchen knife. At the time of the injury, he did not seek medical attention even though it was fairly deep. On the 3rd day following the injury, he became concerned about the condition of the wound and the way he was feeling.

(BONNINSTUDIO/
iStock/Thinkstock)

Subjective Data
• Reports a fever and has had a general feeling of malaise
• Reports pain in the area of the cut and the entire left lower arm

Objective Data
• 4-cm area around cut is hot, erythematous, and edematous with redness extending both up and down his left arm
• Temp: 100.8°F (38.2°C)

Questions

1. **Choose the most likely options for the information missing from the statements below by selecting from the options provided.**

The nurse expects the HCP to diagnose W.B. with _____**1**_____. The 2 most common causative agents are _____**2**_____ and_____**2**_____. The main tissues affected by this type of infection are _____**3**_____. If left untreated, this infection can progress to _____**4**_____ and _____**4**_____.

Options for 1	Options for 2	Options for 3	Options for 4
Erysipelas	Human papillomavirus	Dermis	Gangrene
Folliculitis	*Candida albicans*	Epidermis	Melanoma
Cellulitis	*Enterococcus faecalis*	Adipose	Basal cell carcinoma
Furuncle	Streptococci	Sebaceous glands	Septicemia
Actinic keratosis	Varicella-zoster virus	Subcutaneous	Sézary syndrome
Shingles	*Staphylococcus aureus*	Connective	Dysplastic Nevi

2. What would the nurse do to treat W.B.'s cut?

Use an X to indicate whether the nursing action is <u>Indicated</u> (necessary), <u>Contraindicated</u> (could be harmful), or <u>Non-Essential</u> (makes no difference or is unnecessary).

Nursing Action	Indicated	Contraindicated	Non-Essential
Measure the size and depth of the cut			
Cleanse the wound with alcohol			
Use sterile saline to flush the wound			
Apply a clean dressing to the wound			
Arrange for casting of the arm			
Use an arm sling to elevate the extremity			
Pack the cut with xeroform gauze			

3. What instructions would the nurse include when doing discharge teaching with W.B. about caring for his wound and infection? **Select all that apply.**

_____A. The extremity should be immobilized and not be used to prevent the spread of the infection.

_____B. Take the antibiotics until the swelling and redness disappear.

_____C. Apply ice packs for pain.

_____D. Apply warm moist compresses several times a day until the redness and swelling disappear.

_____E. Elevate the extremity above the level of your heart as often as possible to reduce swelling.

_____F. Apply fluorouracil ointment to the cut 3 times per day.

_____G. Protect the cut from sun exposure.

_____H. Report temperatures greater than 101° (38.3°C) to your HCP.

_____I. Report any foul odor from the wound to your HCP.

4. What assessment findings would indicate to the nurse that the infection is progressing and complications are developing? **Indicate which assessment finding in the far-left column corresponds to the potential complications associated with this type of infection. Note that some assessment findings may not be used.**

Assessment Finding	Potential Complication from Infection	Appropriate Assessment Finding for Complication
Tachycardia	Sepsis	
Absent radial pulse	Gangrene	
Decreased blood pressure		
Leukocytosis		
Anemia		
Fingers are cold and numb		
Confusion		
Arm is pale		
Hemorrhage		

1. Which type of burn injury would cause myoglobinuria, long bone fractures, dysrhythmias, and/or cardiac arrest?
   a. Thermal
   b. Electrical
   c. Chemical
   d. Smoke and inhalation

2. Which characteristics accurately describe chemical burns? **Select all that apply.**
   a. Metabolic asphyxiation may occur.
   b. Metabolic acidosis occurs immediately following the burn.
   c. The visible skin injury does not often represent the full extent of tissue damage.
   d. Lavaging with large amounts of water is important to stop the burning process with these injuries.
   e. Alkaline substances that cause these burns continue to cause tissue damage even after being neutralized.

3. What would the nurse expect to find when assessing a patient's full-thickness burn injury during the emergent phase?
   a. Leathery, dry, hard skin
   b. Red, fluid-filled vesicles
   c. Massive edema at the injury site
   d. Serous exudate on a shiny, dark brown wound

4. A patient has the following mixed deep partial-thickness and full-thickness burn injuries: face, anterior neck, right anterior trunk, and anterior surfaces of the right arm and lower leg.
   a. According to the Lund-Browder chart, what is the extent of the patient's burns?
      _____% total body surface area (TBSA)
   b. According to the rule of nines chart, what is the extent of the patient's burns?
      _____% TBSA
   c. Is it possible to determine the actual extent and depth of burn injury during the emergent phase of the burn? Why or why not?

5. Beginning with number 1 for the first action, number the following actions in the order they would be done in the emergency management for any burn type.
   _____ a. Establish and maintain an airway.
   _____ b. Assess for other associated injuries.
   _____ c. Establish an IV line with a large-gauge needle.
   _____ d. Remove the patient from the burn source and stop the burning process.

6. The patient was admitted to the burn center with a full-thickness burn 42 hours after the thermal burn occurred. Which phase of burn management would the nurse implement for this patient's care?
   a. Acute
   b. Emergent
   c. Postacute
   d. Rehabilitative

7. What laboratory results would most likely occur during the early emergent phase of burn injury?
   a. ↑ Hematocrit (Hct), ↓ serum albumin, ↓ serum Na, ↑ serum K.
   b. ↓ Hct, ↓ serum albumin, ↓ serum Na, ↓ serum K.
   c. ↓ Hct, ↑ serum albumin, ↑ serum Na, ↑ serum K.
   d. ↑ Hct, ↑ serum albumin, ↓ serum Na, ↓ serum K.

8. What is the initial cause of hypovolemia during the emergent phase of burn injury?
   a. Increased capillary permeability
   b. Loss of sodium to the interstitium
   c. Decreased vascular oncotic pressure
   d. Fluid loss from denuded skin surfaces

9. How is the immune system altered in a burn injury?
   a. Bone marrow stimulation
   b. Increase in immunoglobulin levels
   c. Impaired function of white blood cells (WBCs)
   d. Overwhelmed by microorganisms entering denuded tissue

10. What clinical manifestation would the nurse expect to find during the emergent phase in a patient with a full-thickness burn over the lower half of the body?
    a. Fever
    b. Shivering
    c. Severe pain
    d. Unconsciousness

11. A patient has a 20% TBSA deep partial-thickness and full-thickness burn to the right anterior chest and entire right arm. What is most important for the nurse to assess in this patient?
    a. Presence of pain
    b. Swelling of the arm
    c. Formation of eschar
    d. Presence of pulses in the arms

12. Which burn patient should have orotracheal or endotracheal intubation?
    a. Carbon monoxide poisoning
    b. Electrical burns causing dysrhythmias
    c. Thermal burn injuries to the face, neck, or airway
    d. Respiratory distress from eschar formation around the chest

13. A patient is admitted to the emergency department at 10:15 PM following a flame burn at 9:30 PM. The patient has 40% TBSA deep partial-thickness and full-thickness burns and weighs 132 lb.
    a. According to the Parkland (Baxter) formula, the type of fluid prescribed for the patient would be
       _____, and the total amount to be given during the first 24 hours would be _____ mL.
    b. The schedule for the fluid administration would be _____ mL between _____ and _____ (time),
       _____ mL between _____ and _____, and _____ mL between _____ and _____.
    c. Colloidal solutions are given in the second 24 hours. Based on the patient's body weight, what amount of these solutions will be given during this time?
    d. The adequacy of the patient's fluid replacement is determined by_____ and
       _____.

14. A patient's deep partial-thickness facial burns are treated with the open method. What would the nurse do when caring for the patient?
    a. Ensure that sterile water is used in the debridement tank.
    b. Wear a cap, mask, gown, and gloves during patient contact.
    c. Use sterile gloves to remove the dressings and wash the wounds.
    d. Apply topical antimicrobial ointment with clean gloves to prevent wound trauma.

15. A patient with deep partial-thickness burns over 45% of his trunk and legs, is going for debridement in the shower trolley 48 hours postburn. What is the drug of choice to control the patient's pain during this activity?
    a. IV morphine
    b. Midazolam
    c. IM meperidine
    d. Long-acting oral morphine

16. The nurse assesses that bowel sounds are absent and abdominal distention is present in a patient 12 hours postburn. The nurse notifies the health care provider and anticipates doing what action next?
    a. Withhold all oral intake except water.
    b. Insert a nasogastric tube for decompression.
    c. Administer a H₂-histamine blocker, such as ranitidine (Zantac).
    d. Give nutrition supplements through a feeding tube placed in the duodenum.

17. How would the nurse position the patient with ear, face, and neck burns?
    a. Prone
    b. On the side
    c. Without pillows
    d. With extra padding around the head

18. What factors increase nutrition needs of the patient during the emergent and acute phases of burn injury? **Select all that apply.**
    a. Electrolyte imbalance
    b. Core temperature elevation
    c. Calories and protein used for tissue repair
    d. Hypometabolic state secondary to decreased gastrointestinal function
    e. Massive catabolism characterized by protein breakdown and increased gluconeogenesis

19. At the end of the emergent phase and the initial acute phase of burn injury, a patient has a serum sodium level of 152 mEq/L (152 mmol/L) and a serum potassium level of 2.8 mEq/L (2.8 mmol/L). What could have caused these imbalances?
    a. Free oral water intake
    b. Prolonged hydrotherapy
    c. Mobilization of fluid and electrolytes in the acute phase
    d. Excessive fluid replacement with dextrose in water without potassium supplementation

20. A burn patient has a clinical problem of impaired mobility due to limited range of motion (ROM) resulting from pain. What is the best nursing intervention for this patient?
    a. Have the patient perform ROM exercises when pain is not present.
    b. Provide analgesic medications before physical activity and exercise.
    c. Teach the patient the importance of exercise to prevent contractures.
    d. Arrange for the physical therapist to encourage exercise during hydrotherapy.

21. What change causes the nurse to initially suspect the possibility of sepsis in a burn patient?
    a. Vital signs
    b. Urinary output
    c. Gastrointestinal function
    d. Burn wound appearance

22. Identify 1 major complication of burns that is believed to be stress related that may occur in each of these systems during the acute burn phase.

Body System	Complication
Neurologic	
Gastrointestinal	
Endocrine	

23. Complete the following sentences.
    a. A permanent skin graft that may be available for the patient with large body surface area burns who has limited skin for donor harvesting is _____.
    b. Early excision and grafting of burn wounds involve excising _____ down to clean viable tissue and applying a(n) _____ whenever possible.
    c. Blebs can be removed from facial skin grafts by _____.

24. The burn patient has developed an increasing dread of painful dressing changes. What would be the most appropriate treatment to ask the health care provider to prescribe?
    a. Midazolam to be used with morphine before dressing changes
    b. Buprenorphine to be given with morphine before dressing changes
    c. Morphine in a dosage range so that more may be given before dressing changes
    d. Patient-controlled analgesia so that the patient may have control of analgesic administration

25. During the rehabilitation phase of a burn injury, what can control the contour of the scarring?
    a. Pressure garments
    b. Avoidance of sunlight
    c. Splinting joints in extension
    d. Application of emollient lotions

26. A 24-year-old female patient does not want the wound cleansing and dressing change to take place. She asks, "What difference will it make anyway?" What would the nurse encourage the patient to do?
    a. Have the wound cleaned and the dressing changed.
    b. Have a snack before having the treatments completed.
    c. Talk about what is troubling her with the nurse and/or her family.
    d. Call the chaplain to come and talk to her and convince her to have the care.

27. The nurse has received the change-of-shift report on a group of patients. Beginning with number 1 as the top priority, indicate the order in which the nurse would see the patients.
    _____ a. A 40-year-old female who is returning from the PACU after surgical debridement of her back and legs
    _____ b. A 76-year-old male with partial-thickness burns of his arms and abdomen who is reporting severe pain
    _____ c. A 62-year-old female who was just admitted following partial-thickness burns to her anterior chest, face, and neck
    _____ d. An 18-year-old male with full-thickness burns of his lower extremities who is refusing to go for his scheduled dressing change

CASE STUDY Electrical Burn Patient

(vystek-photographie/ iStock/Thinkstock)

Patient Profile
D.K. is a 30-year-old woman who was holding an umbrella in a thunderstorm and is now being admitted to the ED after being struck by lightning. She sustained partial- and full-thickness burns to anterior and posterior hands and forearms bilaterally, in addition to the anterior chest. She was briefly unconscious and only remembers waking up with people standing around her.

Subjective Data
- Reports tightness and pain in her hands and forearms
- Reports feeling like her heart is racing
- Reports chest pressure

Objective Data
- Upon admission, alert and oriented x3, GCS 15
- BP: 98/45 mm Hg, HR 110 beats/min and irregular, RR 28 breaths/min, Temperature 99.5°F (37.5°C), SpO$_2$ 98% on 10 L/min nonrebreather mask

Questions
1. **Complete the following sentences by choosing the most likely option for the missing information from the lists of options provided.**
   Using the Rule of Nines, the nurse calculates the TBSA is approximately _____**1**_____. Using the Lund-Browder chart, the nurse calculates the TBSA to be _____**2**_____. The patient weighs 165 lbs. The nurse plans to administer lactated Ringer's between _____**3**_____ mL over 24 hours. The nurse will administer _____**4**_____ mL in the first 8 hours, ____**5**____ mL during the next 8 hours and repeat this amount during the last 8 hours. The nurse knows that the hourly urine output for this patient should be between ____**6**____ mL to ____**7**___ mL.

Options for 1	Options for 2	Options for 3	Options 4
4.5%	3%	3750-4050	1125
9%	6%	900-1350	1068
13.5%	9%	1800-2700	1950
18%	12%	450-675	280

Options for 1	Options for 2	Options for 3	Options 4
27%	18%	2025-2250	2550
36%	25%	4800-5400	562

Options for 5	Options for 6	Options for 7
562	30	50
975	38	60
1275	45	75
534	50	80
281	75	100
140	100	125

2. What interventions would the nurse implement to treat D.K.'s burn injury during the emergent phase of care? **Use an X to indicate whether the nursing action is <u>Indicated</u> (appropriate or necessary), <u>Contraindicated</u> (<u>could be harmful</u>), or <u>Non-Essential</u> (<u>makes no difference or is unnecessary</u>).**

Nursing Action	Indicated	Contraindicated	Non-Essential
Continuous cardiac monitoring			
Collect urine for a urinalysis			
Place an oropharyngeal airway			
Collect blood for coagulation studies			
Administer lactated Ringer's IV bolus			
Perform 12-lead ECG			
Insert an indwelling urinary catheter			
Perform active ROM exercises			

3. D.K. is at increased risk of developing complications from the burn injuries. **Indicate which assessment finding listed in the far-left column is applicable to each potential complication from burn injuries.**

Assessment Finding	Potential Complication from Burn Injury	Appropriate Assessment Finding for Complication
Myoglobinuria	Acute kidney injury (AKI)	
Elevated troponin levels	Compartment syndrome	
Absent right radial pulse	Myocardial injury	
ST segment elevation		
Pale and cool right hand		
Urine output 25 mL/hr		
Frequent premature ventricular contractions (PVCs)		
Creatinine 2.8 mg/dL		

4. D.K. has transitioned to the acute phase of burn care. **Use an X to indicate whether the assessment finding indicates whether treatment has been <u>Effective</u> (meets expected outcomes), <u>Ineffective</u> (<u>did not meet outcomes</u>), or <u>Unrelated</u> (<u>is not related to expected outcomes</u>).**

Assessment Finding	Effective	Ineffective	Unrelated
Headache 4 out of 10			
MAP 66 mm Hg			
Urine output 40 mL/hr			
1+ radial pulses			
HR 82 beats/min			
5/5 dorsi plantar flexion			
Irregular heart rhythm			
Temperature 38.3°C			

5. What information will the nurse include when doing discharge teaching with D.K.? **Select all that apply.**

_____A. You will need to work with physical therapy.

_____B. You may need skin grafting surgery in the future.

_____C. You will have to continue taking anticoagulants.

_____D. Eat a low protein diet.

_____E. You may want to join a support group for burn victims.

_____F. Take your antibiotics until they are gone.

_____G. Report any pain to your HCP.

_____H. Report a temperature greater than 100°F (37.8°C) to your HCP.

_____I. A home health nurse will come to your home to help change your dressings.

Assessment: Respiratory System

1. Map the pathway of air after it is inspired through the nose. Number 1 is the first organ after the environment, and number 13 is the last organ before the alveoli.

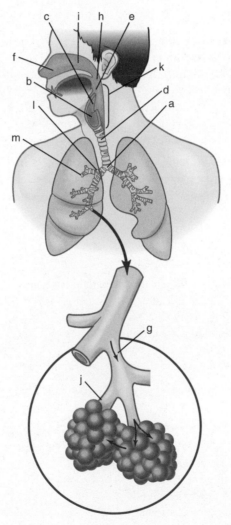

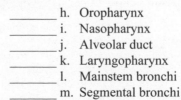

_____ a. Carina

_____ b. Larynx

_____ c. Glottis

_____ d. Trachea

_____ e. Epiglottis

_____ f. Nasal cavity

_____ g. Bronchioles

_____ h. Oropharynx

_____ i. Nasopharynx

_____ j. Alveolar duct

_____ k. Laryngopharynx

_____ l. Mainstem bronchi

_____ m. Segmental bronchi

2. A 92-year-old female patient is being admitted to the emergency department with severe shortness of breath. Being aware of the patient's condition, what approach would the nurse use to assess the patient's lungs? **Select all that apply.**
   a. Apex to base
   b. Base to apex
   c. Lateral sequence
   d. Anterior then posterior
   e. Posterior then anterior

3. What keeps alveoli from collapsing?
   a. Carina
   b. Surfactant
   c. Empyema
   d. Thoracic cage

4. What accurately describes the alveolar sacs?
   a. Line the lung pleura
   b. Warm and moisturize inhaled air
   c. Terminal structures of the respiratory tract
   d. Contain dead air that is not available for gas exchange

5. What covers the larynx during swallowing?
   a. Trachea
   b. Epiglottis
   c. Turbinates
   d. Parietal pleura

6. A 75-year-old patient who is breathing room air has the following arterial blood gas (ABG) results: pH 7.40, partial pressure of oxygen in arterial blood (PaO_2) 74 mm Hg, arterial oxygen saturation (SaO_2) 92%, partial pressure of carbon dioxide in arterial blood ($PaCO_2$) 40 mm Hg. What is the most appropriate action by the nurse?
   a. Document the results in the patient's record.
   b. Repeat the ABGs within an hour to validate the findings.
   c. Encourage deep breathing and coughing to open the alveoli.
   d. Initiate pulse oximetry for continuous monitoring of the patient's oxygen status.

7. A patient's ABG results include a PaO_2 of 88 mm Hg and a $PaCO_2$ of 38 mm Hg, and mixed venous blood gas results include a partial pressure of oxygen in venous blood (PvO_2) of 40 mm Hg and partial pressure of carbon dioxide in venous blood ($PvCO_2$) of 46 mm Hg. What do these findings indicate?
   a. Impaired cardiac output
   b. Unstable hemodynamics
   c. Inadequate delivery of oxygen to the tissues
   d. Normal capillary oxygen–carbon dioxide exchange

8. During peripheral pulse oximetry (SpO_2) monitoring, the patient has a decrease from 95% to 85% over several hours. What is the first action the nurse should take?
   a. Order stat ABGs to confirm the SpO_2 with a SaO_2.
   b. Start O_2 administration by nasal cannula at 2 L/min.
   c. Check the position of the probe on the finger or earlobe.
   d. Notify the health care provider regarding the change from baseline PaO_2.

9. Pulse oximetry may not be a reliable indicator of oxygen saturation in which patient?
   a. Patient with a fever
   b. Patient who is anesthetized
   c. Patient in hypovolemic shock
   d. Patient receiving O_2 therapy

10. A 73-year-old patient has a SpO_2 of 70%. What assessment would the nurse consider before making a judgment about the adequacy of the patient's oxygenation?
    a. What the oxygenation status is with a stress test
    b. Trend and rate of development of the hyperkalemia
    c. Comparison of patient's SpO_2 values with normal values
    d. Comparison of patient's current vital signs with normal vital signs

11. Which values indicate a need for the use of continuous oxygen therapy?
    a. SpO_2 of 92%; PaO_2 of 65 mm Hg
    b. SpO_2 of 95%; PaO_2 of 70 mm Hg
    c. SpO_2 of 90%; PaO_2 of 60 mm Hg
    d. SpO_2 of 88%; PaO_2 of 55 mm Hg

12. Why does a patient's respiratory rate increase when there is an excess of CO_2 in the blood?
    a. CO_2 displaces oxygen on hemoglobin, leading to a decreased PaO_2.
    b. CO_2 causes an increase in the amount of hydrogen ions available in the body.
    c. CO_2 combines with water to form carbonic acid, which lowers the pH of cerebrospinal fluid.
    d. CO_2 directly stimulates chemoreceptors in the medulla to increase respiratory rate and volume.

13. Which respiratory defense mechanism is most impaired by smoking?
    a. Cough reflex
    b. Filtration of air
    c. Mucociliary clearance
    d. Reflex bronchoconstriction

14. Which age-related changes in the respiratory system cause decreased secretion clearance? **Select all that apply.**
    a. Decreased force of cough
    b. Decreased functional cilia
    c. Decreased chest wall compliance
    d. Small airway closure earlier in expiration
    e. Decreased functional immunoglobulin A (IgA)

15. Identify 1 specific finding identified by the nurse during assessment of each of the patient's functional health patterns that indicates a risk factor for respiratory problems or a patient response to an actual respiratory problem.

Functional Health Pattern	Risk Factor for or Response to Respiratory Problem
Health perception–health management	
Nutritional-metabolic	
Elimination	
Activity-exercise	
Sleep-rest	
Cognitive-perceptual	
Self-perception–self-concept	
Role-relationship	
Sexuality-reproductive	
Coping–stress tolerance	
Value-belief	

16. The abnormal assessment findings of dullness and hyperresonance are found with which assessment technique?
    a. Inspection
    b. Palpation
    c. Percussion
    d. Auscultation

17. Palpation is the assessment technique used to find which abnormal assessment findings? Select all that apply.
    a. Stridor
    b. Finger clubbing
    c. Tracheal deviation
    d. Limited chest expansion
    e. Increased tactile fremitus
    f. Use of accessory muscles

18. How does the nurse assess the patient's chest expansion?
    a. Put the palms of the hands against the chest wall.
    b. Put the index fingers on either side of the trachea.
    c. Place the thumbs at the midline of the lower chest.
    d. Place 1 hand on the lower anterior chest and 1 hand on the upper abdomen.

19. When does the nurse record the presence of an increased anteroposterior (AP) diameter of the chest?
    a. There is a prominent protrusion of the sternum.
    b. The width of the chest is equal to the depth of the chest.
    c. There is equal but diminished movement of the 2 sides of the chest.
    d. The patient cannot fully expand the lungs because of kyphosis of the spine.

20. The patient is admitted with pneumonia and the nurse hears a grating sound when assessing the patient. How would the nurse document this sound?
    a. Stridor
    b. Bronchophony
    c. Course crackles
    d. Pleural friction rub

21. Match the descriptions or possible causes with the appropriate abnormal assessment findings.

    Assessment Finding   **Description or Possible Cause**
    _____ a. Finger clubbing   1. Lung consolidation with fluid or exudate
    _____ b. Stridor   2. Air trapping
    _____ c. Wheezes   3. Atelectasis
    _____ d. Pleural friction rub   4. Interstitial edema
    _____ e. Increased tactile fremitus   5. Bronchoconstriction
    _____ f. Hyperresonance   6. Partial obstruction of trachea or larynx
    _____ g. Fine crackles   7. Chronic hypoxemia
    _____ h. Absent breath sounds   8. Pleurisy

22. A nurse has been caring for a patient with tuberculosis (TB) and has a TB skin test performed. When is the nurse considered infected?
    a. There is no redness or induration at the injection site.
    b. There is an induration of only 5 mm at the injection site.
    c. A negative skin test is followed by a negative chest x-ray.
    d. Testing causes a 10-mm red, indurated area at the injection site.

23. What is a primary nursing responsibility after obtaining a blood specimen for ABGs?
    a. Add heparin to the blood specimen.
    b. Apply pressure to the puncture site for 2 full minutes.
    c. Take the specimen immediately to the laboratory in an iced container.
    d. Avoid any changes in oxygen intervention for 15 minutes following the procedure.

24. What should the nurse do when preparing a patient for a pulmonary angiogram?
    a. Assess the patient for iodine allergy.
    b. Implement NPO orders for 6 to 12 hours before the test.
    c. Explain the test before the patient signs the informed consent form.
    d. Inform the patient that radiation isolation for 24 hours after the test is necessary.

25. The nurse is preparing the patient for and will assist the health care provider with a thoracentesis in the patient's room. Number the following actions in the order the nurse should complete them. Use 1 for the first action and 7 for the last action.
    _____ a. Verify breath sounds in all fields.
    _____ b. Obtain the supplies that will be used.
    _____ c. Send labeled specimen containers to the laboratory.
    _____ d. Direct the family members to the waiting room.
    _____ e. Observe for signs of hypoxia during the procedure.
    _____ f. Instruct the patient not to talk during the procedure.
    _____ g. Position the patient sitting upright with the elbows on an over-the-bed table.

26. After which diagnostic study would the nurse observe the patient for symptoms of a pneumothorax?
    a. Thoracentesis
    b. Pulmonary function test
    c. Ventilation-perfusion scan
    d. Positron emission tomography (PET) scan

27. The health care provider orders a pulmonary angiogram for a patient admitted with dyspnea and hemoptysis. Which problem is this test most commonly used as a diagnostic measure?
    a. TB   c. Airway obstruction
    b. Lung cancer   d. Pulmonary embolism

28. Match the following pulmonary capacities and function tests with their descriptions.

    Pulmonary Capacity or
    Function Test   **Description**
    _____ a. VT   1. Amount of air exhaled in first second of forced vital capacity
    _____ b. RV   2. Maximum amount of air lungs can contain
    _____ c. TLC   3. Volume of air inhaled and exhaled with each breath
    _____ d. VC   4. Maximum amount of air that can be exhaled after maximum inspiration
    _____ e. FVC   5. Amount of air that can be quickly and forcefully exhaled after maximum inspiration
    _____ f. PEFR   6. Maximum rate of airflow during forced expiration
    _____ g. FEV$_1$ 7. Amount of air remaining in lungs after forced expiration
    _____ h. FRC   8. Volume of air in lungs after normal exhalation

Supporting Ventilation

1. Identify the *a, b, c, d,* and *e* labels on the chest drainage devices pictured below (note that only Figure B has an *e* label).

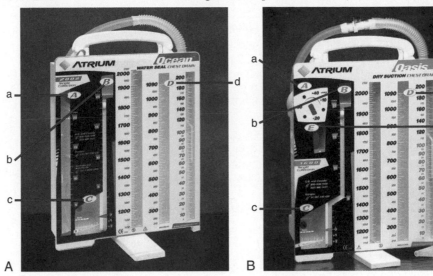

a. _____
b. _____
c. _____
d. _____
e. _____

2. Describe the function of each chamber.

Chamber	Function
Water-seal	
Suction control	
Collection	
Suction monitor bellows	

3. When would the nurse check for leaks in the chest tube and pleural drainage system?
   a. There is continuous bubbling in the water-seal chamber.
   b. There is constant bubbling of water in the suction control chamber.
   c. Fluid in the water-seal chamber fluctuates with the patient's breathing.
   d. The water levels in the water-seal and suction control chambers are decreased.

4. An assistive personnel (AP) is taking care of a patient with a chest tube. What action by the AP would cause the nurse to intervene?
   a. Loops the drainage tubing on the bed.
   b. Secures the drainage container in an upright position.
   c. Strips or milks the chest tube to promote drainage.
   d. Reminds the patient to cough and deep breathe every 2 hours.

5. Which chest surgery is used for the stripping of a fibrous membrane?
   a. Lobectomy
   b. Decortication
   c. Thoracotomy
   d. Wedge resection

6. How would the nurse explain to the patient and family the purpose of video-assisted thoracic surgery (VATS)?
   a. Removal of a lung
   b. Removal of 1 or more lung segments
   c. Removal of lung tissue by multiple wedge excisions
   d. Inspection, diagnosis, and management of intrathoracic injuries

7. After a thoracotomy, the patient is having difficulty coughing because of pain and positioning. What action would the nurse take?
   a. Have the patient drink 16 oz of water before attempting to deep breathe.
   b. Auscultate the lungs before and after deep breathing and coughing regimens.
   c. Place the patient in the Trendelenburg position for 30 minutes before the coughing exercises.
   d. Medicate the patient with analgesics 20 to 30 minutes before assisting to cough and deep breathe.

8. What advantage does a tracheostomy have over an endotracheal (ET) tube for long-term management of an upper airway obstruction?
   a. A tracheostomy is safer to perform in an emergency.
   b. An ET tube has a higher risk of tracheal pressure necrosis.
   c. A tracheostomy tube allows for more comfort and mobility.
   d. An ET tube is more likely to lead to lower respiratory tract infection.

9. What are the characteristics of a fenestrated tracheostomy tube? **Select all that apply.**
   a. The cuff passively fills with air.
   b. Cuff pressure monitoring is not required.
   c. It has 2 tubings with one opening just above the cuff.
   d. Patient can speak with an attached air source with the cuff inflated.
   e. Airway obstruction is likely if the exact steps are not followed to produce speech.
   f. Airflow around the tube and through the window allows speech when the cuff is deflated and the plug is inserted.

10. During care of a patient with a cuffed tracheostomy, the nurse notes that the tracheostomy tube has an inner cannula. To care for the tracheostomy appropriately, what would the nurse do?
    a. Deflate the cuff, then remove and suction the inner cannula.
    b. Remove the inner cannula and replace it per institutional guidelines.
    c. Remove the inner cannula if the patient shows signs of airway obstruction.
    d. Keep the inner cannula in place at all times to prevent dislodging the tracheostomy tube.

11. What actions prevent the dislodgement of a tracheostomy tube in the first 3 days after its placement? **Select all that apply.**
    a. Provide tracheostomy care every 24 hours.
    b. Keep the patient in the semi-Fowler's position at all times.
    c. Keep a same-size or larger replacement tube at the bedside.
    d. Tracheostomy ties are not changed for 24 hours after tracheostomy procedure.
    e. Suction the tracheostomy tube when there is a moist cough or a decreased arterial oxygen saturation by pulse oximetry (SpO_2).
    f. A physician performs the first tracheostomy tube change 2 days after the tracheostomy.

12. When planning care for a patient with a tracheostomy, who has been stable and is to be discharged later in the day, what interventions can the registered nurse (RN) delegate to the licensed practical/vocational nurse (LPN/VN)? **Select all that apply.**
    a. Suction the tracheostomy.
    b. Provide tracheostomy care.
    c. Determine the need for suctioning.
    d. Assess the patient's swallowing ability.
    e. Teach the patient about home tracheostomy care.

13. What would the nurse include in the plan of care for a patient with a cuffed tracheostomy tube?
    a. Change the tube every 3 days.
    b. Monitor cuff pressure every 8 hours.
    c. Perform mouth care every 12 hours.
    d. Assess arterial blood gases every 8 hours.

14. A patient's tracheostomy tube becomes dislodged with vigorous coughing. What would the nurse do first?
    a. Attempt to replace the tube.
    b. Notify the health care provider.
    c. Place the patient in high Fowler's position.
    d. Ventilate the patient with a manual resuscitation bag until the health care provider arrives.

15. A comatose patient with a possible cervical spine injury is intubated with a nasal endotracheal (ET) tube. What would the nurse recognize as a disadvantage of a nasal ET tube in comparison with an oral ET tube?
    a. Requires the placement of a bite block
    b. Is more likely to cause laryngeal trauma
    c. Requires greater respiratory effort in breathing
    d. Requires the placement of an additional airway to keep the trachea open

16. When preparing a patient in the ICU for oral ET intubation, what would the nurse do that is most important for successful intubation?
    a. Place the patient supine with the head extended and the neck flexed.
    b. Tell the patient that the tongue must be extruded while the tube is inserted.
    c. Position the patient supine with the head hanging over the edge of the bed to align the mouth and trachea.
    d. Inform the patient that while it will not be possible to talk during insertion of the tube, speech will be possible after it is correctly placed.

17. A patient has an oral ET tube inserted to relieve an upper airway obstruction and to facilitate secretion removal. Using number 1 as the first priority, number the following responsibilities of the nurse immediately following placement of the tube.
    _____a. Suction the tube to remove secretions.
    _____b. X-ray confirmation of the ET tube placement.
    _____c. Place an end tidal CO_2 detector on the ET tube.
    _____d. Secure the ET tube to the face with adhesive tape.
    _____e. Assess for bilateral breath sounds and symmetric chest movement.

18. What complication does the nurse minimize the risk of when using the minimal occluding volume technique to inflate the cuff on an ET tube?
    a. Infection
    b. Hypoxemia
    c. Tracheal damage
    d. Accidental extubation

19. When suctioning an ET tube, the nurse would use a suction pressure of _____ mm Hg.

20. When would the nurse suction a patient's ET tube?
    a. When the patient has peripheral wheezes in all lobes
    b. When the patient has not been suctioned for the past 2 hours
    c. When the nurse auscultates adventitious sounds over the central airways
    d. When the nurse assesses a need to stimulate the patient to cough and deep breathe

21. What action would the nurse include in the plan of care for the patient with an ET tube?
    a. Check the cuff pressure every hour.
    b. Keep a tracheostomy tray at the bedside.
    c. Hyperoxygenate before and after suctioning.
    d. Reuse the suction catheter at the bedside for 24 hours.

22. While suctioning the ET tube of a spontaneously breathing patient, the nurse notes that the patient develops bradycardia with premature ventricular contractions. What would the nurse do first?
    a. Stop the suctioning and assess the patient for spontaneous respirations.
    b. Attempt to suction the patient again with reduced suction pressure and pass time.
    c. Stop the suctioning and ventilate the patient with slow, small-volume breaths using a bag-valve-mask (BVM) device.
    d. Stop suctioning and ventilate the patient with a BVM device with 100% oxygen until the HR returns to baseline.

23. What precautions would the nurse take during mouth care and repositioning of an oral ET tube to prevent and detect tube dislodgement? **Select all that apply.**
    a. Confirm bilateral breath sounds after care.
    b. Use suction pressures less than 120 mm Hg.
    c. Use humidified inspired gas to help thin secretions.
    d. One staff member holds the tube and another performs care.
    e. Move secretions into larger airways with turning every 2 hours.

24. What are appropriate nursing interventions to decrease the risk for aspiration for a patient with an oral ET tube? **Select all that apply.**
    a. Assess gag reflex.
    b. Suction the patient's mouth frequently.
    c. Ensure that the cuff is properly inflated.
    d. Keep the ventilator tubing cleared of condensed water.
    e. Raise the head of the bed 30 to 45 degrees unless the patient is unstable.

25. A patient who is orally intubated and mechanically ventilated patient is restless and very anxious. The oxygen saturation is greater than 92%. What interventions would most likely decrease the risk of accidental extubation? **Select all that apply.**
    a. Administer sedatives.
    b. Have a caregiver stay with the patient.
    c. Obtain an order and apply soft wrist restraints.
    d. Remind the patient that he needs the tube inserted to breathe.
    e. Move the patient to an area close to the nurses' station for closer observation.

26. Patients with which conditions are most likely to require mechanical ventilation? **Select all that apply.**
    a. Sleep apnea
    b. Cystic fibrosis
    c. Acute kidney injury
    d. Type 2 diabetes
    e. Acute respiratory distress syndrome (ARDS)

27. What characteristics describe positive pressure ventilators? **Select all that apply.**
    a. Require an artificial airway
    b. Applied to outside of the body
    c. Most similar to physiologic ventilation
    d. Most frequently used with acutely ill patients
    e. Used in the home for neuromuscular or nervous system disorders

28. What is included in the description of positive pressure ventilation? **Select all that apply.**
    a. Peak inspiratory pressure is predetermined
    b. Consistent volume is delivered with each breath
    c. Increased risk for hyperventilation and hypoventilation
    d. Preset volume of gas delivered with variable pressure based on compliance
    e. Volume delivered varies based on selected pressure and patient lung compliance

29. Which mode of ventilation is used with critically ill patients and allows the patient to self-regulate the rate and depth of spontaneous respirations, but may also deliver a preset volume and frequency of breaths?
    a. Assist-control ventilation (ACV)
    b. Pressure support ventilation (PSV)
    c. Pressure control ventilation (PCV)
    d. Synchronized intermittent mandatory ventilation (SIMV)

30. A patient in acute respiratory failure is receiving ACV with a positive end-expiratory pressure (PEEP) of 10 cm H_2O. What sign alerts the nurse to undesirable effects of increased airway and thoracic pressure?
    a. Decreased BP
    b. Decreased partial pressure of oxygen in arterial blood (PaO_2)
    c. Increased crackles
    d. Decreased spontaneous respirations

31. What factor is commonly responsible for sodium and fluid retention in the patient on mechanical ventilation?
    a. Increased release of antidiuretic hormone (ADH)
    b. Increased release of atrial natriuretic factor
    c. Increased insensible water loss via the airway
    d. Decreased renal perfusion with release of renin

32. The registered nurse (RN) caring for a stable patient on mechanical ventilation in a long-term acute care facility plans the interventions listed below. Indicate whether each intervention must be done by the RN or if it could be delegated to the licensed practical nurse (LPN) or assistive personnel (AP), who would report back to the RN.
    _____a. Give routinely scheduled enteral medications.
    _____b. Administer sedatives, analgesics, and paralytic medications.
    _____c. Give enteral nutrition through a gastrostomy tube.
    _____d. Obtain vital signs and measure urine output.
    _____e. Teach the patient and caregiver about mechanical ventilation and weaning.
    _____f. Assist the respiratory therapist with repositioning and securing the ET tube.
    _____g. Auscultate breath sounds and respiratory effort.
    _____h. Perform passive or active range-of-motion (ROM) exercises.
    _____i. Maintain appropriate cuff inflation on the ET tube.
    _____j. Provide personal hygiene and skin care.

33. A patient receiving mechanical ventilation is very anxious and agitated, which necessitates the use of neuromuscular blocking agents to promote ventilation. What would the nurse recognize about the care of this patient?
    a. The patient will be sedated and unaware of the details of care.
    b. Encourage caregivers to provide stimulation and diversion.
    c. Always address the patient and provide explanations of care given.
    d. Communication will not be possible with the use of neuromuscular blocking agents.

34. A patient develops anemia while receiving prolonged mechanical ventilation. The patient is having difficulty being weaned from the ventilator related to a recurrent pneumonia and early fatigue during weaning trials. What is contributing to the patient's prolonged recovery?
    a. Hypoxemia
    b. Enteral feeding
    c. Inadequate nutrition
    d. Decreased activity level

35. What assessment finding leads the nurse to determine that alveolar hypoventilation is occurring in a patient on a ventilator?
    a. The patient develops dysrhythmias.
    b. Auscultation reveals an air leak around the ET tube cuff.
    c. ABG results show a $PaCO_2$ of 32 mm Hg and a pH of 7.47.
    d. The patient tries to breathe faster than the ventilator setting.

36. What action would the nurse take when weaning a patient from a ventilator?
    a. Decrease the delivered fractional inspired oxygen concentration (FiO_2) concentration
    b. Intermittent trials of spontaneous ventilation followed by ventilatory support to provide rest
    c. Substitute ventilator support with a manual resuscitation bag if the patient becomes hypoxemic
    d. Implement weaning procedures around the clock until the patient does not experience ventilatory fatigue

37. A patient is to be discharged home with mechanical ventilation. Before discharge, what is most important for the nurse to do for the patient and caregiver?
    a. Teach the caregiver to care for the patient with a home ventilator.
    b. Help the caregiver plan for placement of the patient in a long-term care facility.
    c. Stress the advantages for the patient in being cared for in their home environment.
    d. Have the caregiver arrange for around-the-clock home health nurses for the first several weeks.

CASE STUDY   Mechanical Ventilation Patient

(ajr_images/
iStock/
Thinkstock)

Patient Profile

D.V., 42-years-old, has a history of human immunodeficiency virus (HIV) infection with the development of manifestations of acquired immunodeficiency syndrome (AIDS) 2 years ago. He has been hospitalized and treated twice for *Pneumocystis jiroveci* pneumonia and is now admitted to ICU with suspected cryptococcal meningitis. ET intubation with assist-control mechanical ventilation at 12 breaths/min, 15 cm H_2O PEEP, and FiO_2 of 50% is established.

Subjective Data

• A friend reports that D.V. had 2 generalized tonic-clonic seizures in the 2 hours before admission

Objective Data

• Glasgow Coma Scale (GCS) score: 6
• Weight 65.9 kg, height 6 ft 1 in
• Vital signs: temp 102.2°F (39°C), HR 80 beats/min, RR 26 breaths/min, BP 100/46 mm Hg
• ABGs: pH 7.26, $PaCO_2$ 32 mm Hg, PaO_2 65 mm Hg, HCO_3^- 16 mEq/L, SaO_2 92%
• Other laboratory tests: glucose 228 mg/dL (12.6 mmol/L), lactate 3 mEq/L (3 mmol/L), white blood cells (WBCs) 18,500/µL
• Skin warm and dry
• Indwelling urinary catheter inserted with 30 mL returned

Questions

1. What effects of PEEP would the nurse expect? **Use an X to indicate if the assessment finding is Expected (a side effect of PEEP) or Unexpected (is not a side effect of PEEP).**

Assessment Finding	Expected	Unexpected
Increase in SpO_2		
Decrease in blood pressure		
Increase in cardiac output (CO)		
Decrease in intracranial pressure (ICP)		
Increase in PaO_2		
Increase in systemic vascular resistance		
Decrease in functional residual capacity (FRC)		

2. What nursing interventions specific to ET intubation and mechanical ventilation would the nurse include in D.V.'s plan of care? **Use an X to indicate whether the nursing action is Indicated (is appropriate or necessary), Contraindicated (could be harmful), or is Non-essential (makes no difference or is unnecessary).**

Nursing Action	Indicated	Contraindicated	Non-Essential
Assess the need for ETT suction every 4 hours			
Insert an oropharyngeal airway to prevent patient from biting the ETT			
Auscultate bowel sounds			
Monitor $EtCO_2$			
Document the RASS score while on sedation			
Explain procedures while patient is receiving sedation and neuromuscular blockades			
Use 4-point restraints while intubated			
Monitor for new heart murmurs			

3. What does the nurse know is true about assist-control (AC) ventilation? **Select all that apply.**
_____A. The patient can determine their V_T.
_____B. The patient's RR will never be below the set respiratory rate.
_____C. A spontaneous breath will receive the preset V_T.
_____D. The potential for hyperventilation exists.
_____E. It is the least common mode of mechanical ventilation.
_____F. AC needs a set peak inspiratory pressure.
_____G. It is preferred in patients without acute lung injury or ARDS.
_____H. It is considered volume control, not pressure control.
_____ I. It is preferred in patients with spontaneous ventilation.

4. What interventions would the nurse include in D.V.'s plan of care to reduce the risk of ventilator-associated pneumonia (VAP)? **Use an X to indicate if the nursing action is Indicated (is necessary or appropriate), Contraindicated (could be harmful), or Non-essential (makes no difference or is unnecessary).**

Nursing Action	Indicated	Contraindicated	Non-Essential
Perform oral care once daily with chlorhexidine			
Extubate as soon as medically possible			
Obtain sputum cultures			
Put patient on contact isolation			
Keep HOB elevated 30-45°			
Monitor urine output hourly			
Drain ventilator tubing condensation away from the patient			
Keep the patient on bedrest			
Change the ventilator circuit tubing every 48 hours			

5. D.V. is placed on a weaning trial. What assessment information does not support weaning and extubating the patient? **Highlight the information in the Nurse's Note below that does not support weaning D.V. from mechanical ventilation.**

NURSE'S NOTE:

GCS 12. Patient opens eyes to name and follows simple commands. Breath sounds clear with bibasilar rhonchi. Tracheal secretions are thin and white. Vital signs: HR 103 beats/min, RR 32 breaths/min, BP 128/78 mm Hg, SpO_2 93%, temperature 100.4°F (38°C). Ventilator settings: SIMV, RR 6 breaths/min, FiO_2 40%, PEEP 10 mm Hg, PS +10. ABG results: pH 7.30, $PaCO_2$ 40 mm Hg, PaO_2 75 mm Hg, HCO_3^- 20 mEq/L. V_T 395 mL, NIP is -15 mm Hg. Bowel sounds hypoactive. Urine output: amber, 40 mL/hr. Peripheral pulses 2+, pitting edema BLE +2. Skin warm and moist.

29

Upper Respiratory Problems

1. A patient develops epistaxis after removal of a nasogastric tube. What would the nurse do?
   a. Pinch the soft part of the nose.
   b. Position the patient on the side.
   c. Have the patient hyperextend the neck.
   d. Apply an ice pack to the back of the neck.

2. The nurse receives a report on a patient who underwent posterior nasal packing for epistaxis earlier in the day. What patient assessment would the nurse perform first?
   a. Patient's temperature
   b. Level of the patient's pain
   c. Drainage on the nasal dressing
   d. Oxygen saturation by pulse oximetry

3. What would the nurse teach the patient with intermittent allergic rhinitis is the most effective way to decrease allergic symptoms?
   a. Undergo weekly immunotherapy.
   b. Identify and avoid triggers of the allergic reaction.
   c. Use cromolyn nasal spray prophylactically year-round.
   d. Use over-the-counter antihistamines and decongestants during an acute attack.

4. During assessment of the patient with a viral upper respiratory infection, the nurse recognizes that antibiotics may be indicated based on what finding?
   a. Cough and sore throat
   b. Copious nasal discharge
   c. Temperature of 100°F (38°C)
   d. Dyspnea and severe sinus pain

5. A 36-year-old patient with type 1 diabetes asks the nurse whether an influenza vaccine is necessary every year. What is the best response by the nurse?
   a. "You should get the inactivated influenza vaccine that is injected every year."
   b. "Only health care workers in contact with high-risk patients should be immunized each year."
   c. "An annual vaccination is not necessary because previous immunity will protect you for several years."
   d. "Antiviral drugs, such as zanamivir (Relenza), eliminate the need for vaccine except in the older adult."

6. A patient with an acute pharyngitis is seen at the clinic with fever and severe throat pain that affects swallowing. On inspection, the throat is reddened and edematous with patchy yellow exudates. What management would the nurse anticipate?
   a. Treatment with antibiotics
   b. Treatment with antifungal agents
   c. A throat culture or rapid strep antigen test
   d. Treatment with medication only if the pharyngitis does not resolve in 3 to 4 days

7. While the nurse is feeding a patient, the patient appears to choke on the food. Which symptoms indicate to the nurse that the patient has a partial airway obstruction? **Select all that apply.**
   a. Stridor
   b. Cyanosis
   c. Wheezing
   d. Bradycardia
   e. Rapid respiratory rate

8. When obtaining a health history from a patient with possible cancer of the mouth, what would the nurse expect the patient to report?
   a. Long-term denture use
   b. Heavy tobacco and/or alcohol use
   c. Persistent swelling of the neck and face
   d. Chronic herpes simplex infections of the mouth and lips

9. What treatment would the nurse expect to treat a patient diagnosed with an early vocal cord tumor?
   a. Radiation therapy that preserves the quality of the voice.
   b. A hemilaryngectomy that prevents the need for a tracheostomy.
   c. A radical neck dissection that removes possible sites of metastasis.
   d. A total laryngectomy to prevent development of second primary cancers.

10. During preoperative teaching with the patient scheduled for a total laryngectomy, what would the nurse include?
    a. The postoperative use of nonverbal communication techniques
    b. Techniques that will be used to alleviate a dry mouth and prevent stomatitis
    c. The need for frequent, vigorous coughing in the first 24 hours postoperatively
    d. Self-help groups and community resources for patients with cancer of the larynx

11. When assessing the patient following a total laryngectomy and radical neck dissection, what would the nurse expect to find?
    a. A closed-wound drainage system
    b. A nasal ET tube in place
    c. A nasogastric tube with orders for tube feedings
    d. A tracheostomy tube and mechanical ventilation

12. What would the nurse include in discharge teaching for the patient after a total laryngectomy?
    a. How to use esophageal speech to communicate
    b. How to use a mirror when performing tracheostomy suctioning
    c. The necessity of never covering the laryngectomy stoma
    d. The need to use baths instead of showers for personal hygiene

13. What is the most normal functioning method of speech restoration for the patient with a total laryngectomy?
    a. Esophageal speech
    b. A transesophageal puncture
    c. An electrolarynx held to the neck
    d. An electrolarynx placed in the mouth

CASE STUDY   Rhinoplasty

Patient Profile

F.N. is a 28-year-old male who sustained a displaced nasal fracture, 3 rib fractures, and a comminuted fracture of the right tibia in an automobile crash 5 days ago. An open reduction and internal fixation of the right tibia were performed on the day of the trauma. F.N. is now scheduled for a rhinoplasty to reestablish an adequate airway and improve cosmetic appearance.

(g-stockstudio/
iStock/
Thinkstock)

Subjective Data
- Reports facial pain at a level of 6 on a 0-10 scale
- Expresses concern about his facial appearance
- Reports a dry mouth

Objective Data
- RR 24 breaths/min
- HR 68 beats/min
- Bilateral ecchymosis of eyes (raccoon eyes)
- Periorbital and facial edema reduced by about half since second hospital day
- Has been NPO since midnight in preparation for surgery

Questions

1. F.N. has the potential to develop complications from sustained injuries and subsequent treatment. **Indicate which nursing action listed in the far-left column is applicable to prevent each potential complication. Note that some actions may be used for more than one complication while others may not be used.**

Nursing Action	Potential Complication	Appropriate Nursing Action for Complication
Ambulate the patient at least 3x per day	Infection	
Have the patient use the incentive spirometer 10x/hr while awake	Venous Thromboembolism	
Place the patient on neutropenic precautions	Atelectasis	
Have the patient deep breath and cough		
Apply ice to the nasal fracture		
Perform sterile dressing changes to the tibia		
Apply sequential compression devices to BLE while patient is in bed		

2. **Complete the following sentences by choosing the most likely option for the missing information from the lists of options provided.** Nasal fracture is the most common facial fracture and the ____**1**____ most common fracture of any bone. Periorbital bruising bilaterally, called raccoon eyes, suggests a ____**2**____ fracture. A meningeal tear can cause ____**3**____ to drain from the nose which should be analyzed for the presence of ____**4**____ to confirm the fluid type. Complications of this type of fracture include ____**5**____, ____**5**____, and ____**5**____. Surgical reconstruction can occur after the edema subsides. **A** ____**6**____ corrects the nasal septum while a ____**6**____ is a surgical reconstruction to repair deformities and improve airway passages.

Options for 1	Options for 2	Options for 3	Options for 4
1st	Nasal	Soft tissue fluid	WBCs
2nd	Periorbital	Blood	Glucose
3rd	Facial	Salivary fluid	Sodium
4th	Temporal bone	Cerebrospinal fluid	RBCs
5th	Basilar skull	Mucus	Antibodies
6th	Frontal bone	Purulent fluid	Platelets

Options for 5	Options for 6
Airway obstruction	Blepharoplasty
Crepitus	Rhinoplasty
Epistaxis	Abdominoplasty
Blindness	Septoplasty
Septal hematoma	Mammoplasty
Anosmia	Angioplasty

3. Below is the nurse's most recent assessment of F.N. What is the nurse's priority when planning care for F.N.?

NURSE'S NOTES:

A&O x3. Reports headache 5 on 0-10 pain scale. Reports sharp pain when taking deep breaths. Vital signs: HR 78 beats/min, RR 26 breaths/min, BP 125/83 mm Hg, SpO$_2$ 91% on room air, temperature 38.1°C. Bibasilar breath sounds are diminished without adventitious sounds. Surgical dressing on the right leg is 25% saturated with serous drainage. RLE cool and pale, LLE warm and pink, dorsalis pedis pulses +1 bilaterally. Patient denies any numbness or tingling in the lower extremities.

Based on the nurse's notes above, choose the most likely options for the information missing from the statement below by selecting from the list of options provided.

The nurse will implement the use of _____ due to signs of _____, which is a result of _____ sustained in the motor vehicle accident 5 days ago.

Options:	
Nasal fracture	Opioids
Tibial fracture	Incentive spirometry
Atelectasis	Antibiotics

Options:	
Acute Pain	Infection
Rib fractures	Trauma

4. What interventions would the nurse implement to treat F.N. postoperatively? **Use an X to indicate whether the nursing action is Indicated (appropriate or necessary), Contraindicated (could be harmful), or Non-Essential (makes no difference or is unnecessary).**

Nursing Action	Indicated	Contraindicated	Non-Essential
Keep the head of the bed less than 30 degrees			
Apply heat packs to nose			
Apply nasal sling with gauze under the nose			
Avoid stimulating the patient			
Apply ice to periorbital areas			
Pinch nostrils for scant sanguineous drainage			
Insert a nasopharyngeal airway to maintain airway patency			

5. What discharge teaching would the nurse provide F.N. upon discharge to home? Select all that apply.
   _____A. Perform nasal rinses starting the day after surgery.
   _____B. Lie down and hyperextend your neck if you have nosebleeds.
   _____C. Report any change in vision to your HCP.
   _____D. You can use over-the-counter phenylephrine nasal spray to treat minor bleeding.
   _____E. Use frozen vegetables or crushed ice to apply to the bridge of the nose for the next 72 hours.
   _____F. Sleep propped up with pillows to decrease swelling.
   _____G. You may take steamy hot showers if you prefer.
   _____H. Don't blow your nose for the next 2 weeks.
   _____ I. You may take aspirin for pain.
   _____J. Don't lift anything heavier than 10 pounds.

30

Lower Respiratory Problems

1. How do microorganisms reach the lungs and cause pneumonia? **Select all that apply.**
   a. Aspiration
   b. Lymphatic spread
   c. Inhalation of microbes in the air
   d. Touch contact with the infectious microbes
   e. Hematogenous spread from infections elsewhere in the body

2. Why is the classification of pneumonia as community-acquired pneumonia (CAP) or hospital-acquired pneumonia (HAP) clinically useful?
   a. Atypical pneumonia syndrome is more likely to occur in HAP.
   b. Diagnostic testing does not have to be used to identify causative agents.
   c. Causative agents can be predicted, and empiric treatment is often effective.
   d. IV antibiotic therapy is necessary for HAP, but oral therapy is adequate for CAP.

3. The microorganisms *Pneumocystis jiroveci* (PJP) and cytomegalovirus (CMV) are associated with which type of pneumonia?
   a. Necrotizing pneumonia
   b. Opportunistic pneumonia
   c. HAP
   d. CAP

4. Which microorganisms are associated with both CAP and HAP? **Select all that apply.**
   a. *Klebsiella*
   b. *Acinetobacter*
   c. *Staphylococcus aureus*
   d. *Mycoplasma pneumoniae*
   e. *Pseudomonas aeruginosa*
   f. *Streptococcus pneumoniae*

5. Using number 1 as the first stage and 4 as the last state, place the most common pathophysiologic stages of pneumonia in order.
   _____ a. Macrophages lyse the debris and normal lung tissue and function is restored.
   _____ b. Mucus production increases and can obstruct airflow and further decrease gas exchange.
   _____ c. Inflammatory response in the lungs with neutrophils is activated to engulf and kill the offending organism.
   _____ d. Increased capillary permeability contributes to alveolar filling with organisms and neutrophils leading to hypoxia.

6. When obtaining a health history from a 76-year-old patient with suspected CAP, what would the nurse expect the patient or caregiver to report?
   a. Confusion
   b. A recent loss of consciousness
   c. An abrupt onset of fever and chills
   d. A gradual onset of headache and sore throat

7. What is the initial antibiotic treatment for pneumonia based on?
   a. The severity of symptoms
   b. The presence of characteristic leukocytes
   c. Gram stains and cultures of sputum specimens

    d. History and physical examination and characteristic chest x-ray findings

8. A patient with a stroke has developed a fever and adventitious lung sounds. Which intervention would the nurse implement first?
    a. Anterior/posterior and lateral chest x-rays
    b. Start IV levofloxacin 500 mg every 24 hr now
    c. Complete blood count (CBC) with differential
    d. Sputum specimen for Gram stain and culture and sensitivity

9. Identify 4 clinical situations in which hospitalized patients are at risk for aspiration pneumonia and 1 nursing intervention for each situation that is indicated to prevent pneumonia.

Clinical Situation	Nursing Intervention

10. Which assessment finding in a patient with pneumonia would most concern the nurse?
    a. Arterial oxygen saturation by pulse oximetry (SpO_2) of 86%
    b. Crackles in both lower lobes
    c. Temperature of 101.4°F (38.6°C)
    d. Production of greenish purulent sputum

11. A patient with pneumonia is having difficulty clearing the airway because of pain, fatigue, and thick secretions. What is an expected outcome for this patient?
    a. SpO_2 is 90%
    b. Lungs clear to auscultation
    c. Patient tolerates walking in hallway
    d. Patient takes 3 to 4 shallow breaths before coughing to minimize pain

12. During an annual health assessment of a 66-year-old patient at the clinic, the patient tells the nurse he has not had the pneumonia vaccine. What would the nurse advise him is the best way for him to prevent pneumonia?
    a. Obtain a pneumococcal vaccine now and get a booster 12 months later.
    b. Seek medical care and antibiotic therapy for all upper respiratory infections.
    c. Obtain the pneumococcal vaccine if he is exposed to individuals with pneumonia.
    d. Obtain only the influenza vaccine every year because he should have immunity to the pneumococcus because of his age.

13. What is a cause of a resurgence in tuberculosis (TB) resulting from the emergence of multidrug-resistant (MDR) strains of *Mycobacterium tuberculosis*?
    a. A lack of effective means to diagnose TB
    b. Poor compliance with drug therapy in patients with TB
    c. Indiscriminate use of antitubercular drugs in treatment of other infections
    d. Increased population of immunosuppressed persons with acquired immunodeficiency syndrome (AIDS)

14. A patient diagnosed with class 3 TB 1 week ago is admitted to the hospital with symptoms of chest pain and coughing. What nursing action has the highest priority?
    a. Administering the patient's antitubercular drugs
    b. Admitting the patient to an airborne infection isolation room
    c. Preparing the patient's room with suction equipment and extra linens
    d. Placing the patient in an intensive care unit, where he can be closely monitored

15. When obtaining a health history from a patient suspected of having early TB, what manifestations would the nurse ask the patient about?
    a. Chest pain, hemoptysis, and weight loss
    b. Fatigue, low-grade fever, and night sweats
    c. Cough with purulent mucus and fever with chills
    d. Pleuritic pain, nonproductive cough, and temperature elevation at night

16. Which medications would be used in 4-drug treatment for the initial phase of TB? **Select all that apply.**
    a. Isoniazid
    b. Levofloxacin
    c. Pyrazinamide
    d. Rifampin (Rifadin)
    e. Rifabutin (Mycobutin)
    f. Ethambutol (Myambutol)

17. A patient with active TB continues to have positive sputum cultures after 6 months of treatment because he cannot remember to take the medications. What action would the nurse take?
    a. Arrange for directly observed therapy (DOT) by a public health nurse.
    b. Schedule the patient to come to the clinic every day to take the medication.
    c. Have a patient who has recovered from TB tell the patient about his successful treatment.
    d. Schedule more teaching sessions so that the patient will understand the risks of noncompliance.

18. To reduce the risk for many occupational lung diseases, what is the most important measure the occupational nurse would promote?
    a. Maintaining smoke-free work environments for all employees
    b. Using masks and effective ventilation systems to reduce exposure to irritants
    c. Inspection and monitoring of workplaces by national occupational safety agencies
    d. Requiring periodic chest x-rays and pulmonary function tests for exposed employees

19. During a health promotion program, why would the nurse plan to target women in a discussion of lung cancer prevention? **Select all that apply.**
    a. Women develop lung cancer at a younger age than do men.
    b. More women die from lung cancer than die from breast cancer.
    c. Women have a worse prognosis from lung cancer than do men.
    d. Black women have a higher rate of lung cancer than other ethnic groups.
    e. Nonsmoking women are at greater risk for developing lung cancer than nonsmoking men are.

20. A patient with a 40 pack-year smoking history has recently stopped smoking because of the fear of developing lung cancer. The patient asks the nurse what he can do to learn about whether he develops lung cancer. What is the best response by the nurse?
    a. "You should get a chest x-ray every 6 months to screen for any new growths."
    b. "It would be very rare for you to develop lung cancer now that you have stopped smoking."
    c. "You should monitor for any persistent cough, wheezing, or difficulty breathing, which could indicate tumor growth."
    d. "Adults aged 55 to 77 years with a history of heavy smoking who quit in the past 15 years should be screened yearly with low-dose CT."

21. A patient with a lung mass found on chest x-ray is undergoing further testing. The nurse explains that a definitive diagnosis of lung cancer can be confirmed using which diagnostic test?
    a. Lung biopsy
    b. Lung tomograms
    c. Pulmonary angiography
    d. CT scans

22. Match the following treatments for lung cancer with their descriptions.

Description	Treatment
_____ a. Considered primary treatment for small cell lung cancer (SCLC)	1. Surgical therapy
_____ b. Drug activated by laser light that destroys cancer cells	2. Radiation therapy
_____ c. Electric current heats and destroys tumor cells	3. Chemotherapy
_____ d. Palliative treatment for airway collapse or external compression	4. Prophylactic cranial radiation
_____ e. Best procedure for cure of early non-small cell lung cancer (NSCLC)	5. Bronchoscopic laser
_____ f. Medications that block molecules involved in tumor growth	6. Photodynamic therapy
_____ g. Palliative treatment by bronchoscope to remove obstructing bronchial tumors	7. Airway stenting
_____ h. Used to treat both NSCLC and SCLC	8. Radiofrequency ablation
_____ i. Used to prevent metastasis to the brain with SCLC	9. Biologic and targeted therapy
_____ j. Used with early-stage lung cancers when patient is not a surgical candidate	10. Stereotactic radiotherapy

23. A patient with advanced lung cancer refuses pain medication, saying, "I deserve everything this cancer can give me." How would the nurse respond?
    a. "Would talking to a counselor help you?"
    b. "Can you tell me what the pain means to you?"
    c. "Are you using the pain as a punishment for your smoking?"
    d. "Pain control will help you deal more effectively with your feelings."

24. A male patient has chronic obstructive pulmonary disease (COPD) and is a smoker. The nurse notices respiratory distress and no breath sounds over the left chest. Which type of pneumothorax would the nurse suspect?
    a. Tension pneumothorax
    b. Iatrogenic pneumothorax
    c. Traumatic pneumothorax
    d. Spontaneous pneumothorax

25. What assessment finding would indicate the presence of a tension pneumothorax in a patient with chest trauma?
    a. Dull percussion sounds on the injured side
    b. Severe respiratory distress and tracheal deviation
    c. Muffled and distant heart sounds with decreasing BP
    d. Decreased movement and diminished breath sounds on the affected side

26. Following a motor vehicle accident, what would the nurse recognize as a distinctive sign of flail chest in a patient?
    a. Severe hypotension
    b. Chest pain over ribs
    c. Absence of breath sounds
    d. Paradoxical chest movement

27. Match the following restrictive lung conditions with the mechanisms that cause decreased vital capacity (VC) and decreased total lung capacity (TLC).

Restrictive Lung Condition	Causative Mechanism
_____ a. Pleurisy	1. Paralysis of respiratory muscles
_____ b. Empyema	2. Presence of collapsed, airless alveoli
_____ c. Atelectasis	3. Spinal angulation restricting ventilation
_____ d. Kyphoscoliosis	4. Central depression of respiratory rate and depth
_____ e. Pleural effusion	5. Excessive scar tissue in connective tissue in lungs
_____ f. Muscular dystrophy	6. Lung expansion restricted by fluid in pleural space
_____ g. Obesity-hypoventilation syndrome	7. Lung expansion restricted by pus in intrapleural space
_____ h. Opioid and sedative overdose	8. Inflammation of the pleura restricting lung movement
_____ i. Idiopathic pulmonary fibrosis	9. Excess fat restricts chest wall and diaphragmatic excursion

28. Two days after undergoing pelvic surgery, a patient develops marked dyspnea and anxiety. What would be the nurse's first action?
    a. Raise the head of the bed.
    b. Notify the health care provider.
    c. Take the patient's pulse and blood pressure.
    d. Determine the patient's SpO_2 with an oximeter.

29. A pulmonary embolus is suspected in a patient with a deep vein thrombosis who develops dyspnea, tachycardia, and chest pain. Which diagnostic test would the nurse expect?
    a. D-dimer
    b. Chest x-ray
    c. Spiral (helical) CT scan
    d. Ventilation-perfusion lung scan

30. Which condition contributes to secondary pulmonary arterial hypertension by causing pulmonary capillary and alveolar damage?
    a. COPD
    b. Sarcoidosis
    c. Pulmonary fibrosis
    d. Pulmonary embolism

31. While caring for a patient with idiopathic pulmonary arterial hypertension (IPAH), the nurse observes that the patient has exertional dyspnea and chest pain in addition to fatigue. What are these symptoms related to?
    a. Decreased left ventricular output
    b. Right ventricular hypertrophy and failure
    c. Increased systemic arterial blood pressure
    d. Development of alveolar interstitial edema

32. What is a primary treatment goal for cor pulmonale?
    a. Controlling dysrhythmias
    b. Dilating the pulmonary arteries
    c. Strengthening the cardiac muscle
    d. Treating the underlying pulmonary condition

33. Six days after a heart-lung transplant, the patient develops a low-grade fever, dyspnea, and decreased SpO_2. What would the nurse recognize this may indicate?
    a. A normal response to extensive surgery
    b. A frequently fatal cytomegalovirus infection
    c. Acute rejection that will be treated with corticosteroids
    d. Bronchiolitis obliterans, which plugs terminal bronchioles

---

CASE STUDY Pulmonary Hypertension

(DragonImages/
iStock/Thinkstock)

Patient Profile

T.S. is a 54-year-old female patient who was diagnosed with idiopathic pulmonary arterial hypertension at the age of 44 years. At that time, she presented to her primary care HCP with a history of increasing fatigue and recent onset of swelling in her feet and ankles. A chest x-ray showed severe cardiomegaly with pulmonary congestion. She underwent a right-sided cardiac catheterization, which showed very high pulmonary artery pressures. Since then she has been treated with several drugs, but her pulmonary hypertension has never been controlled and her peripheral edema has progressively worsened.

Subjective Data
• Reports shortness of breath at rest and exercise intolerance to the extent that she had to quit her job
• Recently divorced from her husband
• Has 2 children: a 15-year-old girl and a 13-year-old boy

Objective Data
• 3 + pitting edema bilaterally from her feet to her knees
• RR: 28 breaths/min at rest
• HR: 92 beats/min

Questions
1. What additional assessment findings would indicate cor pulmonale?
   Use an X to indicate whether the assessment finding is Expected (a clinical manifestation of cor pulmonale) or Unrelated (not related to cor pulmonale).

Assessment Finding	Expected	Unrelated
Syncope		
Jugular venous distention		
Hepatomegaly		
Crackles in the lungs		
Renal insufficiency		
Weight gain		
Confusion		

2. What drugs may be prescribed to treat T.S.'s pulmonary arterial hypertension? **Choose the most likely options for the information missing from the table below by selecting from the lists of options provided.**

Drug	Dose, Route, Frequency	Drug Class	Mechanism of Action or Indication
1	200 mg PO once daily	Calcium channel blocker	Lowers PA pressure
Sildenafil	20 mg PO three times per day	2	Relaxes smooth muscle in lung vasculature
Iloprost	3	Vasodilator	4
Bosentan	125 mg PO twice daily	Endothelin Receptor Antagonist	5
6	7	Loop diuretic	Peripheral edema
Warfarin	5 mg PO once daily	8	Prevent VTE

Options for 1 and 6:	Options for 2 and 8:
Diltiazem	ACE inhibitor
Bumetanide	Phosphodiesterase Enzyme Inhibitor
Furosemide	Angiotensin receptor blockade
Nimodipine	Unfractionated heparin
Spironolactone	Vitamin K antagonist
Digoxin	Vasoconstrictor

Options for 3 and 7:	Options for 4 and 5:
150 mg PO once daily	Blocks constriction of pulmonary artery
7.5 mcg inhaled every 2 hours	Strengthens cardiac contractility
500 mg PO twice daily	Dilates systemic and PA vasculature
40 mg PO once daily	Reduces SVR
10 mg PO three times per day	Increases PA pressure
2.5 mcg inhaled every 4 hours	Decreases venous return

3. What preoperative teaching would the nurse include when preparing T.S. for a transplant procedure? **Use an X to indicate if the teaching statement is Indicated (appropriate or necessary), Contraindicated (is not appropriate or incorrect), or Non-essential (is unnecessary).**

Teaching	Indicated	Contraindicated	Non-Essential
You will not be a candidate if you have had cancer within the past 2 years.			
You may travel while waiting to be notified about an organ.			
You will need to take immunosuppressants for the rest of your life.			
There is a low risk of postoperative complications.			
Lung transplant recipients are prioritized based on a lung allocation score.			
You will need adequate financial resources to afford post-transplant care and drugs.			
You will be considered permanently disabled and will not be able to be employed.			

4. **Choose the most likely options for the information missing in the statements below by selecting from the lists of options provided.**
A single-lung transplant involves a _____1_____ incision on the affected side of the chest. There are 3 anastomoses: _____2_____, _____2_____, and _____2_____. In a double-lung transplant, the incision is made across the _____3_____ and the donor lungs are implanted separately. A median sternotomy is used for a _____4_____ transplant procedure. Those who urgently need a transplant and are unlikely to survive while waiting on the transplant list may be eligible for a _____5_____ transplantation. These come from _____6_____.

Options for 1:	**Options for 2:**	**Options for 3:**
Tracheotomy	Pulmonary veins	Abdomen
Thoracotomy	Aorta	Neck
Laparotomy	Bronchus	Back
Craniotomy	Superior vena cava	Sternum
Sternotomy	Pulmonary artery	Intercostal
Fasciotomy	Alveolar	Breast

Options for 4:	**Options for 5:**	**Options for 6:**
Single-lung	Alveolar	Friends
Lobar	Heart	Unrelated donors
Heart-lung	Bronchus	Cadavers
Lung-kidney	Lobar	Animals
Lung-liver	Pulmonary artery	Relatives
Lobar	Stem cell	Donor Network

5. What instructions would the nurse include when doing discharge teaching with T.S.? **Select all that apply.**

_____A. Acute rejection is fairly common in the first year after transplant.

_____B. Acute rejection will be diagnosed through a surgical incision to obtain a lung biopsy.

_____C. Dyspnea is expected after a lung transplant and doesn't need to be reported to the HCP.

_____D. You will need to perform home spirometry to monitor trends in lung function.

_____E. You should enroll in a rehabilitation program to improve physical endurance.

_____F. You should avoid crowded events.

_____G. You will not be allowed to travel on airplanes.

_____H. Deep breathing and coughing will be important to maintain clear lungs.

Obstructive Pulmonary Diseases

1. What would the nurse teach a patient with intermittent asthma about identifying specific triggers of asthma?
   a. Food and drug allergies do not cause respiratory symptoms.
   b. Exercise-induced asthma is seen only in persons with sensitivity to cold air.
   c. Asthma attacks are psychogenic in origin and can be controlled with relaxation techniques.
   d. Viral upper respiratory infections are a common precipitating factor in acute asthma attacks.

2. A patient is admitted to the emergency department with an acute asthma attack. Which assessment finding most concerns the nurse?
   a. The presence of a pulsus paradoxus
   b. Markedly decreased breath sounds with no wheezing
   c. A respiratory rate of 34 breaths/min and increased pulse and BP
   d. Use of accessory muscles of respiration and a feeling of suffocation

3. A patient with asthma has the following arterial blood gas (ABG) results early in an acute asthma attack: pH 7.48, partial pressure of carbon dioxide in arterial blood ($PaCO_2$) 30 mm Hg, partial pressure of oxygen in arterial blood (PaO_2) 78 mm Hg. What is the most appropriate action by the nurse?
   a. Prepare the patient for mechanical ventilation.
   b. Have the patient breathe in a paper bag to raise the $PaCO_2$.
   c. Document the findings and monitor the ABGs for a trend toward acidosis.
   d. Reduce the patient's oxygen flow rate to keep the PaO_2 at the current level.

4. Indicate the role or relationship of the following agents to asthma.

Agent	Role or Relationship to Asthma
Salicylic acid	
Nonselective β-adrenergic blockers	
Beer and wine	

5. What finding indicates marked bronchoconstriction with air trapping and hyperinflation of the lungs in a patient with asthma?
   a. Arterial oxygen saturation (SaO_2) of 85%
   b. Peak (expiratory) flow meter (PEF) rate of < 200 L/min
   c. Forced expiratory volume in 1 second (FEV_1) of 85% of predicted
   d. Chest x-ray showing a flattened diaphragm

6. Which medication would the nurse anticipate being used first in the emergency department for relief of severe respiratory distress related to asthma?
   a. Prednisone orally
   b. Tiotropium inhaler
   c. Fluticasone inhaler
   d. Albuterol nebulizer

7. Which medications are the most effective in improving asthma control by reducing bronchial hyperresponsiveness, blocking the late-phase reaction, and inhibiting migration of inflammatory cells? **Select all that apply.**
   a. Zileuton (Zyflo CR)
   b. Omalizumab (Xolair)
   c. Fluticasone (Flovent HFA)
   d. Salmeterol (Serevent)
   e. Montelukast (Singulair)
   f. Budesonide
   g. Beclomethasone (Qvar)
   h. Theophylline
   i. Mometasone (Asmanex Twisthaler)

8. When teaching the patient about going from a metered-dose inhaler (MDI) to a dry powder inhaler (DPI), which patient statement indicates to the nurse that the patient needs more teaching?
   a. "I do not need to use the spacer like I used to."
   b. "I will hold my breath for 10 seconds or longer if I can."
   c. "I will not shake this inhaler like I did with my old inhaler."
   d. "I will store it in the bathroom, so I will be able to clean it when I need to."

9. The nurse recognizes that additional teaching about medications is necessary when the patient with moderate asthma makes which statements? **Select all that apply.**
   a. "If I can't afford all of my medicines, I will only use the salmeterol (Serevent)."
   b. "I will stay inside if there is a high pollen count to prevent having an asthma attack."
   c. "I will rinse my mouth after using fluticasone (Flovent HFA) to prevent oral candidiasis."
   d. "I must have omalizumab (Xolair) injected every 2 to 4 weeks because inhalers don't help my asthma."
   e. "I can use my inhaler 3 times, every 20 minutes, before going to the hospital if my peak flow has not improved."
   f. "My gastroesophageal reflux disease (GERD) medications will help my asthma, and my asthma medications will help my GERD."

10. To decrease the patient's sense of panic during an acute asthma attack, what is the best action by the nurse?
    a. Leave the patient alone to rest in a quiet, calm environment.
    b. Stay with the patient and encourage slow, pursed-lip breathing.
    c. Reassure the patient that the attack can be controlled with treatment.
    d. Let the patient know that frequent monitoring is being done by measuring vital signs and arterial oxygen saturation by pulse oximetry (SpO_2).

11. When teaching the patient with mild asthma about the use of the peak flow meter, what would the nurse teach the patient to do?
    a. Always carry the flowmeter in case an asthma attack occurs.
    b. Use the flowmeter to check the status of the patient's asthma every time the patient takes quick-relief medication.
    c. Follow the written asthma action plan (e.g., take quick-relief medication) if the expiratory flow rate is in the yellow zone.
    d. Use the flowmeter by emptying the lungs, closing the mouth around the mouthpiece, and inhaling through the meter as quickly as possible.

12. Which patient statement indicates to the nurse that additional teaching is necessary?
    a. "I should exercise every day if my symptoms are controlled."
    b. "I may use over-the-counter bronchodilator drugs occasionally if I develop chest tightness."
    c. "I should inform my spouse about my medications and how to get help if I have a severe asthma attack."
    d. "A diary to record my medication use, symptoms, PEF rates, and activity levels will help in adjusting my therapy."

13. Tobacco smoke causes defects in multiple areas of the respiratory system. What is a long-term effect of smoking?
    a. Bronchospasm and hoarseness
    b. Decreased mucus secretions and cough
    c. Increased function of alveolar macrophages
    d. Increased risk of infection and hyperplasia of mucous glands

14. Indicate whether the following manifestations are most characteristic of asthma (A), chronic obstructive pulmonary disease (COPD) (C), or both (B).
    _____ a. Wheezing
    _____ b. Weight loss
    _____ c. Barrel chest
    _____ d. Polycythemia
    _____ e. Cor pulmonale
    _____ f. Flattened diaphragm
    _____ g. Decreased breath sounds
    _____ h. Increased total lung capacity
    _____ i. Frequent sputum production
    _____ j. Increased fractional exhaled nitric oxide (FENO)

15. What causes pulmonary vasoconstriction leading to the development of cor pulmonale in the patient with COPD?
    a. Increased viscosity of the blood
    b. Alveolar hypoxia and hypercapnia
    c. Long-term low-flow oxygen therapy
    d. Administration of high concentrations of oxygen

16. In addition to smoking cessation, what treatment is included to slow the progression of COPD?
    a. Use of bronchodilator drugs
    b. Use of inhaled corticosteroids
    c. Lung volume reduction surgery
    d. Prevention of respiratory tract infections

17. Which method of low, constant oxygen administration is the safest system to use for a patient with COPD exacerbation?
    a. Venturi mask
    b. Nasal cannula
    c. Simple face mask
    d. Nonrebreather mask

18. What characteristic describes a partial rebreather mask?
    a. Used for long-term O_2 therapy
    b. Reservoir bag conserves oxygen
    c. Provides highest oxygen concentrations
    d. Most comfortable and causes the least restriction on activities

19. A patient with COPD is being discharged with home O_2 therapy provided by an O_2 concentrator with a portable unit. In preparing the patient to use the equipment, what would the nurse teach the patient?
    a. The portable unit will last about 6 to 8 hours.
    b. The unit is strictly for portable and emergency use.
    c. The unit concentrates O_2 from the air, providing a continuous O_2 supply.
    d. Weekly delivery of 1 large cylinder of O_2 will be needed for a 7- to 10-day supply of O_2.

20. Which breathing technique to promote exhalation of CO_2 would the nurse teach the patient with moderate COPD?
    a. Huff coughing
    b. Thoracic breathing
    c. Pursed lip breathing
    d. Diaphragmatic breathing

21. What would the nurse include when planning to do postural drainage for the patient with COPD?
    a. Schedules the procedure 1 hour before and after meals
    b. Has the patient cough before positioning to clear the lungs
    c. Assesses the patient's tolerance for dependent (head-down) positions
    d. Ensures that percussion and vibration are done before positioning the patient

22. Which diet modification helps meet the nutrition needs of patients with COPD?
    a. Eating a high-carbohydrate, low-fat diet
    b. Avoiding foods that require a lot of chewing
    c. Preparing most foods of the diet to be eaten hot
    d. Drinking fluids with meals to promote digestion

23. The nurse is caring for a patient with COPD. Which intervention could be delegated to assistive personnel (AP)?
    a. Assist the patient to get out of bed.
    b. Auscultate breath sounds every 4 hours.
    c. Plan patient activities to minimize exertion.
    d. Teach the patient pursed-lip breathing technique.

24. Which medication is a long-acting β_2-adrenergic agonist and DPI that is used only for COPD?
    a. Roflumilast (Daliresp)
    b. Salmeterol (Serevent)
    c. Ipratropium (Atrovent HFA)
    d. Levalbuterol (Xopenex)

25. During an acute exacerbation of mild COPD, the patient is severely short of breath. The nurse identifies impaired respiratory function as the clinical problem, due to alveolar hypoventilation and anxiety. What is the best nursing action?
    a. Prepare and administer routine bronchodilator medications.
    b. Perform chest physiotherapy to promote removal of secretions.
    c. Administer oxygen at 5 L/min until the shortness of breath is relieved.
    d. Position the patient upright with the elbows resting on the over-the-bed table.

26. The husband of a patient with severe COPD tells the nurse that he and his wife have not had any sexual activity since she was diagnosed with COPD because she becomes too short of breath. How would the nurse respond?
    a. "You need to discuss your feelings and needs with your wife so that she knows what you expect of her."
    b. "There are other ways to maintain intimacy besides sexual intercourse that will not make her short of breath."
    c. "You should explore other ways to meet your sexual needs since your wife is no longer capable of sexual activity."
    d. "Would you like me to talk with you and your wife about some modifications that can be made to maintain sexual activity?"

27. What would the nurse include when teaching the patient with COPD about the need for physical exercise?
    a. All patients with COPD should be able to increase walking gradually up to 20 minutes per day.
    b. A bronchodilator inhaler should be used to relieve exercise-induced dyspnea immediately after exercise.
    c. Shortness of breath is expected during exercise but should return to baseline within 5 minutes after the exercise.
    d. Monitoring the heart rate before and after exercise is the best way to determine how much exercise can be tolerated.

28. The patient has had COPD for years, and ABGs usually show hypoxemia ($PaO_2 < 60$ mm Hg or $SaO_2 < 88\%$) and hypercapnia ($PaCO_2 > 45$ mm Hg). Which ABG results show movement toward respiratory acidosis and worsening hypoxemia indicating respiratory failure?
    a. pH 7.35, PaO_2 62 mm Hg, $PaCO_2$ 45 mm Hg
    b. pH 7.34, PaO_2 45 mm Hg, $PaCO_2$ 65 mm Hg
    c. pH 7.42, PaO_2 90 mm Hg, $PaCO_2$ 43 mm Hg
    d. pH 7.46, PaO_2 92 mm Hg, $PaCO_2$ 32 mm Hg

29. Pulmonary rehabilitation (PR) is designed to reduce symptoms and improve the patient's quality of life. Along with improving exercise capacity, what are anticipated results of PR? **Select all that apply.**
    a. Decreased FEV_1
    b. Decreased depression
    c. Increased oxygen need
    d. Decreased fear of exercise
    e. Decreased hospitalizations

30. What is the pathophysiologic mechanism of cystic fibrosis that leads to obstructive lung disease?
    a. Fibrosis of mucous glands and destruction of bronchial walls
    b. Destruction of lung parenchyma from inflammation and scarring
    c. Production of secretions low in sodium chloride and resulting thickened mucus
    d. Increased serum levels of pancreatic enzymes that are deposited in the bronchial mucosa

31. What is the most effective treatment for cystic fibrosis?
    a. Heart-lung transplant
    b. Administration of prophylactic antibiotics
    c. Administration of nebulized bronchodilators
    d. Vigorous and consistent airway clearance techniques

32. What problem makes it difficult to meet the developmental tasks of young adults with cystic fibrosis?
    a. They eventually need a lung transplant.
    b. They must also adapt to a chronic disease.
    c. Any children they have will develop cystic fibrosis.
    d. Their illness keeps them from becoming financially independent.

33. In an adult patient with bronchiectasis, what is a health history likely to reveal?
    a. Chest trauma
    b. Childhood asthma
    c. Smoking or oral tobacco use
    d. Recurrent lower respiratory tract infections

34. When planning care for the patient with bronchiectasis, which nursing intervention is the priority?
    a. Relieve or reduce pain
    b. Prevent paroxysmal coughing
    c. Prevent spread of the disease to others
    d. Promote drainage and removal of mucus

35. A 30-year-old white female patient with a parent with obstructive pulmonary disease is most likely to be diagnosed with which disease?
    a. COPD
    b. Asthma
    c. Cystic fibrosis
    d. α_1-Antitrypsin (AAT) deficiency

CASE STUDY Asthma

Patient Profile

E.S. is a 35-year-old mother of 2 school-age boys who arrives via ambulance in the emergency department (ED) with severe wheezing, dyspnea, and anxiety. She was in the ED 6 hours earlier with an asthma attack. An IV was started in her left forearm with normal saline infusing at 100 mL/hr.

(Wavebreakmedia/
iStock/Thinkstock)

Subjective Data

- Treated during previous ED visit with nebulized albuterol and responded quickly
- Allergic to cigarette smoke
- Began to have increasing tightness in her chest and shortness of breath when she returned home after her previous ED visit
- Used the albuterol several times after she returned home with no relief
- Diagnosed with asthma 2 years ago
- Does not have a health care provider and is not taking any medications

Objective Data

Physical Examination

- Sitting upright and using accessory muscles to breathe
- Talks in 1- to 3-word sentences
- RR: 34 breaths/min and shallow
- Audible wheezing
- Auscultation of lung fields reveals absent breath sounds in lower lobes
- HR: 126 beats/min
- Appears to be extremely anxious and restless

Diagnostic Studies

- ABGs: pH 7.46, $PaCO_2$ 36 mm Hg, PaO_2 66 mm Hg, SpO_2 88%
- Chest x-ray: bilateral lung hyperinflation with lower lobe atelectasis
- CBC with differential and electrolytes: within normal limits

Questions

1. What additional assessment information would the nurse obtain? **Use an X to indicate if the information is <u>Related</u> (necessary) or is <u>Unrelated</u> (unnecessary).**

Assessment Information	Related	Unrelated
Peak expiratory flow rate		
Jugular vein distention		
Blood cultures		
Serum IgE levels		
History of heartburn		
Recent urinary tract infection		
History of migraines		

2. What nursing interventions would the nurse include in E.S.'s plan of care? **Use an X to indicate whether the nursing action is <u>Indicated</u> (necessary or appropriate), <u>Contraindicated</u> (could be harmful), or is <u>Non-essential</u> (makes no difference or is unnecessary).**

Nursing Action	Indicated	Contraindicated	Non-Essential
Administer oxygen via non-rebreather mask			
Administer labetalol to treat tachycardia			
Have the patient breathe into a paper bag			
Administer lorazepam for anxiety			
Administer albuterol/ipratropium nebulizer			
Obtain a spiral CT scan			
Administer hydrocortisone			

3. What data indicate that E.S. is experiencing a severe or life-threatening asthma attack? **Use an X to indicate whether the assessment data indicates a Severe (life-threatening) asthma attack or if it indicates a Mild to Moderate asthma attack.**

Assessment Data	Mild to Moderate	Severe
Sitting upright		
Use of accessory muscles		
Audible Wheezing		
PaCO$_2$ 36 mm Hg		
HR 126 beats/min		
1- to 3-word sentences		
Breath sounds absent in bilateral bases		
Dyspnea		
SpO$_2$ 88%		

4. There are a number of medications that can be prescribed to treat patients with asthma to reduce the risk of asthma attacks. **Choose the most likely options for the information missing from the table below by selecting from the lists of options provided.**

Drug	Drug Class	Mechanism of Action	Nursing Consideration
Albuterol	4	Bronchodilation	8
1	Anticholinergic	6	May cause dizziness
Fluticasone	5	Reduces inflammation	9
2	Leukotriene modifier	Reduces breathing problems associated with allergies	Fatigue and headaches have been reported
3	ICS/LABA	Combo inhaled corticosteroid and long acting beta-adrenergic	10
Omalizumab	Monoclonal antibody	7	May cause arthralgia

Options for 1, 2, and 3	Options for 4 and 5	Options for 6 and 7
Ipratropium	β$_1$-Adrenergic Agonist	Anti-IgE
Beclomethasone	Anti-Interleukin 5	Vasodilator
Montelukast	Anticholinergic	Bronchodilator
Advair	β$_2$-Adrenergic Agonist	Decreases leukotrienes
Theophylline	Corticosteroid	Anti-IgG
Carvedilol	Methylxanthine	Antiinflammatory

Options for 8, 9 and 10:
May cause hypotension
Don't use in an acute asthma attack
May cause hoarseness
Rinse mouth after use to prevent fungal infections
Tachycardia is a side effect
May cause changes in sleep patterns

5. What information would the nurse include when doing discharge teaching with E.S.? **Select all that apply.**

_____A. You need to measure your peak flow daily.

_____B. You don't need to carry your inhaler if your peak flow is in the green zone.

_____C. You should wear a MedicAlert bracelet.

_____D. Use Asthma Control Test online to determine good control.

_____E. You don't need to take the inhaled corticosteroid medication if you are not wheezing.

_____F. You should be tested for allergies.

_____G. There are asthma support groups available online and in the community.

_____H. Even if you are well controlled, asthma symptoms may wake you up during the night.

Acute Respiratory Failure and Acute Respiratory Distress Syndrome

1. When the nurse is explaining respiratory failure to the patient's family, what is the most accurate description to use?
   a. The absence of effective ventilation
   b. Any problem in which part of the airway is obstructed
   c. An episode of acute hypoxemia caused by a lung problem
   d. Inadequate gas exchange arising from problems with oxygenation or ventilation

2. Which descriptions are characteristic of hypoxemic respiratory failure? **Select all that apply.**
   a. Referred to as ventilatory failure
   b. Main problem is inadequate O_2 transfer
   c. Risk of inadequate O_2 saturation of hemoglobin exists
   d. Body is unable to compensate for acidemia of increased partial pressure of carbon dioxide in arterial blood ($PaCO_2$)
   e. Most often caused by ventilation-perfusion (V/Q) mismatch and shunt
   f. Exists when partial pressure of oxygen in arterial blood (PaO_2) is less than 60 mm Hg, even when O_2 is given at 60% or more

3. Which explanation is accurate when teaching the patient with an intrapulmonary shunt about what is happening?
   a. This occurs when an obstruction impairs the flow of blood to the ventilated areas of the lung.
   b. This occurs when blood passes through an anatomic channel in the heart and bypasses the lungs.
   c. This occurs when blood flows through the capillaries in the lungs without taking part in gas exchange.
   d. Gas exchange across the alveolar capillary interface is decreased by thickened or damaged alveolar membranes.

4. When the V/Q lung scan results show a mismatch ratio that is greater than 1, which condition would be suspected?
   a. Pain
   b. Atelectasis
   c. Pulmonary embolus
   d. Ventricular septal defect

5. Which physiologic mechanism of hypoxemia occurs with pulmonary fibrosis?
   a. Anatomic shunt
   b. Diffusion limitation
   c. Intrapulmonary shunt
   d. V/Q mismatch ratio of less than 1

6. Which patient with the following manifestations is most likely to develop hypercapnic respiratory failure?
   a. Rapid, deep respirations in response to pneumonia
   b. Slow, shallow respirations because of sedative overdose
   c. Large airway resistance because of severe bronchospasm
   d. Poorly ventilated areas of the lung due to pulmonary edema

7. Which arterial blood gas (ABG) results would indicate acute respiratory failure in a patient with chronic lung disease?
   a. PaO_2 52 mm Hg, $PaCO_2$ 56 mm Hg, pH 7.4
   b. PaO_2 46 mm Hg, $PaCO_2$ 52 mm Hg, pH 7.36
   c. PaO_2 48 mm Hg, $PaCO_2$ 54 mm Hg, pH 7.38
   d. PaO_2 50 mm Hg, $PaCO_2$ 54 mm Hg, pH 7.28

8. The patient is being admitted to the intensive care unit (ICU) with hypercapnic respiratory failure. Which assessment findings would the nurse expect? **Select all that apply.**
   a. Cyanosis
   b. Metabolic acidosis
   c. Morning headache
   d. Respiratory acidosis
   e. Use of tripod position
   f. Rapid, shallow respirations

9. Which assessment finding would cause the nurse to suspect the early onset of hypoxemia?
   a. Restlessness
   b. Hypotension
   c. Central cyanosis
   d. Dysrhythmias

10. Which changes of aging contribute to the increased risk for respiratory failure in older adults ? **Select all that apply.**
    a. Alveolar dilation
    b. Increased delirium
    c. Changes in vital signs
    d. Increased infection risk
    e. Decreased respiratory muscle strength
    f. Diminished elastic recoil within the airways

11. The nurse determines that a patient in respiratory distress is developing respiratory fatigue and is at risk of respiratory arrest when the patient displays which behavior?
    a. Cannot breathe unless he is sitting upright
    b. Uses the abdominal muscles during expiration
    c. Has an increased inspiratory-expiratory (I/E) ratio
    d. Has a change in respiratory rate from rapid to slow

12. A patient has a PaO_2 of 50 mm Hg and a $PaCO_2$ of 42 mm Hg because of an intrapulmonary shunt. Which is the best therapy for this patient?
    a. Positive pressure ventilation
    b. O_2 therapy at a fractional inspired O_2 concentration (FIO_2) of 100%
    c. Applying O_2 per nasal cannula at 1 to 3 L/min
    d. Clearing airway secretions with coughing and suctioning

13. A patient with a massive hemothorax and pneumothorax has absent breath sounds in the right lung. To promote improved V/Q matching, how would the nurse position the patient?
    a. On the left side
    b. On the right side
    c. In a reclining chair bed
    d. Supine with the head of the bed elevated

14. A patient in hypercapnic respiratory failure has impaired airway clearance caused by increasing exhaustion. What is an appropriate nursing intervention for this patient?
    a. Inserting an oral airway
    b. Performing augmented coughing
    c. Teaching the patient huff coughing
    d. Teaching the patient slow pursed-lip breathing

15. The patient with a history of heart failure and acute respiratory failure has thick secretions that is difficult to cough up. Which intervention would best help mobilize the secretions?
    a. Give more IV fluid.
    b. Perform postural drainage.
    c. Provide O_2 by aerosol mask.
    d. Suction nasopharyngeal airways.

16. After endotracheal intubation and mechanical ventilation have been initiated, a patient in respiratory failure becomes very agitated and is breathing asynchronously with the ventilator. What would the nurse to do first?
    a. Evaluate the patient's pain level, ABGs, and electrolyte values.
    b. Sedate the patient to unconsciousness to eliminate patient awareness.
    c. Give as-needed vecuronium to promote synchronous ventilations.
    d. Slow the ventilator's rate of ventilations to allow for the patient to spontaneously breathe.

17. What is the main reason that hemodynamic monitoring is used in severe respiratory failure?
    a. To detect V/Q mismatches
    b. To continuously measure the arterial BP
    c. To evaluate oxygenation and ventilation status
    d. To evaluate cardiac status and blood flow to tissues

18. Patients with acute respiratory failure will need drug therapy to meet their individual goals. Which drugs reduce pulmonary congestion? **Select all that apply.**
    a. Morphine
    b. Ceftriaxone
    c. Nitroglycerin
    d. Furosemide (Lasix)
    e. Albuterol (Ventolin HFA)
    f. Methylprednisolone (Solu-Medrol)

19. The nurse recognizes that noninvasive positive pressure ventilation (NIPPV) may be used for which patient in acute respiratory failure?
    a. Is comatose and has high oxygen requirements
    b. Has copious secretions that require frequent suctioning
    c. Responds to hourly bronchodilator nebulization treatments
    d. Is alert and cooperative but has increasing respiratory exhaustion

20. The patient progressed from acute lung injury to acute respiratory distress syndrome (ARDS). The patient is on a ventilator and receiving propofol (Diprivan) for sedation and fentanyl (Sublimaze) to decrease anxiety, agitation, and pain to decrease the work of breathing, O_2 consumption, carbon dioxide production, and risk of injury. What intervention may be recommended when caring for this patient?
    a. A sedation holiday
    b. Monitoring for hypermetabolism
    c. Keeping his legs still to avoid dislodging the airway
    d. Repositioning him every 4 hours to decrease agitation

21. Although ARDS may result from direct or indirect lung injury from systemic inflammatory response syndrome (SIRS), the nurse is aware that ARDS most likely occurs from what?
    a. Sepsis
    b. Oxygen toxicity
    c. Prolonged hypotension
    d. Cardiopulmonary bypass

22. What are the main pathophysiologic changes that occur in the injury or exudative phase of ARDS? **Select all that apply.**
    a. Atelectasis
    b. Shortness of breath
    c. Interstitial and alveolar edema
    d. Hyaline membranes line the alveoli
    e. Influx of neutrophils, monocytes, and lymphocytes

23. In patients with ARDS who survive the acute phase of lung injury, what manifestations are seen when they progress to the fibrotic phase?
    a. Chronic pulmonary edema and atelectasis
    b. Resolution of edema and healing of lung tissue
    c. Continued hypoxemia because of diffusion limitation
    d. Increased lung compliance caused by the breakdown of fibrotic tissue

24. When caring for the patient with ARDS, what is the most characteristic sign the nurse would expect the patient to exhibit?
    a. Refractory hypoxemia
    b. Bronchial breath sounds
    c. Progressive hypercapnia
    d. Increased pulmonary artery wedge pressure (PAWP)

25. Which findings would lead the nurse to suspect the early stage of ARDS in a seriously ill patient?
    a. Develops respiratory acidosis
    b. Exhibits dyspnea and restlessness
    c. Has diffuse crackles and wheezing
    d. Has a decreased PaO_2 and an increased $PaCO_2$

26. A patient with ARDS is at risk for infection. To detect the presence of infections commonly associated with ARDS, what would the nurse monitor?
    a. Gastric aspirate for pH and blood
    b. Quality, quantity, and consistency of sputum
    c. Subcutaneous emphysema of the face, neck, and chest
    d. Mucous membranes of the oral cavity for open lesions

27. The best patient response to treatment of ARDS occurs when initial management includes what?
    a. Treatment of the underlying condition
    b. Administration of prophylactic antibiotics
    c. Treatment with diuretics and mild fluid restriction
    d. Endotracheal intubation and mechanical ventilation

28. When mechanical ventilation is used for the patient with ARDS, what is the reason for applying positive end-expiratory pressure (PEEP)?
    a. Prevent alveolar collapse and open collapsed alveoli
    b. Permit smaller tidal volumes with permissive hypercapnia
    c. Promote complete emptying of the lungs during exhalation
    d. Permit extracorporeal oxygenation and carbon dioxide removal outside the body

29. Which finding causes the nurse to suspect that a patient on mechanical ventilation is experiencing negative effects from PEEP?
    a. Increasing PaO_2
    b. Decreasing blood pressure
    c. Decreasing heart rate (HR)
    d. Increasing central venous pressure (CVP)

30. Prone positioning is considered for a patient with ARDS who has not responded to other measures to increase PaO_2. How does this position improve the PaO_2?
    a. It increases the mobilization of pulmonary secretions.
    b. It decreases the workload of the diaphragm and intercostal muscles.
    c. It promotes opening of atelectatic alveoli in the upper part of the lung.
    d. It promotes perfusion of nonatelectatic alveoli in the anterior part of the lung.

31. Calculate the P/F ratios for the following patients:
    a. FiO_2 is 60% and a PaO_2 of 70 mm Hg; P/F ratio = _____
    b. FiO_2 is 40% and a PaO_2 of 80 mm Hg; P/F ratio = _____
    c. FiO_2 is 35% and a PaO_2 of 95 mm Hg; P/F ratio = _____
    d. Which patient is most likely to be diagnosed with ARDS?

32. The nurse understands that patients diagnosed with ARDS may be allowed to have permissive hypercapnia. Which patient would the nurse recognize as being contraindicated for this condition?
    a. A patient with a C5 spinal cord injury
    b. A patient with opacities on chest x-ray and a P/F ratio of 225
    c. A patient who has metabolic acidosis from acute kidney injury
    d. A patient with increased intracranial pressure after blunt trauma to the skull

33. The nurse caring for a patient diagnosed with ARDS understands that low tidal volume ventilation will be prescribed while the patient is on mechanical ventilation. Using this knowledge, what is the most appropriate tidal volume if the patient weighs 175 lbs.?
    a. 700 mL
    b. 800 mL
    c. 525 mL
    d. 477 mL

CASE STUDY   Acute Respiratory Failure

Patient Profile
P.C. is a 75-year-old married woman with severe oxygen- and corticosteroid-dependent chronic obstructive pulmonary disease (COPD). She is admitted to the medical ICU in acute respiratory failure with pneumonia.

(TatyanaGl/
iStock/Thinkstock)

Subjective Data
- Reports increasing shortness of breath, increased purulent sputum, and difficulty breathing with minimal exertion

Objective Data
- ABGs on oxygen 2 L/min: pH 7.3, $PaCO_2$ 55 mm Hg, PaO_2 60 mm Hg, HCO_3^- 20 mEq/L, SaO_2 84%
- Awake, alert, and oriented
- Sitting in tripod position and using pursed-lip breathing
- Vital signs: HR 105 beats/min, BP 155/88 mm Hg, RR 32/min, Temp. 38.1°C

Interprofessional Care
- O_2 at 2 L/min per NIPPV
- Ipratropium/albuterol nebulization every hour PRN
- IV ciprofloxacin
- IV methylprednisolone (Solu-Medrol)

Questions
1. **Choose the most likely options for the information missing from the statements below by selecting from the lists of options provided.**
   Based on the following assessment data: _____1_____, _____1_____, and _____1_____, the nurse identifies that P.C. is experiencing _____2_____respiratory failure caused by_____3_____. The nurse documents the ABG result as _____4_____ with hypoxemia and assigns _____5_____ as the priority clinical problem.

Options for 1	Options for 2	Options for 3	Options for 4
Purulent sputum	Hypoxemic	COPD	Respiratory alkalosis
pH 7.3	Hypercapnic	Corticosteroids	Metabolic acidosis
Tripod positioning	Alveolar hyperventilation	Pneumonia	Respiratory acidosis
SaO_2 84%	Diffusion-related	Smoking	Respiratory alkalosis
Shortness of breath	Alveolar hypoventilation	Bronchitis	Combined acidosis
Pursed-lip breathing	Chronic	Emphysema	Combined alkalosis

Options for 5
Activity intolerance
Infection
Anxiety
Impaired respiratory function
ARDS
Fatigue

2. The nurse performs an assessment several hours after being admitted to the ICU.

   For each assessment finding, use an X to indicate whether the intervention was Effective (helped to meet expected outcomes), Ineffective (did not help to meet expected outcomes), or Unrelated (not related to the expected outcomes).

Assessment Finding	Effective	Ineffective	Unrelated
Temp 38.5°C			
Bilateral +1 edema in ankles			
SpO$_2$ 92%			
No JVD			
Reports pain during inspiration			
Voiding 100 mL/hr			
Ambulates in hallway			
EtCO$_2$ 48 mm Hg			

3. Use an X to indicate whether the nursing actions listed below are **Indicated** (appropriate or necessary), **Contraindicated** (could be harmful), or **Non-essential** (makes no difference or is unnecessary).

Nursing Action	Indicated	Contraindicated	Non-Essential
Keep the HOB greater than 30 degrees			
Place the patient on Droplet Precautions			
Perform FSBG checks every 4 hours			
Place the patient on a fluid restriction			
Educate the patient about the incentive spirometer			
Use a non-rebreather mask to deliver oxygen			
Weigh the patient daily			

4. **Choose the most likely options for the information missing from the statements below by selecting from the lists of options provided.**

   When administering albuterol, the nurse expects _____**1**_____ and _____**1**_____ as possible side effects. The nurse will monitor for _____**2**_____ when administering corticosteroids. If the patient experiences anxiety, _____**3**_____ can be administered. Ciprofloxacin is a _____**4**_____ which is a class of antibiotics often used to treat pneumonia.

Options for 1	Options for 2	Options for 3	Options for 4
Hypotension	Hypoglycemia	Opioids	Cephalosporin
Bradycardia	Hypokalemia	Barbiturates	Penicillin
Tachycardia	Hypernatremia	Hypnotics	Fluoroquinolone
Tachypnea	Hyperkalemia	Sedatives	Macrolide
Hypertension	Hypocalcemia	Benzodiazepines	Sulfonamide

5. When doing discharge teaching with P.C., what information would the nurse include? **Select all that apply.**

   _____A. Increase fluid intake to 3 L/day

   _____B. Stop taking the corticosteroids in 1 week

   _____C. Continue taking the antibiotics until they are gone

   _____D. Only use the albuterol inhaler prior to exercise

   _____E. Report any signs of infection to your HCP

   _____F. Stop using your home oxygen

   _____G. Ambulate only to use the bathroom, otherwise rest

   _____H. Get an annual influenza vaccine

33

Assessment: Hematologic System

1. What are the characteristics of neutrophils? **Select all that apply.**
   a. Also known as "segs"
   b. Band is an immature cell
   c. First white blood cells (WBCs) at injury site
   d. Arise from megakaryocyte
   e. Increased in individuals with allergies
   f. 65% to 75% of WBCs

2. An increase in which blood cell indicates an increased rate of erythropoiesis?
   a. Basophil
   b. Monocyte
   c. Reticulocyte
   d. Lymphocyte

3. Which cells are classified as granulocytes? **Select all that apply.**
   a. Basophil
   b. Monocyte
   c. Eosinophil
   d. Neutrophil
   e. Lymphocyte
   f. Thrombocyte

4. After a woman had a right breast mastectomy, her right arm became severely swollen. What hematologic problem caused this?
   a. Lymphedema
   b. Right-sided heart failure
   c. Wound on her right hand
   d. Refusal to use her right arm

5. Which nutrients are essential for red blood cell (RBC) production? **Select all that apply.**
   a. Iron
   b. Folic acid
   c. Vitamin C
   d. Vitamin D
   e. Vitamin B_{12}
   f. Carbohydrates

6. Number the components of normal hemostasis in the order of occurrence, beginning with 1 for the first component and ending with 6 for the last component.
   a. _____ Adhesion
   b. _____ Activation of the clotting cascade
   c. _____ Aggregation
   d. _____ Blood clot formation
   e. _____ Clot retraction and dissolution
   f. _____ Vascular injury, vasoconstriction, and subendothelial exposure

7. Which component of normal hemostasis involves the processes of proteins C and S and plasminogen?
   a. Activation of the clotting cascade
   b. Aggregation
   c. Bood clot formation
   d. Clot retraction and dissolution

8. A patient who was in a car accident had abdominal trauma. Which organs may be damaged and contribute to altered function of the hematologic system? **Select all that apply.**
   a. Liver
   b. Spleen
   c. Stomach
   d. Gallbladder
   e. Lymph nodes

9. What would the nurse monitor the patient for when laboratory test results show increased fibrin split products (FSPs)?
   a. Fever
   b. Bleeding
   c. Faintness
   d. Thrombotic episodes

10. When reviewing the results of an 83-year-old patient's diagnostic studies, which finding would most concern the nurse?
    a. Platelets 150,000/μL
    b. Serum iron 50 mcg/dL
    c. Partial thromboplastin time (PTT) 60 seconds
    d. Erythrocyte sedimentation rate (ESR) 35 mm in 1 hour

11. A patient with a bone marrow disorder has an overproduction of myeloblasts. The nurse would expect the results of a complete blood count (CBC) to include an increase in which cell types? **Select all that apply.**
    a. Basophils
    b. Eosinophils
    c. Monocytes
    d. Neutrophils
    e. Lymphocytes

12. During the nursing assessment of a patient with anemia, what specific information would the nurse ask the patient about?
    a. Stomach surgery
    b. Recurring infections
    c. Corticosteroid therapy
    d. Oral contraceptive use

13. Identify 1 specific finding identified by the nurse during assessment of cach of the patient's functional health patterns that indicates a risk factor for hematologic problems or a patient response to an actual hematologic problem.

Functional Health Pattern	Risk Factor or Response to Hematologic Problem
Health perception–health management	
Nutritional-metabolic	
Elimination	
Activity-exercise	
Sleep-rest	
Cognitive-perceptual	
Self-perception–self-concept	
Role-relationship	
Sexuality-reproductive	
Coping–stress tolerance	
Value-belief	

14. Using light pressure with the index and middle fingers, the nurse cannot palpate any of the patient's superficial lymph nodes. Based on this assessment, what action would the nurse take?
    a. Record this finding as normal
    b. Reassess the lymph nodes using deeper pressure
    c. Ask the patient about any history of radiation therapy
    d. Notify the health care provider (HCP) that x-rays of the nodes will be necessary

15. During physical assessment of a patient with thrombocytopenia, what would the nurse expect to find?
    a. Sternal tenderness
    b. Petechiae and purpura
    c. Jaundiced sclera and skin
    d. Tender enlarged lymph nodes

16. A patient with a hematologic disorder has a smooth, shiny, red tongue. Which laboratory result would the nurse expect?
    a. Neutrophils 45%
    b. Hemoglobin (Hgb) 9.6 g/dL (96 g/L)
    c. WBC count 13,500/μL
    d. RBC count 6.4×10^6/μL

17. A patient is being treated with chemotherapy. Which laboratory result would cause the nurse to revise the care plan?
    a. WBC count 4000/μL
    b. RBC count 4.3×10^6/μL
    c. Platelets 50,000/μL
    d. Hematocrit (Hct) 39%

18. Identify a possible etiology for the abnormal laboratory findings.

Laboratory Finding	Possible Etiology
Serum iron 40 mcg/dL (7 μmol/L)	
ESR 30 mm/hr	
Increased band neutrophils	
Activated partial thromboplastin time 60 sec	
Indirect bilirubin 2.0 mg/dL (34 μmol/L)	
Bence Jones protein in urine	

19. If a patient with blood type O Rh$^+$ is given AB Rh$^-$ blood, what would the nurse expect to happen?
    a. The patient's Rh factor will react with the RBCs of the donor blood.
    b. The anti-A and anti-B antibodies in the patient's blood will hemolyze the donor blood.
    c. The anti-A and anti-B antibodies in the donor blood will hemolyze the patient's blood.
    d. No adverse reaction is expected because the patient has no antibodies against the donor blood.

20. A patient is undergoing a contrast CT scan of the spleen. What is most important for the nurse to ask the patient about before the test?
    a. Iodine sensitivity
    b. Prior blood transfusions
    c. Phobia of confined spaces
    d. Internal metal implants or appliances

21. When teaching a patient about a bone marrow examination, what would the nurse explain?
    a. The procedure will be done under general anesthesia because it is so painful.
    b. The patient will not have any pain after the area at the puncture site is anesthetized.
    c. The patient will experience a brief, very sharp pain during aspiration of the bone marrow.
    d. There will be no pain during the procedure, but an ache will be present several days afterward.

22. What is a lymph node biopsy used to diagnose?
    a. Leukemia
    b. Cause of lymphedema
    c. Hemorrhagic tendencies
    d. Neoplastic cells in lymph nodes

23. The patient's laboratory results show a marked decrease in RBCs, WBCs, and platelets. What term would the nurse use when reporting the results to the HCP?
    a. Hemolysis
    b. Leukopenia
    c. Pancytopenia
    d. Thrombocytosis

24. Molecular cytogenetics and gene analysis may be done to diagnose, stage, and help determine treatment options for various hematologic disorders. Which sites are preferred to obtain the sample for this testing? **Select all that apply.**
    a. Skin sample
    b. Lymph node
    c. Bone marrow
    d. Arterial blood
    e. Inner cheek mucosa

34

Hematologic Problems

1. Match each of the anemic states with both the etiologic and morphologic classifications (answers may be used more than once).

Type or Cause of Anemia	Etiology	Morphology
Malaria		
Thalassemia		
Acute trauma		
Aplastic anemia		
Pernicious anemia		
Sickle cell anemia		
Anemia of gastritis		
Anemia of leukemia		
Iron-deficiency anemia		
Anemia of renal injury		
Glucose-6-phosphate dehydrogenase (G6PD)		
Anemia associated with prosthetic heart valve		

Etiologic	Morphologic
1. Decreased red blood cell (RBC) production	4. Normocytic, normochromic
2. Blood loss	5. Macrocytic, normochromic
3. Increased RBC destruction	6. Microcytic, hypochromic

2. A patient with a hemoglobin (Hgb) level of 7.8 g/dL (78 g/L) has cardiac palpitations, a heart rate of 102 beats/min, and an increased reticulocyte count. Considering the severity of anemia, what other manifestation would the nurse expect the patient to exhibit?
   a. Pallor
   b. Dyspnea
   c. A smooth tongue
   d. Sensitivity to cold

3. A 76-year-old woman has an Hgb of 7.3 g/dL (73 g/L) and is experiencing ataxia, confusion, weakness, and fatigue on admission to the hospital. What is the priority nursing intervention for this patient?
   a. Provide a darkened, quiet room.
   b. Have the family stay with the patient.
   c. Keep top bedside rails up and call bell in close reach.
   d. Question the patient about possible causes of anemia.

4. During the physical assessment of a patient with severe anemia, which finding would most concern the nurse?
   a. Anorexia
   b. Bone pain
   c. Hepatomegaly
   d. Dyspnea at rest

5. Which anemia is manifested with pancytopenia?
   a. Thalassemia
   b. Aplastic anemia
   c. Megaloblastic anemia
   d. Anemia of chronic disease

6. Which descriptions are characteristic of iron-deficiency anemia? **Select all that apply.**
   a. Lack of intrinsic factor
   b. Autoimmune-related disease
   c. Most common type of anemia
   d. Associated with chronic blood loss
   e. May occur with removal of the stomach
   f. May occur with removal of the duodenum

7. A 20-year-old female patient is in the emergency department for anorexia and fatigue. She takes phenytoin (Dilantin) for a seizure disorder and oral contraceptives. For which type of anemia is this patient most at risk?
   a. Aplastic anemia
   b. Hemolytic anemia
   c. Iron-deficiency anemia
   d. Folic acid deficiency anemia

8. Explain the following laboratory findings in anemia.

Laboratory Finding	Explanation
Reticulocyte counts are increased in chronic blood loss but decreased in cobalamin (vitamin B_{12}) deficiency.	
Bilirubin levels are increased in sickle cell anemia but are normal in acute blood loss.	
Mean corpuscular volume (MCV) is increased in folic acid deficiency but decreased in iron-deficiency anemia.	

9. What would the nurse include when teaching the patient about a new prescription for oral iron supplements?
   a. Increase fluid and dietary fiber intake
   b. Take the iron preparations with meals
   c. Use enteric-coated preparations taken with orange juice
   d. Report the presence of black stools to the health care provider

10. When teaching the patient about pernicious anemia, what would the nurse state is deficient?
    a. Folic acid
    b. Intrinsic factor
    c. Extrinsic factor
    d. Cobalamin intake

11. During the assessment of a patient with cobalamin deficiency, what manifestation would the nurse expect?
    a. Icteric sclera
    b. Hepatomegaly
    c. Paresthesia of the hands and feet
    d. Intermittent heartburn with acid reflux

12. Which patient statement indicates to the nurse that teaching about pernicious anemia has been effective?
    a. "This condition can kill me unless I take injections of the vitamin for the rest of my life."
    b. "My symptoms can be completely reversed after I take a cobalamin (vitamin B_{12}) supplement."
    c. "If my anemia does not respond to cobalamin therapy, my only other alternative is a bone marrow transplant."
    d. "The least expensive and most convenient treatment of pernicious anemia is to use a diet with foods high in cobalamin."

13. Which anemia is a strict vegetarian at greatest risk of developing?
    a. Thalassemia
    b. Iron-deficiency anemia
    c. Folic acid deficiency anemia
    d. Cobalamin deficiency anemia

14. A patient with aplastic anemia has impaired oral mucous membranes. This problem can be related to the effects of what deficiencies? **Select all that apply.**
    a. RBCs
    b. Ferritin
    c. Platelets
    d. Coagulation factor VIII
    e. White blood cells (WBCs)

15. Nursing interventions for the patient with aplastic anemia are directed toward the prevention of which complications?
    a. Fatigue and dyspnea
    b. Hemorrhage and infection
    c. Thromboemboli and gangrene
    d. Cardiac dysrhythmias and heart failure

16. Which statements describe anemia related to blood loss? **Select all that apply.**
    a. A major concern is prevention of shock.
    b. This anemia is most frequently treated with increased dietary iron intake.
    c. In addition to the general symptoms of anemia, this patient also manifests jaundice.
    d. A patient who has acute blood loss may have postural hypotension and increased heart rate.
    e. Initial clinical symptoms are the most reliable way to evaluate the effect and degree of blood loss.

17. What causes anemia in sickle cell disease?
    a. Intracellular hemolysis of sickled RBCs
    b. Accelerated breakdown of abnormal RBCs
    c. Autoimmune antibody destruction of RBCs
    d. Isoimmune antibody-antigen reactions with RBCs

18. A patient with sickle cell anemia asks the nurse why the sickling crisis does not stop when oxygen therapy is started. Which explanation would the nurse give to the patient?
    a. Sickling occurs in response to decreased blood viscosity, which is not affected by oxygen therapy.
    b. When RBCs sickle, they occlude small vessels, which causes more local hypoxia and more sickling.
    c. The primary problem during a sickle cell crisis is destruction of the abnormal cells, resulting in fewer RBCs to carry oxygen.
    d. Oxygen therapy does not alter the shape of the abnormal erythrocytes but only allows for increased oxygen concentration in hemoglobin.

19. What nursing intervention is indicated for the patient in sickle cell crisis?
    a. Frequent ambulation
    b. Application of antiembolism hose
    c. Restriction of sodium and oral fluids
    d. Administration of large doses of continuous opioid analgesics

20. What would the nurse include when providing discharge teaching to a patient with newly diagnosed sickle cell disease?
    a. Limit fluid intake
    b. Avoid humid weather
    c. Eliminate exercise from the lifestyle
    d. Seek early medical intervention for upper respiratory infections

21. Which statements accurately describe thrombocytopenia? **Select all that apply.**
    a. Patients with platelet deficiencies can have internal or external hemorrhage.
    b. The most common acquired thrombocytopenia is thrombotic thrombocytopenic purpura (TTP).
    c. Immune thrombocytopenic purpura (ITP) is characterized by increased platelet destruction by the spleen.
    d. TTP is characterized by decreased platelets, decreased RBCs, and enhanced aggregation of platelets.
    e. A classic clinical manifestation of thrombocytopenia that the nurse would expect to find on physical examination of the patient is ecchymosis.

22. A 45-year-old patient has symptoms including arthralgia, impotence, weight loss, and liver enlargement. His laboratory results include an elevated serum iron, total iron binding capacity (TIBC), and serum ferritin levels. Which disorder does this describe and which treatment will be used?
    a. Thalassemia; combination chemotherapy
    b. Hemochromatosis; deferoxamine (Desferal)
    c. Myelodysplastic syndrome; blood transfusions
    d. Delayed transfusion reaction; deferasirox (Exjade)

23. In providing care for a patient hospitalized with an acute exacerbation of polycythemia vera, the nurse gives priority to which activity?
    a. Maintaining protective isolation
    b. Promoting leg exercises and ambulation
    c. Protecting the patient from injury or falls
    d. Promoting hydration with a large oral fluid intake

24. A patient has a platelet count of 50,000/μL and is diagnosed with ITP. What does the nurse anticipate initial treatment will include?
    a. Splenectomy
    b. Corticosteroids
    c. Administration of platelets
    d. Immunosuppressive therapy

25. A patient is admitted to the hospital for evaluation and treatment of thrombocytopenia. Which action is most important for the nurse to implement?
    a. Taking the temperature every 4 hours to assess for fever
    b. Maintaining the patient on strict bed rest to prevent injury
    c. Monitoring the patient for headaches, vertigo, or confusion
    d. Removing the oral crusting and scabs with a soft brush 4 times a day

26. The nurse caring for a patient with heparin-induced thrombocytopenia (HIT) identifies risk for hemorrhaging as the priority clinical problem. Identify at least 5 nursing interventions that would be implemented.
    a.
    b.
    c.
    d.
    e.

27. When reviewing the laboratory results of a patient with hemophilia A, what would the nurse expect?
    a. An absence of factor IX
    b. A decreased platelet count
    c. A prolonged bleeding time
    d. A prolonged partial thromboplastin time (PTT)

28. A patient with hemophilia comes to the clinic for treatment. What intervention would the nurse anticipate?
    a. Whole blood
    b. Thromboplastin
    c. Coagulation factor
    d. Fresh frozen plasma

29. A patient with hemophilia is hospitalized with acute knee pain and swelling. What is an appropriate nursing intervention?
    a. Wrapping the knee with an elastic bandage
    b. Placing the patient on bed rest and applying ice to the joint
    c. Administering nonsteroidal antiinflammatory drugs (NSAIDs) as needed for pain
    d. Gently performing range-of-motion (ROM) exercises to the knee to prevent adhesions

30. Which bleeding disorder affects both genders, is autosomal dominant, and will have laboratory results showing prolonged bleeding time?
    a. Hemophilia A
    b. Hemophilia B
    c. Thrombocytopenia
    d. von Willebrand disease

31. Beginning with 1 as the first event and 7 as the last event, number the events that occur in disseminated intravascular coagulation (DIC).
    a. _____ Activation of fibrinolytic system
    b. _____ Uncompensated hemorrhage
    c. _____ Widespread fibrin and platelet deposition in capillaries and arterioles
    d. _____ Release of fibrin-split products
    e. _____ Fibrinogen converted to fibrin
    f. _____ Inhibition of normal blood clotting
    g. _____ Production of intravascular thrombin

32. A patient has a WBC count of 2300/μL and a neutrophil percentage of 40%. Answer the following questions.
    a. Does the patient have leukopenia?
    b. What is the patient's absolute neutrophil count?
    c. Does the patient have neutropenia?
    d. Is the patient at risk for developing a bacterial infection? If so, why?

33. What is the most important method to identify the presence of infection in a neutropenic patient?
    a. Frequent temperature monitoring
    b. Routine blood and sputum cultures
    c. Assessing for redness and swelling
    d. Monitoring WBC count

34. What is a major method of preventing infection in the patient with neutropenia?
    a. Prophylactic antibiotics
    b. A diet that eliminates fresh fruits and vegetables
    c. High-efficiency particulate air (HEPA) filtration
    d. Strict hand washing by all persons in contact with the patient

35. How does myelodysplastic syndrome (MDS) differ from acute leukemia?
    a. MDS has a slower disease progression.
    b. MDS does not result in bone marrow failure.
    c. MDS is a clonal disorder of hematopoietic cells.
    d. MDS affects only the production and function of platelets and WBCs.

36. Which leukemia is seen in 80% of adults with acute leukemia and exhibits proliferation of precursors of granulocytes?
    a. Hairy cell leukemia
    b. Biphenotypic leukemia
    c. Acute lymphocytic leukemia (ALL)
    d. Acute myelogenous leukemia (AML)

37. Which statements accurately describe chronic lymphocytic leukemia (CLL)? **Select all that apply.**
    a. Most common leukemia of adults in Western countries
    b. Only cure is bone marrow transplant
    c. Neoplasm of activated B lymphocytes
    d. Increased incidence in survivors of atomic bombs
    e. Philadelphia chromosome is a diagnostic hallmark
    f. Mature-appearing but functionally inactive lymphocytes

38. What is the underlying cause of lymphadenopathy, splenomegaly, and hepatomegaly in leukemia?
    a. The development of infection at these sites
    b. Increased compensatory production of blood cells by these organs
    c. Infiltration of the organs by increased numbers of WBCs in the blood
    d. Normal hypertrophy of the organs in an attempt to destroy abnormal cells

39. A patient with AML is considering a hematopoietic stem cell transplant and asks the nurse what is involved. How would the nurse respond?
    a. "Your bone marrow is destroyed by radiation, and new bone marrow cells from a matched donor are injected into your bones."
    b. "A specimen of your bone marrow may be aspirated and treated to destroy any leukemic cells and then reinfused when your disease becomes worse."
    c. "Leukemic cells and bone marrow stem cells are eliminated with chemotherapy and/or total-body radiation, and new bone marrow cells from a donor are infused."
    d. "During chemotherapy and/or total-body irradiation to destroy all of your blood cells, you may be given transfusions of RBCs and platelets to prevent complications."

40. Indicate whether the following characteristics are associated with Hodgkin's lymphoma (HL), non-Hodgkin's lymphoma (NHL), or both (B).
    a. _____ Affects all ages
    b. _____ Presence of Reed-Sternberg cells
    c. _____ Associated with Epstein-Barr virus
    d. _____ Multiple histopathologic classifications
    e. _____ Originates in lymph nodes in most patients
    f. _____ Often widely disseminated at time of diagnosis
    g. _____ Treated with chemotherapy and possibly radiation
    h. _____ Ingested alcohol-induced pain at the site of disease
    i. _____ Primary initial clinical manifestation is painless lymph node enlargement

41. What characteristics must the nurse be aware of when planning care for the patient with Hodgkin's lymphoma?
    a. Staging of Hodgkin's lymphoma is not important to predict prognosis.
    b. Management of the patient being treated for Hodgkin's lymphoma includes measures to prevent infection.
    c. Hodgkin's lymphoma is characterized by proliferation of malignant activated B cells that destroy the kidneys.
    d. An important nursing intervention in the care of patients with Hodgkin's lymphoma is increasing fluids to manage hypercalcemia.

42. Following a splenectomy for the treatment of ITP, what laboratory test result would the nurse expect?
    a. Decreased RBCs
    b. Decreased WBCs
    c. Increased platelets
    d. Increased immunoglobulins

43. A 60-year-old male farmer is diagnosed with multiple myeloma. He has pain in his ribs with movement and his diagnostic studies show hypercalcemia. What nursing interventions would be included in the plan of care? **Select all that apply.**
    a. Provide privacy
    b. Complete bed rest
    c. Adequate hydration
    d. Prepare for dialysis
    e. Assess for infection
    f. Encourage ambulation

44. While receiving a unit of packed RBCs, the patient develops chills and a temperature of 102.2°F (39°C). What is the nurse's priority?
    a. Stop the transfusion and instill normal saline.
    b. Notify the health care provider and the blood bank.
    c. Add a leukocyte reduction filter to the blood administration set.
    d. Recognize this as a mild allergic transfusion reaction and slow the transfusion.

45. A patient with thrombocytopenia with active bleeding is to receive 2 units of platelets. To administer the platelets, what would the nurse do?
    a. Check for ABO compatibility.
    b. Agitate the bag periodically during the transfusion.
    c. Take vital signs every 15 minutes during the procedure.
    d. Refrigerate the second unit until the first unit has transfused.

46. Which type of transfusion reaction occurs with leukocyte or plasma protein incompatibility and may be avoided with leukocyte reduction filters?
    a. Allergic reaction
    b. Acute hemolytic reaction
    c. Febrile, nonhemolytic reaction
    d. Massive blood transfusion reaction

47. Which characteristics are related to an acute hemolytic transfusion reaction? **Select all that apply.**
    a. ABO incompatibility
    b. Hypothermia common
    c. Destruction of donor RBCs
    d. Acute kidney injury occurs
    e. Hypocalcemia and hyperkalemia
    f. Epinephrine used for severe reaction

48. The nurse is preparing to administer a blood transfusion. Number the actions in order of priority, 1 is the first action and 10 is the last action.
    a. _____ Verify the order for the transfusion.
    b. _____ Ensure that the patient has a patent 16- to 22-gauge IV.
    c. _____ Prime the transfusion tubing and filter with normal saline.
    d. _____ Verify that the physician has discussed risks, benefits, and alternatives with the patient.
    e. _____ Obtain the blood product from the blood bank.
    f. _____ Ask another licensed person (nurse or MD) to assist in verifying the product identification and the patient identification.
    g. _____ Document outcomes in the patient record. Document vital signs, names of personnel, and starting and ending times.
    h. _____ Adjust the infusion rate and continue to monitor the patient every 30 minutes for up to an hour after the product is infused.
    i. _____ Infuse the first 50 mL over 15 minutes, staying with the patient.
    j. _____ Obtain the patient's vital signs before starting the transfusion.

CASE STUDY   Disseminated Intravascular Coagulation (DIC)

Patient Profile

N.T., a 35-year-old mother of 2, is admitted in active labor to the labor and delivery department for delivery of her third child. She delivers a 9-lb boy following an unusually difficult and prolonged labor.

(Huntstock/Thinkstock)

Objective Data

- During her recovery period, N.T. continues to have heavy uterine bleeding and a boggy fundus
- Her skin is pale and diaphoretic
- BP: 70/40 mm Hg
- HR: 150 beats/min
- Although the placenta appeared intact on examination, she is suspected of having retained placental fragments, causing DIC.

Questions

1. Use an X to indicate whether the laboratory results below are **Expected** (finding that occurs in DIC), **Unexpected** (finding that does not occur in DIC), or **Unrelated** (finding that isn't applicable to DIC).

Laboratory Result	Expected	Unexpected	Unrelated
Decreased fibrinogen levels			
Decreased fibrin split products			
Normal PTT			
Hypocalcemia			
Decreased Factor VIII levels			
Increased INR			
Hyperkalemia			
Increased antithrombin III levels			
Thrombocytopenia			
Increased hematocrit			

2. Use an X to indicate whether the nursing actions below are **Indicated** (appropriate or necessary), **Contraindicated** (could be harmful), or **Non-essential** (makes no difference or is unnecessary) for the care of this patient.

Nursing Action	Indicated	Contraindicated	Non-Essential
Transfuse a pack of platelets			
Warfarin 5 mg PO twice daily			
Oxygen 6 L/min via simple face mask			
Administer 2 units of fresh frozen plasma (FFP)			
Acetaminophen 650 mg per rectum			
Monitor for oozing around invasive catheters			
Administer ondansetron 4 mg IV			
Massage the fundus			
Administer 1000 mL D_5W bolus			
Apply a cooling blanket			

3. **Choose the most likely options for the information missing from the statements below by selecting from the lists of options provided.**

The nurse would monitor for additional signs of DIC which include _____1_____, _____1_____, and _____1_____. _____2_____ may be used to treat clotting as long as it outweighs the risk of bleeding. _____3_____ would be administered to increase fibrinogen levels while fresh frozen plasma increases levels of _____4_____. Based on the objective data, the nurse assigns the clinical problem of _____5_____ as the priority.

Options for 1	Options for 2	Options for 3	Options for 4
Decreased LOC	Warfarin	Platelets	Protein C
Hyperglycemia	Alteplase	PRBCs	Antithrombin
Ecchymosis	Urokinase	Cryoprecipitate	Fibrinogen
Oliguria	Heparin	FFP	Protein S
Hyperemia	Apixaban	Whole blood	Platelets
Leukopenia	Dabigatran	Albumin	Schistocytes

Options for 5
Anxiety
Acute pain
Impaired tissue perfusion
Fatigue
Impaired cognition
Impaired urinary elimination

4. When the nurse plans care for N.T., what interventions would be included to decrease the risk of bleeding? Select all that apply.

_____A. Use a draw sheet to move patient up in bed
_____B. Use the IM route to administer medications
_____C. Use soft-bristled toothbrush for mouth care
_____D. Use Excedrin for reports of a headache
_____E. Apply an ice pack after giving a subcutaneous injection
_____F. Use tampons for vaginal bleeding
_____G. Do occult testing on all stools
_____H. Report any changes in vision

5. The health care provider orders 2 units of PRBCs, 2 units of FFP, and 1 unit of cryoprecipitate to be transfused for N.T. The nurse is preparing to administer the blood products.

Use an X to indicate whether the nursing actions below are <u>Indicated</u> (appropriate or necessary), <u>Contraindicated</u> (could be harmful), or <u>Non-essential</u> (makes no difference or is unnecessary) regarding the preparation and administration of these blood products.

Nursing Action	Indicated	Contraindicated	Non-Essential
Make sure the patient has at least 2 20-gauge IV sites			
Spike both PRBCs and transfuse simultaneously			
Use plasmalyte to prime the Y-type blood tubing			
The RN and the AP checks all the blood products			
The nurse checks ABO compatibility for the cryo-precipitate before administration			
Stay with the patient for the first 15 minutes of the PRBC transfusion			
Infuse FFP over 30 minutes			
Transfuse the blood products using an IO route			
Stop the blood transfusion if the patient reports SOB			
Perform a passive leg raise prior to the infusion of these blood products			

Assessment: Cardiovascular System

1. Using the list of terms, identify the structures in the illustration below.

Terms

Chordae tendineae
Mitral valve
Pulmonic (semilunar) valve
Papillary muscle

Tricuspid valve
Interventricular septum
Aortic (semilunar) valve

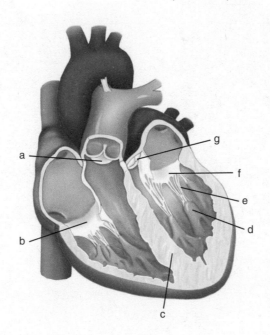

a. _____

b. _____

c. _____

d. _____

e. _____

f. _____

g. _____

2. Using the list of terms, identify the structures in the illustrations below by placing the correct term in the corresponding answer blank at the bottom of the page. **(Some terms will be used more than once.)**

Terms

Left anterior descending artery
Aorta
Circumflex artery
Coronary sinus
Great cardiac vein
Left atrium
Left coronary artery
Left marginal artery
Left ventricle
Middle cardiac vein

Posterior descending artery
Posterior vein
Pulmonary trunk
Right atrium
Right coronary artery
Right marginal artery
Right ventricle
Small cardiac vein
Superior vena cava

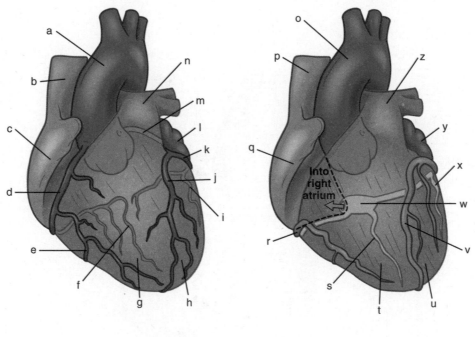

a. _____   n. _____

b. _____   o. _____

c. _____   p. _____

d. _____   q. _____

e. _____   r. _____

f. _____   s. _____

g. _____   t. _____

h. _____   u. _____

i. _____   v. _____

j. _____   w. _____

k. _____   x. _____

l. _____   y. _____

m. _____   z. _____

3. Which arteries are the major providers of coronary circulation? **Select all that apply.**
   a. Left marginal artery
   b. Right marginal artery
   c. Left circumflex artery
   d. Right coronary artery
   e. Posterior descending artery
   f. Left anterior descending artery

4. Number in sequence the path of the action potential along the conduction system of the heart.
   _____ a. Atrioventricular (AV) node
   _____ b. Purkinje fibers
   _____ c. Internodal pathways
   _____ d. Bundle of His
   _____ e. Ventricular cells
   _____ f. Sinoatrial (SA) node
   _____ g. Right and left atrial cells
   _____ h. Right and left bundle branches

5. Using the illustration below, locate and letter the following normal electrocardiographic (ECG) pattern deflections and indicate where to locate and measure the intervals.
   P
   PR interval
   Q
   QRS interval
   QT interval
   R
   S
   T
   U

   a. _____   f. _____

   b. _____   g. _____

   c. _____   h. _____

   d. _____   i. _____

   e. _____

6. Match the cardiac activity and time frames characteristic of the waveforms of the ECG. (**Answers may be used more than once.**)

   Cardiac Characteristics
   _____ a. Measured from beginning of P wave to beginning of QRS complex
   _____ b. Repolarization of the ventricles
   _____ c. 0.12 to 0.20 sec
   _____ d. 0.16 sec
   _____ e. Time of depolarization and repolarization of ventricles
   _____ f. ≤0.12 sec
   _____ g. Depolarization from the AV node throughout ventricles
   _____ h. 0.06 to 0.12 sec

   Cardiac Waveforms
   1. P wave
   2. PR interval
   3. QRS interval
   4. T wave
   5. QT interval

7. When considering each situation, indicate the stroke volume factor (i.e., preload, afterload, or contractility) and how that factor of stroke volume is primarily affected (i.e., increased or decreased) in addition to whether cardiac output (CO) is increased or decreased.

Situation	Stroke Volume Factor	Cardiac Output
Valsalva maneuver		
Venous dilation		
Hypertension		
Administration of epinephrine		
Obstruction of pulmonary artery		
Hemorrhage		

8. Which effects result from sympathetic nervous system stimulation of β-adrenergic receptors? **Select all that apply.**
   a. Vasoconstriction
   b. Increased heart rate
   c. Decreased heart rate
   d. Increased rate of impulse conduction
   e. Decreased rate of impulse conduction
   f. Increased force of cardiac contraction

9. What are the age-related physiologic changes in the older adult that result in the following cardiovascular problems?

Cardiovascular Problem	Physiologic Change
Widened pulse pressure	
Decreased cardiac reserve	
Increased cardiac dysrhythmias	
Decreased response to sympathetic stimulation	
Aortic or mitral valve murmurs	

10. During an assessment of the cardiovascular system, what is a significant finding in the health history of a patient?
    a. Metastatic cancer
    b. Calcium supplementation
    c. Frequent viral pharyngitis
    d. Frequent use of recreational drugs

11. Identify 1 specific finding identified by the nurse during assessment of each of the patient's functional health patterns that indicates a risk factor for cardiovascular disease or a patient response to an actual cardiovascular problem.

Functional Health Pattern	Risk Factor for or Response to Cardiovascular Problem
Health perception–health management	
Nutritional-metabolic	
Elimination	
Activity-exercise	
Sleep-rest	
Cognitive-perceptual	
Self-perception–self-concept	
Role-relationship	
Sexuality-reproductive	
Coping–stress tolerance	
Value-belief	

12. When palpating the patient's popliteal pulse, the nurse feels a vibration at the site. How would the nurse document this finding?
    a. Thready, weak pulse
    b. Bruit at the artery site
    c. Bounding pulse volume
    d. Thrill of the popliteal artery

13. Using the illustration below, identify the following points or locations that are inspected and palpated on the chest wall.

    Angle of Louis   Mitral area (apex) and point of maximal impulse (PMI)
    Aortic area   Pulmonic area
    Erb's point   Tricuspid area

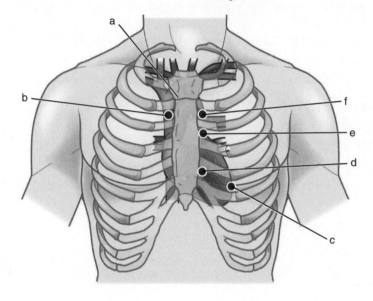

    a. _____   d. _____
    b. _____   e. _____
    c. _____   f. _____

14. Indicate whether the following are characteristic of the first heart sound (S_1) or the second heart sound (S_2).
    _____ a. Soft lub sound
    _____ b. Sharp dub sound
    _____ c. Indicates beginning of systole
    _____ d. Indicates the onset of diastole
    _____ e. Loudest at pulmonic and aortic areas
    _____ f. Loudest at tricuspid and mitral areas

15. What sounds can be auscultated in a patient with cardiac valve problems? **Select all that apply**.
    a. Arterial bruit
    b. Heart murmurs
    c. Pulsus alternans
    d. Third heart sound (S_3)
    e. Pericardial friction rub
    f. Fourth heart sound (S_4)

16. The nursing student is seeking assistance in hearing the patient's abnormal heart sounds. What would the nurse tell the student to do for a more effective assessment?
    a. Use the diaphragm of the stethoscope with the patient prone.
    b. Use the diaphragm of the stethoscope with the patient supine.
    c. Use the bell of the stethoscope with the patient leaning forward.
    d. Use the bell of the stethoscope with the patient on the right side.

17. Which finding is associated with a blue color around the lips and conjunctiva?
    a. Finger clubbing
    b. Central cyanosis
    c. Peripheral cyanosis
    d. Delayed capillary filling time

18. A patient is scheduled for exercise nuclear imaging stress testing. What does this test involve?
    a. IV administration of a radioisotope at the maximum heart rate during exercise to identify the heart's response to physical stress.
    b. Placement of electrodes inside the right-sided heart chambers through a vein to record the electrical activity of the heart directly.
    c. Exercising on a treadmill or stationary bicycle with continuous ECG monitoring to detect ischemic changes in the heart during exercise.
    d. Placement of a small transducer in 4 positions on the chest to record the direction and flow of blood through the heart by the reflection of sound waves.

19. Which action would be the highest priority for the nurse caring for a patient immediately following a transesophageal echocardiogram (TEE)?
    a. Monitor the ECG.
    b. Monitor pulse oximetry.
    c. Assess vital signs (BP, HR, RR, temperature).
    d. Maintain NPO status until gag reflex has returned.

20. Which method is used to evaluate the ECG responses to normal activity over a period of 1 or 2 days?
    a. Serial ECGs
    b. Holter monitoring
    c. 6-minute walk test
    d. Event monitor or loop recorder

21. When caring for a patient after a cardiac catheterization with coronary angiography, which finding would most concern the nurse?
    a. Swelling at the catheter insertion site
    b. Development of raised wheals on the patient's trunk
    c. Absence of pulses distal to the catheter insertion site
    d. Patient pain at the insertion site at 4 on a scale of 0 to 10

22. A female patient has a total cholesterol level of 232 mg/dL (6.0 mmol/L) and a high-density lipoprotein (HDL) of 65 mg/dL (1.68 mmol/L). A male patient has a total cholesterol level of 200 mg/dL (5.172 mmol/L) and an HDL of 32 mg/dL (0.83 mmol/L). Based on these results, which patient has the highest cardiac risk?
    a. The man, because his HDL is lower
    b. The woman, because her HDL is higher
    c. The woman, because her cholesterol is higher
    d. The man, because his cholesterol-to-HDL ratio is higher

23. Increases in which blood studies are diagnostic for acute coronary syndrome (ACS)? **Select all that apply.**
    a. Copeptin
    b. Creatine kinase (CK-MM)
    c. Cardiac troponin T (cTnT)
    d. B-type natriuretic peptide (BNP)
    e. High-sensitivity C-reactive protein (hs-CRP)
    f. Lipoprotein-associated phospholipase A_2 (Lp-PLA$_2$)

24. What factor will cause a decrease in cardiac output (CO)?
    a. Decreased afterload
    b. Decreased heart rate (HR)
    c. Increased stroke volume (SV)
    d. Decreased systemic vascular resistance (SVR)

25. The patient with shortness of breath is scheduled for an impedance cardiography to differentiate if the cause is cardiac or pulmonary. How would the nurse best explain this test to the patient?
    a. It is an invasive method of measuring CO.
    b. Electricity is transmitted through the bones in the chest.
    c. It will be most effective when the patient has generalized edema.
    d. Thoracic fluid status is determined by changes in impedance with each heartbeat.

26. The patient has an increased preload which supports an increase in CO. What nursing action contributes to an increased preload?
    a. Diuretic administration
    b. Dopamine administration
    c. Increased fluid administration
    d. Calcium channel blocker administration

27. During hemodynamic monitoring, the nurse finds that the patient has a decreased CO with unchanged pulmonary artery wedge pressure (PAWP), HR, and SVR. What would the nurse identify has decreased?
    a. Preload
    b. Afterload
    c. Contractility
    d. Stroke volume

28. Before assessing hemodynamic measurements, what would the nurse do to reference the monitoring equipment?
    a. Position the stopcock nearest the transducer level with the phlebostatic axis.
    b. Place the transducer on the left side of the chest at the fourth intercostal space.
    c. Confirm that when pressure in the system is zero, the equipment is functioning.
    d. Place the patient in a left lateral position with the transducer level with the top surface of the mattress.

29. Which statement is accurate in describing advanced cardiac technology?
    a. A pulmonary artery flow–directed catheter has a balloon at the distal tip that floats into the left atrium.
    b. In the absence of mitral valve impairment, the left ventricular end-diastolic pressure is reflected by the cardiac index.
    c. The pressure obtained when the balloon of the pulmonary artery catheter is inflated reflects the preload of the left ventricle.
    d. When a patient has an arterial catheter placed for arterial blood gas (ABG) sampling, the low-pressure alarm must be activated to detect functioning of the line.

30. When preparing the patient for insertion of a pulmonary artery catheter, what would the nurse do?
    a. Place the patient in high Fowler's position.
    b. Obtain an informed consent from the patient.
    c. Perform an Allen test to confirm adequate ulnar artery perfusion.
    d. Ensure that the patient has continuous electrocardiographic (ECG) monitoring.

31. What is a rationale for using arterial pressure–based CO (APCO) monitoring instead of a pulmonary artery catheter?
    a. Dysrhythmia   c. Less invasive technique
    b. Atrial fibrillation   d. Mechanical atrial or mitral valve

32. A patient in the ICU with hemodynamic monitoring has the following values:
    BP: 90/68 mm Hg
    HR: 124 beats/min
    PAWP: 22 mm Hg
    CO: 3.2 L/min
    Right atrial pressure (central venous pressure [CVP]): 14 mm Hg
    Pulmonary artery pressure: 38/20 mm Hg
    a. Calculate the additional values that can be determined from these findings.
    Mean arterial pressure (MAP) _____
    Pulmonary artery mean pressure (PAMP) _____
    SV _____
    SVR _____
    b. What interpretation can the nurse make about the patient's circulatory status and cardiac function from these values?

33. A patient has central venous oxygen saturation/mixed venous oxygen saturation ($ScvO_2/SvO_2$) of 52%, CO of 4.8 L/min, arterial oxygen saturation by pulse oximetry (SpO_2) of 95%, and an unchanged hemoglobin level. What would the nurse consider as the cause?
    a. Dysrhythmias
    b. Pain or movement
    c. Pulmonary edema
    d. Septic shock

34. The nurse observes a PAWP waveform on the monitor when the balloon of the patient's pulmonary artery catheter is deflated. What would the nurse recognize about this situation?
    a. The patient is at risk for embolism because of occlusion of the catheter with a thrombus.
    b. The patient is developing pulmonary edema that has increased the pulmonary artery pressure.
    c. The patient is at risk for an air embolus because the injected air cannot be withdrawn into the syringe.
    d. The catheter must be immediately repositioned to prevent pulmonary infarction or pulmonary artery rupture.

Hypertension

1. In the regulation of normal blood pressure (BP), indicate whether the following mechanisms increase BP by increasing cardiac output (CO), increasing systemic vascular resistance (SVR), or increasing both, and identify how these mechanisms cause the increase.

	Increasing Cardiac Output	Increasing Systemic Vascular Resistance	Mechanisms Causing Increases
β_1-Adrenergic stimulation			
α_1-Adrenergic stimulation			
α_2-Adrenergic stimulation			
Endothelin release			
Angiotensin II			
Aldosterone release			
Antidiuretic hormone (ADH) release			

2. A patient is given an α_1-adrenergic agonist and experiences a reflex bradycardia. What normal mechanism of BP control is stimulated in this situation?

3. A patient uses a mixed β-adrenergic blocking drug for treatment of migraine headaches. What effect may this drug have on BP and why?

4. What are nonmodifiable risk factors for primary hypertension? **Select all that apply.**
   a. Age
   b. Obesity
   c. Gender
   d. Ethnicity
   e. Genetic link

5. A patient diagnosed with secondary hypertension asks why it is called secondary and not primary. What is the best explanation by the nurse?
   a. Secondary has a more gradual onset than primary hypertension.
   b. Secondary does not cause the target organ damage that occurs with primary hypertension.
   c. Secondary has a specific cause, such as renal disease, that can often be treated by medicine or surgery.
   d. Secondary is caused by age-related changes in BP regulatory mechanisms in people over 65 years of age.

6. What early manifestation(s) is the patient with primary hypertension likely to report?
   a. No symptoms
   b. Cardiac palpitations
   c. Dyspnea on exertion
   d. Dizziness and vertigo

7. What is the main cause of target organ damage in hypertension?
   a. Increased fluid pressure exerted against organ tissue
   b. Atherosclerotic changes in vessels that supply the organs
   c. Erosion and thinning of blood vessels in organs from constant pressure
   d. Increased hydrostatic pressure causing leakage of plasma into organ interstitial spaces

8. The patient who is being admitted has had a history of uncontrolled hypertension. Which organ is most likely to be damaged by an increased SVR?
   a. Brain
   b. Heart
   c. Retina
   d. Kidney

9. Identify the significance of the following laboratory study results when found in patients with hypertension.

Laboratory Studies	Significance
Blood urea nitrogen (BUN): 48 mg/dL (17.1 mmol/L) Creatinine: 4.3 mg/dL (380 mmol/L)	
Serum K^+: 3.1 mEq/L (3.1 mmol/L)	
Serum uric acid: 9.2 mg/dL (547 mmol/L)	
Fasting blood glucose: 183 mg/dL (10.2 mmol/L)	
Low-density lipoproteins (LDL): 154 mg/dL (4.0 mmol/L)	

10. A 42-year-old man has been diagnosed with primary hypertension with an average BP of 162/92 mm Hg on 3 consecutive clinic visits. What are 4 priority lifestyle modifications that should be explored in the initial treatment of the patient?
    a.
    b.
    c.
    d.

11. What is the primary BP effect of β-adrenergic blockers, such as atenolol (Tenormin)?
    a. Vasodilation of arterioles by blocking movement of calcium into cells
    b. Decrease Na^+ and water reabsorption by blocking the effect of aldosterone
    c. Decrease CO by decreasing rate and strength of the heart and renin secretion by the kidneys
    d. Vasodilation caused by inhibiting sympathetic outflow from the central nervous system (CNS)

12. The patient asks the nurse about valsartan (Diovan), the new medication prescribed for blood pressure. What would the nurse tell the patient is the action of this medication?
    a. Prevents the conversion of angiotensin I to angiotensin II
    b. Acts directly on smooth muscle of arterioles to cause vasodilation
    c. Decreases extracellular fluid volume by increasing Na^+ and Cl^- excretion with water
    d. Vasodilation, prevents the action of angiotensin II, and promotes increased salt and water excretion

13. Which drug would include teaching that incorporates eating diet sources of potassium?
    a. Enalapril
    b. Labetalol
    c. Spironolactone
    d. Hydrochlorothiazide

14. A patient with stage 2 hypertension who is taking chlorothiazide (Diuril) and lisinopril (Zestril) has prazosin (Minipress) added to the medication regimen. What is most important for the nurse to teach the patient to do?
    a. Weigh every morning to monitor for fluid retention.
    b. Change position slowly and avoid prolonged standing.
    c. Use sugarless gum or candy to help relieve dry mouth.
    d. Take the pulse daily to note any slowing of the heart rate.

15. A 38-year-old man is treated for hypertension with triamterene and hydrochlorothiazide and metoprolol (Lopressor). Four months after his last clinic visit, his BP returns to pretreatment levels, and he admits he has not been taking his medication regularly. What is the nurse's best response to this patient?
    a. "Try to always take your medication when you carry out another daily routine so that you do not forget to take it."
    b. "You probably would not need to take medications for hypertension if you exercise more and stop smoking."
    c. "The drugs you are taking cause impaired sexual function in many patients. Are you experiencing any problems in this area?"
    d. "You need to remember that hypertension can only be controlled with medication, not cured, so you must always take your medication."

16. A 78-year-old patient is admitted with a BP of 180/98 mm Hg. Which age-related physical changes may contribute to this patient's hypertension? **Select all that apply**.
    a. Decreased renal function
    b. Increased baroreceptor reflexes
    c. Increased peripheral vascular resistance
    d. Increased adrenergic receptor sensitivity
    e. Increased collagen and stiffness of the myocardium
    f. Loss of elasticity in large arteries from arteriosclerosis

17. What would the nurse emphasize when teaching a patient who is newly prescribed clonidine (Catapres)?
    a. The drug should never be stopped abruptly.
    b. The drug should be taken early in the day to prevent nocturia.
    c. The first dose should be taken when the patient is in bed for the night.
    d. Because aspirin will decrease the drug's effectiveness, acetaminophen should be used instead.

18. What is included in the correct technique for BP measurements?
    a. Always take the BP in both arms.
    b. Position the patient supine for all readings.
    c. Place the cuff loosely around the upper arm.
    d. Take readings at least 2 times at least 1 minute apart.

19. The unit is very busy and short staffed. What could the RN delegate to the assistive personnel (AP)?
    a. Administer antihypertensive medications to stable patients.
    b. Obtain orthostatic BP readings for older patients.
    c. Check BP readings for the patient receiving IV sodium nitroprusside.
    d. Teach about home BP monitoring and use of automatic BP monitoring equipment.

20. Which manifestation is an indication that a patient is having a hypertensive emergency?
    a. Symptoms of a stroke with an elevated BP
    b. A systolic BP (SBP) > 180 mm Hg and a diastolic BP (DBP) > 110 mm Hg
    c. A sudden rise in BP accompanied by neurologic impairment
    d. A severe elevation of BP that occurs over several days or weeks

21. Which drugs are most commonly used to treat hypertensive crises?
    a. Labetalol and bumetanide (Bumex)
    b. Esmolol (Brevibloc) and captopril (Captopril)
    c. Enalaprilat (Vasotec) and minoxidil (Minoxidil)
    d. Fenoldopam (Corlopam) and sodium nitroprusside (Nitropress)

22. A patient has a BP of 222/148 mm Hg and confusion, nausea, and vomiting. Which goal would the nurse try to achieve by titrating medications?
    a. Decrease the mean arterial pressure (MAP) to 129 mm Hg
    b. Lower the BP to the patient's normal within the second to third hour
    c. Decrease the SBP to 160 mm Hg and the DBP to 100 mm Hg as quickly as possible
    d. Reduce the SBP to 158 mm Hg and the DBP to 90 mm Hg within the first 2 hours

23. What nursing responsibility is included in the management of the patient with hypertensive urgency?
    a. Monitoring hourly urine output for drug effectiveness
    b. Titrating IV drug dosages based on BP and HR measurements every 2 to 3 minutes
    c. Providing continuous electrocardiographic (ECG) monitoring to detect side effects of the drugs
    d. Instructing the patient to follow up with a health care provider within 24 hours after outpatient treatment

CASE STUDY   Primary Hypertension

(jeffwqc/iStock/
Thinkstock)

Patient Profile

K.J. is a 66-year-old woman with no history of hypertension. She came to the doctor's office for a flu shot.

Subjective Data

- Reports she has gained 20 lbs over the past year since her husband died
- Has never smoked and doesn't use alcohol
- Takes 1 multivitamin per day
- Eats a lot of canned food
- Does not exercise

Objective Data

- Height: 5 ft 4 in (162.6 cm)
- Weight: 180 lbs (77.1 kg)
- BP: 170/86 mm Hg
- Physical examination shows no abnormalities
- Serum potassium: 3.3 mEq/L (3.3 mmol/L)

The health care provider diagnoses stage 2 hypertension and prescribes lifestyle modifications.

Questions

1. How would the nurse correctly measure K.J.'s blood pressure? **Select all that apply.**

_____A. Rest the arm below level of the heart

_____B. Measure and record BP in both arms

_____C. Take the BP measurement using an oscillometric device

_____D. Use the arm with the lowest BP

_____E. Use the right cuff size for the patient's arm

_____F. Ask her to remain quiet during the measurements

_____G. Have her rest for at least 10 minutes before BP measurements

_____H. Legs should be uncrossed during the measurement

2. There are many medications to treat hypertension. **Match each Drug (Column A) to its correct Drug Class (Column B) placing the answers in Column C.**

Drug (Column A)	Drug Class (Column B)	Correct Drug for Drug Class (Column C)
Triamterene	Dihydropyridine	
Lisinopril	Mixed α- and β-blocker	
Metoprolol	ACE inhibitor	
Hydralazine	Angiotensin II receptor blocker	
Nicardipine	Cardioselective β-blocker	
Diltiazem	Potassium-sparing diuretic	
Losartan	Non-dihydropyridine	
Carvedilol	Direct vasodilator	

3. What nursing actions would the nurse implement to help K.J. reduce her blood pressure? **Use an X to indicate if the nursing action is <u>Indicated</u> (appropriate or necessary), <u>Contraindicated</u> (could be harmful), or <u>Non-essential</u> (makes no difference or is unnecessary).**

Nursing Action	Indicated	Contraindicated	Non-Essential
Obtain a referral for a dietician			
Encourage K.J. to use a salt substitute			
Encourage K.J. to exercise for 20 minutes once per week			
Advise K.J. that she can drink 2 glasses of red wine per day			
Refer K.J. to an occupational therapist			

Nursing Action	Indicated	Contraindicated	Non-Essential
Teach her that she will be able to stop taking antihypertensive medications once her BP is < 120/80 mm Hg			
Have her monitor BP at home and keep a record			

4. What patient statements indicate teaching about BP management has been effective? **Use an X to indicate if the patient statement is <u>Effective</u> (indicates understanding), <u>Ineffective</u> (indicates further teaching is necessary), or <u>Unrelated</u> (isn't related to BP management).**

Patient Statement	Effective	Ineffective	Unrelated
"I will read labels on foods that I buy."			
"Training for a half marathon is good exercise."			
"I will work with a physical therapist to increase my exercise tolerance."			
"I will weigh myself daily and report any weight gain."			
"I will eat more fiber or take a fiber supplement."			
"I will add up my daily salt intake and consume no more than 3 grams per day."			
"I can have one alcoholic beverage per day."			
"Grief counseling may be an option for me."			

5. The following antihypertensive medications have special nursing considerations. **Match each Drug (Column A) to its correct Nursing Consideration (Column B) placing the answers in Column C.**

Drug (Column A)	Nursing Consideration (Column B)	Correct Nursing Consideration for Drug (Column C)
Fenoldopam	Monitor thiocyanate levels	
Hydralazine	May cause daytime drowsiness	
Nifedipine	Use cautiously in patients with glaucoma	
Methyldopa	May increase serum creatinine levels	
Verapamil	Don't use sublingual in hypertensive emergencies	
Captopril	Don't use in 2nd degree or 3rd degree heart blocks	
Propranolol	Contraindicated in patients with CAD	
Sodium nitroprusside	Contraindicated in patients with asthma history	

37

Coronary Artery Disease and Acute Coronary Syndrome

1. Which patient is most likely to be in the fibrous stage of development of coronary artery disease (CAD)?
   a. Age 40 years, thrombus adhered to the coronary artery wall
   b. Age 50 years, rapid onset of disease with hypercholesterolemia
   c. Age 32 years, thickened coronary arterial walls with narrowed vessel lumen
   d. Age 19 years, high low-density lipoprotein (LDL) cholesterol, lipid-filled smooth muscle cells

2. What statement accurately describes the pathophysiology of CAD?
   a. Partial or total occlusion of the coronary artery occurs during the stage of raised fibrous plaque.
   b. Endothelial changes are caused by chemical irritants, such as hyperlipidemia or tobacco use.
   c. Collateral circulation in the coronary circulation is more likely to be present in the young patient with CAD.
   d. The leading theory of atherogenesis proposes that infection and fatty dietary intake are the basic underlying causes of atherosclerosis.

3. Which patient does the nurse identify as having the greatest risk for CAD?
   a. A white man, age 54 years, who is a smoker and has a stressful lifestyle
   b. A white woman, age 75 years, with a BP of 172/100 mm Hg and who is physically inactive
   c. An Asian woman, age 45 years, with a cholesterol level of 240 mg/dL and a BP of 130/74 mm Hg
   d. An obese Hispanic man, age 65 years, with a cholesterol level of 195 mg/dL and a BP of 128/76 mm Hg

4. What would the nurse emphasize when teaching women about the risks and incidence of CAD?
   a. Smoking is not as significant a risk factor for CAD in women as it is in men.
   b. Women seek treatment sooner than do men when they have symptoms of CAD.
   c. Estrogen replacement therapy in postmenopausal women decreases the risk of CAD.
   d. CAD is the leading cause of death in women, with a higher mortality rate after myocardial infarction (MI).

5. Which characteristics are associated with LDLs? **Select all that apply.**
   a. Increases with exercise
   b. Contains the most cholesterol
   c. Has an affinity for arterial walls
   d. Carries lipids away from arteries to liver
   e. High levels correlate most closely with CAD
   f. The higher the level, the lower the risk for CAD

6. Which serum lipid elevation, along with high LDL, is strongly associated with CAD?
   a. Apolipoproteins
   b. Fasting triglycerides
   c. Total serum cholesterol
   d. High-density lipoprotein (HDL)

7. The nurse reviews the following laboratory results for 4 patients. Which patient would the nurse identify as having the greatest risk for CAD and teach first about prevention?
   a. Total cholesterol: 152 mg/dL, triglycerides: 148 mg/dL, LDL: 148 mg/dL, HDL: 52 mg/dL
   b. Total cholesterol: 160 mg/dL, triglycerides: 102 mg/dL, LDL: 138 mg/dL, HDL: 56 mg/dL
   c. Total cholesterol: 200 mg/dL, triglycerides: 150 mg/dL, LDL: 160 mg/dL, HDL: 48 mg/dL
   d. Total cholesterol: 250 mg/dL, triglycerides: 164 mg/dL, LDL: 172 mg/dL, HDL: 32 mg/dL

8. The nurse is encouraging a sedentary patient, with major risks for CAD, to perform physical exercise on a regular basis. In addition to decreasing the risk factor of physical inactivity, the nurse tells the patient that exercise will directly contribute to reducing which risk factors?
   a. Diabetes and hypertension
   b. Hyperlipidemia and obesity
   c. Increased serum lipids and stressful lifestyle
   d. Hypertension and increased serum homocysteine

9. During a routine health examination, a 48-year-old patient is found to have a total cholesterol level of 224 mg/dL (5.8 mmol/L) and an LDL level of 140 mg/dL (3.6 mmol/L). What diet changes would the nurse teach the patient to make? **Select all that apply.**
   a. Use fat-free milk
   b. Abstain from alcohol use
   c. Reduce red meat in the diet
   d. Eliminate intake of simple sugars
   e. Avoid foods prepared with egg yolks

10. The nurse would teach which patients to make diet changes to reduce the risk of CAD?
    a. Patients who have had an MI
    b. All patients to reduce CAD risk
    c. Those with 2 or more risk factors for CAD
    d. Those with a cholesterol level > 200 mg/dL (5.2 mmol/L)

11. A 62-year-old woman smokes a pack of cigarettes per day and has a BP 138/88 mm Hg. She has no symptoms of CAD, but a recent LDL level was 154 mg/dL (3.98 mmol/L). Based on these findings, which treatment plan would the nurse expect would be used first?
    a. Diet and drug therapy
    b. Exercise instruction only
    c. Diet therapy and smoking cessation
    d. Drug therapy and smoking cessation

12. What are manifestations of acute coronary syndrome (ACS)? **Select all that apply.**
    a. Dysrhythmia
    b. Stable angina
    c. Unstable angina
    d. ST-segment-elevation myocardial infarction (STEMI)
    e. Non–ST-segment-elevation myocardial infarction (NSTEMI)

13. Myocardial ischemia occurs because of increased oxygen demand and decreased oxygen supply. What factors and disorders result in increased oxygen demand? **Select all that apply.**
    a. Hypovolemia or anemia
    b. Increased cardiac workload with aortic stenosis
    c. Narrowed coronary arteries from atherosclerosis
    d. Angina in the patient with atherosclerotic coronary arteries
    e. Left ventricular hypertrophy caused by chronic hypertension
    f. Sympathetic nervous system stimulation by drugs, emotions, or exertion

14. What causes the pain that occurs with myocardial ischemia?
    a. Death of myocardial tissue
    b. Dysrhythmias caused by cellular irritability
    c. Lactic acid accumulation during anaerobic metabolism
    d. Increased pressure in the ventricles and pulmonary vessels

15. What types of angina can occur in the patient who does not have CAD? **Select all that apply.**
    a. Silent ischemia
    b. Nocturnal angina
    c. Prinzmetal's angina
    d. Microvascular angina
    e. Chronic stable angina

16. Which characteristics describe unstable angina? **Select all that apply.**
    a. Usually precipitated by exertion
    b. New-onset angina with minimal exertion
    c. Occurs only when the person is recumbent
    d. Characterized by increased duration or severity
    e. Usually occurs in response to coronary artery spasm

17. Tachycardia that is a response of the sympathetic nervous system to the pain of ischemia is detrimental because it increases oxygen demand and
    a. increases cardiac output.
    b. causes reflex hypotension.
    c. may lead to atrial dysrhythmias.
    d. impairs perfusion of the coronary arteries.

18. Which effects contribute to making nitrates the first-line therapy for the treatment of angina? **Select all that apply.**
    a. Decrease preload
    b. Decrease afterload
    c. Dilate coronary arteries
    d. Decrease heart rate (HR)
    e. Prevent thrombosis of plaques
    f. Decrease myocardial contractility

19. The patient who has used sublingual nitroglycerin (NTG) and long-acting nitrates now has an ejection fraction of 38% and is considered at a high risk for a cardiac event. Which medication would be added first to vasodilate and reduce ventricular remodeling?
    a. Captopril
    b. Clopidogrel
    c. Diltiazem
    d. Metoprolol

20. When teaching a patient with angina about taking sublingual NTG tablets, what would the nurse include?
    a. Lie or sit and place 1 tablet under the tongue when chest pain occurs.
    b. Take the tablet with a large amount of water so it will dissolve right away.
    c. If 1 tablet does not relieve the pain in 15 minutes, go to the hospital.
    d. If the tablet causes dizziness and a headache, stop the medication and call the doctor or go to the hospital.

21. The nurse is teaching an older adult with CAD about the treatment for angina. What instructions would the nurse include?
    a. Sit for 2 to 5 minutes before standing when getting out of bed
    b. Exercise only twice a week to avoid unnecessary strain on the heart
    c. Lifestyle changes are not as necessary as they would be in a younger person
    d. Aspirin therapy is contraindicated in older adults because of the risk for bleeding

22. Why must unstable angina be identified and rapidly treated?
    a. The pain may be severe and disabling.
    b. Electrocardiogram (ECG) changes and dysrhythmias may occur during an attack.
    c. Rupture of unstable plaque may cause complete thrombosis of the vessel lumen.
    d. Spasm of a major coronary artery may cause total occlusion of the vessel with progression to MI.

23. A patient is reporting chest pain. What would cause the nurse to suspect the patient is experiencing stable angina rather than a myocardial infarction?
    a. The pain is relieved by NTG.
    b. The pain is described as a sensation of tightness or squeezing.
    c. The pain does not radiate to the neck, back, or arms.
    d. The pain is precipitated by physical or emotional exertion.

24. A patient admitted to the hospital for evaluation of chest pain has normal serum cardiac biomarkers 4 hours after the onset of pain. What noninvasive diagnostic test can be used to differentiate angina from other types of chest pain?
    a. 12-lead ECG
    b. Exercise stress test
    c. Coronary angiogram
    d. Transesophageal echocardiogram

25. A 52-year-old man is in the emergency department reporting severe chest pain. What assessment finding leads the nurse to believe the patient is experiencing a myocardial infarction?
    a. He has pale, cool, clammy skin.
    b. He reports nausea and vomited once at home.
    c. He says he is anxious and has a feeling of impending doom.
    d. He reports he has had no relief of the pain with rest or position change.

26. At what point in the healing process of the myocardium following an infarct does early scar tissue result in an unstable heart wall?
    a. 2 to 4 days after MI
    b. 4 to 10 days after MI
    c. 10 to 14 days after MI
    d. 6 weeks after MI

27. What would the nurse do to detect and treat the most common complication of MI?
    a. Measure hourly urine output.
    b. Auscultate the lungs for crackles.
    c. Use continuous cardiac monitoring.
    d. Take vital signs every 2 hours for the first 8 hours.

28. While assessing the patient who had an MI, the nurse auscultates crackles in the lungs and an S_3 heart sound. Which complication would the nurse suspect?
    a. Pericarditis
    c. Ventricular aneurysm
    b. Heart failure
    d. Papillary muscle dysfunction

29. In the patient who reports chest pain, which results can distinguish unstable angina from an MI?
    a. ECG changes present at the onset of the pain
    b. A chest x-ray showing left ventricular hypertrophy
    c. Serum troponin levels increased 4 to 6 hours after the onset
    d. Creatine kinase MB (CK-MB) elevations that peak 6 hours after the infarct

30. A second 12-lead ECG performed on a patient 4 hours after the onset of chest pain reveals ST segment elevation. What does this finding indicate?
    a. Transient ischemia typical of unstable angina
    b. Lack of permanent damage to myocardial cells
    c. MI associated with prolonged and complete coronary thrombosis
    d. MI associated with transient or incomplete coronary artery occlusion

31. What phrase describes transmyocardial laser revascularization (TMR)?
    a. Structure applied to hold vessels open
    b. Requires anticoagulation following the procedure
    c. Laser-created channels in the heart muscle to allow blood flow to ischemic areas
    d. Surgical construction of new vessels to carry blood beyond obstructed coronary artery

32. Which treatment is used first for the patient with a confirmed MI to open the blocked artery within 90 minutes of arrival to a health care facility?
    a. TMR
    c. Coronary artery bypass graft (CABG)
    b. Stent placement
    d. Percutaneous coronary intervention (PCI)

33. In planning care for a patient who has just returned to the unit following a PCI, which activity can the nurse delegate to assistive personnel (AP)?
    a. Monitor the IV fluids and measure urine output.
    b. Check vital signs and report changes in HR, BP, or pulse oximetry.
    c. Explain to the patient the need for frequent vital signs and pulse checks.
    d. Assess circulation to the extremity used by checking pulses, skin temperature, and color.

34. A patient is scheduled to have CABG surgery. How would the nurse explain the procedure?
    a. A synthetic graft will be used as a tube for blood flow from the aorta to a coronary artery distal to an obstruction.
    b. A stenosed coronary artery will be resected, and a synthetic arterial tube graft will be inserted to replace the diseased artery.
    c. The internal mammary artery will be detached from the chest wall and attached to a coronary artery distal to the stenosis.
    d. Reversed segments of a saphenous artery from the aorta will be anastomosed to the coronary artery distal to an obstruction.

35. What initial treatment would the nurse expect when caring for a patient with a NSTEMI?
    a. PCI
    c. Acute intensive drug therapy
    b. CABG
    d. Reperfusion therapy with thrombolytics

36. During treatment with reteplase (Retavase) for a patient with a STEMI, which finding would most concern the nurse?
    a. Oozing of blood from the IV site
    b. BP of 102/60 mm Hg with an HR of 78 bpm
    c. Decrease in the responsiveness of the patient
    d. Intermittent accelerated idioventricular rhythms

37. The nurse evaluates that thrombolytic therapy for the treatment of an MI has not been successful based on which manifestation?
    a. Continues to have chest pain
    b. Develops gastrointestinal (GI) bleeding
    c. Has a marked increase in CK-MB levels within 3 hours of therapy
    d. Develops premature ventricular contractions and ventricular tachycardia during treatment

38. The patient diagnosed with an MI is experiencing chest pain that is not relieved with IV NTG. Which medication would the nurse expect to be used next?
    a. IV morphine sulfate
    b. Calcium channel blockers
    c. IV administration of amiodarone
    d. Angiotensin-converting enzyme (ACE) inhibitors

39. What is the rationale for giving docusate sodium (Colace) to a patient after an MI?
    a. Relieves cardiac workload
    b. Minimizes vagal stimulation
    c. Controls ventricular dysrhythmias
    d. Prevents the binding of fibrinogen to platelets

40. A patient who has hypertension just had an MI. Which type of medication would the nurse expect to administer with the goal of decreasing cardiac workload?
    a. ACE inhibitor
    b. β-adrenergic blocker
    c. Calcium channel blocker
    d. Angiotensin II receptor blocker (ARB)

41. A patient with an MI is exhibiting anxiety while being taught about possible lifestyle changes. Which patient statement indicates to the nurse that the anxiety is relieved?
    a. "I'm going to take this recovery one step at a time."
    b. "I feel much better and am ready to get on with my life."
    c. "How soon do you think I will be able to go back to work?"
    d. "I know you are doing everything possible to save my life."

42. A patient hospitalized for evaluation of unstable angina reports severe chest pain. Prioritize the following interventions from 1 (highest priority) to 6 (lowest priority). All interventions are available to the nurse.
    a. Notify the provider.
    b. Obtain a 12-lead ECG.
    c. Check the patient's vital signs.
    d. Apply oxygen per nasal cannula.
    e. Perform a focused assessment of the chest.
    f. Assess pain (PQRST) and medicate as ordered.

43. Which statement indicates the patient is experiencing anger as the psychologic response to an acute MI?
    a. "Yes, I'm having a little chest pain. It's no big deal."
    b. "I don't think I can take care of myself at home yet."
    c. "What's going to happen if I have another heart attack?"
    d. "I hope my wife is happy after harping about my eating habits."

44. Which activity would the nurse and patient identify as a moderate-energy activity during rehabilitation after an MI?
    a. Golfing
    b. Walking at 5 mph
    c. Cycling at 13 mph
    d. Mowing the lawn using a push lawnmower

45. A 58-year-old patient is in a cardiac rehabilitation program. Which sign or symptom would the nurse teach the patient is a reason to stop exercising?
    a. Pain or dyspnea develop
    b. The HR exceeds 150 bpm
    c. The respiratory rate increases to 30
    d. The HR is 30 bpm over the resting HR

46. What is the nurse's best approach when counseling the patient about sexual activity following an MI?
    a. Wait for the patient to ask about resuming sexual activity.
    b. Discuss sexual activity while teaching about other physical activity.
    c. Have the patient ask the health care provider when sexual activity can be resumed.
    d. Inform the patient that impotence is a common long-term complication following an MI.

47. What advice about sexual activity would the nurse give to a male patient who had an MI?
    a. The patient should use the superior position.
    b. Prophylactic NTG may be used if angina occurs.
    c. Foreplay may cause too great an increase in HR.
    d. Performance can be enhanced with the use of sildenafil (Viagra).

48. A patient is hospitalized after a successful resuscitation of an episode of sudden cardiac death (SCD). During the care of the patient, what nursing intervention is most important?
    a. Continuous ECG monitoring
    b. Auscultation of the carotid arteries
    c. Frequent assessment of heart sounds
    d. Monitoring airway status and respirations

CASE STUDY   Coronary Artery Disease

Patient Profile
H.C., a 67-year-old Navajo woman, comes to the emergency department with a burning sensation in her epigastric area extending into her sternum.

(Katrina Brown/
Hemera/Thinkstock)

Subjective Data
• Has had unexplained fatigue
• Has had chest pain with activity that is relieved with rest for the past 3 months
• Has had type 2 diabetes since age 35 yrs
• Uses albuterol to treat asthma
• Has a smoking history of 1 pack a day for 27 yrs
• No regular exercise program
• Expresses frustration with physical problems
• Reluctant to get medical therapy because it will interfere with her life
• Has no health insurance

Objective Data
• Anxious, clenching fists
• Appears overweight and withdrawn

Questions
1. Use an X to indicate whether the nursing actions below are **Indicated (appropriate or necessary)**, **Contraindicated (could be harmful)**, or **Non-essential (makes no difference or is unnecessary)** for the patient's care at this time.

Nursing Action	Indicated	Contraindicated	Non-Essential
Apply supplemental oxygen			
Perform a pain assessment using PQRST			
Perform a head-to-toe assessment			
Obtain a 12-lead ECG			
Obtain a chest x-ray			
Administer NTG 0.4 mg SL			
Administer a non-cardioselective beta blocker			

2. For each drug listed in the table below, select the drug's **Purpose** and **Common Side/Adverse Effect** from the options provided.

Drug	Purpose	Common Side/Adverse Effect
Metoprolol		
Atorvastatin		
Morphine sulfate		
Captopril		
Aspirin		

Options for Purpose	Options for Common Side/Adverse Effect
Prevent ventricular remodeling	Muscle pain, tenderness, or weakness
Prevent platelet aggregation	Bradycardia
Decrease myocardial oxygen consumption	Persistent cough
Increase ventricular filling time	Black tarry stools
Prevent atherosclerosis	Decreased respiratory effort

3. For each assessment finding below, put an X in the column consistent with **stable angina**, **unstable angina**, or **myocardial infarction**. Findings may support more than 1 option. Each column must have at least 1 option selected.

Patient Findings	Stable Angina	Unstable Angina	Myocardial Infarction
Chest pain with activity that is relieved with rest			
Chest pain at rest			
ST segment elevation			
Elevated cardiac biomarkers			
Ventricular remodeling			

4. H.C. has been admitted to the telemetry floor for a cardiac work-up. Which assessment findings require immediate follow-up by the nurse? **Select all that apply.**
_____A. Temperature of 100°F (37.8°C)
_____B. Bibasilar crackles in the lungs
_____C. Reports nausea
_____D. O_2 saturation 96% on 2 L/min nasal cannula
_____E. Troponin 0.8 ng/mL
_____F. Intermittent low back pain
_____G. Heart rate 105 beats/min
_____H. Productive cough

5. H.C. presses the call light and reports to the nurse that she is having chest pain and difficulty catching her breath. During the nurse's assessment, H.C. reports her pain to be 7/10 radiating to her jaw, she is diaphoretic, anxious, O_2 saturation is 95% on room air, HR 115 beats/min, BP 150/90 mm Hg, and RR 30 breaths/min and shallow. **From the options provided below, insert the correct choices for each category into their respective columns. Not all options will be used.**

Potential Conditions	Actions to Take	Parameters to Monitor

Options for Potential Conditions	Options for Actions to Take	Options for Parameters to Monitor
Heart failure	Apply nasal cannula at 2 L/min	Urinary output
Unstable angina	Administer albuterol 2 puffs	Temperature
Acute renal injury	Draw blood cultures	ECG rhythm
Acute coronary syndrome	Administer lorazepam 0.5 mg PO	Pain level
Anaphylactic reaction	Administer 0.4 mg NTG SL	Arterial blood gasses
Panic attack	Administer 500 mL normal saline bolus IV	Glucose level
Sepsis	Administer hydralazine 5 mg IV	Lung sounds
Hypertensive crisis	Perform 12-lead ECG	Cardiac enzymes
Pulmonary embolism	Administer diphenhydramine 25 mg IV	Peripheral pulses
Asthma attack	Administer aspirin 325 mg chewed	Vital signs

Heart Failure

1. Which statements accurately describe heart failure (HF)? **Select all that apply.**
   a. A common cause of HF with preserved ejection fraction (HFpEF) is left ventricular dysfunction.
   b. A primary risk factor for HF is coronary artery disease (CAD).
   c. Systolic failure results in a normal left ventricular ejection fraction.
   d. HF with reduced ejection fraction (HFrEF) is characterized by abnormal resistance to ventricular filling.
   e. Hypervolemia precipitates HF by decreasing cardiac output and increasing oxygen consumption.

2. Describe how each of the following compensatory mechanisms of HF increases cardiac output and identify at least 1 effect of the mechanism that is detrimental to cardiac function.

Compensatory Mechanism	↑ Cardiac Output	Detrimental Effect
Cardiac dilation		
Cardiac hypertrophy		
Neurohormonal response		
Renin-angiotensin-aldosterone system		
Antidiuretic hormone (ADH)		
Sympathetic nervous system		

3. What describes the action of natriuretic peptides and nitric oxide in response to HF?
   a. Excretion of potassium
   b. Increased release of ADH
   c. Vasodilation and decreased BP
   d. Decreased glomerular filtration rate and edema

4. The acronym FACES is used to help teach patients to identify early symptoms of HF. What does this acronym stand for?
   a. Frequent activity leads to cough in the elderly and swelling
   b. Factors of risk: activity, cough, emotional upsets, salt intake
   c. Follow activity plan, continue exercise, and know signs of problems
   d. Fatigue, limitation of activities, chest congestion/cough, edema, shortness of breath

5. What is the pathophysiologic mechanism that results in pulmonary edema from left-sided HF?
   a. Increased right ventricular preload
   b. Increased pulmonary hydrostatic pressure
   c. Impaired alveolar oxygen and carbon dioxide exchange
   d. Increased lymphatic flow of pulmonary extravascular fluid

6. Which initial physical assessment finding would the nurse expect to be present in a patient with acute left-sided HF?
   a. Bubbling crackles and tachycardia
   b. Hepatosplenomegaly and tachypnea
   c. Peripheral edema and cool, diaphoretic skin
   d. Frothy, blood-tinged sputum and distended jugular veins

7. The nurse assesses the patient with chronic biventricular HF for paroxysmal nocturnal dyspnea (PND). What question would the nurse ask?
   a. Do you wake feeling restless or confused?
   b. Do you frequently urinate during the night?
   c. Do you have any swelling in your legs?
   d. Do you wake in a panic with a feeling of suffocation?

8. The nurse reviews the following vital signs recorded by assistive personnel (AP) on a patient with acute decompensated heart failure (ADHF): BP 98/60 mm Hg, heart rate (HR) 102 beats/min, respiratory rate (RR) 24, temperature 98.2°F (36.7°C), arterial oxygen saturation by pulse oximetry (SpO_2) 84% on 2 L/min via nasal cannula.
   a. Which of these findings is of highest priority?
   b. What would the nurse do next?

9. A patient with chronic HF has atrial fibrillation and a left ventricular ejection fraction (LVEF) of 18%. To decrease the risk of complications from these conditions, what drug would the nurse anticipate administering?
   a. Diuretic
   b. Anticoagulant
   c. β-Adrenergic blocker
   d. Potassium supplement

10. Which diagnostic test is most useful in differentiating dyspnea related to pulmonary effects of HF from dyspnea related to pulmonary disease?
    a. Exercise stress testing
    b. Cardiac catheterization
    c. B-type natriuretic peptide (BNP) levels
    d. Determination of blood urea nitrogen (BUN)

11. Which medication improves hypertension and angina in black patients with HFrEF?
    a. Captopril
    b. Nitroglycerin
    c. Spironolactone (Aldactone)
    d. Isosorbide dinitrate and hydralazine (BiDil)

12. A patient is admitted to the emergency department with ADHF. Which IV medication would the nurse expect to administer first?
    a. Digoxin (Lanoxin)
    b. Morphine sulfate
    c. Nesiritide (Natrecor)
    d. Furosemide (Lasix)

13. The patient with chronic HF is being discharged with a diuretic, a renin-angiotensin-aldosterone system (RAAS) inhibitor, and a β-adrenergic blocker. Which medication would not be included for this patient?
    a. Dopamine
    b. Losartan (Cozaar)
    c. Carvedilol (Coreg)
    d. Hydrochlorothiazide

14. In the patient with HF, which medications or treatments require careful monitoring of the patient's serum potassium level to prevent further cardiac dysfunction? **Select all that apply.**
    a. Enalapril (Vasotec)
    b. Furosemide (Lasix)
    c. Nesiritide (Natrecor)
    d. Spironolactone (Aldactone)
    e. Metoprolol CR/XL (Toprol XL)

15. A patient with chronic HF is treated with hydrochlorothiazide, digoxin, and lisinopril. To prevent the risk of digitalis toxicity, what is most important to monitor?
    a. HR
    b. Potassium levels
    c. BP
    d. Gastrointestinal function

16. The health care provider prescribes spironolactone (Aldactone) for the patient with chronic HF. What diet modifications, related to the use of this drug, would the nurse include in patient teaching?
    a. Decrease both sodium and potassium intake.
    b. Increase calcium intake and decrease sodium intake.
    c. Decrease sodium intake and increase potassium intake.
    d. Decrease sodium intake by using salt substitutes for seasoning.

17. The nurse monitors the patient receiving treatment for ADHF with the knowledge that marked hypotension is most likely to occur with the IV administration of which medication?
    a. Milrinone
    b. Furosemide
    c. Nitroglycerin
    d. Nitroprusside

18. A 2400-mg sodium diet is prescribed for a patient with chronic HF. The nurse recognizes that additional teaching is necessary when the patient makes which statement?
    a. "I should limit my milk intake to 2 cups a day."
    b. "I can eat fresh fruits and vegetables without worrying about sodium content."
    c. "I can eat most foods as long as I do not add salt when cooking or at the table."
    d. "I need to read the labels on prepared foods and medicines for their sodium content."

19. List 4 cardiovascular conditions that may lead to HF and what can be done to prevent the development of HF in each condition.

Cardiovascular Condition Leading to HF	Preventive Measures

20. What assessment findings indicate that treatment of HF has been successful?
    a. Weight loss and diuresis
    b. Warm skin and less fatigue
    c. Clear lung sounds and decreased HR
    d. Absence of chest pain and improved level of consciousness (LOC)

21. Which statement by the patient with chronic HF would cause the nurse to determine that additional discharge teaching is needed?
    a. "I will call my health clinic if I wake up breathless at night."
    b. "I will look for sodium content on labels of foods and over-the-counter medicines."
    c. "I plan to organize my household tasks so I don't have to constantly go up and down the stairs."
    d. "I should weigh myself every morning and go on a diet if I gain more than 2 or 3 pounds in 2 days."

22. The evaluation team for cardiac transplantation is evaluating patients. Which patient is most likely to receive the greatest benefit from a new heart?
    a. A 24-year-old man with Down syndrome who has received excellent care from parents in their 60s
    b. A 46-year-old single woman with a limited support system who has alcohol-induced cardiomyopathy
    c. A 60-year-old man with inoperable CAD who has not been compliant with lifestyle changes and rehabilitation programs
    d. A 52-year-old woman with end-stage CAD who has limited financial resources but is emotionally stable and has strong social support

23. When planning long-term goals for the patient who had a heart transplant, what would the nurse consider is the most common cause of death in heart transplant patients during the first year?
    a. Infection
    b. HF
    c. Embolization
    d. Malignant conditions

24. A patient with which disorder would benefit most from the use of the intraaortic balloon pump (IABP)?
    a. An insufficient aortic valve
    b. A dissecting thoracic aortic aneurysm
    c. Generalized peripheral vascular disease
    d. Acute myocardial infarction (MI) with cardiogenic shock

25. Which statement about the function of the IABP is accurate?
    a. Deflation of the balloon allows the HR to increase.
    b. A primary effect of the IABP is increased systolic blood pressure.
    c. The rapid deflation of the intraaortic balloon causes a decreased preload.
    d. During intraaortic counterpulsation, the balloon is inflated during diastole.

26. What would the nurse do to prevent arterial trauma during the use of the IABP?
    a. Reposition the patient every 2 hours.
    b. Check the site for bleeding every hour.
    c. Prevent hip flexion of the cannulated leg.
    d. Cover the insertion site with an occlusive dressing.

27. A patient who is hemodynamically stable has an order to wean the IABP. How would the nurse accomplish this?
    a. Decrease the augmentation pressure to zero.
    b. Stop the machine since hemodynamic parameters are satisfactory.
    c. Stop the infusion flow through the catheter when weaning is initiated.
    d. Change the pumping ratio from 1 : 1 to 1 : 2 or 1 : 3 until the balloon is removed.

28. What are ventricular assist devices (VADs) designed to do for the patient? **Select all that apply.**
    a. To support a patient with renal failure or liver failure unrelated to a cardiac event
    b. Support circulation when patients cannot be weaned from cardiopulmonary bypass
    c. Partially or totally support circulation temporarily until a donor heart can be obtained
    d. Provide permanent, total circulatory support for a patient with limited life expectancy
    e. Reverse the effects of circulatory failure in patients with acute MI in cardiogenic shock

---

CASE STUDY Acute Decompensated Heart Failure

(Ljupco/iStock/ Thinkstock)

Patient Profile

L.J. is a 63-year-old man who has a history of hypertension, chronic HF, and sleep apnea. He has been smoking 2 packs of cigarettes a day for 40 years and has refused to quit. Three days ago, he had an onset of flu with fever, pharyngitis, and malaise. He has not taken his antihypertensive medications or his medications to control his HF for 4 days. Today he has been admitted to the hospital intensive care unit with ADHF.

Subjective Data
- Is very anxious and asks, "Am I going to die?"
- Denies pain but says that he feels like he cannot get enough air
- Says his heart feels like it is "running away"
- After being weighed, he reports, "That is more than I usually weigh."
- Reports that he is so exhausted he can't eat or drink by himself

Objective Data
- Height: 5 ft 10 in (175 cm)
- Weight: 210 lbs (95.5 kg)
- Vital signs: Temp 99.6°F (37.6°C), HR 118 beats/min and irregular, RR 34, BP 90/58 mm Hg
- Cardiovascular: Distant S_1, S_2; S_3, S_4 present; point of maximal impulse (PMI) at sixth intercostal space (ICS) and faint; bilateral jugular vein distention; all peripheral pulses are 1 + and there is peripheral edema; initial cardiac monitoring indicates atrial fibrillation with a ventricular rate of 132 beats/min
- Respiratory: Pulmonary crackles, decreased breath sounds right lower lobe, coughing frothy, blood-tinged sputum; SpO_2 82% on room air
- Gastrointestinal: Bowel sounds present; hepatomegaly 4 cm below costal margin
- Laboratory work and diagnostic testing are scheduled

Questions

1. What clinical manifestations of right-sided and left-sided HF is L.J. experiencing?

Use an X to indicate whether the assessment finding is a manifestation of <u>Right-sided HF</u>, <u>Left-sided HF</u>, <u>Both</u> right-sided and left-sided HF or <u>Unrelated</u> to heart failure.

Assessment Finding	Right-sided HF	Left-sided HF	Both	Unrelated
JVD				
Weight gain				
Pharyngitis				
Dyspnea				
Peripheral edema				
PMI displacement				
Hepatomegaly				
HR 118 beats/min				
BP 90/58 mm Hg				
Sleep apnea				
SpO$_2$ 82%				
Blood-tinged frothy sputum				

2. What nursing interventions are appropriate for L.J. at the time of his admission?

Use an X to indicate if the nursing action is <u>Indicated</u> (necessary or appropriate), <u>Contraindicated</u> (could be harmful), or <u>Non-Essential</u> (makes no difference or is unnecessary).

Nursing Action	Indicated	Contraindicated	Non-Essential
Obtain a 12-lead ECG			
Facilitate an echocardiogram			
Offer ice chips			
Administer oxygen			
Place the patient in the supine position with legs raised			
Administer furosemide 20 mg IV			
Place sequential compression devices on BLE			
Administer 0.4 mg nitroglycerin SL			
Insert an indwelling urinary catheter			

3. L.J has been prescribed the following medications to improve his condition.

Choose the most likely options for the information missing from the table by selecting from the lists of options provided.

Drug	Dose, Route, Frequency	Drug Class	Indication
1	1 mg PO once daily	Loop diuretic	4
Metoprolol	2	β-Adrenergic blocker	Reverses cardiac remodeling
Benazepril	6	3	Decreases afterload
Digoxin	0.25 mg PO once daily	7	8
5	150 mg PO twice daily	Anticoagulant	Atrial fibrillation

Options for 1 and 5	Options for 2 and 6	Options for 3 and 7	Options for 4 and 8
Bumetanide	150 mg PO twice daily	Angiotensin receptor blockade	Reverses cardiac remodeling
Dabigatran	50 mg PO once daily	Cardiac glycoside	Atrial fibrillation
Benazepril	0.25 mg PO once daily	Loop diuretic	Decreases afterload
Digoxin	1 mg PO once daily	β-Adrenergic blocker	Positive inotrope
Metoprolol	5 mg PO once daily	ACE inhibitor	Decreases preload
Valsartan	40 mg PO twice daily	Anticoagulant	Vasodilates

4. What assessment findings indicate treatment has been effective in improving L.J.'s heart failure?

For each assessment finding, use an X to indicate whether the interventions were <u>Effective</u> (helped to meet expected outcomes), <u>Ineffective</u> (did not help to meet expected outcomes), or <u>Unrelated</u> (not related to the expected outcomes).

Assessment Finding	Effective	Ineffective	Unrelated
EF 55%			
CVP 12 mm Hg			
MAP 55 mm Hg			
Urine output 100 mL/hr			
Temperature 99.0°F (37.2°C)			
Creatinine 2.5			
PAWP 8 mm Hg			
SVR 1000 dynes/sec/cm^5			
Normal skin turgor			

5. What information would the nurse include in L.J.'s discharge teaching? **Select all that apply.**

_____A. Read food labels to reduce sodium in your diet.

_____B. Restrict the amount of sodium to 2500 mg per day.

_____C. Weigh yourself daily and report weight gain > 3–5 lbs. in a week.

_____D. Get an annual influenza vaccine.

_____E. Restrict your activity level to walking around the house.

_____F. Quit smoking all tobacco products.

_____G. You can try vaping to offset the nicotine craving.

_____H. Implement methods to reduce stress.

1. What accurately describes electrocardiographic (ECG) monitoring?
   a. Depolarization of the cells in the ventricles produces the T wave on the ECG.
   b. An abnormal cardiac impulse that arises in the atria, ventricles, or atrioventricular (AV) junction can create a premature beat that is known as "an artifact."
   c. Lead placement for V_1 includes 1 lead each for right arm, right leg, left arm, and left leg with the fifth lead on the fourth intercostal space to the right of the sternal border.
   d. If the sinoatrial (SA) node fails to discharge an impulse or discharges very slowly, a secondary pacemaker in the AV node is able to discharge at a rate of 30 to 40 times per minute.

2. What accurately describes the PR interval? **Select all that apply.**
   a. 0.16 seconds
   b. < 0.12 seconds
   c. 0.06 to 0.12 seconds
   d. 0.12 to 0.20 seconds
   e. Time of depolarization and repolarization of ventricles
   f. Measured from beginning of P wave to beginning of QRS complex

3. A patient with a regular heart rate (HR) has 4 QRS complexes between every 3-second marker on the ECG paper. Calculate the patient's HR.
   _____bpm

4. The ECG pattern of a patient with a regular HR reveals 20 small squares between each R-R interval. What is the patient's HR?
   _____bpm

5. What describes the SA node's ability to discharge an electrical impulse spontaneously?
   a. Excitability
   b. Contractility
   c. Conductivity
   d. Automaticity

6. What describes the refractory phase?
   a. Abnormal electrical impulses
   b. Period in which heart tissue cannot be stimulated
   c. Areas of the heart do not repolarize at the same rate because of depressed conduction
   d. Sodium migrates rapidly into the cell, so it is positive compared to the outside of the cell

7. The patient's PR interval comprises 6 small boxes on the ECG graph. What does the nurse determine that this indicates?
   a. A normal finding
   b. A problem with ventricular depolarization
   c. A disturbance in the repolarization of the atria
   d. A problem with conduction from the SA node to the ventricular cells

8. The nurse plans close monitoring for the patient during electrophysiologic study (EPS) because this study
   a. requires the use of dyes that irritate the myocardium.
   b. causes myocardial ischemia, resulting in dysrhythmias.
   c. involves the use of anticoagulants to prevent thrombus and embolism.
   d. induces dysrhythmias that may require cardioversion or defibrillation to correct.

9. How would the nurse interpret the ECG rhythm strip with a regular PR interval but a blocked QRS complex?
   a. Asystole
   b. Atrial fibrillation
   c. First-degree AV block
   d. Type II second-degree AV block

10. After defibrillation, the advanced cardiac life support (ACLS) nurse says that the patient has pulseless electrical activity (PEA). What is most important for the nurse to understand about this rhythm?
    a. The HR is 40 to 60 bpm.
    b. Hypoxemia and hypervolemia are common with PEA.
    c. There is dissociated activity of the ventricle and atrium.
    d. There is electrical activity with no mechanical response.

11. The nurse is evaluating the telemetry ECG rhythm strip. How would the nurse document the distorted P wave causing an irregular rhythm?
    a. Atrial flutter
    b. Sinus bradycardia
    c. Premature atrial contraction (PAC)
    d. Paroxysmal supraventricular tachycardia (PSVT)

12. A patient with an acute myocardial infarction (MI) develops the following ECG pattern: atrial rate of 82 bpm and regular; ventricular rate of 46 bpm and regular; P wave and QRS complex are normal but there is no relationship between the P wave and the QRS complex. How would the nurse interpret this dysrhythmia and what treatment is expected?
    a. Sinus bradycardia treated with atropine
    b. Third-degree heart block treated with a pacemaker
    c. Atrial fibrillation treated with electrical cardioversion
    d. Type I second-degree AV block treated with observation

13. Which rhythm abnormality has an *increased* risk of ventricular tachycardia and ventricular fibrillation?
    a. PAC
    b. Premature ventricular contraction (PVC) on the T wave
    c. Accelerated idioventricular rhythm
    d. PVC couplet

14. A patient with an acute MI has sinus tachycardia of 126 bpm. The nurse recognizes that if this dysrhythmia is not treated, what is the *worst* thing the patient is likely to experience?
    a. Hypertension
    b. Escape rhythms
    c. Ventricular tachycardia
    d. An increase in infarct size

15. A patient with no history of heart disease has a rhythm strip that shows an occasional distorted P wave followed by normal AV and ventricular conduction. About what would the nurse question the patient?
    a. The use of caffeine
    b. The use of sedatives
    c. Any aerobic training
    d. Holding of breath during exertion

16. A patient's rhythm strip indicates a normal HR and rhythm with normal P waves and QRS complexes, but the PR interval is 0.26 second. What is the most appropriate action by the nurse?
    a. Continue to assess the patient.
    b. Administer atropine per protocol.
    c. Prepare the patient for synchronized cardioversion.
    d. Prepare the patient for placement of a temporary pacemaker.

17. In the patient with a dysrhythmia, which assessment indicates decreased cardiac output (CO)?
    a. Hypertension and bradycardia
    b. Chest pain and decreased mentation
    c. Abdominal distention and hepatomegaly
    d. Bounding pulses and a ventricular heave

18. A patient with an acute MI is having multifocal PVCs and couplets. He is alert and has a BP reading of 118/78 mm Hg with an irregular pulse of 86 beats/min. What is the priority nursing action at this time?
    a. Continue to assess the patient.
    b. Ask the patient to perform Valsalva maneuver.
    c. Prepare to administer antidysrhythmic drugs per protocol.
    d. Be prepared to administer cardiopulmonary resuscitation (CPR).

19. Which rhythm pattern finding is indicative of PVCs?
    a. A QRS complex > 0.12 second followed by a P wave
    b. Continuous wide QRS complexes with a ventricular rate of 160 bpm
    c. P waves hidden in QRS complexes with a regular rhythm of 120 bpm
    d. Saw-toothed P waves with no measurable PR interval and an irregular rhythm

20. In the patient experiencing ventricular fibrillation (VF), what is the rationale for using defibrillation?
    a. Enhance repolarization and relaxation of ventricular myocardial cells
    b. Provide an electrical impulse that stimulates normal myocardial contractions
    c. Depolarize the cells of the myocardium to allow the SA node to resume pacemaker function
    d. Deliver an electrical impulse to the heart at the time of ventricular contraction to convert the heart to a sinus rhythm

21. What action is included in the nurse's responsibilities in preparing to administer defibrillation?
    a. Applying gel pads to the patient's chest
    b. Setting the defibrillator to deliver 50 joules
    c. Setting the defibrillator to a synchronized mode
    d. Sedating the patient with midazolam before defibrillation

22. While providing discharge instructions to the patient who had an implantable cardioverter-defibrillator (ICD) inserted, what would the nurse teach the patient is most important to do if the ICD fires?
    a. Lie down.
    b. Call the cardiologist.
    c. Push the reset button on the pulse generator.
    d. Immediately take a dose of their antidysrhythmic medication.

23. A patient with a sinus node dysfunction has a permanent pacemaker inserted. Before discharge, what would the nurse include when teaching the patient?
    a. Avoid cooking with microwave ovens.
    b. Avoid standing near antitheft devices in doorways.
    c. Use mild analgesics to control the chest spasms caused by the pacing current.
    d. Start lifting the arm above the shoulder right away to prevent a "frozen shoulder."

24. A patient on the telemetry unit goes into VF and is unresponsive. Following initiation of the emergency call system (Code Blue), what would the nurse do next?
    a. Begin CPR.
    b. Get the crash cart.
    c. Administer amiodarone IV.
    d. Defibrillate with 360 joules.

25. The use of radiofrequency catheter ablation therapy to "burn" areas of the cardiac conduction system is indicated for the treatment of which problem?
    a. Sinus arrest
    b. Heart blocks
    c. Tachydysrhythmias
    d. Premature ventricular beats

26. A patient with chest pain that is unrelieved by nitroglycerin is admitted to the coronary care unit for observation and diagnosis. While the patient has continuous ECG monitoring, what finding would most concern the nurse?
    a. Occasional PVCs
    b. QRS complex change
    c. ST segment elevation
    d. A PR interval of 0.18 second

27. A 54-year-old patient who has no structural heart disease has an episode of syncope. A head-up tilt-test is performed to rule out cardioneurogenic syncope. What will the patient experience if cardioneurogenic syncope is the problem?
    a. No change in HR or BP
    b. Palpitations and dizziness
    c. Tachydysrhythmias and chest pain
    d. Marked bradycardia and hypotension

28. The patient is brought to the emergency department with acute coronary syndrome (ACS). What changes would the nurse expect to see on the ECG if only myocardial injury has occurred?
    a. Absent P wave
    b. A wide QT interval
    c. Tall, peaked T wave
    d. ST-segment elevation

29. Identify the following cardiac rhythms using the systematic approach to assessing cardiac rhythms found in Table 39.3 and information in Table 39.7 in the textbook. All rhythm strips are 6 seconds.

a.

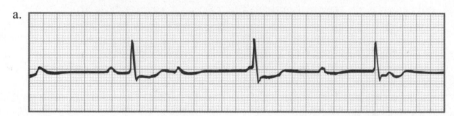

b.

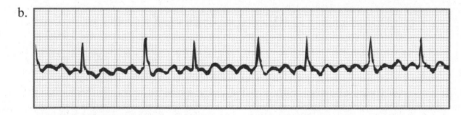

c.

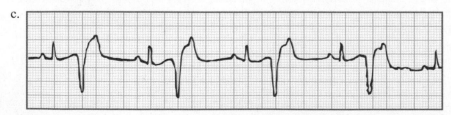

d.

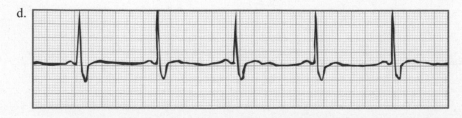

e.

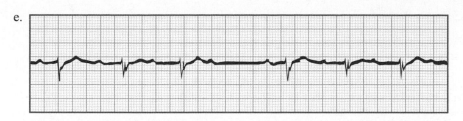

f.

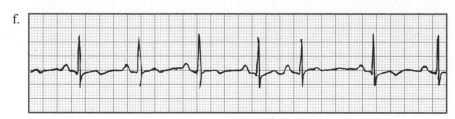

g.

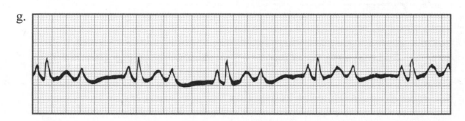

h.

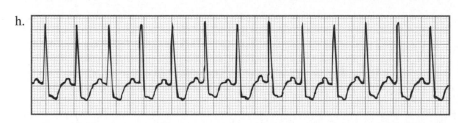

i.

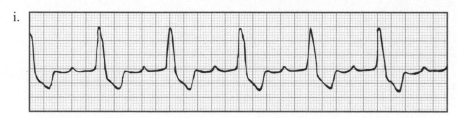

j.

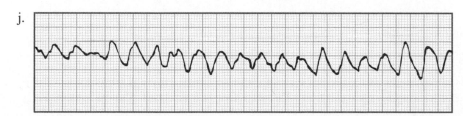

k.

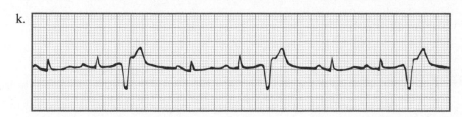

l.

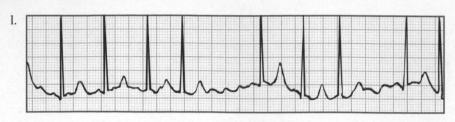

m.

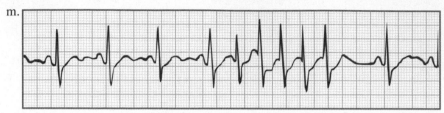

n.

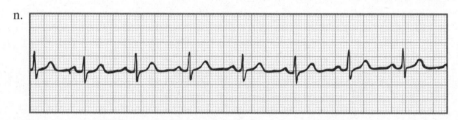

o.

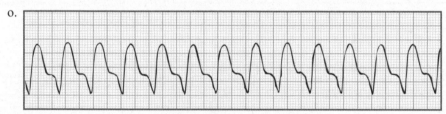

CASE STUDY   Dysrhythmia

(Dmitry Berkut/
iStock/Thinkstock)

Patient Profile
R.S. is a 78-year-old woman who is admitted to the telemetry unit with a diagnosis of new-onset atrial fibrillation.

Subjective Data
- Has a history of hypothyroidism and hypertension
- Has no history of atrial fibrillation
- Is taking levothyroxine (Synthroid) and enalapril (Vasotec)
- Reports palpitations, dizziness, shortness of breath, and mild chest pressure
- Has been drinking more coffee since her husband died last month

Objective Data
Physical Examination
- Alert, anxious, older woman
- Vital signs: BP 100/70 mm Hg, HR 150 beats/min, RR 32 breaths/min
- Lungs: bibasilar crackles
- Heart: S_1 and S_2, irregular

Diagnostic Study
- 12-lead ECG: atrial fibrillation with an uncontrolled ventricular response

Interprofessional Care
- Continuous ECG monitoring
- Discontinue enalapril (Vasotec)
- IV diltiazem (Cardizem) bolus and then IV infusion
- Digoxin
- Enoxaparin (Lovenox)
- Warfarin (Coumadin)

Questions

1. What nursing interventions would be included in the initial management of R.S.? **Use an X to indicate whether the nursing actions below are Anticipated (appropriate or likely necessary), Contraindicated (could be harmful), or Non-essential (makes no difference or is unnecessary).**

Nursing Action	Anticipated	Contraindicated	Non-Essential
Ambulate the patient to the bathroom			
Apply oxygen via simple mask			
Facilitate an echocardiogram			
Draw cardiac enzymes			
Administer 1 mg atropine			
Position the head of bed at 45 degrees			
Administer 500 mL 0.9% normal saline bolus			

2. Indicate which nursing action listed in the far-left column is appropriate for each potential complication. Note that not all actions will be used.

Nursing Action	Potential Complication	Appropriate Nursing Action for Potential Complication
12-lead ECG	Pulmonary edema	
Incentive spirometer 10x per hour	Angina	
Chest x-ray	Embolus	
Furosemide 20 mg IV		
Nitroglycerin 0.4 mg SL		
Warfarin 5 mg PO		
Perform a neurological assessment every hour.		

3. R.S. is scheduled for electrical cardioversion. What nursing actions would the nurse perform when preparing, assisting, and recovering R.S.? **Select all that apply.**
_____A. Establish IV access
_____B. Apply multifunction pads attached to the defibrillator
_____C. Make sure synchronization is turned off
_____D. Set the defibrillator machine to 150 joules
_____E. Assess the skin for burns
_____F. Administer PO sedation as ordered
_____G. Make sure all health care personnel are clear before discharging the energy
_____H. Have the patient void before the procedure
_____I. If the patient remains in atrial fibrillation, start CPR

4. What findings would indicate that therapies, including medications and cardioversion, were effective? **For each assessment finding, use an X to indicate whether the interventions were Effective (helped to meet expected outcomes), Ineffective (did not help to meet expected outcome), or Unrelated (not related to the expected outcomes).**

Assessment finding	Effective	Ineffective	Unrelated
HR 98 beats/min			
Rhythm is irregular			
Patient is oriented x3			
Breath sounds are clear			
Urine output is 100 mL/hr			
Patient reports palpitations			
Patient stands at the bedside without dizziness			

5. Choose the most likely options for the information missing from the table below by selecting from the lists of options provided.

Medication	Dose, Route, Frequency	Drug Class	Indication
Levothyroxine	2	Synthetic thyroid hormone replacement	hypothyroidism
1	0.25 mg IV once daily	Cardiac glycoside	Atrial fibrillation
Enalapril	10 mg PO once daily	6	hypertension
Diltiazem	4	Calcium channel blocker	3
5	40 mg SQ every 12 hours	7	Risk of thrombus secondary to atrial fibrillation

Options for 1 and 5	Options for 2 and 4	Options for 3	Options for 6 and 7
Levothyroxine	40 mg SQ every 12 hours	Hypothyroidism	Loop diuretic
Enalapril	125 mcg once daily	Pulmonary edema	Calcium channel blocker
Diltiazem	0.25 mg/kg IV once	Hypertension	Anticoagulant
Digoxin	0.25 mg IV once	Heart rate control	ACE inhibitor
Enoxaparin	20 mg once daily	Atrial fibrillation	Cardiac glycoside
Furosemide	10 mg PO once daily	Thrombus risk	Synthetic hormone

Inflammatory and Structural Heart Disorders

1. A 20-year-old patient has acute infective endocarditis. What topics would the nurse ask the patient about during the health history? **Select all that apply.**
   a. Renal dialysis
   b. IV drug use
   c. Recent dental work
   d. Cardiac catheterization
   e. Recent urinary tract infection

2. A patient has an admitting diagnosis of acute left-sided infective endocarditis. What is the best test to confirm this diagnosis?
   a. Three blood cultures
   b. Complete blood count
   c. Cardiac catheterization
   d. Transesophageal echocardiogram

3. Which manifestation of infective endocarditis is a result of fragmentation and microembolization of vegetative lesions?
   a. Petechiae
   b. Roth's spots
   c. Osler's nodes
   d. Splinter hemorrhages

4. Which statement describes Janeway's lesions as manifestations of infective endocarditis?
   a. Hemorrhagic retinal lesions
   b. Black longitudinal streaks in nail beds
   c. Painful red or purple lesions on fingers or toes
   d. Flat, red, painless spots on the palm of hands and soles of feet

5. A patient with infective endocarditis of a prosthetic mitral valve develops left hemiparesis and vision changes. What would the nurse expect to be included in interprofessional care?
   a. Embolectomy
   b. Surgical valve replacement
   c. Administration of anticoagulants
   d. Higher-than-usual antibiotic dosages

6. A patient with aortic valve endocarditis develops dyspnea, crackles in the lungs, and restlessness. What complication would the nurse suspect?
   a. Pulmonary embolization from valve vegetations
   b. Vegetative embolization to the coronary arteries
   c. Valvular incompetence with resulting heart failure
   d. Nonspecific manifestations that accompany infectious diseases

7. A patient hospitalized for 1 week with subacute infective endocarditis is afebrile and has no signs of heart damage. Discharge with outpatient antibiotic therapy is planned. During discharge planning with the patient, what is it most important for the nurse to do?
   a. Plan how his needs will be met while he continues on bed rest.
   b. Encourage the use of diversional activities to relieve boredom and restlessness.
   c. Teach the patient to avoid crowds and exposure to upper respiratory infections.
   d. Assess the patient's home environment in terms of family assistance and hospital access.

8. What would the nurse teach the patient who has endocarditis about preventing recurrence of the infection?
   a. Start on antibiotic therapy when exposed to persons with infections.
   b. Take one aspirin a day to prevent vegetative lesions from forming around the valves.
   c. Always maintain continuous antibiotic therapy to prevent the development of any systemic infection.
   d. Obtain prophylactic antibiotic therapy before certain invasive medical or dental procedures (e.g., dental cleaning).

9. A patient is admitted to the hospital with a suspected acute pericarditis. What is the best method for the nurse to use when assessing for the presence of a pericardial friction rub?
   a. Timing the sounds with the respiratory pattern
   b. Place the bell of the stethoscope at the apical area of the heart
   c. Use the diaphragm of the stethoscope to auscultate for a high-pitched continuous rumbling sound
   d. Place the stethoscope at the lower left sternal border, patient leaning forward and holding breath

10. A patient with acute pericarditis has markedly distended jugular veins, decreased BP, tachycardia, tachypnea, and muffled heart sounds. What does the nurse recognize as the cause of these manifestations?
    a. The pericardial space is obliterated with scar tissue and thickened pericardium.
    b. Excess pericardial fluid compresses the heart and prevents adequate diastolic filling.
    c. The parietal and visceral pericardial membranes adhere to each other, preventing normal myocardial contraction
    d. Fibrin accumulation on the visceral pericardium infiltrates the myocardium, creating myocardial dysfunction.

11. Which statements explain the measurement of pulsus paradoxus with cardiac tamponade? **Select all that apply.**
    a. A difference of < 10 mm Hg occurs.
    b. A difference of > 10 mm Hg occurs.
    c. It is measured with an automatic sphygmomanometer.
    d. Rapidly inflate the cuff until you hear sounds throughout the respiratory cycle.
    e. Subtract the number when sounds are heard in the respiratory cycle from the number when the first Korotkoff sound during expiration is heard.

12. The patient with acute pericarditis is having a pericardiocentesis. What complication would the nurse monitor the patient for after surgery?
    a. Pneumonia
    b. Pneumothorax
    c. Myocardial infarction (MI)
    d. Cerebrovascular accident (CVA)

13. A patient with acute pericarditis has pain from pericardial inflammation. What is the best nursing intervention for the patient?
    a. Administer opioids as prescribed on a round-the-clock schedule.
    b. Promote progressive relaxation exercises with the use of deep, slow breathing.
    c. Position the patient on the right side with the head of the bed elevated 15 degrees.
    d. Position the patient in Fowler's position with a padded table for the patient to lean on.

14. When obtaining a nursing history for a patient with myocarditis, what would the nurse question the patient about?
    a. Prior use of digoxin for treatment of cardiac problems
    b. Recent symptoms of a viral illness, such as fever and malaise
    c. A history of coronary artery disease (CAD) with or without an MI
    d. A recent streptococcal infection requiring treatment with penicillin

15. What is the most important role of the nurse in preventing rheumatic fever?
    a. Teach patients with infective endocarditis to adhere to antibiotic prophylaxis.
    b. Identify patients with valvular heart disease who are at risk for rheumatic fever.
    c. Encourage the use of antibiotics for treatment of all infections involving a sore throat.
    d. Promote the early diagnosis and immediate treatment of group A streptococcal pharyngitis.

16. What manifestations strongly support a diagnosis of acute rheumatic fever?
    a. Carditis, polyarthritis, and erythema marginatum
    b. Polyarthritis, chorea, and decreased antistreptolysin-O titer
    c. Organic heart murmurs, fever, and elevated erythrocyte sedimentation rate (ESR)
    d. Positive C-reactive protein, elevated white blood cells (WBCs), and subcutaneous nodules

17. When teaching the patient with acute rheumatic fever, identify the rationale for the use of each drug in the patient's treatment plan.

Drug	Rationale for Use
Antibiotics	
Aspirin	
Corticosteroids	
Nonsteroidal antiinflammatory drugs (NSAIDs)	

18. A patient with rheumatic heart disease with carditis asks the nurse how long activity will be restricted. What is the best answer by the nurse?
    a. "Full activity will be allowed as soon as acute symptoms have subsided."
    b. "Bed rest will be continued until symptoms of heart failure are controlled."
    c. "Nonstrenuous activities can be performed as soon as antibiotics are started."
    d. "Bed rest must be maintained until antiinflammatory therapy has been discontinued."

19. What effect does valvular regurgitation have on a patient?
    a. It causes a pressure gradient difference across an open valve.
    b. A pericardial friction rub is heard on the right sternal border of the chest.
    c. It leads to decreased flow of blood and hypertrophy of the preceding chamber.
    d. There is a backward flow of blood and volume overload in the preceding chamber.

20. A registered nurse (RN) is working with a licensed practical nurse/licensed vocational nurse (LPN/VN) in caring for a group of patients on a cardiac telemetry unit. Which nursing activity could be delegated to the LPN?
    a. Explain the reason for planning frequent periods of rest.
    b. Evaluate the patient's understanding of his disease process.
    c. Monitor BP, heart rate (HR), respiratory rate (RR), and arterial oxygen saturation by pulse oximetry (SpO$_2$) before, during, and after ambulation.
    d. Teach the patient which activities to choose that will gradually increase endurance.

21. Which statement accurately describes mitral valve prolapse?
    a. Rapid onset prevents left chamber dilation
    b. May be caused by pulmonary hypertension
    c. Buckling of valve into left atrium during ventricular systole
    d. Rapid development of pulmonary edema and cardiogenic shock

22. Which cardiac valve disorder causes a sudden onset of cardiovascular collapse?
    a. Mitral valve stenosis
    b. Tricuspid valve disease
    c. Pulmonic valve stenosis
    d. Acute aortic regurgitation

23. The patient is admitted with angina, syncope, and dyspnea on exertion. During the assessment, the nurse auscultates a systolic murmur with a prominent S_4. What does the nurse consider as the cause?
    a. Mitral valve stenosis
    b. Aortic valve stenosis
    c. Acute mitral valve regurgitation
    d. Chronic mitral valve regurgitation

24. Which drugs would the nurse expect to be prescribed for patients with a mechanical valve replacement?
    a. Oral nitrates
    b. Anticoagulants
    c. Atrial antidysrhythmics
    d. β-adrenergic blocking agents

25. A patient with symptomatic mitral valve prolapse has atrial and ventricular dysrhythmias. In addition to monitoring for decreased cardiac output related to the dysrhythmias, what is an important nursing intervention related to the dysrhythmias?
    a. Monitor breathing pattern related to hypervolemia.
    b. Encourage calling for assistance when getting out of bed.
    c. Give sleeping pills to decrease paroxysmal nocturnal dyspnea.
    d. Teach the patient exercises to prevent recurrence of dysrhythmias.

26. Which patients would the nurse expect to be scheduled for percutaneous transluminal balloon valvuloplasty?
    a. Any patient with aortic regurgitation
    b. Older patients with aortic regurgitation
    c. Older patients with stenosis of any valve
    d. Young adult patients with mild mitral valve stenosis

27. A patient is scheduled for an open surgical valvuloplasty of the mitral valve. What information about this surgery would the nurse use to plan care?
    a. Cardiopulmonary bypass is not required with this procedure.
    b. Valve repair is a palliative measure, while valve replacement is curative.
    c. The operative mortality rate is lower in valve repair than in valve replacement.
    d. Patients with valve repair do not need postoperative anticoagulation as do those who have valve replacement.

28. In which patient would a mechanical prosthetic valve be preferred over a biologic valve for valve replacement?
    a. 41-year-old man with peptic ulcer disease
    b. 22-year-old woman who wants to have children
    c. 35-year-old man with a history of seasonal asthma
    d. 62-year-old woman with early Alzheimer's disease

29. Which statement by a patient after mechanical valve replacement indicates to the nurse that further instruction is needed?
    a. "I may begin an exercise program to gradually increase my cardiac tolerance."
    b. "I will always need to have my blood checked once a month for its clotting function."
    c. "I will take prophylactic antibiotics before I have dental or invasive medical procedures."
    d. "The biggest risk I have during invasive health procedures is bleeding because of my anticoagulants."

30. A patient is admitted with symptoms of cardiomyopathy (CMP) following radiation therapy. Which type of CMP would the nurse suspect?
    a. Dilated
    b. Restrictive
    c. Takotsubo
    d. Hypertrophic

31. Which statements accurately describe dilated CMP? **Select all that apply.**
    a. Characterized by ventricular stiffness
    b. The least common type of CMP
    c. The hyperdynamic systolic function creates a diastolic failure
    d. Echocardiogram reveals cardiomegaly with thin ventricular walls
    e. Often follows an infective myocarditis or exposure to toxins or drugs
    f. Differs from chronic heart failure in that there is no ventricular hypertrophy

32. What would the nurse include when planning care for the patient with hypertrophic CMP?
    a. Ventricular pacing
    b. Administration of vasodilators
    c. Teach the patient to avoid strenuous activity and dehydration
    d. Surgery for cardiac transplantation will have to be done soon

33. When providing discharge teaching for any patient with CMP, what would the nurse teach the patient to do? **Select all that apply.**
    a. Eat a low-sodium diet.
    b. Go to the gym every day.
    c. Engage in stress reduction activities.
    d. Abstain from alcohol and caffeine intake.
    e. Avoid strenuous activity and allow for periods of rest.
    f. Suggest that caregivers learn cardiopulmonary resuscitation (CPR).

CASE STUDY Infective Endocarditis

Patient Profile

N.B. is a 60-year-old man who is hospitalized with a suspected stroke.

(Michael Blann/
Photodisc/
Thinkstock)

Subjective Data
- Laparoscopic cholecystectomy a few weeks ago
- Reports 6 out of 10 chest pain

Objective Data
- Neurologic signs typical of a stroke (paralysis on right side involving right arm and leg, slurred speech)
- Petechiae over the chest
- Crescendo-decrescendo murmur present
- Vital signs: HR 101 beats/min, RR 26 breaths/min, BP 105/66 mm Hg, SpO$_2$ 96% on 4 L/min nasal cannula, Temp: 103°F (39.4°C)

Questions
1. The following diagnostic tests were ordered.

Highlight or place a check mark next to the findings that require the nurse to follow-up.

Diagnostic Test	Results
Blood cultures	No growth
C-reactive protein	Increased
Echocardiogram	Vegetation on aortic valve
Chest x-ray	No signs of infiltrates or consolidation, cardiac silhouette normal
12-lead EKG	2nd degree Type II AV block
WBC	12800/µL
Neutrophils	8500/mm^3
Hemoglobin	10.5 g/dL
Platelet count	250,000/mm^3

Diagnostic Test	Results
Serum lactate	20 mg/dL
Serum potassium	4.7 mEq/L
Creatinine	1.5 mg/dL
BUN	20 mg/dL
Troponins	0.25 ng/mL

2. What clinical problems would the nurse include when planning interventions?

Indicate which nursing intervention in the left column is appropriate for the clinical problem. Note that not all nursing interventions will be used.

Nursing Intervention	Clinical Problem	Appropriate Nursing Intervention for Clinical Problem
Every 2-hour turning schedule while on bedrest	Hyperthermia	
Administer antibiotics as ordered	Infection	
Advocate for a physical therapy consult	Impaired mobility	
Administer acetaminophen 650 mg PR q. 8 hours PRN		
Obtain a dietary consult		
Monitor temperature every 4 hours		
Apply sequential compression devices		
Administer 500 mL 0.9% normal saline bolus		
Obtain blood glucose before meals		

3. **Choose the most likely options for the information missing from the statements below by selecting from the lists of options provided.**

The microorganism that causes infective endocarditis in about 50% of the cases is _____**1**_____. The petechiae on N.B.'s chest is caused by _____**2**_____. If the aortic valve is involved, the nurse may assess _____**3**_____ during the physical assessment. Most patients present with _____**3**_____. Approximately _____**4**_____ of patients with infective endocarditis will need valve replacement surgery. Left-sided vegetations can cause _____**5**_____, _____**5**_____, and ____**5**_____ while right-sided vegetations can cause _____**5**_____.

Options for 1	Options for 2	Options for 3
Eikenella	Bacteremia	Pericardial friction rub
Haemophilus	Vegetations	ST segment elevation
Streptococcus viridans	Pericardial effusions	Murmurs
Staphylococcus aureus	Microthrombi	Janeway's lesions
Actinobacillus	Hemorrhage	Fever
Cardiobacterium	Pulmonary hypertension	Osler's nodes

Options for 4	Options for 5
10.5%	Renal failure
55%	Liver failure
90%	Cerebrovascular accident
30%	Myocardial infarction
75%	Limb infarction
25%	Pulmonary emboli

4. **For each assessment finding, use an X to indicate whether the implemented interventions by the nurse were Effective (helped to meet expected outcomes), Ineffective (did not help to meet expected outcomes), or Unrelated (not related to the expected outcomes).**

Assessment Finding	Effective	Ineffective	Unrelated
Temperature 37.9°C			
Urine output > 1 mL/kg/hour			
Positive Trousseau sign			
Crackles auscultated in bilateral bases			
Respiratory rate 18 breaths/min			
Bilateral lower extremities cool and pale with > 3 sec capillary refill			
Urine ketones are negative			

5. What would the nurse include when doing discharge teaching with N.B.? **Select all that apply.**

_____A. "You would be on complete bedrest, unless using the bathroom."

_____B. "You need to report any difficulty breathing to your health care provider."

_____C. "Notify your health care provider if you have signs of a cold."

_____D. "You will be prescribed nitroglycerin tablets to treat chest pain."

_____E. "You would wear elastic compression stockings, like TED hose."

_____F. "You would restrict your fluid intake to 1000 mL/day."

_____G. "You do not need to share your medical condition with other health care providers, like your dentist."

_____H. "It is a good idea to wear a mask when in public or group settings."

41

Vascular Disorders

1. When obtaining a health history from a 72-year-old man with peripheral arterial disease (PAD) of the lower extremities, which condition would the nurse consider is related?
   a. Venous thrombosis
   b. Venous stasis ulcers
   c. Pulmonary embolism
   d. Coronary artery disease (CAD)

2. A 45-year-old patient with chronic arterial disease has a brachial systolic blood pressure (SBP) of 132 mm Hg and an ankle SBP of 102 mm Hg.

   What is the ankle-brachial index? _____

   What does this ankle-brachial index indicate? (mild/moderate/severe arterial disease) _____
   _____.

3. Following teaching about medications for PAD, the nurse determines that additional instruction is needed when the patient states:
   a. "I can take 1 aspirin a day to prevent clotting in my legs."
   b. "The lisinopril I use for my blood pressure may help me walk further without pain."
   c. "I will need to have frequent blood tests to evaluate the effect of the pentoxifylline I will be taking."
   d. "Cilostazol will help me increase my walking distance and speed and help prevent pain in my legs."

4. A patient with PAD has a clinical problem of ineffective tissue perfusion. What would be included in the teaching plan for this patient? **Select all that apply.**
   a. Apply cold compresses when the legs become swollen.
   b. Wear protective footwear and avoid hot or cold extremes.
   c. Walk at least 30 minutes per day, at least 3 times per week.
   d. Use nicotine replacement therapy as a substitute for smoking.
   e. Inspect lower extremities for pulses, temperature, and any injury.

5. When teaching the patient with PAD about modifying risk factors associated with the condition, what would the nurse emphasize?
   a. Amputation is the ultimate outcome if the patient does not alter lifestyle behaviors.
   b. Modifications will reduce the risk of other atherosclerotic conditions, such as stroke.
   c. Risk-reducing behaviors started after angioplasty can stop the progression of the disease.
   d. Maintenance of normal body weight is the most important factor in controlling arterial disease.

6. During care of the patient following femoral bypass graft surgery, what assessment finding would the nurse immediately notify the health care provider (HCP)?
   a. Fever and redness at the incision site
   b. 2 + edema of the extremity and pain at the incision site
   c. A loss of palpable pulses and numbness and tingling of the feet
   d. Increasing ankle-brachial indices and serous drainage from the incision

7. A patient has atrial fibrillation and develops an acute arterial occlusion at the iliac artery bifurcation. What are the 6 *Ps* of acute arterial occlusion?
   a.
   b.
   c.
   d.
   e.
   f.

8. Which conditions characterize critical limb ischemia? **Select all that apply.**
   a. Cold feet
   b. Arterial leg ulcers
   c. Venous leg ulcers
   d. Gangrene of the leg
   e. No palpable peripheral pulses
   f. Rest pain lasting more than 2 weeks

9. What are characteristics of vasospastic disease (Raynaud's phenomenon)? **Select all that apply.**
   a. Predominant in young females
   b. May be associated with autoimmune disorders
   c. Precipitated by exposure to cold, caffeine, and tobacco
   d. Involves small cutaneous arteries of the fingers and toes
   e. Inflammation of small and medium-sized arteries and veins
   f. Episodes involve white, blue, and red color changes of fingertips

10. Which aneurysm is uniform in shape and a circumferential dilation of the artery?
    a. False aneurysm
    b. Pseudoaneurysm
    c. Saccular aneurysm
    d. Fusiform aneurysm

11. A surgical repair is planned for a patient who has a 5.5-cm abdominal aortic aneurysm (AAA). When assessing the patient, what would the nurse expect to find?
    a. Hoarseness and dysphagia
    b. Severe back pain with flank ecchymosis
    c. Presence of a bruit in the periumbilical area
    d. Weakness in the lower extremities progressing to paraplegia

12. A thoracic aortic aneurysm is identified when a patient has a routine chest x-ray. Which test would the nurse anticipate to determine the size and structure of the aneurysm?
    a. Angiography
    b. Ultrasonography
    c. Echocardiography
    d. CT scan

13. A patient with a small AAA is not a good surgical candidate. What would the nurse teach the patient is the best way to prevent expansion of the lesion?
    a. Avoid strenuous physical exertion.
    b. Control hypertension with prescribed therapy.
    c. Comply with prescribed anticoagulant therapy.
    d. Maintain a low-calcium diet to prevent calcification of the vessel.

14. During preoperative preparation of the patient scheduled for an AAA, why would the nurse obtain a baseline patient assessment?
    a. All physiologic processes will be changed postoperatively.
    b. The cause of the aneurysm is a systemic vascular disease.
    c. Surgery will be canceled if any physiological function is not normal.
    d. BP and heart rate (HR) will be maintained well below baseline levels during the postoperative period.

15. Which surgical therapy for an AAA is most likely to have the postoperative complication of renal injury?
    a. Open aneurysm repair (OAR) above the level of the renal arteries
    b. Excising only the weakened area of the artery and suturing the artery closed
    c. Bifurcated graft used in aneurysm repair when the AAA extends into the iliac arteries
    d. Endovascular graft procedure with an aortic graft inside the aneurysm via the femoral artery

16. What would the nurse include when teaching a patient preparing for AAA repair surgery?
    a. Prepare the bowel on the night before surgery with laxatives or an enema.
    b. Use moisturizing soap to clean the skin three times the day before surgery.
    c. Eat a high-protein and high-carbohydrate breakfast to help with healing postoperatively.
    d. Take the prescribed oral antibiotic the morning of surgery before going to the operating room.

17. During the acute postoperative period following repair of an AAA, which patient goal would the nurse ensure is achieved?
    a. Hypothermia is maintained to decrease oxygen need.
    b. IV fluids are given to maintain urine output of 100 mL/hr.
    c. BP and all peripheral pulses are assessed at least every hour.
    d. BP is kept lower than baseline to prevent leaking at the incision line.

18. Following an ascending aortic aneurysm repair, what assessment finding would the nurse immediately report to the HCP?
    a. Shallow respirations and poor coughing
    b. Decreased drainage from the chest tubes
    c. A change in level of consciousness and inability to speak
    d. Lower extremity pulses that are decreased from the preoperative baseline

19. Which assessment finding would alert the nurse that the patient may have graft thrombosis after an AAA repair?
    a. Dysrhythmias or chest pain
    b. Absent bowel sounds, abdominal distention, or diarrhea
    c. Increased temperature and increased white blood cell count
    d. Decreased pulses and cool, painful extremities below the level of repair

20. A patient who is status-post repair of an AAA has been receiving IV fluids at 125 mL/hr continuously for the last 12 hours. Urine output for the last 4 hours has been 60 mL, 42 mL, 28 mL, and 20 mL, respectively. What action would the nurse take?
    a. Monitor for a couple more hours.
    b. Contact the HCP and report the decrease in urine output.
    c. Send blood for electrolytes, blood urea nitrogen (BUN), and creatinine.
    d. Decrease the rate of infusion to prevent blood leakage at the suture line.

21. Following discharge teaching with a male patient with an AAA repair, the nurse determines that further instruction is needed when the patient makes which statement?
    a. "I should avoid heavy lifting for 6 weeks."
    b. "I may have some sexual dysfunction because of the surgery."
    c. "I should maintain a low-fat and low-cholesterol diet to help keep the new graft open."
    d. "I will take the pulses in my legs and let the doctor know if they get too fast or too slow."

22. During the assessment of the patient with a type B aortic dissection, what would the nurse expect the patient to manifest?
    a. Altered level of consciousness (LOC) with dizziness and weak carotid pulses
    b. A cardiac murmur characteristic of aortic valve insufficiency
    c. Severe "ripping" back or abdominal pain with decreased urine output
    d. Severe hypertension and orthopnea and dyspnea of pulmonary edema

23. A patient with a type A dissection of the arch of the aorta has a decreased LOC and weak carotid pulses. What would the nurse anticipate that initial treatment of the patient will include?
    a. Immediate surgery to replace the torn area with a graft
    b. Administration of anticoagulants to prevent embolization
    c. Administration of packed red blood cells (RBCs) to replace blood loss
    d. Giving antihypertensives to maintain a mean arterial pressure of 70 to 80 mm Hg

24. What indicates to the nurse that treatment for the patient with an uncomplicated aortic dissection is successful?
    a. Pain is relieved.
    b. Surgical repair is completed.
    c. BP is increased to normal range.
    d. Renal output is maintained at 30 mL/hr.

25. What are characteristics of PAD? **Select all that apply.**
    a. Pruritus
    b. Thickened, brittle nails
    c. Dull ache in calf or thigh
    d. Decreased peripheral pulses
    e. Pallor on elevation of the legs
    f. Ulcers over bony prominences on toes and feet

26. The patient is diagnosed with a superficial vein thrombosis (SVT). Which characteristic would the nurse know about SVT?
    a. Embolization to lungs may result in death.
    b. Clot may extend to deeper veins if untreated.
    c. Vein is tender to pressure and there is edema.
    d. Typically found in the iliac, inferior, or superior vena cava.

27. The nurse receives report about a 68-year-old female being admitted after a lengthy hip replacement surgery. Her history includes smoking and taking hormone therapy. What risk factors increase her risk for developing venous thromboembolism (VTE) related to Virchow's triad? **Select all that apply.**
    a. Smoking
    b. IV therapy
    c. Dehydration
    d. Estrogen therapy
    e. Orthopedic surgery
    f. Prolonged immobilization

28. The patient comes to the HCP office with pain, edema, and warm skin on her lower left leg. What test would the nurse expect to be ordered first?
    a. Duplex ultrasound
    b. Complete blood count (CBC)
    c. Magnetic resonance angiography
    d. Computed venography (phlebogram)

29. What care could the registered nurse (RN) delegate to the assistive personnel (AP) for a patient with VTE?
    a. Assess the patient's use of herbs.
    b. Measure the patient for elastic compression stockings.
    c. Remind the patient to flex and extend the legs and feet every 2 hours.
    d. Teach the patient to call emergency response system with signs of pulmonary embolus.

30. To help prevent embolization of a thrombus in a patient with acute VTE and severe edema and limb pain, what would the nurse teach the patient to do first?
    a. Dangle on the edge of the bed q2–3hr.
    b. Ambulate around the bed 3 to 4 times a day.
    c. Keep the affected leg elevated above the level of the heart.
    d. Maintain bed rest until edema is relieved and anticoagulation is established.

31. Which indirect thrombin inhibitor is only given subcutaneously and does not need routine coagulation tests?
    a. Warfarin (Coumadin)
    b. Unfractionated heparin
    c. Hirudin derivatives (bivalirudin [Angiomax])
    d. Low-molecular-weight heparin (enoxaparin [Lovenox])

32. Which characteristics describe the anticoagulant warfarin (Coumadin)? **Select all that apply.**
    a. Vitamin K is the antidote
    b. Protamine sulfate is the antidote
    c. May be given orally or subcutaneously
    d. May be given intravenously or subcutaneously
    e. Monitor dosage using international normalized ratio (INR)
    f. Monitor dosage using activated partial thromboplastin time (aPTT)

33. The patient with VTE is receiving therapy with heparin and asks the nurse whether the drug will dissolve the clot in her leg. What is the best response by the nurse?
    a. "This drug will break up and dissolve the clot so that circulation in the vein can be restored."
    b. "The purpose of the heparin is to prevent growth of the clot or formation of new clots where the circulation is slowed."
    c. "Heparin won't dissolve the clot, but it will inhibit the inflammation around the clot and delay the development of new clots."
    d. "The heparin will dilate the vein, preventing turbulence of blood flow around the clot that may cause it to break off and travel to the lungs."

34. A patient with VTE being discharged on long-term warfarin (Coumadin) therapy is taught about prevention and continuing treatment of VTE. The nurse determines that discharge teaching has been effective when the patient makes which statement?
    a. "I should expect that Coumadin will cause my stools to be somewhat black."
    b. "I should avoid all dark green and leafy vegetables while I am taking Coumadin."
    c. "Massaging my legs several times a day will help increase my venous circulation."
    d. "Swimming is a good activity to include in my exercise program to increase my circulation."

35. What would the nurse teach the patient with any venous disorder is the best way to prevent venous stasis and increase venous return?
    a. take short walks.
    b. sit with the legs elevated.
    c. frequently rotate the ankles.
    d. always wear elastic compression stockings.

36. Number the processes, from 1 (the first process) to 9 (the last process), that occur as venous stasis leads to varicose veins and venous leg ulcers.
    _____ a. Veins dilate
    _____ b. Edema forms
    _____ c. Ulceration occurs
    _____ d. Venous pressure increases
    _____ e. Capillary pressure increases
    _____ f. Venous blood flow backs up
    _____ g. Additional venous distention occurs
    _____ h. Venous valves become incompetent
    _____ i. Blood supply to local tissues decreases

37. What is the most important measure in the treatment of venous leg ulcers?
    a. Elevation of the affected leg
    b. Application of topical antibiotics
    c. Graduated compression stockings
    d. Application of moist to dry dressings

CASE STUDY   Abdominal Aortic Aneurysm

Patient Profile

C.S. is a 73-year-old man who was brought to the local ED reporting severe back pain.

(deeepblue/
iStock/Thinkstock)

Subjective Data

* Has a known AAA, which has been followed with yearly abdominal ultrasound testing
* Has smoked a pack of cigarettes per day for 52 years
* Has had occasional bouts of angina for the past 3 years

Objective Data

* Has a pulsating abdominal mass
* HR 114 beats/min, BP 88/68 mm Hg
* Extremities are cool and clammy
* Dorsalis pedis pulses 2+ bilaterally

Questions

1. What diagnostic tests would the nurse anticipate? **Use an X to indicate whether the tests below are** <u>Anticipated</u> **(appropriate or necessary) or** <u>Non-essential</u> **(makes no difference or is unnecessary).**

Diagnostic Test	Anticipated	Non-Essential
Abdominal CT scan		
Echocardiogram		
Complete blood count (CBC)		
Coagulation studies (PTT/PT/INR)		
Blood glucose		
Abdominal x-ray		
Cholesterol studies		
12-lead ECG		
BUN and creatinine		
Liver function tests		

2. Diagnostic tests reveal that C.S. has a 6 cm abdominal aortic aneurysm (AAA) that is leaking requiring emergency surgery using an open repair. What would the nurse anticipate to prepare C.S. for surgery?

   Use an X to indicate whether the actions below are <u>Anticipated</u> **(appropriate or necessary),** <u>Contraindicated</u> **(could be harmful or not appropriate), or** <u>Non-essential</u> **(makes no difference or is unnecessary).**

Surgical Preparation	Anticipated	Contraindicated	Non-Essential
The nurse keeps the patient NPO.			
The nurse provides informed consent.			
The HCP orders 1000 mL of 0.9% NSS.			
The nurse inserts an indwelling urinary catheter.			
The nurse obtains an order to insert a nasogastric tube.			
The nurse gets the surgical consent signed by the patient.			
The nurse ambulates the patient to the bathroom prior to transfer to the OR suite.			
The nurse performs an abdominal assessment.			

Surgical Preparation	Anticipated	Contraindicated	Non-Essential
The nurse documents a baseline creatinine level.			
The nurse requests an order for an enema.			
The HCP orders to type and crossmatch 4 units of PRBCs.			

3. C.S. is status-post an open repair to repair the AAA. The nurse documents the following nurse's note.

Highlight the findings in the nurse's note that the nurse would report to the health care provider.

NURSE'S NOTES:

The patient is AO x3. He reports 3 out of 10 abdominal pain. Lung sounds with scattered rhonchi in all fields. Bowel sounds absent. NG tube is connected to LIWS, with 50 mL blood-tinged drainage. The abdominal dressing is CDI. Capillary refill is < 3 sec in BUE and > 3 sec in BLE. Radial pulses 3+, dorsalis pedis pulses are not palpable but present by doppler. The patient can move BLE but reports numbness and tingling. Skin is warm and dry in BUE but cool and pale in BLE. The urine output is 25 mL/hr and is tea-colored. Vital signs: HR 82 beats/min, RR 14 breaths/min, BP 100/58 mm Hg, SpO_2 96% on 4L/min nasal cannula, Temp. 37.5°C.

4. The nurse is teaching C.S. about anticoagulation therapy following open repair of the AAA. **Complete the following by choosing the most likely options for the missing information from the lists of options provided.**

The health care provider has prescribed _____1_____ which is a low-molecular weight type of heparin. The nurse teaches the patient that the _____2_____ will be monitored at regular intervals. The medication will be administered through the _____3_____ route. If necessary, _____4_____ can be administered as an antidote to reverse the effects of the medication.

Options for 1	Options for 2	Options for 3	Options for 4
Heparin sodium	aPTT	IV push	Idarucizumab
Betrixaban	INR	Oral	Vitamin K
Warfarin	Factor Xa	Subcutaneous	Protamine sulfate
Bivalirudin	CBC	IV infusion	Andexanet alfa
Dabigatran	ACT	Intradermal	Fresh frozen plasma
Enoxaparin	D-dimer	IVPB	Kcentra

5. What would the nurse include when teaching the patient how to prevent future abdominal aortic aneurysms? **Select all that apply.**

_____A. Limit your caffeine to 1 cup per day
_____B. Consider a smoking cessation program
_____C. Avoid all alcohol consumption
_____D. Restrict your sodium to 1500 mg per day
_____E. Eat foods that increase your low-density lipoprotein level
_____F. Don't abruptly stop the antihypertensive medication
_____G. Monitor your blood glucose levels 4 times/day
_____H. Increase your exercise to at least 3 times/week

Shock, Sepsis, and Multiple Organ Dysfunction Syndrome

1. What is the key factor in describing any type of shock?
   a. Hypoxemia
   b. Hypotension
   c. Vascular collapse
   d. Decreased tissue perfusion

2. What type of shock occurs in a patient with pulmonary embolism or abdominal compartment syndrome?
   a. Distributive shock
   b. Obstructive shock
   c. Cardiogenic shock
   d. Hypovolemic shock

3. What physical problems can precipitate hypovolemic shock? **Select all that apply.**
   a. Burns
   b. Ascites
   c. Vaccines
   d. Insect bites
   e. Hemorrhage
   f. Ruptured spleen

4. A 70-year-old patient with malnourishment and a history of type 2 diabetes is admitted from the nursing home with pneumonia and tachypnea. Which kind of shock is this patient most likely to develop?
   a. Septic shock
   b. Neurogenic shock
   c. Cardiogenic shock
   d. Anaphylactic shock

5. Which hemodynamic monitoring description of the identified shock is accurate?
   a. Tachycardia with hypertension is characteristic of neurogenic shock.
   b. Increased pulmonary artery wedge pressure (PAWP) and a decreased cardiac output (CO) occur in cardiogenic shock.
   c. Anaphylactic shock is characterized by increased systemic vascular resistance (SVR), decreased CO, and decreased PAWP.
   d. In septic shock, bacterial endotoxins cause vascular changes that result in increased SVR, decreased CO, and increased heart rate.

6. In the compensatory stage of hypovolemic shock, after the sympathetic nervous system activates the α-adrenergic stimulation, what organs experience decreased blood flow? **Select all that apply.**
   a. Skin
   b. Brain
   c. Heart
   d. Kidneys
   e. Gastrointestinal (GI) tract

7. As the body continues to try to compensate for hypovolemic shock, there is increased angiotensin II from the activation of the renin-angiotensin-aldosterone system. What physiologic change occurs related to the increased angiotensin II?
   a. Vasodilation
   b. Decreased BP and CO
   c. Aldosterone release results in sodium and water excretion
   d. Antidiuretic hormone (ADH) release increases water reabsorption

8. What clinical manifestations would the nurse observe when a patient is in the compensatory stage of shock? **Select all that apply.**
   a. Pale and cool
   b. Unresponsive
   c. Lower BP than baseline
   d. Moist crackles in the lungs
   e. Hyperactive bowel sounds
   f. Tachypnea and tachycardia

9. Which laboratory test result indicates sepsis as a cause of shock?
   a. Hypokalemia
   b. Thrombocytopenia
   c. Decreased hemoglobin
   d. Increased blood urea nitrogen (BUN)

10. Progressive tissue hypoxia leading to anaerobic metabolism and metabolic acidosis is characteristic of the progressive stage of shock. What changes in the heart contribute to tissue hypoxia?
    a. Coronary artery constriction causes decreased perfusion.
    b. Cardiac vasoconstriction decreases blood flow to pulmonary capillaries.
    c. Increased capillary permeability and profound vasoconstriction cause increased hydrostatic pressure.
    d. Decreased perfusion occurs, leading to dysrhythmias, decreased CO, and decreased oxygen delivery to cells.

11. A patient with severe trauma has been treated for hypovolemic shock. What assessment finding is consistent with the refractory stage of shock?
    a. A respiratory alkalosis with a pH of 7.46
    b. Marked hypotension and refractory hypoxemia
    c. Unresponsiveness that responds only to painful stimuli
    d. Profound vasoconstriction with absent peripheral pulses

12. A patient with acute pancreatitis has hypovolemic shock. Which order would the nurse implement first?
    a. Start 1000 mL of normal saline at 500 mL/hr.
    b. Obtain blood cultures before starting IV antibiotics.
    c. Draw blood for hematology and coagulation factors.
    d. Apply high-flow oxygen (100%) with a non-rebreather mask.

13. What abnormal finding would the nurse expect to find in early compensatory shock?
    a. Metabolic acidosis
    b. Increased serum sodium
    c. Decreased blood glucose
    d. Increased serum potassium

14. In late refractory shock in a patient with massive thermal burns, what would the nurse expect the patient's laboratory results to show?
    a. Respiratory alkalosis
    b. Decreased potassium
    c. Increased blood glucose
    d. Increased ammonia (NH_3) levels

15. A patient with hypovolemic shock is receiving lactated Ringer's solution for fluid replacement therapy. During this therapy, which laboratory result is most important for the nurse to monitor?
    a. Serum pH
    b. Serum sodium
    c. Serum potassium
    d. Hemoglobin (Hgb) and hematocrit (Hct)

16. What hemodynamic monitoring parameter indicates that administering a large amount of crystalloid fluids to a patient in septic shock has been effective?
    a. CO of 2.6 L/min
    b. Central venous pressure (CVP) of 15 mm Hg
    c. PAWP of 4 mm Hg
    d. Heart rate (HR) of 106 beats/min

17. The nurse is caring for a patient in cardiogenic shock. What change in hemodynamic monitoring indicates that the metabolic demands of turning and moving the patient exceed the oxygen supply?
    a. Venous oxygen saturation (SvO_2) from 62% to 54%
    b. CO from 4.2 L/min to 4.8 L/min
    c. Stroke volume (SV) from 52 to 68 mL/beat
    d. SVR from 1300 dyne/sec/cm^5 to 1120 dyne/sec/cm^5

18. What would the nurse assess the patient for during administration of IV norepinephrine (Levophed)?
    a. Hypotension
    b. Marked diuresis
    c. Metabolic alkalosis
    d. Decreased tissue perfusion

19. When administering any vasoactive drug during the treatment of shock, what would the nurse recognize as the goal of the therapy?
    a. Increasing urine output to 50 mL/hr
    b. Constriction of vessels to maintain BP
    c. Maintaining a MAP greater than 65 mm Hg
    d. Dilating vessels to improve tissue perfusion

20. Identify 2 medical therapies that are specific to each of the following types of shock.

Type of Shock	Medical Therapies
Cardiogenic	
Hypovolemic	
Septic	
Anaphylactic	

21. Identify 4 drugs and their actions that are used in the treatment of cardiogenic shock but are not generally used for other types of shock.

Drug	Action

22. What is the priority nursing responsibility in the prevention of shock?
    a. Frequently monitoring all patients' vital signs
    b. Using aseptic technique for all invasive procedures
    c. Being aware of the potential for shock in all patients at risk
    d. Teaching patients health promotion activities to prevent shock

23. Which indicators of tissue perfusion would the nurse monitor in critically ill patients? **Select all that apply.**
    a. Skin
    b. Urine output
    c. Level of consciousness
    d. Activities of daily living
    e. Vital signs, including pulse oximetry
    f. Peripheral pulses with capillary refill

24. A patient in the progressive stage of shock has rapid, deep respirations. Which arterial blood gas (ABG) values are consistent with compensation for metabolic acidosis?
    a. pH 7.42, partial pressure of oxygen in arterial blood (PaO_2) 80 mm Hg
    b. pH 7.48, PaO_2 69 mm Hg
    c. pH 7.38, partial pressure of carbon dioxide in arterial blood ($PaCO_2$) 30 mm Hg
    d. pH 7.32, $PaCO_2$ 48 mm Hg

25. Which interventions would be implemented for a patient experiencing anaphylactic shock? **Select all that apply.**
    a. Antibiotics
    b. Vasodilators
    c. Antihistamines
    d. Oxygen supplementation
    e. Colloid volume expansion
    f. Crystalloid volume expansion

26. A patient in shock is expressing anxiety about their condition and fear of possibly dying. What is an appropriate nursing intervention?
    a. Administer antianxiety agents.
    b. Allow caregivers to visit as much as possible.
    c. Call a member of the clergy to visit the patient.
    d. Inform the patient of the current plan of care and its rationale.

27. Which statement describes systemic inflammatory response syndrome (SIRS) and/or multiple organ dysfunction syndrome (MODS)?
    a. MODS may occur independently from SIRS.
    b. All patients with septic shock develop MODS.
    c. The GI system is often the first to show evidence of dysfunction in SIRS and MODS.
    d. A common initial mediator that causes endothelial damage leading to SIRS is endotoxin.

28. What mechanism that can trigger SIRS is related to myocardial infarction or pancreatitis?
    a. Abscess formation
    b. Microbial invasion
    c. Global perfusion deficits
    d. Ischemic or necrotic tissue

29. Since mechanical tissue trauma can trigger SIRS, the nurse will include assessing for SIRS as part of the plan of care for patients with which types of problems? **Select all that apply.**
    a. Burns
    b. Crush injuries
    c. Viral infections
    d. Fungal infections
    e. Surgical procedures

30. Which intervention may prevent GI bacterial and endotoxin translocation in a critically ill patient with SIRS?
    a. Early enteral feedings
    b. Surgical removal of necrotic tissue
    c. Aggressive multiple antibiotic therapy
    d. Strict aseptic technique in all procedures

31. A patient with a gunshot wound to the abdomen is being treated for hypovolemic and septic shock. To monitor the patient for early organ damage associated with MODS, what is most important for the nurse to assess?
    a. Urine output
    b. Breath sounds
    c. Peripheral circulation
    d. CVP

32. Which patient manifestations confirm the development of MODS?
    a. Upper GI bleeding, Glasgow Coma Scale (GCS) score of 7, and Hct of 25%
    b. Elevated serum bilirubin, serum creatinine of 3.8 mg/dL, and platelet count of 15,000/μL
    c. Urine output of 30 mL/hr, BUN of 45 mg/dL, and white blood cell (WBC) count of 1120/μL
    d. Respiratory rate of 45 breaths/min, $PaCO_2$ of 60 mm Hg, and chest x-ray with bilateral diffuse patchy infiltrates

---

CASE STUDY Septic Shock

(shironosov/
iStock/Thinkstock)

Patient Profile
A.M. is an 81-year-old man who was brought to the emergency department (ED) via an ambulance from a local nursing home. He was found by the nurses on their 6:00 AM rounds to be very confused, restless, and hypotensive.

Health History
A.M. has type 1 diabetes and a history of prostate cancer, myocardial infarction, and heart failure. He has been a resident of the nursing home for 2 years. His wife had to place him because she could no longer take care of him at home. He has had an indwelling urinary catheter in place for 5 days because of difficulty voiding. Until today, A.M. has been oriented and cooperative. His current medications are metoprolol (Lopressor), lisinopril (Zestril), hydrochlorothiazide, isosorbide (Isordil), and insulin.

Subjective Data
• Denies any pain or discomfort

Objective Data
• Neurologic: lethargic, confused to place and time, easily arousable, does not follow commands; moves all extremities in response to stimuli
• Cardiovascular: BP 80/60 mm Hg; HR 112 beats/min and regular; Axillary temp 103°F (40°C); heart sounds normal without murmurs or S_3, S_4; peripheral pulses weak and thready
• Skin: warm, dry, flushed
• Respiratory: RR 34 breaths/min and shallow; breath sounds audible in all lobes with bilateral bibasilar crackles
• GI/GU: abdomen soft with hypoactive bowel sounds; urinary catheter in place draining scant, purulent urine

Interprofessional Care

In the ED, 2 16-gauge IVs were inserted, and 700 mL of normal saline was given over the first hour. The patient was placed on 40% oxygen via simple face mask. The urinary catheter was removed, and the tip cultured; blood cultures were drawn at 2 intervals. A new urinary catheter was inserted. A.M. was started on IV antibiotics and transferred to the intensive care unit (ICU) with a diagnosis of septic shock resulting from gram-negative sepsis.

- In the ICU, a pulmonary artery catheter was inserted in addition to an arterial line.
- The patient was intubated and placed on mechanical ventilation.
- ABG results: pH 7.25, PaO_2 60 mm Hg, $PaCO_2$ 28 mm Hg, HCO_3^- 12 mEq/L, SaO_2 82%
- Hemodynamic pressures were CVP 0 mm Hg, pulmonary artery mean pressure (PAMP) 5 mm Hg, PAWP 4 mm Hg, CO 2.5 L/min, and SVR 650 dynes/sec/cm^{-5}

Laboratory Tests

WBC: 21,000/µL
Na^+: 133 mEq/L
K^+: 4.5 mEq/L
Cl^-: 96 mEq/L
Glucose: 230 mg/dL
Creatinine: 1.7 mg/dL
Hgb: 12 g/dL; Hct: 36%

Questions

1. Choose the most likely options for the information missing from the table below by selecting from the lists of options provided.

Medication	Dose, Route, Frequency	Drug Class	Indication
3	10 mg three times daily	1	Angina
Metoprolol	2	Beta blocker	Heart rate control
Hydrochlorothiazide	25 mg once daily	1	4
3	20 mg twice daily	ACE inhibitor	Heart failure

Options for 1	Options for 2	Options for 3	Options for 4
Beta-blocker	10 mg twice daily	Isosorbide	Angina
ACE inhibitor	25 mg twice daily	Glucophage	Bradycardia
Thiazide diuretic	100 mg once daily	Lisinopril	Hypertension
Nitrate	10 mg once daily	Nitroglycerin	Hypotension
Angiotensin-receptor blockade	12.5 mg twice daily	Furosemide	Chronic kidney disease
Loop diuretic	15 mg three times daily	Losartan	Diabetes

2. For each assessment finding, choose the main cause(s). There may be more than one cause for each assessment finding.

Assessment Finding	Cause	Appropriate Cause(s) for Assessment Finding
Decreased level of consciousness	Metabolic acidosis	
Warm, dry, and flushed skin	Gram-negative infection	
Tachycardia	Impaired tissue perfusion	
Tachypnea	Vasodilation	
Fever		
Decreased SVR		
Increased CO		
Oliguria		
Leukocytosis		

3. **Use an X to indicate whether the nursing actions below are <u>Anticipated</u> (appropriate or necessary), <u>Contraindicated</u> (could be harmful), or <u>Non-essential</u> (makes no difference or is unnecessary).**

Nursing Actions	Anticipated	Contraindicated	Non-Essential
Administer KCL 40 mEq IVPB over 1 hour.			
Advocate for physical therapy.			
Monitor vital signs every hour.			

Nursing Actions	Anticipated	Contraindicated	Non-Essential
Provide oral care every 4 hours and PRN.			
Administer antibiotics as prescribed.			
Administer nitroglycerin IV infusion.			
Frequent FSBG monitoring.			
Administer norepinephrine to keep MAP ≥ 65 mm Hg.			
Complete a diet assessment.			
Transfuse 1 unit PRBC over 2 hours.			
Obtain an order for an echocardiogram.			

4. Based on the assessment findings once A.M. was transferred to the ICU, what priority actions would the nurse take to help stabilize him? **Select all that apply.**

_____A. Administer 30 mL/kg of isotonic crystalloid
_____B. Perform neurologic assessments once every 4 hours
_____C. Increase the respiratory rate on the ventilator to correct the $PaCO_2$
_____D. Administer phenylephrine to increase BP
_____E. Increase the FiO_2 on the ventilator to correct the PaO_2
_____F. Administer sodium nitroprusside to decrease the SVR
_____G. Administer regular insulin to treat hyperglycemia
_____H. Administer a beta-blocker to treat tachycardia
_____I. Administer norepinephrine to increase the SVR
_____J. Monitor serum lactate levels

5. **Complete the following statement by choosing the most likely option for the missing information from the lists of options provided.**

Goals for stabilizing A.M. include maintaining the _____1_____ between 8-12 mm Hg and the _____1_____ equal to or greater than 65 mm Hg. _____2_____ would be used as prophylaxis for stress ulcers while _____3_____ would be used to prevent VTE. _____3_____ would be used to increase O_2 delivery and increase SvO_2. Giapreza is a(n) _____4_____ that is used to increase BP, MAP, and SVR.

Options for 1	Options for 2	Options for 3	Options for 4
Systemic vascular resistance	Histamine-receptor blockades	Dobutamine	ACE inhibitor
Mean arterial pressure	Antacids	Enoxaparin	Angiotensin-receptor blockade
Pulmonary artery wedge pressure	Proton pump inhibitors	Norepinephrine	Vasopressor
Central venous pressure	Cytoprotective agents	Vasopressin	Inotrope
Cardiac output	Antiemetics	Warfarin	α-Adrenergic agonist
Stroke volume	Prokinetic agents	Aspirin	Angiotensin II

Assessment: Gastrointestinal System

1. Identify the structures in the illustration below:

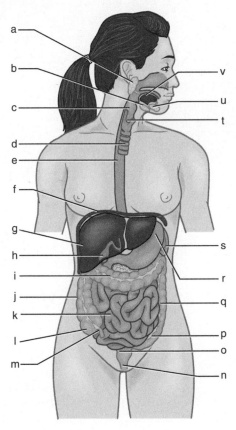

a. _____
b. _____
c. _____
d. _____
e. _____
f. _____
g. _____
h. _____
i. _____
j. _____
k. _____

l. _____
m. _____
n. _____
o. _____
p. _____
q. _____
r. _____
s. _____
t. _____
u. _____
v. _____

2. Identify the structures in the illustration below using these terms.

Terms

Ampulla of Vater	Gallbladder	Pancreas (tail)
Common bile duct	Left lobe of liver	Right hepatic duct
Cystic duct	Main pancreatic duct	Right lobe of liver
Duodenum	Pancreas (head)	Sphincter of Oddi

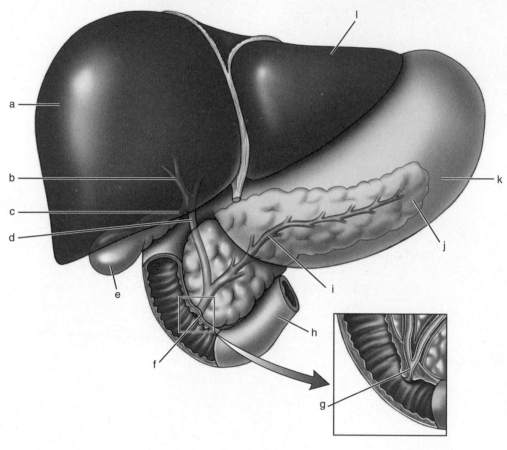

a. _____   h. _____
b. _____   i. _____
c. _____   j. _____
d. _____   k. _____
e. _____   l. _____
f. _____   m. _____
g. _____

3. A patient receives atropine, an anticholinergic drug, in preparation for surgery. Which action would the nurse expect this drug to have on the gastrointestinal (GI) tract?
   a. Increases gastric emptying
   b. Relaxes pyloric and ileocecal sphincters
   c. Decreases secretions and peristaltic action
   d. Stimulates the nervous system of the GI tract

4. After eating, a patient with an inflamed gallbladder has pain caused by contraction of the gallbladder. What causes this to occur?
   a. Production of bile by the liver
   b. Production of secretin by the duodenum
   c. Release of gastrin from the stomach antrum
   d. Production of cholecystokinin by the duodenum

5. When caring for a patient who has had most of their stomach surgically removed, what is important for the nurse to teach the patient?
   a. Extra iron will need to be taken to prevent anemia.
   b. Avoid foods with lactose to prevent bloating and diarrhea.
   c. Lifelong supplementation of cobalamin (vitamin B_{12}) will be needed.
   d. Because of the absence of digestive enzymes, protein malnutrition is likely.

6. A 68-year-old patient is in the office for a physical. The patient states they no longer has regular bowel movements. Which suggestion by the nurse would be most helpful to the patient?
   a. Take an additional laxative to stimulate defecation.
   b. Eat less acidic foods to enable the GI system to increase peristalsis.
   c. Eat less food at each meal to prevent feces from backing up due to slowed peristalsis.
   d. Attempt defecation after breakfast because gastrocolic reflexes increase colon peristalsis at that time.

7. Which digestive substances are active, or activated, in the stomach? **Select all that apply.**
   a. Bile
   b. Pepsin
   c. Gastrin
   d. Maltase
   e. Secretin
   f. Amylase

8. What problem would the nurse assess the patient for if the patient was on prolonged antibiotic therapy?
   a. Coagulation problems
   b. Elevated serum ammonia levels
   c. Impaired absorption of amino acids
   d. Increased mucus and bicarbonate secretion

9. How will an obstruction at the ampulla of Vater affect the digestion of all nutrients?
   a. Bile is responsible for emulsification of all nutrients and vitamins.
   b. Intestinal digestive enzymes are released through the ampulla of Vater.
   c. Both bile and pancreatic enzymes enter the duodenum at the ampulla of Vater.
   d. Gastric contents can only pass to the duodenum when the ampulla of Vater is open.

10. A patient has increased red blood cell (RBC) destruction from a mechanical heart valve prosthesis. Describe what happens to the bilirubin that is released from the breakdown of hemoglobin (Hgb) from the RBCs.

11. What is a manifestation of age-related changes in the GI system that the nurse may find in an older patient?
    a. Gastric hyperacidity
    b. Intolerance to fatty foods
    c. Yellowish tinge to the skin
    d. Reflux of gastric contents into the esophagus

12. Identify 1 specific finding identified by the nurse during assessment of each of the patient's functional health patterns that indicates a risk factor for GI problems or the response of the patient to a GI disorder.

Functional Health Pattern	Risk Factor for or Response to GI Problem
Health perception–health management	
Nutritional-metabolic	
Elimination	
Activity-exercise	
Sleep-rest	
Cognitive-perceptual	
Self-perception–self-concept	
Role-relationship	
Sexuality-reproductive	
Coping–stress tolerance	
Value-belief	

13. What is a normal finding during physical assessment of the mouth?
    a. A red, slick appearance of the tongue
    b. Uvular deviation to the side on saying "Ahh"
    c. A thin, white coating of the dorsum of the tongue
    d. Scattered red, smooth areas on the dorsum of the tongue

14. What is a normal finding on physical examination of the abdomen?
    a. Auscultation of bruits
    b. Observation of visible pulsations
    c. Percussion of liver dullness in the left midclavicular line
    d. Palpation of the spleen 1 to 2 cm below the left costal margin

15. A patient is admitted to the hospital with left upper quadrant (LUQ) pain. What organ may be the source of the pain?
    a. Liver
    b. Pancreas
    c. Appendix
    d. Gallbladder

16. What characterizes auscultation of the abdomen?
    a. The presence of borborygmi indicates hyperperistalsis.
    b. The bell of the stethoscope is used to auscultate high-pitched sounds.
    c. High-pitched, rushing, and tinkling bowel sounds are heard after eating.
    d. Absence of bowel sounds for 1 minute in each quadrant is reported as abnormal.

17. Following auscultation of the abdomen, what would be the nurse's next action?
    a. Lightly percuss over all 4 quadrants.
    b. Have the patient empty their bladder.
    c. Inspect perianal and anal areas for color, masses, rashes, and scars.
    d. Perform deep palpation to delineate abdominal organs and masses.

18. In the table below, indicate with an X which preparations are required for each of the diagnostic procedures listed.

Diagnostic Procedure	NPO up to 8 hours or More	Bowel Emptying with Laxatives, Enemas, or Both	Informed Consent	Determine Allergy to Iodine
Upper GI series				
Barium enema				
Percutaneous transhepatic cholangiogram				
Gallbladder ultrasound				
Hepatobiliary scintigraphy				
Esophagogastroduodenoscopy				
Colonoscopy				
Endoscopic retrograde cholangiopancreatography (ERCP)				

19. A patient's serum liver enzyme tests reveal an elevated aspartate aminotransferase (AST). What would the nurse recognize about an elevated AST?
    a. It eliminates infection as a cause of liver damage.
    b. It is diagnostic for liver inflammation and damage.
    c. Tissue damage in organs other than the liver may be identified.
    d. Nervous system symptoms related to hepatic encephalopathy may be the cause.

20. Which nursing actions are indicated for a liver biopsy? **Select all that apply.**
    a. Observe for white stools.
    b. Monitor for rectal bleeding.
    c. Monitor for internal bleeding.
    d. Position to right side after test.
    e. Ensure bowel preparation was done.
    f. Check coagulation status before test.

21. After which diagnostic procedure, is it necessary for the nurse to check for the return of the gag reflex and monitor for LUQ pain, nausea, and vomiting?
    a. ERCP
    b. Colonoscopy
    c. Defecography
    d. Barium swallow

Nutrition Problems

1. A 30-year-old man's diet consists of 3000 calories with 120 g of protein, 160 g of fat, and 270 g of carbohydrate. He weighs 176 lbs and is 5 ft 11 inches tall.
   a. Indicate what percentage of total calories each of the nutrients contributes to this man's diet.

Nutrient	Percentage of Total Calories from Nutrient
Protein	
Fat	
Carbohydrates	

   b. How does his percentage of nutrients compare to the Dietary Reference Intake recommendations for each nutrient?
   c. How many calories would be recommended for him as an average adult?
   d. Using MyPlate as a guide, what changes could the nurse suggest to bring this man's diet more in line with nutrition recommendations?

2. Which statement accurately describes vitamin deficiencies?
   a. Vitamin deficiencies in adults are always clinically manifested by disorders of the skin.
   b. Surgery on the GI tract causing impaired absorption contributes to vitamin deficiencies.
   c. The two nutrients most often lacking in the diet of a vegan are vitamin B_6 and folic acid.
   d. Vitamin imbalances occur frequently in the United States because of excessive fat intake.

3. What is the most common cause of chronic disease-related or secondary protein-calorie malnutrition in the United States?
   a. The unavailability of foods high in protein
   b. A lack of knowledge about nutrition needs
   c. A lack of money to purchase high-protein foods
   d. A problem with ingestion, digestion, absorption, or metabolism

4. Describe the metabolism of nutrients used for energy during starvation within the given approximate time frames.

Time Frame	Metabolism of Nutrients
First 18 hours	
18 hours to 5 to 9 days	
9 days to 6 weeks	
Over 6 weeks	

5. What may occur with failure of the sodium-potassium pump during severe protein depletion?
   a. Ascites
   b. Anemia
   c. Hyperkalemia
   d. Hypoalbuminemia

6. What contributes to increased protein-calorie needs?
   a. Surgery
   b. Vegan diet
   c. Lowered temperature
   d. Cultural or religious beliefs

7. During assessment of the patient with protein-calorie malnutrition, what would the nurse expect to find? **Select all that apply.**
   a. Frequent cold symptoms
   b. Decreased bowel sounds
   c. Cool, rough, dry, scaly skin
   d. A flat or concave abdomen
   e. Prominent bony structures
   f. Decreased reflexes and lack of attention

8. Which problem has the highest risk for malnutrition related to decreased ingestion?
   a. Tuberculosis infection
   b. Malabsorption syndrome
   c. Treatment of draining decubitus ulcers
   d. Severe anorexia resulting from radiation therapy

9. The nurse monitors the laboratory results of the patient with protein-calorie malnutrition during treatment. Which result indicates an improvement in the patient's condition?
   a. Decreased lymphocytes
   b. Increased serum potassium
   c. Increased serum transferrin
   d. Decreased serum prealbumin

10. To evaluate the long-term effect of nutrition interventions for a patient with protein-calorie malnutrition, what is the best indicator for the nurse to use?
    a. Height and weight
    b. Body mass index (BMI)
    c. Weight in relation to ideal body weight
    d. Midupper arm circumference and triceps skinfold

11. The nurse determines patient teaching about a high-calorie, high-protein diet has been effective when the patient selects which breakfast option from the hospital menu?
    a. Two poached eggs, hash brown potatoes, and whole milk
    b. Two slices of toast with butter and jelly, orange juice, and skim milk
    c. Three pancakes with butter and syrup, 2 slices of bacon, and apple juice
    d. Cream of wheat with 2 tbsp of skim milk powder, one-half grapefruit, and a high-protein milkshake

12. When teaching the older adult about changes in nutrition needs with aging, what would the nurse emphasize?
    a. The need for all nutrients decreases as a person ages.
    b. Fewer calories, but the same or slightly increased amount of protein, are required as one ages.
    c. Fats, carbohydrates, and protein should be decreased, but vitamin and mineral intake should be increased.
    d. High-calorie oral supplements should be taken between meals to ensure that recommended nutrient needs are met.

13. When planning nutrition interventions for a healthy 83-year-old widowed man, what factor does the nurse recognize is most likely to affect his nutrition status?
    a. Living alone on a fixed income
    b. Changes in cardiovascular function
    c. An increase in GI motility and absorption
    d. Snacking between meals, resulting in obesity

14. When considering enteral nutrition (EN) for a patient with severe protein-calorie malnutrition, what is an advantage of a gastrostomy tube versus a nasogastric (NG) tube?
    a. There is less irritation to the nasal and esophageal mucosa.
    b. The patient experiences the sights and smells associated with eating.
    c. Aspiration resulting from reflux of formulas into the esophagus is less common.
    d. Routine checking for placement is not needed because gastrostomy tubes do not become displaced.

15. Identify 2 nursing interventions for each of the following desired outcomes of EN.

Desired Outcome	Nursing Intervention
Prevention of aspiration	
Prevention of diarrhea	
Maintenance of tube patency	
Maintenance of tube placement	
Administration of medication	

16. Indicate whether the following nursing actions must be performed by the registered nurse (RN) or if they can be delegated to a licensed practical nurse/licensed vocational nurse (LPN/VN) or assistive personnel (AP).

_____a. Insert NG tube for stable patients.

_____b. Weigh the patient receiving EN.

_____c. Teach the patient about home gastric tube care.

_____d. Remove an NG tube.

_____e. Provide oral care to the patient with an NG tube.

_____f. Position patient receiving EN.

_____g. Monitor a patient with continuous feeding for complications.

_____h. Respond to infusion pump alarm by reporting it to an RN or LPN/VN.

17. Indicate whether the following characteristics of parenteral nutrition apply to central parenteral nutrition (CPN) or peripheral parenteral nutrition (PPN).

_____a. Limited to 20% glucose

_____b. Tonicity of 1600 mOsm/L

_____c. Nutrients can be infused using smaller volumes

_____d. Supplements inadequate enteral feedings

_____e. Long-term nutrition support

_____f. Increased risk of phlebitis

_____g. May use peripherally inserted central catheter (PICC)

18. What is an indication for parenteral nutrition that is not an appropriate indication for enteral tube feedings?
    a. Head and neck cancer
    b. Hypermetabolic states
    c. Malabsorption syndrome
    d. Protein-calorie malnutrition

19. What nursing interventions are indicated during parenteral nutrition to prevent the following complications?

Complication	Preventive Measure
Infection	
Hyperglycemia	
Air embolism	

20. The nurse is caring for a patient receiving 1000 mL of parenteral nutrition solution over 24 hours. When it is time to change the solution, 150 mL remain in the bag. What is the most appropriate action by the nurse?
    a. Hang the new solution and discard the unused solution.
    b. Open the IV line and rapidly infuse the remaining solution.
    c. Notify the health care provider for instructions regarding the infusion rate.
    d. Wait to change the solution until the remaining solution infuses at the prescribed rate.

21. Identify the following characteristics of eating disorders as being associated with anorexia nervosa (A), bulimia nervosa (B), or both (AB).

_____a. Treated with psychotherapy

_____b. Ignores feelings of hunger

_____c. Binge eating with purging

_____d. Conceals abnormal eating habits

_____e. Concerned about body image

_____f. Self-induced starvation

_____g. Compulsive exerciser

_____h. Broken blood vessels in the eyes

22. An 18-year-old female patient with anorexia nervosa is admitted to the hospital for treatment. On admission, she weighs 82 lb (37 kg) and is 5 ft 3 in (134.6 cm). Her laboratory test results include the following: K^+ 2.8 mEq/L (2.8 mmol/L), hemoglobin (Hgb) 8.9 g/dL (89 g/L), and blood urea nitrogen (BUN) 64 mg/dL (22.8 mmol/L). When planning care for the patient, the nurse gives the highest priority to which clinical problem?

a. Risk for injury due to dizziness and weakness from anemia

b. Nutritionally compromised from inadequate food intake

c. Impaired urinary system function from elevated BUN and renal failure

d. Risk for impaired cardiac function due to dysrhythmias from hypokalemia

---

CASE STUDY Malnutrition

Patient Profile

R.M., a 58-year-old Hispanic widow, recently underwent radiation and chemotherapy following surgery for breast cancer. On a follow-up visit to the clinic, the nurse notes that R.M. appears thinner and more tired than usual.

(Christophe Bourloton/iStock/Thinkstock)

Subjective Data

- Reports no appetite since the treatment for cancer was started
- Feels "weak" and "worn out"
- Thinks the treatment for cancer has not been effective
- Lives alone in an apartment in the inner city
- Is a naturalized citizen from Honduras
- Speaks English but does not read English very well

Objective Data

Physical Examination

- Height: 5 ft, 2 in (155 cm)
- Weight: 92 lbs (41.8 kg)
- Vital signs: BP 98/60 mm Hg, HR 60 beats/min, RR 12 breaths/min
- Ulcerations of her buccal mucosal membranes and tongue

Laboratory Tests

- Serum albumin: 2.8 g/dL (28 g/L)
- Hgb: 10 g/dL (100 g/L)
- Hct: 32%

Questions

1. Based on the information provided, what additional assessment data and clinical manifestations would the nurse consider when planning care for R.M.?

For each data below, use an X to specify whether it is <u>Expected</u> (occurs or will help determine malnutrition), <u>Unexpected</u> (doesn't occur or will not help determine malnutrition), or <u>Unrelated</u> (data that isn't relevant to malnutrition).

Additional Data	Expected	Unexpected	Unrelated
Calculate the patient's BMI			
Obtain a bone density scan			
Obtain a prealbumin level			
Collect a food intake history			

Additional Data	Expected	Unexpected	Unrelated
Obtain coagulation studies			
Peripheral edema in bilateral lower extremities +2 pitting			
Mucous membranes are pink			
Skin is pale			
Hyperactive bowel sounds			

2. **Choose the most likely options for the information missing from the paragraph below by selecting from the lists of options provided.**

When planning care for R.M., the nurse determines _____**1**_____ is the priority clinical problem. The nurse calculates the energy expenditure for R.M. as _____**2**_____. Currently, the patient considers herself as sedentary because of constant fatigue. Considering R.M.'s current health condition, the nurse determines R.M.'s minimal total daily calories should be _____**3**_____. The nurse should advocate for a _____**4**_____ consult.

Options for 1	Options for 2	Options for 3	Options for 4
Risk for infection	900	1123	Physical therapy
Risk for injury	850	1000	Dietary
Fatigue	936	1287	Occupational therapy
Nutritionally compromised	1000	1450	Speech therapy
Impaired Immunity	975	1075	Social work

3. The nurse is recommending vitamins and minerals for R.M. to incorporate into her diet. **For each food option, place an X in the column identifying which mineral or vitamin, is a major source. Food options may contain more than one vitamin or mineral.**

Food Option	Magnesium	B12	Zinc	Calcium	B6	Vitamin E	Vitamin A
Chicken							
Tofu							
Carrots							
Milk							
Spinach							
Legumes							
Salmon							
Meat							
Grains							

4. What would the nurse include when teaching R.M. about her diet? **Select all that apply.**

_____A. Use MyPlate to help plan meals.

_____B. Meals should be high in calories that come from fats.

_____C. Alcohol intake can increase your risk for malnutrition.

_____D. Read food labels when you shop for groceries.

_____E. Keep a journal of your weekly weight.

_____F. If you cannot tolerate high-protein foods, drink high-protein shakes.

_____G. Provide written instructions in English.

_____H. Consider using Meals on Wheels if you are too tired to prepare your meals.

_____I. Drink more water with your meals.

5. If the patient's malnutrition doesn't improve or if she is unable to consume enough calories to improve her nutrition status, R.M. may need parenteral nutrition (PN). What actions would the nurse implement when preparing and administering PN?

For each action below, use an X to specify whether the action would be <u>Indicated</u> (appropriate or necessary), <u>Contraindicated</u> (could be harmful), or is <u>Non-Essential</u> (makes no difference or is unnecessary) when administering PN.

Nursing Action	Indicated	Contraindicated	Non-Essential
Never refrigerate PN.			
Use a 0.22-micron filter during PN infusion.			
Change the IV tubing every 72 hours.			
Monitor potassium levels during PN administration.			
If the PN infusion empties before the next PN bag is ready, administer a 10% dextrose infusion through a peripheral IV catheter.			
Fat emulsion can concurrently be administered with PN.			
Add insulin to the PN if the patient is hyperglycemic.			
2 RNs need to verify the PN label before administration.			
Montior glucose levels during PN infusion.			
Keep the patient NPO.			

Obesity

1. Using the body mass index (BMI) chart (see Fig. 45.7) in the textbook or the BMI formula:

$$BMI\left(kg/m^2\right) = \frac{Weight\left(pounds\right) \times 703}{Height\left(inches\right)^2}$$

   a. Determine the BMI for a patient who is 5 ft 5 in (164 cm) and weighs 202 lb (91.8 kg). What is the patient's weight classification?
   b. Calculate the waist-to-hip ratio of a woman who has a waist measurement of 32 in and a hip measurement of 36 in. What does this value indicate?

2. Which statement about obesity is explained by genetics?
   a. Older obese patients have exacerbated changes of aging.
   b. Android body shape and weight gain are influenced by genetics.
   c. White Americans have a higher incidence of obesity than blacks.
   d. Men have a harder time losing weight as they have more muscle mass.

3. Which patient is at greatest risk for complications of obesity?
   a. A 30-year-old woman who is 5 ft (151 cm) tall, weighs 140 lb (63.6 kg), and carries weight in her thighs
   b. A 56-year-old woman with a BMI of 38 kg/m^2, a waist measurement of 38 in (96 cm), and a hip measurement of 36 in (91 cm)
   c. A 42-year-old man with a waist measurement of 36 in (91 cm) and a hip measurement of 36 in (91 cm) who is 5 ft 6 in (166 cm) tall and weighs 150 lb (68.2 kg)
   d. A 68-year-old man with a waist measurement of 38 in (96 cm) and a hip measurement of 42 in (76 cm) who is 5 ft, 11 in (179 cm) tall and weighs 200 lb (90.9 kg)

4. A woman is 5 ft 6 in (166 cm) tall and weighs 200 lb (90.9 kg) with a waist-to-hip ratio of 0.7. Which problem would the nurse inform the patient she is at greatest risk of developing?
   a. Diabetes
   b. Osteoporosis
   c. Heart disease
   d. Endometrial cancer

5. Before selecting a weight reduction plan with an obese patient, what is most important for the nurse to assess first?
   a. The patient's motivation to lose weight
   b. The length of time that the patient has been obese
   c. Whether financial considerations will affect the patient's choices
   d. The patient's height, weight, BMI, waist-to-hip ratio, and skinfold thickness

6. Which hormones and peptides normally affect appetite? **Select all that apply.**
   a. Leptin
   b. Insulin
   c. Ghrelin
   d. Peptide YY
   e. Neuropeptide Y
   f. Cholecystokinin

7. The nurse is teaching a moderately obese woman about interventions for the management of obesity. Initially, which strategies would support restricting diet intake to below energy requirements? **Select all that apply.**
   a. Limit alcohol
   b. Rest when fatigued
   c. Determine portion sizes
   d. 1800- to 2200-calorie diet
   e. Attend Overeaters Anonymous
   f. Park farther away from destination

8. Which explanation about weight reduction would be included when teaching the obese patient and her obese partner?
   a. Weight gain is caused by psychologic factors.
   b. Daily weighing is recommended to monitor weight loss.
   c. Progressively increasing physical activity helps decrease weight, cholesterol, and BP levels.
   d. Men lose weight less quickly than women because they have a higher percentage of metabolically less active fat.

9. A patient has been on a 1000-calorie diet with a daily exercise routine. In 2 months, the patient has lost 20 lb (9 kg) toward a goal of 50 lb (23 kg), but is now discouraged that no weight has been lost in the last 2 weeks. What would the nurse tell the patient about this plateau?
   a. A steady weight may be caused by water gain from eating foods high in sodium.
   b. Plateaus where no weight is lost normally occur during a weight loss program.
   c. A weight considered by the body to be most efficient for functioning has been reached.
   d. A return to former eating habits is the most common cause of not continuing to lose weight.

10. When teaching a patient about weight reduction diets, what would the nurse teach the patient is an appropriate single serving of a food?
    a. A 6-inch bagel
    b. 1 cup of chopped vegetables
    c. A piece of cheese the size of 3 dice
    d. A chicken breast the size of a deck of cards

11. When medications are used in the treatment of obesity, what is most important for the nurse to teach the patient?
    a. Over-the-counter (OTC) diet aids are safer than other agents and can be useful in controlling appetite.
    b. Drugs should be used only as adjuncts to a diet and exercise program as treatment for a chronic condition.
    c. All drugs used for weight control can affect central nervous system function and should be used with caution.
    d. The primary effect of medications is psychological, controlling the urge to eat in response to feelings of rejection.

12. A patient asks the nurse about taking phentermine and topiramate (Qsymia) for weight loss. What condition would the nurse identify as increasing the risk of side effects?
    a. Glaucoma
    b. Hypertension
    c. Valvular heart disease
    d. Irritable bowel disease

13. The nurse has completed initial instruction with a patient about a weight loss program. Which patient statement indicates to the nurse that the teaching has been effective?
    a. "I will keep a diary of daily weight to illustrate my weight loss."
    b. "I plan to lose 4 lb/week until I have lost the 60 lb I want to lose."
    c. "I should not exercise more than what is required so I don't increase my appetite."
    d. "I plan to join a behavior modification group to help establish long-term behavior changes."

14. A 40-year-old female patient, who has extreme obesity and type 2 diabetes, wants to lose weight. After learning about the surgical procedures, she thinks a combination of restrictive and malabsorptive surgery would be best. Which procedure would the nurse teach her about?
    a. Lipectomy
    b. Sleeve gastrectomy
    c. Roux-en-Y gastric bypass
    d. Adjustable gastric banding

15. What characteristics describe adjustable gastric banding? **Select all that apply.**
    a. 75% of the stomach is removed
    b. Stomach restriction can be reversed
    c. Eliminates hormones that stimulate hunger
    d. Malabsorption of fat-soluble vitamins occurs
    e. Inflatable band allows for modification of gastric stoma size
    f. Stomach with a gastric pouch surgically anastomosed to the jejunum

16. During care of the patient with extreme obesity, what is most important for the nurse to do?
    a. Avoid any reference to the patient's weight to avoid embarrassing the patient.
    b. Emphasize to the patient how important it is to lose weight to maintain health.
    c. Plan for necessary modifications in equipment and nursing techniques before starting care.
    d. Recognize that a full assessment may not be possible because of numerous layers of skinfolds.

17. What physiologic problems is an obese patient with cancer at a greater risk of having? **Select all that apply.**
    a. Tinnitus
    b. Fractures
    c. Sleep apnea
    d. Type 2 diabetes
    e. Trousseau's sign
    f. Gastroesophageal reflux disease (GERD)

18. The nurse is admitting a patient for bariatric surgery. Which finding in a patient's history would be brought to the surgeon's attention before proceeding with further patient preparation?
    a. Hypertension
    b. Untreated depression
    c. Multiple attempts at weight loss
    d. Sleep apnea treated with continuous positive airway pressure (CPAP)

19. What is a postoperative nursing intervention for the obese patient who has had bariatric surgery?
    a. Irrigating and repositioning the nasogastric (NG) tube as needed
    b. Delaying ambulation until the patient has enough strength to support self
    c. Keeping the patient positioned on the side to facilitate respiratory function
    d. Providing adequate support to the incision during coughing and deep breathing

20. What information would be included in the diet teaching for the patient after a Roux-en-Y gastric bypass?
    a. Avoid sugary foods and fluids to prevent dumping syndrome.
    b. Gradually increase the amount of food ingested to preoperative levels.
    c. Maintain a long-term liquid diet to prevent damage to the surgical site.
    d. Consume foods high in complex carbohydrates, protein, and fiber to add bulk to contents.

21. Which female patient is most likely to have metabolic syndrome?
    a. BP 128/78 mm Hg, triglycerides 160 mg/dL, fasting blood glucose 102 mg/dL
    b. BP 142/90 mm Hg, high-density lipoproteins 45 mg/dL, fasting blood glucose 130 mg/dL
    c. Waist circumference 36 in, triglycerides 162 mg/dL, high-density lipoproteins 55 mg/dL
    d. Waist circumference 32 in, high-density lipoproteins 38 mg/dL, fasting blood glucose 122 mg/dL

22. Which teaching points are important when providing information to a patient with metabolic syndrome? **Select all that apply.**
    a. Stop smoking.
    b. Monitor weight daily.
    c. Increase level of activity.
    d. Decrease saturated fat intake.
    e. Reduce weight and maintain lower weight.
    f. Check blood glucose each morning before eating.

23. What is the main underlying risk factor for metabolic syndrome?
    a. Age
    b. Heart disease
    c. Insulin resistance
    d. High cholesterol levels

CASE STUDY   Extreme Obesity

Patient Profile

L.C., a 52-year-old single man, is seeking information at the outpatient clinic about bariatric surgery for his obesity. He reports that he has always been heavy, even as a small child, but he has gained about 100 lb in the last 2 to 3 years. Previous medical evaluations have not indicated any metabolic disease. He says he has sleep apnea and high BP, which he tries to control with sodium restriction. He currently works at a telemarketing center.

(Yurikr/iStock/
Thinkstock)

Subjective Data
- Says he is constantly dieting but eventually hunger takes over and he eats to satisfy his appetite
- Reports that he used fenfluramine (Pondimin) for about 2 months before it was taken off the market, but he lost only about 5 lbs
- Reports being treated for depression, "but only when he felt that he had no quality of life."
- Lives alone in an apartment and has several good friends in the building but rarely socializes with them outside of the complex because of his size

Objective Data
Physical Examination
- Height: 68 in (171 cm)
- Weight: 296 lbs (134.5 kg)
- Vital signs: BP 172/96 mm Hg, HR 88 beats/min, RR 24 breaths/min
- Waist measure: 56 in (141 cm)

Laboratory Tests
- Fasting blood glucose: 146 mg/dL (8.1 mmol/L)
- Total cholesterol: 250 mg/dL (6.5 mmol/L)
- Triglycerides: 312 mg/dL (3.5 mmol/L)
- High-density lipoprotein (HDL): 30 mg/dL (0.77 mmol/L)

Questions

1. What assessment data indicates that L.C. has metabolic syndrome? **Use an X to indicate if the assessment finding Indicates (is diagnostic criteria) metabolic syndrome or if it is Unrelated (is not included as diagnostic criteria) to the presence of metabolic syndrome.**

Assessment Finding	Indicates	Unrelated
Weight 296 lbs (134.5 kg)		
Triglycerides 312 mg/dL		
Height 68 in		
HDL 30 mg/dL		
Fasting blood glucose 146 mg/dL		
HR 88 beats/min		
Waist circumference 56 in		
BP 172/96 mm Hg		
Total cholesterol 250 mg/dL		

2. The nurse is obtaining a history from L.C. What patient statement indicates to the nurse that L.C. has developed one or more complications associated with obesity? **Use an X to indicate if the patient's statement Indicates (is associated) a complication of obesity exists or if the patient's statement is Unrelated (isn't associated) to a complication related to obesity.**

Patient's Statement	Indicates	Unrelated
"I use a CPAP machine when sleeping."		
"I have been prescribed metformin twice daily."		

Patient's Statement	Indicates	Unrelated
"I urinate approximately 550 mL/day."		
"I have chest pain when climbing several flights of stairs."		
"It is harder for me to hear out of my left ear."		
"I have some blood in my stools."		
"I get abdominal pain after eating bread."		

3. **Choose the most likely options for the information missing from the statements below by selecting from the lists of options provided.**

L.C. is considering several surgical options to treat obesity. The nurse explains that _____**1**_____ will encircle the stomach creating a pouch that accommodates up to a maximum of ___**2**___ of capacity. A _____**3**_____ removes about ___**4**___ of the stomach. A _____**5**_____ provides better weight loss than with restrictive procedures; however, _____**6**_____ is common. The least invasive is a _____**7**_____ which uses impulses to the vagus nerve sending the brain a message that the stomach is full.

Options for 1, 3, 5, and 7	Options for 2	Options for 4:	Options for 6
Gastric Plication	30 mL	25%	Gastric ulceration
Gastric Banding	45 mL	50%	Leakage
Roux-en-Y	90 mL	15%	Swallowing difficulty
Gastric Sleeve	100 mL	75%	Heartburn
Gastric Pacemaker	150 mL	35%	Dumping syndrome

4. L.C. undergoes bariatric surgery. Postoperatively, which nursing action would the nurse include in the plan of care? **Use an X to indicate if the nursing action is <u>Indicated</u> (is appropriate or necessary), <u>Contraindicated</u> (could be harmful, or is <u>Non-Essential</u> (is unnecessary or makes no difference).**

Nursing Action	Indicated	Contraindicated	Non-Essential
Keep the HOB at least 45°			
Have the patient splint the incision when coughing			
Have the patient use a straw when drinking liquids			
Initially, allow the patient to drink up to 90 mL			
Keep the patient on bedrest until postop day #2			
Measure abdominal girth			
Palpate peripheral pulses			
Administer IV fluids until the patient is tolerating 500 mL of PO fluids			

5. What information would the nurse provide when discharging L.C. from the acute care setting after having a Roux-en-Y? **Select all that apply.**
_____A. Notify your HCP if the wound edges are separating.
_____B. Don't lift anything heavier than 30 lbs.
_____C. You will need to take cobalamin lifelong.
_____D. Notify your HCP if your stools appear black.
_____E. You may begin soft foods in 10 days.
_____F. Eat slowly and stop when you get full.
_____G. You can drive once you stop taking narcotics for pain.
_____H. Avoid a diet high in carbohydrates.
_____I. If you are dissatisfied you can have surgery to reverse it.

Upper Gastrointestinal Problems

1. What physiologically occurs with vomiting?
   a. The acid–base imbalance most commonly associated with persistent vomiting is metabolic acidosis caused by loss of bicarbonate.
   b. Stimulation of the vomiting center by the chemoreceptor trigger zone (CTZ) is commonly caused by stretch and distention of hollow organs.
   c. Vomiting requires the coordination of activities of structures including the glottis, respiratory expiration, relaxation of the pylorus, and closure of the lower esophageal sphincter (LES).
   d. Immediately before the act of vomiting, activation of the parasympathetic nervous system causes increased salivation, increased gastric motility, and relaxation of the LES.

2. Which laboratory findings would the nurse expect in the patient with persistent vomiting?
   a. ↓ pH, ↑ sodium, ↓ hematocrit
   b. ↑ pH, ↓ chloride, ↓ hematocrit
   c. ↑ pH, ↓ potassium, ↑ hematocrit
   d. ↓ pH, ↓ potassium, ↑ hematocrit

3. A patient who has been vomiting for several days from an unknown cause is admitted to the hospital. What action would the nurse implement first?
   a. Oral administration of broth and tea
   b. IV replacement of fluid and electrolytes
   c. Administration of parenteral antiemetics
   d. Insertion of a nasogastric (NG) tube for suction

4. A patient treated for vomiting is to begin oral intake when the symptoms have subsided. To promote rehydration, the nurse plans to administer which fluid first?
   a. Water
   b. Hot tea
   c. Gatorade
   d. Warm broth

5. Ondansetron (Zofran) is prescribed for a patient with cancer chemotherapy–induced vomiting. What should the nurse understand about this drug?
   a. It is a derivative of cannabis and has a potential for abuse.
   b. It has a strong antihistamine effect that provides sedation and induces sleep.
   c. It is used only when other agents are ineffective because of side effects of anxiety and hallucinations.
   d. It relieves vomiting centrally by action in the vomiting center and peripherally by promoting gastric emptying.

6. Older patients may have cardiac or renal insufficiency and be more susceptible to problems from vomiting and antiemetic drug side effects. What nursing intervention is most important to implement with these patients?
   a. Keep the patient flat in bed to decrease dizziness.
   b. Do hourly visual checks and implement fall precautions.
   c. Give IV fluids as rapidly as possible to prevent dehydration.
   d. Keep the patient NPO until nausea and vomiting have stopped.

7. What are characteristics of gingivitis?
   a. Formation of abscesses with loosening of teeth
   b. Caused by upper respiratory tract viral infection
   c. Shallow, painful vesicular ulcerations of lips and mouth
   d. Infectious ulcers of mouth and lips because of systemic disease

8. Which infection or inflammation is related to systemic disease and cancer chemotherapy?
   a. Parotitis
   b. Stomatitis
   c. Oral candidiasis
   d. Vincent's infection

9. A patient is scheduled for biopsy of a painful tongue ulcer. Based on knowledge of risk factors for oral cancer, what would the nurse specifically ask the patient about when obtaining a history?
   a. Excessive exposure to sunlight
   b. Recurrent herpes simplex infections
   c. Use of any type of tobacco products
   d. Difficulty swallowing and pain in the ear

10. When caring for a patient following a glossectomy with dissection of the floor of the mouth and a radical neck dissection for cancer of the tongue, what is the nurse's main concern?
    a. Achieving pain relief
    b. Maintaining a patent airway
    c. Promoting a positive body image
    d. Giving tube feedings to provide nutrition

11. A patient with oral cancer has a history of heavy smoking, excess alcohol intake, and personal neglect. During the patient's early postoperative course, what would the nurse anticipate that the patient may need?
    a. Oral nutrition supplements
    b. Drug therapy to prevent substance withdrawal symptoms
    c. Counseling about lifestyle changes to prevent recurrence of the tumor
    d. Less pain medication because of cross-tolerance with central nervous system (CNS) depressants

12. The nurse is planning to teach the patient with gastroesophageal reflux disease (GERD) about foods or beverages that decrease LES pressure. What would the nurse include? **Select all that apply.**
    a. Alcohol
    b. Root beer
    c. Chocolate
    d. Citrus fruits
    e. Fatty foods
    f. Cola sodas

13. What would the nurse teach the patient with a hiatal hernia or GERD to do to control symptoms?
    a. Drink 10 to 12 ounces of water with each meal.
    b. Space 6 small meals a day between breakfast and bedtime.
    c. Sleep with the head of the bed elevated on 4- to 6-inch blocks.
    d. Perform daily exercises of toe-touching, sit-ups, and weight lifting.

14. A patient with esophageal cancer is scheduled for a partial esophagectomy. Preoperatively, which nursing intervention is the priority?
    a. Practice turning and deep breathing.
    b. Brush the teeth and mouth well each day.
    c. Teach about postoperative tubes and care.
    d. Encourage a high-calorie, high-protein diet.

15. Following a patient's esophagogastrostomy for cancer of the esophagus, what is most important for the nurse to do?
    a. Report any bloody drainage from the NG tube.
    b. Maintain the patient in semi-Fowler's or Fowler's position.
    c. Monitor for abdominal distention that may disrupt the surgical site.
    d. Expect to find decreased breath sounds bilaterally because of the surgical approach.

16. Which esophageal disorder is described as a precancerous lesion and is associated with GERD?
    a. Achalasia
    b. Barrett's esophagus
    c. Esophageal strictures
    d. Esophageal diverticula

17. What is an accurate description of eosinophilic esophagitis?
    a. Adenocarcinoma or squamous cell tumors of the esophagus
    b. Dilated veins in the esophagus caused by portal hypertension
    c. Inflammation of the esophagus from irritants or acidic gastric reflux
    d. Swelling of the esophagus from an allergic response to food or environmental triggers

18. Which type of gastritis is most likely to occur in a college student who has an isolated drinking binge?
    a. Acute gastritis
    b. Chronic gastritis
    c. Helicobacter pylori gastritis
    d. Autoimmune metaplastic atrophic gastritis

19. What would the nurse include when teaching the patient about managing chronic gastritis?
    a. Maintain a nonirritating diet with 6 small meals a day.
    b. Take antacids before meals to decrease stomach acidity.
    c. Eliminate alcohol and caffeine from the diet when symptoms occur.
    d. Use nonsteroidal antiinflammatory drugs (NSAIDs) instead of aspirin for minor pain relief.

20. Duodenal and gastric ulcers have similar as well as differentiating features. What characteristics are unique to duodenal ulcers? **Select all that apply.**
    a. Pain is relieved with eating food.
    b. They have a high recurrence rate.
    c. Increased gastric acid secretion occurs.
    d. Associated with *Helicobacter pylori* infection.
    e. Hemorrhage, perforation, and obstruction may result.
    f. There is burning and cramping in the midepigastric area.

21. Which patient is at greatest risk of developing a gastric ulcer?
    a. 55-year-old female smoker with nausea and vomiting
    b. 45-year-old female admitted for illicit drug detoxification
    c. 27-year-old male who is being divorced and has back pain
    d. 37-year-old male smoker who was in an accident while looking for a job

22. Corticosteroid medications are associated with the development of peptic ulcers because of which pathophysiologic mechanism?
    a. The enzyme urease is produced.
    b. Secretion of hydrochloric acid is increased.
    c. The rate of mucous cell renewal is decreased.
    d. The synthesis of mucus and prostaglandins is inhibited.

23. Regardless of the precipitating factor, what causes the injury to mucosal cells in peptic ulcers?
    a. Acid back diffusion into the mucosa
    b. The release of histamine from gastrointestinal (GI) cells
    c. Ammonia formation in the mucosal wall
    d. Breakdown of the gastric mucosal barrier

24. What would the nurse include when teaching a patient with newly diagnosed peptic ulcer disease?
    a. Maintain a bland, soft, low-residue diet.
    b. Use alcohol and caffeine in moderation and always with food.
    c. Eat as normally as possible, eliminating foods that cause pain or discomfort.
    d. Avoid milk and milk products because they stimulate gastric acid production.

25. What is the rationale for treating acute exacerbation of peptic ulcer disease with NG intubation?
    a. Stop spillage of GI contents into the peritoneal cavity.
    b. Remove excess fluids and undigested food from the stomach.
    c. Feed the patient the nutrients missing from the lack of ingestion.
    d. Remove stimulation for hydrochloric acid (HCl) acid and pepsin secretion by keeping the stomach empty.

26. Which statements describe the use of antacids for peptic ulcer disease? **Select all that apply.**
    a. Used in patients with verified *H. pylori*
    b. Neutralize HCl in the stomach
    c. Produce quick, short-lived relief of heartburn
    d. Cover the ulcer, protecting it from erosion by acids
    e. High incidence of side effects and contraindications
    f. May be given hourly after an acute phase of GI bleeding

27. Which medications are used to decrease gastric or HCl secretion? **Select all that apply.**
    a. Famotidine (Pepcid)
    b. Sucralfate (Carafate)
    c. Omeprazole (Prilosec)
    d. Misoprostol (Cytotec)
    e. Bethanechol (Urecholine)

28. The nurse determines that teaching for the patient with peptic ulcer disease has been effective when the patient makes which statement?
    a. "I must stop all my medications if I develop any side effects."
    b. "I should continue my treatment regimen as long as I have pain."
    c. "I have learned some relaxation strategies that decrease my stress."
    d. "I can buy whatever antacids are on sale because they all have the same effect."

29. A patient with a history of peptic ulcer disease is hospitalized with symptoms of a perforation. During the initial assessment, what would the nurse expect the patient to report?
    a. Vomiting of bright-red blood
    b. Projectile vomiting of undigested food
    c. Sudden, severe generalized abdominal and back pain
    d. Hyperactive bowel sounds and upper abdominal swelling

30. A patient with a gastric outlet obstruction has been treated with NG decompression. After the first 24 hours, the patient develops nausea and increased upper abdominal bowel sounds. What is the nurse's priority?
    a. Check the patency of the NG tube.
    b. Place the patient in a recumbent position.
    c. Assess the patient's vital signs and circulatory status.
    d. Encourage the patient to deep breathe and consciously relax.

31. When caring for a patient with an acute exacerbation of a peptic ulcer, the nurse finds the patient doubled up in bed with shallow, grunting respirations. Which would the nurse do first?
    a. Irrigate the patient's NG tube.
    b. Notify the health care provider.
    c. Place the patient in high-Fowler's position.
    d. Assess the patient's abdomen and vital signs.

32. Match the descriptions with the following surgical procedures used to treat peptic ulcer disease.

Description	Surgical Procedure
_____a. Often done after vagotomy to increase gastric emptying	1. Billroth I
_____b. Severing of a parasympathetic nerve to decrease gastric secretion	2. Billroth II
_____c. Removal of distal two-thirds of stomach with anastomosis to jejunum	3. Pyloroplasty
_____d. Removal of distal two-thirds of stomach with anastomosis to duodenum	4. Vagotomy

33. Following a Billroth II procedure, a patient develops dumping syndrome. What causes these symptoms?
    a. Distention of the smaller stomach by too much food and fluid intake.
    b. Hyperglycemia caused by uncontrolled gastric emptying into the small intestine.
    c. Irritation of the stomach lining by reflux of bile salts because the pylorus has been removed.
    d. Movement of fluid into the small bowel from concentrated food and fluids moving rapidly into the intestine.

34. Which statement by a patient with dumping syndrome indicates to the nurse that further diet teaching is needed?
    a. "I can eat bread and jam with every meal."
    b. "I should avoid drinking fluids with my meals."
    c. "I should eat smaller meals about 6 times a day."
    d. "I need to lie down for 30 to 60 minutes after my meals."

35. While caring for a patient following a subtotal gastrectomy with a gastroduodenostomy anastomosis, the nurse determines that the NG tube is obstructed. What would the nurse do first?
    a. Replace the tube with a new one.
    b. Irrigate the tube until return can be aspirated.
    c. Reposition the tube and then attempt irrigation.
    d. Notify the surgeon to reposition or replace the tube.

36. A patient with cancer of the stomach at the lesser curvature undergoes a total gastrectomy with an esophagojejunostomy. Postoperatively, what would the nurse teach the patient to expect?
    a. Rapid healing of the surgical wound
    b. Lifelong administration of cobalamin
    c. To be able to return to normal dietary habits
    d. Close follow-up for development of peptic ulcers in the jejunum

37. A patient with peptic ulcer disease has a slow upper GI source of bleeding. What type of bleeding would the nurse expect?
    a. Melena
    b. Occult blood
    c. Coffee-ground emesis
    d. Profuse bright-red hematemesis

38. A patient is admitted to the emergency department with profuse bright-red hematemesis. During the initial care of the patient, what is the nurse's priority?
    a. Establish 2 IV sites with large-gauge catheters.
    b. Perform a focused nursing assessment of the patient's status.
    c. Obtain a thorough health history to assist in determining the cause of the bleeding.
    d. Perform a gastric lavage with cool tap water in preparation for endoscopic examination.

39. A patient with upper GI bleeding and melena is treated with several drugs. Which drug would the nurse recognize as a priority to administer before, during, and potentially after endoscopy?
    a. Oral nizatidine (Axid)
    b. Epinephrine injection
    c. Vasopressin injection
    d. IV esomeprazole (Nexium)

40. What would the nurse emphasize when teaching patients at risk for upper GI bleeding to prevent bleeding episodes?
    a. All stools and vomitus must be tested for the presence of blood.
    b. The use of over-the-counter (OTC) medications of any kind must be avoided.
    c. Antacids can be taken with all prescribed medications to prevent gastric irritation.
    d. Misoprostol (Cytotec) should be used to protect the gastric mucosa in persons with peptic ulcers.

41. Which laboratory result indicates to the nurse that management of the patient with upper GI bleeding is effective?
    a. Hematocrit (Hct) of 35%
    b. Urinary output of 20 mL/hr
    c. Urine specific gravity of 1.030
    d. Decreasing blood urea nitrogen (BUN)

42. A large number of people at a picnic have suddenly developed diarrhea and bloody stools. The public health nurse suspects food poisoning and requests analysis and culture of which food?
    a. Milk
    b. Ground beef
    c. Commercially canned fish
    d. Salads with mayonnaise dressing

CASE STUDY Stomach Cancer

(Azndc/iStock/
Thinkstock)

Patient Profile
S.E. is a 68-year-old retired woman who was diagnosed with stomach cancer 2 weeks ago. The home health nurse assigned to her case reads the following information on her medical record.

Subjective Data
- 6-month history of epigastric discomfort, anorexia, nausea, vomiting, and a 25-lb weight loss
- Reports "stomach problems" for a long time; has had chronic gastritis for 20 years
- Says she was told that the tumor could not be removed because it was too advanced
- Says: "I've always been a strong person, but now I'm just too tired to eat or do anything."

Objective Data
Physical Examination
- Palpable mass in left upper quadrant of the abdomen
- Appears emaciated, with areas of skin discoloration on her forearms

Diagnostic Studies
- Barium swallow, gastroscopy, and biopsy/cytology all confirmed the presence of a well-advanced tumor in the fundus of the stomach

Laboratory Tests
- Decreased hemoglobin and hematocrit
- Serum albumin: 2.4 g/dL (24 g/L)

When the nurse visits S.E., she has just returned from a radiation treatment and is holding a plastic emesis basin and tissues in her lap.

Questions
1. Based on the information provided, use an X to indicate whether the assessment findings listed below are <u>Expected</u> (anticipated but not harmful), <u>Unexpected</u> (a complication or condition that could be harmful), or <u>Unrelated</u> (doesn't apply to this condition).

Assessment finding	Expected	Unexpected	Unrelated
Peripheral neuropathy			
Gastric outlet obstruction			
Fatigue			
Jaundice			
Abdominal pain			
Ascites			
Indigestion			

2. Indicate which assessment data in the left column is most appropriate for the clinical problem. Note that not all assessment data will be used.

Assessment Data	Clinical Problem	Appropriate Assessment Data for Clinical Problem
Palpable abdominal mass	Anemia	
Decreased hemoglobin	Nutritionally compromised	
Decreased serum albumin	Impaired gastrointestinal function	
Weight loss		
Emaciated		
Fatigue		
Nausea and vomiting		

3. **Choose the most likely options for the information missing from the statements below by selecting from the lists of options provided.**

Stomach cancer mostly affects older people. The average age at the time of diagnosis is _____**1**_____. Patients who have stomach cancer have an overall 5-year survival rate of _____**2**_____. Risk factors for stomach cancer include _____**3**_____, _____**3**_____, and _____**3**_____. A(n) _____**4**_____ is the best diagnostic tool to diagnose stomach cancer. A(n)_____**4**_____ can stage the disease while a(n) _____**4**_____ is performed to determine peritoneal spread. _____**5**_____ targets the HER-2 protein and kills the cancer cells.

Options for 1	Options for 2	Options for 3	Options for 4	Options for 5
30	50%	Smoking	Colonoscopy	Ramucirumab
45	32%	Acetaminophen	KUB	Fluorouracil
50	25%	Alcohol	Endoscopy	Carboplatin
68	71%	*H. Pylori*	PET scan	Omeprazole
75	10%	Achlorhydria	Echocardiogram	Trastuzumab
90	15%	Whole grains	Laparoscopy	Famotidine

4. What interventions would the nurse include in the treatment plan for S.E. and her family? **Select all that apply.**
   _____A. Discuss hospice options
   _____B. Encourage small frequent meals
   _____C. Referral for home health care
   _____D. Use medium-bristled toothbrush for mouth care
   _____E. Promote bed rest
   _____F. Encourage high-protein diet by eating smoked meats
   _____G. Provide a list of community agencies
   _____H. Use aloe vera gel for skin care
   _____I. Restrict fluids to decrease the risk of lymphedema

5. The following medications may be used to treat side effects from radiation and chemotherapy treatments.

   Choose the most likely options for the information missing from the table by selecting from the lists of options provided.

Medication	Dose, Route, Frequency	Drug Class	Mechanism of Action
1	10 mg IV every 6 hours PRN	Prokinetic	4
Ondansetron (Zofran)	2	5-HT$_3$ Antagonist	8
Dronabinol (Marinol)	5 mg PO every 4 hours PRN	Cannabinoid	Controls vomiting in medulla oblongata
Prochlorperazine (Compazine)	5 mg IV every 4 hours PRN	3	Blocks dopamine receptors
Scopolamine	1 mg transdermal every 3 days PRN	5	Blocks cholinergic pathway to vomiting center
6	7	Substance P/Neurokinin-1 Receptor Antagonist	Blocks interaction of Substance P at NK-1 receptor

Options for 1 and 6	Options for 2 and 7	Options for 3 and 5
Metoclopramide	5 mg IV every 4 hours PRN	Phenothiazine
Prochlorperazine	80 mg PO once daily	Cannabinoid
Scopolamine	4 mg IV every 6 hours PRN	5-HT$_3$ Antagonist
Dronabinol	10 mg IV every 6 hours PRN	Anticholinergic
Ondansetron	5 mg PO every 4 hours PRN	Substance P/NK-1 Receptor Antagonist
Receptor Antagonist		
Aprepitant	1 mg transdermal every 3 days PRN	Prokinetic

Options for 4 and 8
Blocks dopamine receptors
Blocks cholinergic pathway to vomiting center
Controls vomiting in medulla oblongata
Blocks interaction of Substance P at NK-1 receptor
Blocks action of serotonin
Increases gastric motility and emptying

Lower Gastrointestinal Problems

1. The nurse identifies a need for additional teaching when a patient with acute infectious diarrhea makes which statement?
   a. "I can use A&D ointment or Vaseline jelly around the anal area to protect my skin."
   b. "Gatorade is a good liquid to drink because it replaces the fluid and salts I have lost."
   c. "I may use over-the-counter loperamide or paregoric when I need to control the diarrhea."
   d. "I must wash my hands after every bowel movement to prevent spreading the diarrhea to my family."

2. What is the most important action by the nurse when caring for a patient who has contracted *Clostridium difficile?*
   a. Clean the entire room with ammonia.
   b. Feed the patient yogurt with probiotics.
   c. Wear gloves and wash hands with soap and water.
   d. Teach the family to use alcohol-based hand cleaners.

3. In instituting a bowel training program for a patient with fecal incontinence, what would the nurse plan to do first?
   a. Teach the patient to use a perianal pouch.
   b. Insert a rectal suppository at the same time every morning.
   c. Place the patient on a bedpan 30 minutes before breakfast.
   d. Assist the patient to the bathroom at the time of the patient's normal defecation.

4. During assessment of a patient with chronic constipation, what data obtained during the interview may be a factor contributing to the constipation?
   a. Taking methylcellulose (Citrucel) daily
   b. High dietary fiber with high fluid intake
   c. History of hemorrhoids and hypertension
   d. Suppressing the urge to defecate while at work

5. Which food would the nurse teach the patient with chronic constipation has the most dietary fiber?
   a. Peach
   b. Popcorn
   c. Dried beans
   d. Shredded wheat

6. Which method is preferred for immediate treatment of an acute episode of constipation?
   a. An enema
   b. Increased fluid
   c. Stool softeners
   d. Bulk-forming medication

7. A patient is admitted to the emergency department (ED) with acute abdominal pain. Using 1 as the first priority and 5 as the last priority, number the nursing actions in order of priority.
   _____a. Measurement of vital signs
   _____b. Administration of prescribed analgesics
   _____c. Anticipate orders for diagnostic studies based on manifestations
   _____d. Assessment of the onset, location, intensity, duration, frequency, and character of the pain
   _____e. Assessment of the abdomen for distention, bowel sounds, and pigmentation changes

8. When considering the following causes of acute abdomen, for which problems would surgery be indicated? **Select all that apply.**
   a. Pancreatitis
   b. Acute ischemic bowel
   c. Foreign body perforation
   d. Ruptured ectopic pregnancy
   e. Pelvic inflammatory disease
   f. Ruptured abdominal aneurysm

9. A patient returns to the surgical unit with a nasogastric (NG) tube to low intermittent suction, IV fluids, and a Jackson-Pratt drain at the surgical site following an exploratory laparotomy and repair of a bowel perforation. Four hours after admission, the patient develops nausea and vomiting. What is a priority nursing intervention?
   a. Assess the abdomen for distention and bowel sounds.
   b. Inspect the surgical site and drainage in the Jackson-Pratt.
   c. Check the characteristics of gastric drainage and the patency of the NG tube.
   d. Administer prescribed ondansetron (Zofran) to control the nausea and vomiting.

10. Which intervention would the nurse implement for a postoperative patient who has acute pain from the effects of medication and decreased GI motility as evidenced by abdominal pain and distension with an inability to pass flatus?
   a. Ambulate the patient more frequently.
   b. Assess the abdomen for bowel sounds.
   c. Place the patient in high Fowler's position.
   d. Withhold opioids because they decrease bowel motility.

11. A 22-year-old patient calls the outpatient clinic reporting nausea and vomiting and right lower abdominal pain. What would the nurse advise the patient to do?
   a. Use a heating pad to relax the muscles at the site of the pain.
   b. Drink at least 2 quarts of juice to replace the fluid lost in vomiting.
   c. Take a laxative to empty the bowel before examination at the clinic.
   d. Have the symptoms evaluated right away by a health care provider (HCP) at a hospital's ED.

12. When caring for a patient with irritable bowel syndrome (IBS), what is most important for the nurse to do?
   a. Recognize that IBS is a psychogenic illness that cannot be definitively diagnosed.
   b. Develop a trusting relationship with the patient to provide support and symptomatic care.
   c. Teach the patient that a diet high in fiber will relieve the symptoms of both diarrhea and constipation.
   d. Inform the patient that new medications are available and effective for treatment of IBS manifested by either diarrhea or constipation.

13. A patient with a gunshot wound to the abdomen reports increasing abdominal pain several hours after surgery to repair the bowel. What action would the nurse take first?
   a. Notify the HCP.
   b. Assess the patient's vital signs.
   c. Position the patient with the knees flexed.
   d. Determine the patient's IV intake since the end of surgery.

14. The patient has persistent and continuous pain at McBurney's point. Assessment reveals rebound tenderness and muscle guarding with the patient preferring to lie still with the right leg flexed. What interventions would be included in the plan of care?
   a. Laxatives to move the constipated bowel
   b. NPO status in preparation for possible appendectomy
   c. Parenteral fluids and antibiotic therapy for 6 hours before surgery
   d. NG tube inserted to decompress the stomach and prevent aspiration

15. The patient has peritonitis, which is a major complication of ruptured appendix. What treatment would the nurse plan to include?
   a. Peritoneal lavage
   b. Peritoneal dialysis
   c. IV fluid replacement
   d. Increased oral fluid intake

16. A 20-year-old patient with a history of Crohn's disease comes to the clinic with persistent diarrhea. What are common characteristics of Crohn's disease? **Select all that apply.**
   a. Weight loss
   b. Rectal bleeding
   c. Abdominal pain
   d. Toxic megacolon
   e. Has segmented distribution
   f. Involves the entire thickness of the bowel wall

17. What laboratory findings are expected in a patient with ulcerative colitis due to diarrhea and vomiting?
    a. Increased albumin
    b. Elevated white blood cells (WBCs)
    c. Decreased serum Na^+, K^+, Mg^+, Cl^-, and HCO_3^-
    d. Decreased hemoglobin (Hgb) and hematocrit (Hct)

18. What extraintestinal manifestations are seen in both ulcerative colitis and Crohn's disease?
    a. Celiac disease and gallstones
    b. Peptic ulcer disease and uveitis
    c. Conjunctivitis and colonic dilation
    d. Erythema nodosum and osteoporosis

19. For the patient hospitalized with inflammatory bowel disease (IBD), which treatments would be implemented to rest the bowel? **Select all that apply.**
    a. NPO
    b. IV fluids
    c. Bed rest
    d. Sedatives
    e. NG suction
    f. Parenteral nutrition

20. The medications prescribed for the patient with IBD include cobalamin and iron injections. What is the reason for using these drugs?
    a. Alleviate stress
    b. Combat infection
    c. Correct malnutrition
    d. Improve quality of life

21. Which drug is prescribed to relieve symptoms rather than treat a disease?
    a. Corticosteroids
    b. 6-Mercaptopurine
    c. Antidiarrheal agents
    d. Sulfasalazine (Azulfidine)

22. A patient with ulcerative colitis undergoes the first phase of a total proctocolectomy with ileal pouch and anal anastomosis. During the initial postoperative assessment, what would the nurse expect?
    a. A rectal tube set to low continuous suction
    b. A loop ileostomy with a plastic rod to hold it in place
    c. A colostomy stoma with an NG tube in place to provide pouch irrigations
    d. A permanent ileostomy stoma in the right lower quadrant of the abdomen

23. A patient with ulcerative colitis has a total proctocolectomy with formation of a terminal ileum stoma. What is the most important nursing intervention for this patient postoperatively?
    a. Measure the ileostomy output to determine the status of the patient's fluid balance.
    b. Change the ileostomy appliance every 3 to 4 hours to prevent leakage of drainage onto the skin.
    c. Emphasize that the ostomy is temporary and the ileum will be reconnected when the large bowel heals.
    d. Teach the patient about the high-fiber, low-carbohydrate diet required to maintain normal ileostomy drainage.

24. A patient with inflammatory bowel disease is nutritionally compromised because of decreased nutritional intake and decreased intestinal absorption. Which assessment data is evidence of this problem?
    a. Pallor and hair loss
    b. Frequent diarrhea stools
    c. Anorectal excoriation and pain
    d. Hypotension and urine output below 30 mL/hr

25. A patient is diagnosed with a volvulus. How would the nurse describe this to the patient?
    a. Bowel folding in on itself
    b. Twisting of bowel on itself
    c. Emboli of arterial supply to the bowel
    d. Protrusion of bowel in weak or abnormal opening

26. The patient comes to the ED with intermittent crampy abdominal pain, nausea, projectile vomiting, and dehydration. The nurse suspects a GI obstruction. Based on the manifestations, what area of the bowel would the nurse suspect is obstructed?
    a. Large intestine
    b. Esophageal sphincter
    c. Distal small intestine
    d. Proximal small intestine

27. What is an important nursing intervention for a patient with a small bowel obstruction who has an NG tube?
    a. Offer ice chips to suck as needed
    b. Provide mouth care frequently
    c. Irrigate the tube with normal saline every 8 hours
    d. Keep the patient supine with the head of the bed elevated 30 degrees

28. During a routine colonoscopy on a 56-year-old patient, a rectosigmoidal polyp was identified and removed. The patient asks the nurse if the risk for colon cancer is increased because of the polyp. What is the best response by the nurse?
    a. "It is very rare for polyps to become cancerous, but you should continue to have routine colonoscopies."
    b. "People with polyps have a 100% lifetime risk of developing colorectal cancer and at an earlier age than those without polyps."
    c. "All polyps are abnormal and should be removed, but the risk for cancer depends on the type and if malignant changes are present."
    d. "All polyps are premalignant and a source of most colon cancer. You will need to have a colonoscopy every 6 months to check for new polyps."

29. When obtaining a history from the patient with colorectal cancer, what would the nurse ask the patient about?
    a. Diet intake
    b. Sports involvement
    c. Environmental exposure to carcinogens
    d. Long-term use of nonsteroidal antiinflammatory drugs (NSAIDs)

30. When a patient returns to the clinical unit after an abdominal-perineal resection (APR), what would the nurse expect to assess?
    a. An abdominal dressing
    b. An abdominal wound and drains
    c. A temporary colostomy and drains
    d. A perineal wound, drains, and a stoma

31. The patient with a new ileostomy needs discharge teaching. What would the nurse plan to include?
    a. The pouch can be worn for up to 2 weeks before changing it.
    b. Decrease the amount of fluid intake to decrease the amount of drainage.
    c. The pouch can be removed when bowel movements have been regulated.
    d. If leakage occurs, promptly remove the pouch, clean the skin, and apply a new pouch.

32. When assessing a patient 8 hours after having surgery to create a colostomy, what would the nurse expect?
    a. Hyperactive, high-pitched bowel sounds
    b. A brick-red, puffy stoma that oozes blood
    c. A purplish stoma, shiny and moist with mucus
    d. A small amount of liquid fecal drainage from the stoma

33. The registered nurse (RN) coordinating the care for a patient who is 2 days postoperative following an abdominal-perineal resection (APR) with colostomy may delegate which interventions to the licensed practical nurse (LPN)? **Select all that apply.**
    a. Irrigate the colostomy.
    b. Teach ostomy and skin care.
    c. Assess and document stoma appearance.
    d. Monitor and record the volume, color, and odor of the drainage.
    e. Empty the ostomy bag and measure and record the amount of drainage.

34. A male patient who is scheduled for an abdominal-perineal resection (APR) is worried about his sexuality. What is the best nursing intervention for this patient?
    a. Have the patient's sexual partner reassure the patient that he is still desirable.
    b. Reassure the patient that sexual function will return when healing is complete.
    c. Remind the patient that affection can be expressed in ways other than through sexual intercourse.
    d. Explain that physical and emotional factors can affect sexual function but not necessarily the patient's sexuality.

35. During report, the nurse learns that the patient has a transverse colostomy. What would the nurse expect when providing care for this patient?
    a. Semiliquid stools with increased fluid requirements
    b. Liquid stools in a pouch and increased fluid requirements
    c. Formed stools with a pouch, needing irrigation, but no fluid needs
    d. Semiformed stools in a pouch with the need to monitor fluid balance

36. The nurse plans teaching for the patient with a colostomy, but the patient refuses to look at the nurse or the stoma, stating, "I just can't see myself with this thing." What is the best nursing intervention for this patient?
    a. Encourage the patient to share concerns and ask questions.
    b. Refer the patient to a chaplain to help cope with this situation.
    c. Explain that there is nothing the patient can do about it and must take care of it.
    d. Tell the patient that learning about it will prevent stool leaking and the sounds of flatus.

37. What would the nurse teach the patient with diverticulosis?
    a. Use antibiotics routinely to prevent future inflammation.
    b. Have an annual colonoscopy to detect malignant changes in the lesions.
    c. Maintain a high-fiber diet and encourage fluid intake of at least 2 L daily.
    d. Exclude whole grain breads and cereals from the diet to prevent irritating the bowel.

38. An 82-year-old man is admitted with an acute attack of diverticulitis. What is most important for the nurse to include in his care?
    a. Monitor for signs of peritonitis.
    b. Treat with daily medicated enemas.
    c. Prepare for surgery to resect the involved colon.
    d. Provide a heating pad to apply to the left lower quadrant.

39. The patient calls the clinic and describes a bump at the site of a previous incision that disappears when lying down. Which types of hernia would the nurse suspect? **Select all that apply.**
    a. Ventral
    b. Inguinal
    c. Femoral
    d. Reducible
    e. Incarcerated
    f. Strangulated

40. The patient asks the nurse why surgery is necessary for a femoral, strangulated hernia. What is the nurse's best response?
    a. "The surgery will relieve your constipation."
    b. "The abnormal hernia must be replaced into the abdomen."
    c. "The surgery is needed to allow intestinal flow and prevent necrosis."
    d. "The hernia is because the umbilical opening did not close after birth as it should have."

41. What nursing intervention is indicated for a male patient following an inguinal herniorrhaphy?
    a. Applying heat to the inguinal area
    b. Elevating the scrotum with a scrotal support
    c. Applying a truss to support the operative site
    d. Encouraging the patient to cough and deep breathe

42. How is the most common form of malabsorption syndrome treated?
    a. Administration of antibiotics
    b. Avoidance of milk and milk products
    c. Supplementation with pancreatic enzymes
    d. Avoidance of gluten found in wheat, barley, oats, and rye

43. A patient is diagnosed with celiac disease following a workup for iron-deficiency anemia and decreased bone density. The nurse identifies that additional teaching about disease management is needed when the patient makes which statement?
    a. "I should ask my close relatives to be screened for celiac disease."
    b. "If I do not follow the gluten-free diet, I will likely develop malnutrition."
    c. "I don't need to restrict gluten intake because I don't have diarrhea or bowel symptoms."
    d. "It is going to be hard to follow a gluten-free diet because it is found in so many foods."

44. Which patient is most likely to be diagnosed with short bowel syndrome?
    a. History of ulcerative colitis
    b. Extensive resection of the ileum
    c. Diagnosis of irritable bowel syndrome
    d. Colectomy performed for cancer of the bowel

45. The HCP says the patient has an anorectal abscess. How would the nurse explain this to the patient?
    a. It is an ulcer in the anal wall.
    b. It is a collection of perianal pus.
    c. It is a sacrococcygeal hairy tract.
    d. It is a tunnel from the anus or rectum.

46. A 60-year-old woman is afraid she may have anal cancer. What assessment finding increases her risk for anal cancer?
    a. Alcohol use
    b. Only 1 sexual partner
    c. Human papillomavirus (HPV)
    d. Use of a condom with sexual intercourse

47. Following a hemorrhoidectomy, what would the nurse advise the patient to do?
    a. Use daily laxatives to facilitate bowel emptying.
    b. Use ice packs to the perineum to prevent swelling.
    c. Avoid having a bowel movement for several days until healing occurs.
    d. Take warm sitz baths several times a day to promote comfort and cleaning.

CASE STUDY　Cancer of the Rectum

(monkey businessimages/ iStock/Thinkstock)

Patient Profile

C.D. is a 58-year-old married insurance salesman with a history of polyps, obesity, smoking, and eating fast food. C.D. has undergone an abdominal-perineal resection (APR) for stage III rectal cancer. He is 1 day postoperative on the general surgical unit.

Subjective Data

- Reports pain in his abdominal and perineal incisions that is not well controlled even with the patient-controlled analgesia (PCA) machine
- Wants to know when he can smoke and get back to eating his meat and potatoes
- Jokes about his stoma winking at him when the dressings are removed the first time and an ostomy bag is applied
- Refers to his stoma as "Jake"
- Tells his wife that "Jake" will be watching her. Wife is crying.

Objective Data

- Body mass index of 32 kg/m²
- Rose-colored stoma on left lower quadrant of abdomen; ostomy bag contains small amount of pink mucus drainage
- Midline abdominal incision; no signs of infection; sutures intact
- Perineal incision partially closed; 2 Penrose drains with bulky gauze dressings with a large amount of serosanguineous drainage
- PCA programmed on demand to administer 1 mg morphine sulfate every 10 minutes, 17 attempts in the past hour

Questions

1. C.D. has several risk factors associated with the development of colorectal cancer. What symptoms may have alerted C.D. to seek medical care? **Use an X to indicate whether the sign or symptom is Related to colorectal cancer or is Unrelated.**

Sign or Symptom	Related	Unrelated
Hematochezia		
Constipation		
Nausea and vomiting		
Dyspnea on exertion		
Abdominal pain or discomfort		
Fatigue		
Weight gain		

2. What interventions would the nurse include in C.D.'s plan of care postoperatively? **Use an X to indicate whether the nursing action is Indicated (appropriate or necessary), Contraindicated (could be harmful), or is Non-essential (unnecessary or makes no difference).**

Nursing Action	Indicated	Contraindicated	Non-Essential
Keep the patient on bedrest			
Tell the patient's wife that the stoma is temporary			
Report stoma drainage of 50 mL over 24 hours to the HCP			
Ask the patient to report flatus			
Advance diet to soft food once bowel sounds are normal			
Apply a transparent ostomy pouch over the stoma			
Perform daily weights			

3. A student nurse working with C.D. asks the primary nurse what the differences are between a colostomy and an ileostomy. **Use an X to indicate if the description applies to a Colostomy, Ileostomy, or Both.**

Description	Colostomy	Ileostomy	Both
Stool is semiformed			
An ostomy pouch is worn			
Stool is more like liquid			
Passage of stool cannot be regulated			
May be temporary or permanent			
Stoma may arise from the transverse colon			
Stoma arises from the ileum			
Dietary restrictions will apply due to the risk of obstruction			

4. What assessment findings indicate to the nurse that C.D. and his wife are adjusting to the colostomy? **Use an X to indicate if the assessment finding indicates Effective coping (meeting expected outcomes), Ineffective coping (not meeting expected outcomes), or is Unrelated (not related to expected outcomes).**

Assessment Finding	Effective	Ineffective	Unrelated
Wife is emotional			
C.D. calls the stoma "Jake"			
His wife is asking questions about stoma care			
C.D. says the stoma is "winking"			
C.D. says he knows he will have to change his diet			
Attempts to use the PCA 17 times during the last hour			
C.D. asks for a nicotine patch while in the hospital			

5. What instructions will the nurse include when doing discharge teaching with C.D. and his wife? **Select all that apply.**
_____A. You can continue to smoke cigarettes as long as you reduce the number of times you smoke per day.
_____B. Drink at least 3 liters per day to prevent dehydration.
_____C. Refrain from heavy lifting for 2 weeks.
_____D. There are community support groups that can help you adjust to having a stoma.
_____E. Avoid gas forming foods like beans and cabbage.
_____F. Asparagus and garlic can cause diarrhea.
_____G. You can get the stoma wet while taking a shower or when you swim.
_____H. Sexual problems do not occur with this type of surgery.

48

Liver, Biliary Tract, and Pancreas Problems

1. The patient has a diagnosis of a biliary obstruction from gallstones. What type of jaundice is the patient experiencing, and what serum bilirubin results would be expected?
   a. Hemolytic jaundice with normal conjugated bilirubin
   b. Posthepatic icterus with decreased unconjugated bilirubin
   c. Obstructive jaundice with increased unconjugated and conjugated bilirubin
   d. Hepatocellular jaundice with decreased conjugated bilirubin in severe disease

2. The patient had a blood transfusion reaction. What is the best explanation the nurse can give the patient as to why hemolytic jaundice is present?
   a. A malaria parasite has broken apart red blood cells (RBCs)
   b. It results from liver's altered ability from hepatocellular disease
   c. Jaundice results from decreased flow of bile through the liver or biliary system
   d. It is caused by increased breakdown of RBCs that increases serum unconjugated bilirubin

3. The patient returned from a 6-week mission trip to Somalia with reports of nausea, malaise, fatigue, and achy muscles. Which type of hepatitis is this patient most likely to have contracted?
   a. Hepatitis B (HBV)
   b. Hepatitis C (HCV)
   c. Hepatitis D (HDV)
   d. Hepatitis E (HEV)

4. Which type of hepatitis is a DNA virus, can be transmitted via exposure to infectious blood or body fluids, is required for HDV to replicate, and increases the risk of hepatocellular cancer for the chronic carrier?
   a. HAV
   b. HBV
   c. HCV
   d. HEV

5. Serologic findings in viral hepatitis include both the presence of viral antigens and antibodies produced in response to the virus. After vaccination, what laboratory result indicates that the person is immune to HBV?
   a. Anti-HBc immunoglobulin (Ig)G
   b. Surface antigen HBs Ag
   c. Surface antibody anti-HBs
   d. Core antigen anti-HBc IgM

6. The patient asks why the serologic test of HBV DNA quantitation is being done. What is the nurse's best explanation about the test?
   a. Shows an ongoing infection with HBV
   b. Indicates co-infection with HBV and HDV
   c. Determines any previous infection or immunization to HBV
   d. Indicates viral replication and effectiveness of therapy for chronic HBV

7. Although HAV antigens are not tested in the blood, they stimulate specific IgM and IgG antibodies. Which antibody indicates there is acute HAV infection?
   a. Anti-HBc IgG
   b. Anti-HBc IgM
   c. Anti-HAV IgG
   d. Anti-HAV IgM

8. What test will be done before prescribing treatment for the patient testing positive for HCV?
   a. Anti-HCV
   b. HCV genotyping
   c. FibroSure (FibroTest)
   d. HCV RNA quantitation

9. What causes the systemic effects of viral hepatitis?
   a. Toxins produced by the infected liver
   b. Impaired portal circulation from fibrosis
   c. Cholestasis from chemical hepatotoxicity
   d. Complement system activation by antigen-antibody complexes

10. During the incubation period of viral hepatitis, what would the nurse expect the patient to report?
    a. Dark urine and easy fatigability
    b. No symptoms except diagnostic results
    c. Anorexia and right upper quadrant discomfort
    d. Constipation or diarrhea with light-colored stools

11. The occurrence of acute liver failure is most common in which situation?
    a. A person with hepatitis A
    b. A person with hepatitis C
    c. Antihypertensive medication use
    d. Use of acetaminophen with alcohol use

12. Following a needle stick, what is used as prophylaxis against HBV?
    a. Interferon
    b. HBV vaccine
    c. Hepatitis B immune globulin (HBIG)
    d. HBIG and HBV vaccine

13. The family members of a patient with hepatitis A ask if there is anything that will prevent them from developing the disease. What is the best response by the nurse?
    a. "No immunization is available for hepatitis A, nor are you likely to get the disease."
    b. "Those who have had household or close contact with the patient should receive IG."
    c. "All family members should receive the hepatitis A vaccine to prevent or modify the infection."
    d. "Only those people who have had sexual contact with the patient need immunization."

14. A patient diagnosed with chronic hepatitis B asks about drug therapy to treat the disease. What is the most appropriate response by the nurse?
    a. "Only chronic hepatitis C is treatable and primarily with antiviral agents and interferon."
    b. "There are no specific drug therapies that are effective for treating acute viral hepatitis."
    c. "Lamivudine (Epivir) and interferon both decrease viral load and help prevent complications."
    d. "No drugs are used for the treatment of viral hepatitis because of the risk of additional liver damage."

15. The nurse identifies a need for further teaching when the patient with acute hepatitis B makes which statement?
    a. "I should avoid alcohol completely for at least a year."
    b. "I must avoid all physical contact with my family until the jaundice is gone."
    c. "I should use a condom to prevent spread of the disease to my sexual partner."
    d. "I will need to rest several times a day, gradually increasing my activity as I tolerate it."

16. What nursing intervention that promotes healing in the patient with viral hepatitis is the most challenging?
    a. Providing adequate nutritional intake
    b. Promoting strict bed rest during the icteric phase
    c. Providing pain relief without using liver-metabolized drugs
    d. Providing quiet diversional activities during periods of fatigue

17. When caring for a patient with autoimmune hepatitis, what would the nurse understand is different when compared to a patient who has viral hepatitis?
    a. Does not manifest hepatomegaly or jaundice
    b. Experiences less liver inflammation and damage
    c. Is treated with corticosteroids or other immunosuppressive agents
    d. Is an older adult who has used a wide variety of prescription and over-the-counter drugs

18. The patient has been newly diagnosed with Wilson's disease. D-penicillamine, a chelating agent, has been prescribed. What assessment finding would the nurse expect?
    a. Pruritus
    b. Acute kidney injury
    c. Corneal Fleischer rings
    d. Increased serum iron levels

19. A patient, who has a history of ulcerative colitis for several years, presents with jaundice and itching, steatorrhea, and liver enlargement. What would the nurse expect is the most likely diagnosis?
    a. Cirrhosis
    b. Acute liver failure
    c. Hepatorenal syndrome
    d. Primary sclerosing cholangitis

20. An older woman with cirrhosis has anemia. What pathophysiologic changes may contribute to this patient's anemia? **Select all that apply.**
    a. Vitamin B deficiencies
    b. Stretching of liver capsule
    c. Vascular congestion of spleen
    d. Decreased prothrombin production
    e. Decreased bilirubin conjugation and excretion

21. A patient was diagnosed with nonalcoholic fatty liver disease (NAFLD). What treatment measures would the nurse plan to teach the patient? **Select all that apply.**
    a. Weight loss
    b. Diabetes management
    c. Ulcerative colitis dietary changes
    d. Diet management of hyperlipidemia
    e. Maintaining blood pressure with increased sodium and fluid intake

22. Which etiologic manifestations related to esophageal varices occur in the patient with cirrhosis?
    a. Jaundice, peripheral edema, and ascites from increased intrahepatic pressure and dysfunction
    b. Loss of the small bile ducts and cholestasis and cirrhosis in patients with other autoimmune disorders
    c. Development of collateral channels of circulation in inelastic, fragile esophageal veins as a result of portal hypertension
    d. Scarring and nodular changes in the liver lead to compression of the veins and sinusoids, causing resistance of blood flow through the liver from the portal vein

23. Which conditions contribute to the formation of abdominal ascites?
    a. Esophageal varices contribute to 80% of variceal hemorrhages
    b. Increased colloidal oncotic pressure caused by decreased albumin production
    c. Hypoaldosteronism causes increased sodium reabsorption by the renal tubules
    d. Blood flow through the portal system is obstructed, which causes portal hypertension

24. What laboratory test results would the nurse expect in a patient with cirrhosis?
    a. Serum albumin: 7.0 g/dL (70 g/L)
    b. Total bilirubin: 3.2 mg/dL (54.7 mmol/L)
    c. Serum cholesterol: 260 mg/dL (6.7 mmol/L)
    d. Aspartate aminotransferase (AST): 6.0 U/L (0.1 mkat/L)

25. Malnutrition can be a major problem for patients with cirrhosis. Which nursing intervention can help improve nutrient intake?
    a. Oral hygiene before meals and snacks
    b. Provide all foods the patient likes to eat
    c. Improve oral intake by feeding the patient
    d. Limit snack offers to when the patient is hungry

26. What must the patient with cirrhosis be monitored for when being treated with diuretics to treat ascites? **Select all that apply.**
    a. Gastrointestinal (GI) bleeding
    b. Hypokalemia
    c. Renal function
    d. Body image disturbances
    e. Increased clotting tendencies

27. What manifestation does the nurse recognize as an early sign of hepatic encephalopathy?
    a. Manifests asterixis
    b. Becomes unconscious
    c. Has increasing oliguria
    d. Impaired computational skills

28. To treat a cirrhotic patient with hepatic encephalopathy, lactulose, rifaximin (Xifaxan), and a proton pump inhibitor are ordered. The patient's family wants to know why the laxative is ordered. What is the best explanation the nurse can give to the family?
    a. Use reduces portal venous pressure.
    b. It will eliminate blood from the GI tract.
    c. It traps ammonia and eliminates it in the feces.
    d. It decreases bacteria to decrease ammonia formation.

29. The patient has hepatic encephalopathy. What is a priority nursing intervention to keep the patient safe?
    a. Turn the patient every 3 hours.
    b. Encourage increasing ambulation.
    c. Assist the patient to the bathroom.
    d. Prevent constipation to reduce ammonia production.

30. A patient with advanced cirrhosis is nutritionally compromised because of anorexia and an inadequate food intake. What would be an appropriate midday snack for the patient?
    a. Peanut butter and salt-free crackers
    b. A fresh tomato sandwich with salt-free butter
    c. Popcorn with salt-free butter and herbal seasoning
    d. Canned chicken noodle soup with low-protein bread

31. The patient with liver failure had a liver transplant. What would the nurse teach the patient about self-care after the transplant?
    a. Alcohol intake is now okay.
    b. HBIG will be required to prevent rejection.
    c. Elevate the head 30 degrees to improve ventilation when sleeping.
    d. Monitor closely for infection because of the immunosuppressive medication.

32. When treating a patient with bleeding esophageal varices, what is the most important nursing action?
    a. Prepare the patient for immediate portal shunting surgery.
    b. Perform guaiac testing on all stools to detect occult blood.
    c. Maintain the patient's airway and prevent aspiration of blood.
    d. Monitor for the cardiac effects of IV vasopressin and nitroglycerin.

33. A patient with cirrhosis and esophageal varices that are refractory to treatment undergoes a splenorenal shunt. What would the nurse expect the patient to experience?
    a. An improved survival rate
    b. Decreased serum ammonia levels
    c. Improved metabolism of nutrients
    d. Improved hemodynamic function and renal perfusion

34. In discussing long-term management with the newly diagnosed patient with alcoholic cirrhosis, what would the nurse teach the patient?
    a. A daily exercise regimen is important to increase the blood flow through the liver.
    b. Cirrhosis can be reversed if the patient follows a regimen of proper rest and nutrition.
    c. Abstinence from alcohol is the most important factor in improvement of the patient's condition.
    d. The only over-the-counter analgesic that you should take for minor aches and pains is acetaminophen.

35. A patient is hospitalized with metastatic cancer of the liver. The nurse plans care for the patient based on what knowledge?
    a. Chemotherapy is highly successful in the treatment of liver cancer.
    b. The patient will undergo surgery to remove the involved portions of the liver.
    c. Supportive care that is appropriate for all patients with severe liver damage is indicated.
    d. Metastatic cancer of the liver is more responsive to treatment than primary carcinoma of the liver.

36. A patient with cirrhosis asks the nurse about the possibility of a liver transplant. What is the best response by the nurse?
    a. "If you are interested in a transplant, you really should talk to your doctor about it."
    b. "Liver transplants are indicated only in young people with irreversible liver disease."
    c. "Rejection is such a problem in liver transplants that it is seldom attempted in patients with cirrhosis."
    d. "Cirrhosis is an indication for transplantation in some cases. Have you talked to your doctor about this?"

37. Which complication of acute pancreatitis requires prompt surgical drainage to prevent sepsis?
    a. Tetany
    b. Pseudocyst
    c. Pleural effusion
    d. Pancreatic abscess

38. What would the nurse expect when assessing a patient with acute pancreatitis?
    a. Hyperactive bowel sounds
    b. Hypertension and tachycardia
    c. A temperature greater than 102°F (38.9°C)
    d. Severe left upper quadrant (LUQ) or midepigastric pain

39. Combined with clinical manifestations, what is the laboratory finding that is most commonly used to diagnose acute pancreatitis?
    a. Increased serum calcium
    b. Increased serum amylase
    c. Increased urinary amylase
    d. Decreased serum glucose

40. What treatment measure is used in managing the patient with acute pancreatitis?
    a. Surgery to remove the inflamed pancreas
    b. Pancreatic enzyme supplements administered with meals
    c. Nasogastric (NG) suction to prevent gastric contents from entering the duodenum
    d. Endoscopic pancreatic sphincterotomy using endoscopic retrograde cholangiopancreatography (ERCP)

41. A patient with acute pancreatitis has acute pain from distention of the pancreas and peritoneal irritation. In addition to effective use of analgesics, what would the nurse include in the plan of care?
    a. Provide diversional activities to distract the patient from the pain.
    b. Provide small, frequent meals to increase the patient's tolerance to food.
    c. Position the patient on the side with the head of the bed elevated 45 degrees for pain relief.
    d. Ambulate the patient every 3 to 4 hours to increase circulation and decrease abdominal congestion.

42. The nurse determines that further discharge instruction is needed when the patient with acute pancreatitis makes which statement?
    a. "I will look for fat in my stools."
    b. "I must not use alcohol to prevent future attacks of pancreatitis."
    c. "I shouldn't eat any salty foods or foods with high amounts of sodium."
    d. "I will not need to monitor my blood glucose levels when I am at home."

43. What is the patient with chronic pancreatitis more likely to have than the patient with acute pancreatitis?
    a. Has acute abdominal pain
    b. The need to abstain from alcohol
    c. Malabsorption and diabetes
    d. Require a high-carbohydrate, high-protein, low-fat diet

44. What information would the nurse include when teaching a patient with chronic pancreatitis about measures to prevent further attacks? **Select all that apply.**
    a. Avoid nicotine
    b. Eat bland foods
    c. Observe stools for steatorrhea
    d. Eat high-fat, low-protein, high-carbohydrate meals
    e. Take prescribed pancreatic enzymes immediately after meals.

45. What risk factor is associated with pancreatic cancer?
    a. Alcohol intake
    b. Cigarette smoking
    c. Exposure to asbestos
    d. Intake of spoiled milk products

46. In a radical pancreaticoduodenectomy (Whipple procedure) for treatment of pancreatic cancer, what is resected that most affects the patient's nutrition status?
    a. Duodenum
    b. Part of the stomach
    c. Head of the pancreas
    d. Common bile duct and gall bladder

47. Which characteristics are most commonly associated with cholelithiasis? **Select all that apply.**
    a. Obesity
    b. Age over 40 years
    c. Multiparous female
    d. History of excessive alcohol intake
    e. Family history of gallbladder disease
    f. Use of estrogen or oral contraceptives

48. Which factors may be associated with acalculous cholecystitis? **Select all that apply.**
    a. Fasting
    b. Hypothyroidism
    c. Parenteral nutrition
    d. Prolonged immobility
    e. *Streptococcus pneumoniae*
    f. Absence of bile in the intestine

49. A patient with an obstruction of the common bile duct has clay-colored fatty stools. What is the pathophysiologic change that causes this manifestation?
    a. Water-soluble (conjugated) bilirubin in the blood is excreted into the urine.
    b. Absence of bilirubin and bile salts in the small intestine prevents conversion to urobilinogen, fat emulsion, and digestion.
    c. Contraction of the inflamed gallbladder and obstructed ducts is stimulated by cholecystokinin when fats enter the duodenum.
    d. Obstruction of the common duct prevents bile drainage into the duodenum, resulting in congestion of bile in the liver and subsequent absorption into the blood.

50. The patient with suspected gallbladder disease is scheduled for an ultrasound of the gallbladder. What would the nurse teach the patient about this test?
    a. It is noninvasive and is a very reliable method of detecting gallstones.
    b. It is the only test to use when the patient is allergic to contrast medium.
    c. It will outline the gallbladder and the ductal system to enable visualization of stones.
    d. It is an adjunct to liver function tests to determine whether the gallbladder is inflamed.

51. What treatment for acute cholecystitis will prevent further gall bladder stimulation?
    a. NPO with NG suction
    b. Incisional cholecystectomy
    c. Administration of antiemetics
    d. Administration of anticholinergics

52. What would the nurse expect to be included in the patient's plan of care after a laparoscopic cholecystectomy?
    a. Return to work in 2 to 3 weeks
    b. Be hospitalized for 3 to 5 days postoperatively
    c. Have a T-tube placed in the common bile duct to provide bile drainage
    d. Have up to 4 small abdominal incisions covered with small dressings

53. A patient with chronic cholecystitis asks the nurse if continuing a low-fat diet after a cholecystectomy will be necessary. What is the nurse's best response?
    a. "A low-fat diet will prevent the development of further gallstones and should be continued."
    b. "Yes; because you will not have a gallbladder to store bile, you will not be able to digest fats adequately."
    c. "A low-fat diet is recommended for a few weeks after surgery until the intestine adjusts to receiving a continuous flow of bile."
    d. "Removing the gallbladder will eliminate the source of your pain that was associated with fat intake, so you may eat whatever you like."

54. When providing care to a patient after having a cholecystectomy, what would the nurse do to care for the T-tube?
    a. Keep the tube supported and free of kinks.
    b. Attach the tube to low, continuous suction.
    c. Clamp the tube when ambulating the patient.
    d. Irrigate the tube with 10-mL sterile saline every 2 to 4 hours.

55. What instruction would the nurse include when doing discharge teaching for a patient who had a laparoscopic cholecystectomy?
    a. Keep the incision area clean and dry for at least a week.
    b. Report the need to take pain medication for shoulder pain.
    c. Report any bile-colored or purulent drainage from the incisions.
    d. Expect some postoperative nausea and vomiting for several days.

CASE STUDY   Acute Pancreatitis

(9nong/iStock/
Thinkstock)

Patient Profile
V.A. is a 70-year-old man admitted to the hospital with acute pancreatitis.

Subjective Data
- Reports severe abdominal pain in the LUQ radiating to the back
- Reports that he is nauseated and has been vomiting

Objective Data
- Vital signs: Temp 101°F (38.3°C), HR 114 beats/min, RR 26 breaths/min, BP 92/58 mm Hg
- Icteric sclera

Interprofessional Care
- NPO
- NG tube to low intermittent suction (LIS)
- IV therapy with lactated Ringer's solution
- Morphine PCA
- Pantoprazole (Protonix) IV

Questions
1. What additional clinical manifestations associated with acute pancreatitis would the nurse expect? **Use an X to indicate whether the assessment finding is <u>Expected</u> (is a sign or symptom of acute pancreatitis), <u>Unexpected</u> (indicates a complication or severe disease) or is <u>Unrelated</u> (is not associated with acute pancreatitis).**

Assessment Finding	Expected	Unexpected	Unrelated
Decreased or absent bowel sounds			
Palpable epigastric mass			

Assessment Finding	Expected	Unexpected	Unrelated
Crackles in the lungs			
Pleural effusion			
Cullen's sign			
Trousseau's sign			
Grade III/VI murmur			
Increased abdominal girth			

2. What diagnostic results would indicate the presence of acute pancreatitis? **Use an X to indicate whether the diagnostic result is Expected (indicates acute pancreatitis), Unexpected (indicates severe disease or a complication of acute pancreatitis), or is Unrelated (isn't a diagnostic result associated with acute pancreatitis).**

Diagnostic Result	Expected	Unexpected	Unrelated
Serum calcium: 7 mg/dL			
Serum lipase: 600 U/L			
Echocardiogram: EF 40%			
Chest x-ray: whiteout			
WBC count: 20,000/μL			
Serum amylase: 400 U/L			
Hemoglobin 10 g/dL			

3. The HCP has ordered an NG tube to low intermittent suction. What nursing actions will the nurse include in V.A.'s plan of care to insert and manage the nasogastric (NG) tube? **Select all that apply.**

_____A. Use 60 mm Hg suction pressure

_____B. Insert a feeding tube

_____C. Clamp the air vent to prevent reflux of gastric contents

_____D. Choose a 14-Fr or 16-Fr tube

_____E. Keep HOB at least 30°

_____F. Check residuals every 4 hours

_____G. Use a Salem sump tube

_____H. Use pH test paper to check for correct placement

_____I. Inject an air bolus while auscultating over the epigastric area to check placement

4. Indicate which nursing action listed in the far-left column is appropriate for each clinical problem associated with acute pancreatitis.

Nursing Action	Clinical Problem	Appropriate Nursing Action for Each Clinical Problem
Keep patient NPO	Hypotension	
Administer lactated Ringer's solution	Acute Pain	
Administer pantoprazole	Pancreatic Enzyme Production	
Morphine PCA		
Dopamine, if necessary		
NG tube to LIS		
Papaverine, if necessary		
Albumin, if necessary		

5. What assessment findings would indicate to the nurse that V.A.'s condition is improving? **For each assessment finding, use an X to indicate whether the interventions were Effective (helped to meet expected outcomes), Ineffective (did not help to meet expected outcomes), or Unrelated (not related to expected outcomes).**

Assessment Finding	Effective	Ineffective	Unrelated
SpO$_2$ 96% on 3 L/min nasal cannula			
Cheek twitches when tapped			
Flank ecchymosis			
Denies dizziness with position changes			

Assessment Finding	Effective	Ineffective	Unrelated
Reports numbness around lips			
Reports dyspnea on exertion			
Pupils 4 mm equal and reactive			
Denies palpitations			

6. What information would the nurse include when doing discharge teaching with V.A.? **Select all that apply**.
_____A. Don't smoke or use any products that contain nicotine.
_____B. Eat more unsaturated fats.
_____C. Include more carbohydrates in your diet.
_____D. You won't need physical therapy.
_____E. Avoid all alcoholic beverages.
_____F. Report foul-smelling stools to your HCP.
_____G. Eat 3 large meals per day.
_____H. Weight loss is expected and does not need to be reported to your HCP.
_____I. You may develop chronic pancreatitis.

Assessment: Urinary System

1. Using the following list of terms, identify the structures in the illustrations below. (**Some of the terms may be used in both illustrations.**)

Terms

Aorta	Inferior vena cava	Renal pelvis
Bladder	Kidney	Renal artery
Calyx	Left ureter	Renal vein
Cortex	Medulla	Right adrenal gland
Diaphragm	Papilla	Ureter
Fibrous capsule	Pyramid	Urethra

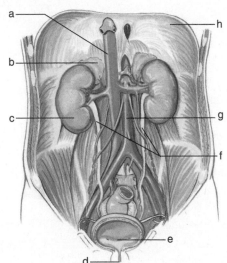

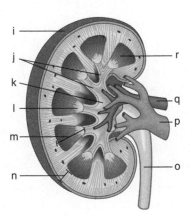

a. _____

b. _____

c. _____

d. _____

e. _____

f. _____

g. _____

h. _____

i. _____

j. _____

k. _____

l. _____

m. _____

n. _____

o. _____

p. _____

q. _____

r. _____

2. Number the following physiologic occurrences in the order they occur in the formation of urine. Begin with 1 for the first occurrence and 6 for the last occurrence.
   a. _____ Blood is filtered in the glomerulus.
   b. _____ Reabsorption of water in the loop of Henle.
   c. _____ Reabsorption of electrolytes, glucose, amino acids, and small proteins in the proximal convoluted tubules.
   d. _____ Acid–base regulation with conservation of bicarbonate (HCO_3^-) and secretion of excess H^+ in the distal convoluted tubules.
   e. _____ Active reabsorption of chloride (Cl^-) ions and passive reabsorption of sodium (Na^+) ions in the ascending loop of Henle.
   f. _____ Ultrafiltrate flows from Bowman's capsule and passes down the tubules without blood cells, platelets, or large plasma proteins.

3. Which important functions of regulation of water balance and acid–base balance occur in the distal convoluted tubules of the nephron? **Select all that apply.**
   a. Secretion of H^+ into filtrate
   b. Reabsorption of water without antidiuretic hormone (ADH)
   c. Reabsorption of Na^+ in exchange for K^+
   d. Reabsorption of glucose and amino acids
   e. Reabsorption of water under ADH influence
   f. Reabsorption of Ca^{+2} under parathormone influence

4. The right atrium myocytes secrete atrial natriuretic peptide (ANP) when there is increased plasma volume. How does ANP produce a large volume of dilute urine? **Select all that apply.**
   a. Inhibits renin
   b. Increases ADH
   c. Inhibits angiotensin II action
   d. Decreases sodium excretion
   e. Increases aldosterone secretion

5. Which statement accurately describes glomerular filtration rate (GFR)?
   a. The primary function of GFR is to excrete nitrogenous waste products.
   b. Decreased permeability in the glomerulus causes loss of proteins into the urine.
   c. The GFR is primarily dependent on adequate blood flow and adequate hydrostatic pressure.
   d. The GFR is decreased when prostaglandins cause vasodilation and increased renal blood flow.

6. A patient with an obstruction of the renal artery causing renal ischemia has hypertension. What factor may have contributed to hypertension in this patient?
   a. Increased renin release
   b. Increased ADH secretion
   c. Decreased aldosterone secretion
   d. Increased synthesis and release of prostaglandins

7. Which clinical situation would cause an increased release of erythropoietin?
   a. Hypoxemia
   b. Hypotension
   c. Hyperkalemia
   d. Fluid overload

8. What common diagnostic studies are done for a patient with severe renal colic? **Select all that apply.**
   a. CT scan
   b. Urinalysis
   c. Cystoscopy
   d. Ureteroscopy
   e. Abdominal ultrasound

9. Which volume of urine in the bladder would cause discomfort and requires urinary catheterization?
   a. 250 mL
   b. 500 mL
   c. 1100 mL
   d. 1500 mL

10. What factor contributes to an increased incidence of urinary tract infections (UTIs) in older women?
    a. Length of the urethra
    b. Larger capacity of bladder
    c. Relaxation of pelvic floor and bladder muscles
    d. Tight muscular support at the urinary sphincter

11. A 78-year-old man asks the nurse why he has to urinate so much at night. What would the nurse explain to the patient that as an older adult may be contributing to his nocturia?
    a. Decreased renal mass
    b. Decreased detrusor muscle tone
    c. Decreased ability to conserve sodium
    d. Decreased ability to concentrate urine

12. List 1 specific finding identified by the nurse during assessment of each of the patient's functional health patterns that indicates a risk factor for urinary problems or a patient response to a urinary disorder.

Functional Health Pattern	Risk Factor for or Response to Urinary Problem
Health perception–health management	
Nutritional-metabolic	
Elimination	
Activity-exercise	
Sleep-rest	
Cognitive-perceptual	
Self-perception–self-concept	
Role-relationship	
Sexuality-reproductive	
Coping–stress tolerance	
Value-belief	

13. What action by the nurse accurately describes the physical assessment of the urinary system?
    a. Auscultates the lower abdominal quadrants for fluid sounds
    b. Palpates an empty bladder at the level of the symphysis pubis
    c. Percusses the kidney with a firm blow at the posterior costovertebral angle
    d. Positions the patient prone to palpate the kidneys with a posterior approach

14. The patient reports "wetting when she sneezes." How should the nurse document this information?
    a. Nocturia
    b. Micturition
    c. Urge incontinence
    d. Stress incontinence

15. The health care provider documented that the patient has urinary retention. What would the nurse expect to find when assessing the patient?
    a. Inability to void
    b. No urine formation
    c. Large amount of urine output
    d. Increased incidence of urination

16. A male patient is admitted with a diagnosis of benign prostatic hyperplasia (BPH). What urination characteristic would the nurse expect to be present?
    a. Oliguria
    b. Hesitancy
    c. Hematuria
    d. Pneumaturia

17. What terminology would the nurse use when documenting that a patient is wetting the bed at night?
    a. Ascites
    b. Dysuria
    c. Enuresis
    d. Urgency

18. If a urine specimen is not processed within 1 hour, what result of the urinalysis may be erroneous?
    a. Glucose
    b. Bacteria
    c. Specific gravity
    d. White blood cells

19. Which urinalysis results, of a freshly voided specimen, most likely indicate a urinary tract infection (UTI)?
    a. Cloudy, yellow; red blood cell (RBC) 5/hpf; white blood cell (WBC) 10/hpf; pH 8.2
    b. Yellow; protein 6 mg/dL; pH 6.8; 10^2 CFU/mL bacteria
    c. Cloudy, brown; ammonia odor; specific gravity 1.030; RBC 18/hpf
    d. Clear; colorless; glucose: trace; ketones: trace; osmolality 500 mOsm/kg (500 mmol/kg)

20. Which urine specific gravity value would indicate to the nurse that the patient is receiving excessive IV fluid therapy?
    a. 1.002
    b. 1.010
    c. 1.025
    d. 1.033

21. After a patient had a renal arteriogram and has returned to the clinical unit, what is the most important action by the nurse?
    a. Observe for gross bleeding in the urine.
    b. Place the patient in high Fowler's position.
    c. Monitor the patient for signs of allergy to the contrast medium.
    d. Assess peripheral pulses in the involved leg every 30 to 60 minutes.

22. Which test is most specific for renal function?
    a. Renal scan
    b. Serum creatinine
    c. Creatinine clearance
    d. Blood urea nitrogen (BUN)

23. What is the most likely reason that a patient has an increased BUN?
    a. Has impaired renal function
    b. Has not eaten enough protein
    c. Has decreased urea in the urine
    d. May have nonrenal tissue hypertrophy

24. What impairment in kidney function would cause the following laboratory results in a patient with kidney disease?

Laboratory Result	Impaired Kidney Function
Serum Ca^{2+}: 7.2 mg/dL (1.8 mmol/L)	
Hemoglobin (Hgb): 9.6 g/dL (96 g/L)	
Serum creatinine: 3.2 mg/dL (283 mmol/L)	

25. Following a renal biopsy, what is the nurse's priority?
    a. Offer warm sitz baths to relieve discomfort.
    b. Test urine for microscopic bleeding with a dipstick.
    c. Expect the patient to experience burning on urination.
    d. Monitor the patient for symptoms of a urinary infection.

26. What steps would the nurse implement to obtain a clean-catch urine specimen from a patient? **Select all that apply.**
    a. Use a sterile container.
    b. The patient must have a full bladder.
    c. Insert a catheter immediately after voiding.
    d. Have the patient void, stop, and then void into the container.
    e. Have the patient clean the meatus before voiding.

27. Which diagnostic study would include assessing for iodine sensitivity, teaching the patient to take a cathartic the night before the procedure, and telling the patient that a warm sensation may occur during the contrast media injection?
    a. Cystometrogram
    b. Renal arteriogram
    c. Kidneys, ureters, bladder (KUB) x-ray
    d. MRI

Renal and Urologic Problems

1. Which classification of urinary tract infection (UTI) is described as infection of the renal parenchyma, renal pelvis, and ureters?
   a. Upper UTI
   b. Lower UTI
   c. Complicated UTI
   d. Uncomplicated UTI

2. While caring for a 77-year-old woman who has an indwelling urinary catheter, the nurse monitors the patient for the development of a UTI. What clinical manifestations would indicate a UTI?
   a. Cloudy urine and fever
   b. Urethral burning and bloody urine
   c. Vague abdominal discomfort and disorientation
   d. Suprapubic pain and slight decline in body temperature

3. A woman with no history of UTI who has urgency, frequency, and dysuria comes to the clinic. A dipstick and microscopic urinalysis indicate bacteriuria. What would the nurse anticipate for this patient?
   a. Obtaining a clean-catch midstream urine specimen for culture and sensitivity
   b. No treatment with medication unless she develops fever, chills, and flank pain
   c. Empirical treatment with trimethoprim-sulfamethoxazole (Bactrim) for 3 days
   d. Need to have a blood specimen drawn for a complete blood count (CBC) and kidney function tests

4. What would the nurse include in the teaching plan for a female patient with a UTI?
   a. Empty the bladder at least 4 times a day.
   b. Drink at least 2 quarts of water every day.
   c. Wait to urinate until the urge is very intense.
   d. Clean the urinary meatus with an antiinfective agent after voiding.

5. What is the most common cause of acute pyelonephritis resulting from an ascending infection from the lower urinary tract?
   a. The kidney is scarred and fibrotic.
   b. The organism is resistant to antibiotics.
   c. There is a preexisting abnormality of the urinary tract.
   d. The patient does not take all of the antibiotics for treatment of a UTI.

6. Which characteristic is more likely associated with acute pyelonephritis than with a lower UTI?
   a. Fever
   b. Dysuria
   c. Urgency
   d. Frequency

7. Which test is required to diagnose pyelonephritis?
   a. Renal biopsy
   b. Blood culture
   c. Intravenous pyelogram (IVP)
   d. Urine for culture and sensitivity

8. A patient with suprapubic pain and symptoms of urinary frequency and urgency has 2 negative urine cultures. Which assessment finding would indicate interstitial cystitis (IC)?
   a. Residual urine greater than 200 mL
   b. A large, atonic bladder on urodynamic testing
   c. A voiding pattern that indicates psychogenic urinary retention
   d. Pain with bladder filling that is transiently relieved by urination

9. When caring for the patient with IC, what would the nurse teach the patient to do?
   a. Avoid foods that make the urine more alkaline.
   b. Use high-potency vitamin therapy to decrease the autoimmune effects of the disorder.
   c. Always keep a voiding diary to document pain, voiding frequency, and patterns of nocturia.
   d. Use the dietary supplement calcium glycerophosphate (Prelief) to decrease bladder irritation.

10. What causes glomerulonephritis characterized by glomerular damage?
    a. Growth of microorganisms in the glomeruli
    b. Release of bacterial substances toxic to the glomeruli
    c. Accumulation of immune complexes in the glomeruli
    d. Hemolysis of red blood cells circulating in the glomeruli

11. What manifestation will indicate the need for restricting dietary protein when managing care for a patient with acute poststreptococcal glomerulonephritis (APSGN)?
    a. Hematuria
    b. Proteinuria
    c. Hypertension
    d. Elevated blood urea nitrogen (BUN)

12. The nurse plans care for the patient with APSGN based on what knowledge?
    a. Most patients with APSGN recover completely or rapidly improve with conservative management.
    b. Chronic glomerulonephritis leading to renal failure is a common sequela to acute glomerulonephritis.
    c. Pulmonary hemorrhage may occur as a result of antibodies also attacking the alveolar basement membrane.
    d. A large percentage of patients with APSGN develop rapidly progressive glomerulonephritis, resulting in kidney failure.

13. What causes edema associated with nephrotic syndrome?
    a. Hypercoagulability
    b. Hyperalbuminemia
    c. Decreased plasma oncotic pressure
    d. Decreased glomerular filtration rate

14. Using numbers 1–8 with number 1 as the first pathologic change, put in order the following ascending pathologic changes that occur in the urinary tract in the presence of a bladder outlet obstruction.
    a. _____ Hydronephrosis
    b. _____ Reflux of urine into ureter
    c. _____ Bladder detrusor muscle hypertrophy
    d. _____ Ureteral dilation
    e. _____ Renal atrophy
    f. _____ Vesicoureteral reflux
    g. _____ Large residual urine in bladder
    h. _____ Chronic pyelonephritis

15. Which infection is asymptomatic at first and then progresses to cystitis, frequent urination, burning when voiding, and epididymitis?
    a. Urosepsis
    b. Urethral diverticula
    c. Goodpasture syndrome
    d. Genitourinary tuberculosis

16. In many cases, what can patients at risk for kidney stones do to prevent them?
    a. Lead an active lifestyle
    b. Limit protein and acidic foods in the diet
    c. Drink enough fluids to produce dilute urine
    d. Take prophylactic antibiotics to control UTIs

17. Which type of urinary tract stones are the most common and often obstruct the ureter?
    a. Cystine
    b. Uric acid
    c. Calcium oxalate
    d. Calcium phosphate

18. A female patient has a UTI and kidney stones. Which type of stone is the most likely cause?
    a. Cystine
    b. Struvite
    c. Uric acid
    d. Calcium phosphate

19. A patient with a history of gout has been diagnosed with kidney stones. Which treatments would the nurse anticipate? **Select all that apply.**
    a. Reduce dietary oxalate
    b. Administer allopurinol
    c. Administer α-penicillamine
    d. Administer thiazide diuretics
    e. Reduce animal protein intake
    f. Reduce intake of milk products

20. Besides being mixed with struvite or oxalate stones, what characteristic is associated with calcium phosphate calculi?
    a. Associated with alkaline urine
    b. Genetic autosomal recessive defect
    c. Three times as common in women as in men
    d. Defective gastrointestinal (GI) and kidney absorption

21. When assessing the patient with a kidney stone passing down the ureter, what would the nurse expect the patient to report?
    a. A history of chronic UTIs
    b. Dull, costovertebral flank pain
    c. Severe, colicky back pain radiating to the groin
    d. A feeling of bladder fullness with urgency and frequency

22. Which foods or drinks should be restricted to prevent calcium oxalate stones?
    a. Milk and milk products
    b. Dried beans and dried fruits
    c. Liver, kidney, and sweetbreads
    d. Spinach, cabbage, and tomatoes

23. Following electrohydraulic lithotripsy for treatment of kidney stones, the patient is at risk for infection. What is the most appropriate nursing intervention?
    a. Monitor for hematuria
    b. Encourage fluid intake of 3 L/day
    c. Apply moist heat to the flank area
    d. Strain all urine through gauze or a special strainer

24. A patient with which condition would benefit from being taught to do self-catheterization?
    a. Renal trauma
    b. Urethral stricture
    c. Renal artery stenosis
    d. Accelerated nephrosclerosis

25. When providing care for the patient with adult-onset polycystic kidney disease, what would the nurse do?
    a. Help the patient cope with the rapid progression of the disease.
    b. Suggest genetic counseling resources for the children of the patient.
    c. Expect the patient to have polyuria and poor concentration ability of the kidneys.
    d. Implement measures for the patient's deafness and blindness in addition to the renal problems.

26. Which disease causes connective tissue changes that cause glomerulonephritis?
    a. Gout
    b. Amyloidosis
    c. Diabetes mellitus
    d. Systemic lupus erythematosus

27. When obtaining a nursing history from a patient with cancer of the urinary system, what would the nurse recognize as a risk factor associated with both kidney cancer and bladder cancer?
    a. Smoking
    b. Family history of cancer
    c. Chronic use of phenacetin
    d. Chronic, recurrent kidney stones

28. Thirty percent of patients with kidney cancer have metastasis at the time of diagnosis. Why does this occur?
    a. The only treatment modalities for the disease are palliative.
    b. Diagnostic tests are not available to detect tumors before they metastasize.
    c. Classic symptoms of hematuria and palpable mass do not occur until the disease is advanced.
    d. Early metastasis to the brain impairs the patient's ability to recognize the seriousness of symptoms.

29. Which characteristics are associated with urge incontinence? **Select all that apply.**
    a. Treated with Kegel exercises
    b. Found following prostatectomy
    c. Common in postmenopausal women
    d. Involuntary urination preceded by urgency
    e. Caused by overactivity of the detrusor muscle
    f. Bladder contracts by reflex, overriding central inhibition

30. The patient has a thoracic spinal cord lesion and incontinence that occurs equally during the day and night. What type of incontinence does this patient have?
    a. Reflex incontinence
    b. Overflow incontinence
    c. Functional incontinence
    d. Incontinence after trauma

31. Which drugs are used to treat overflow incontinence? **Select all that apply.**
    a. Baclofen (Lioresal)
    b. Anticholinergic drugs
    c. α-Adrenergic blockers
    d. 5α-reductase inhibitors
    e. Bethanechol (Urecholine)

32. To assist the patient with stress incontinence, what would the nurse teach the patient to do?
    a. Void every 2 hours to prevent leakage.
    b. Use absorptive perineal pads to contain urine.
    c. Perform pelvic floor muscle exercises 40 to 50 times per day.
    d. Increase intraabdominal pressure during voiding to empty the bladder completely.

33. What nursing care applies to the management of all hospitalized patients with a urinary catheter?
    a. Measuring urine output every 1 to 2 hours to ensure patency
    b. Turning the patient frequently from side to side to promote drainage
    c. Using strict sterile technique during irrigation and obtaining culture specimens
    d. Daily cleaning of the catheter insertion site with soap and water and application of lotion

34. A patient has a right ureteral catheter placed following a lithotripsy for a stone in the ureter. When caring for the patient immediately after the procedure, what is the most appropriate nursing action?
    a. Milk or strip the catheter every 2 hours.
    b. Measure ureteral urinary drainage every 1 to 2 hours.
    c. Encourage ambulation to promote urinary peristaltic action.
    d. Irrigate the catheter with 30-mL sterile saline every 4 hours.

35. What would the nurse expect during assessment of the patient after an open nephrectomy?
    a. Shallow, slow respirations
    b. Clear breath sounds in all lung fields
    c. Decreased breath sounds in the lower left lobe
    d. Decreased breath sounds in the right and left lower lobes

36. What type of continent urinary diversion has an ileal pouch with a stoma for catheterization?
    a. Kock pouch
    b. Ileal conduit
    c. Orthotopic neobladder
    d. Cutaneous ureterostomy

37. A patient with bladder cancer undergoes cystectomy with formation of an ileal conduit. What would the nurse include when planning care during the patient's first postoperative day?
    a. Measure and fit the stoma for a permanent appliance.
    b. Encourage high oral intake to flush mucus from the conduit.
    c. Teach the patient to self-catheterize the stoma every 4 to 6 hours.
    d. Empty the drainage bag every 2 to 3 hours and measure the urinary output.

38. What instructions would the nurse include when developing a teaching plan for the patient with a new ileal conduit?
    a. Clean the skin around the stoma with alcohol every day.
    b. Use a wick to keep the skin dry during appliance changes.
    c. Use sterile supplies and technique during care of the stoma.
    d. Change the appliance every day and wash it with soap and warm water.

39. When working with patients who have urologic problems, which nursing interventions could be delegated to assistive personnel (AP)? **Select all that apply.**
    a. Assess the need for catheterization.
    b. Use bladder scanner to estimate residual urine.
    c. Teach patient pelvic floor muscle (Kegel) exercises.
    d. Insert indwelling catheter for uncomplicated patient.
    e. Assist incontinent patient to commode at regular intervals.
    f. Provide perineal care with soap and water around a urinary catheter.

CASE STUDY   Bladder Cancer

(Szepy/
iStock/Thinkstock)

Patient Profile

P.G. is a married 61-year-old male who works as a bicycle mechanic. He has been healthy all his life until he passed some blood in his urine. He saw a urologist at his wife's insistence. A urine specimen for cytology revealed atypical cells. A diagnosis of bladder cancer was made following a cystoscopy with biopsy of the bladder tissue. The tumor was removed with a transurethral resection and laser cauterization. Intravesical therapy with Bacillus Calmette-Guérin (BCG), a weakened strain of *Mycobacterium bovis*, is planned.

Subjective Data
- Has smoked a pack of cigarettes a day since he was a teenager
- Says he dreads having the chemotherapy because he has heard cancer drugs cause severe side effects

Objective Data
- Cystoscopy and biopsy results: moderately differentiated stage II tumor on the left lateral bladder wall with $T_1N_0M_0$ pathologic stage
- Gross hematuria

Questions

1. What clinical manifestations would the nurse expect in patients with bladder cancer? **Use an X to indicate whether the assessment finding is _Expected_ (a sign or symptom of bladder cancer) or is _Unexpected_ (a sign or symptom not associated with bladder cancer).**

Assessment Finding	Expected	Unexpected
Severe pain in suprapubic region		
Microscopic or gross hematuria		
Urgency		
Frequency		
Bladder distention		
Dribbling		
Pyuria		

2. P.G. undergoes a transurethral resection of the bladder tumor (TURBT). He comes to the PACU with an order for continuous bladder irrigation (CBI) for 4 hours before removing the urinary catheter. What interventions would the nurse expect to include while caring for P.G. in the PACU? **Use an X to indicate whether the nursing action is <u>Indicated</u> (is appropriate or necessary), is <u>Contraindicated</u> (could be harmful), or is <u>Non-Essential</u> (makes no difference or is unnecessary).**

Nursing Action	Indicated	Contraindicated	Non-Essential
Give a B & O suppository for bladder spasms			
Report gross hematuria to the HCP			
Strain (filter) the urine using a paper strainer			
Keep him NPO			
Have the patient void before discharge home			
Use sterile water as the irrigation fluid			
Record the hourly urine output by subtracting the amount of irrigant from the total amount emptied from the urinary bag			
Clamp the irrigation tubing if there are blood clots in the urinary catheter tubing			
Insert a 3-way urinary catheter			

3. What instructions would the nurse include when doing discharge teaching with P.G.? **Select all that apply.**
    _____A. Report dysuria to your HCP.
    _____B. Limit your fluid intake to 1500 mL/day.
    _____C. Try your best to quit smoking.
    _____D. Report urine that is pink to your HCP.
    _____E. You may see brown or red flecks in your urine in about 7 to 10 days.
    _____F. You may have urinary incontinence from this procedure.
    _____G. Increase fiber in your diet or take stool softeners so you don't strain having bowel movements.
    _____H. Avoid coffee and tea as they may irritate your bladder and cause pain.

4. P.G. will receive intravesical therapy to treat any residual cancer cells that surgery may have missed. **Choose the most likely options for the information missing from the statements below by selecting from the lists of options provided.**

    _____1_____ or _____1_____ is placed directly into the bladder through a _____2_____. The drug dwells in the bladder for __3__ hours. The patient may have to change positions every __4__ minutes to wash the solution over the entire bladder. This therapy is usually given __5__ per week for __6__ weeks.

Options for 1:	Options for 2:	Options for 3:	Options for 4:
Radioactive seeds	Urinary catheter	12	60
Chemotherapy	Brachytherapy rod	4–6	5
Immunotherapy	Cystoscopy	2–4	30
Stem cells	Ureteroscopy	1–2	45
Hormone therapy	Cryoprobe	24	15
Targeted drug therapy	Endoscopy	6–8	90

Options for 5:	Options for 6:
Three times	3–4 weeks
Twice	4–6 weeks
Four times	6–12 weeks
Once	1–2 weeks
Five times	6 months
Six times	12 months

5. What statements made by P.G. indicate to the nurse that teaching about intravesical therapy has been effective? **Use an X to indicate whether the patient's statement indicates teaching has been <u>Effective</u> (meets expected outcomes), <u>Ineffective</u> (does not meet expected outcomes), or is <u>Unrelated</u> (doesn't pertain to expected outcomes).**

Patient Statement	Effective	Ineffective	Unrelated
"I will expect hair loss."			
"I may have flu-like symptoms after treatments."			
"I will not be able to swim for several months."			
"I should avoid spicy foods."			
"I can drink wine and beer as long as I stay away from hard-liquor."			
"I should drink water instead of diet soda."			
"I will have annual PSA testing."			

51

Acute Kidney Injury and Chronic Kidney Disease

1. What are intrarenal causes of acute kidney injury (AKI)? **Select all that apply.**
   a. Anaphylaxis
   b. Renal stones
   c. Bladder cancer
   d. Nephrotoxic drugs
   e. Acute glomerulonephritis
   f. Tubular obstruction by myoglobin

2. An 83-year-old female patient was found lying on the bathroom floor. She said she fell 2 days ago and has not been able to take her heart medicine or eat or drink anything since then. What conditions could contribute to the patient developing prerenal AKI? **Select all that apply.**
   a. Anaphylaxis
   b. Renal stones
   c. Hypovolemia
   d. Nephrotoxic drugs
   e. Decreased cardiac output

3. Acute tubular necrosis (ATN) is the most common cause of intrarenal AKI. Which patient is most likely to develop ATN?
   a. Patient with diabetes
   b. Patient with hypertensive crisis
   c. Patient who tried to overdose on acetaminophen
   d. Patient with major surgery who required a blood transfusion

4. A dehydrated patient is in the Injury stage of the RIFLE staging of AKI. What would the nurse anticipate as the first treatment for this patient?
   a. Assessment of daily weight
   b. IV administration of fluid and furosemide (Lasix)
   c. IV administration of insulin and sodium bicarbonate
   d. Urinalysis to check for sediment, osmolality, sodium, and specific gravity

5. What indicates to the nurse that a patient has prerenal oliguria?
   a. Urine testing reveals a low specific gravity.
   b. Causative factor is malignant hypertension.
   c. Urine testing reveals a high sodium concentration.
   d. Reversal of oliguria occurs with fluid replacement.

6. In a patient with AKI, which laboratory urinalysis result indicates tubular damage?
   a. Hematuria
   b. Specific gravity fixed at 1.010
   c. Urine sodium of 12 mEq/L (12 mmol/L)
   d. Osmolality of 1000 mOsm/kg (1000 mmol/kg)

7. What impairment causes metabolic acidosis in the oliguric phase of AKI?
   a. Excretion of sodium
   b. Excretion of bicarbonate
   c. Conservation of potassium
   d. Excretion of hydrogen ions

8. What indicates to the nurse that a patient with AKI is in the recovery phase?
   a. A return to normal weight
   b. A urine output of 3700 mL/day
   c. Decreasing sodium and potassium levels
   d. Decreasing blood urea nitrogen (BUN) and creatinine levels

9. While caring for the patient in the oliguric phase of AKI, when would the nurse notify the health care provider (HCP)?
   a. Urine output is 300 mL/day
   b. Edema occurs in the feet, legs, and sacral area
   c. Cardiac monitor reveals a depressed T wave and elevated ST segment
   d. The patient develops increasing muscle weakness and abdominal cramping

10. What would the nurse consider when caring for the patient with AKI?
    a. The most common cause of death in AKI is irreversible metabolic acidosis.
    b. During the oliguric phase of AKI, daily fluid intake is limited to 1000 mL plus the prior day's measured fluid loss.
    c. Dietary sodium and potassium during the oliguric phase of AKI are managed according to the patient's urinary output.
    d. One of the most important nursing measures in managing fluid balance in the patient with AKI is taking accurate daily weights.

11. A 68-year-old man with a history of heart failure resulting from hypertension has AKI resulting from the effects of nephrotoxic diuretics. Currently, his serum potassium is 6.2 mEq/L (6.2 mmol/L) with cardiac changes, his BUN is 108 mg/dL (38.6 mmol/L), his serum creatinine is 4.1 mg/dL (362 mmol/L), and his serum bicarbonate (HCO_3^-) is 14 mEq/L (14 mmol/L). He is somnolent and disoriented. Which treatment would the nurse expect?
    a. Loop diuretics
    b. Renal replacement therapy
    c. Insulin and sodium bicarbonate
    d. Sodium polystyrene sulfonate (Kayexalate)

12. Prevention of AKI is important because of the high mortality rate. Which patients are at greatest risk for AKI? **Select all that apply.**
    a. An 86-year-old woman scheduled for a cardiac catheterization
    b. A 48-year-old man with multiple injuries from a motor vehicle accident
    c. A 32-year-old woman following a C-section delivery for abruptio placentae
    d. A 64-year-old woman with chronic heart failure admitted with bloody stools
    e. A 58-year-old man with prostate cancer undergoing preoperative workup for prostatectomy

13. A patient on a medical unit has a potassium level of 6.8 mEq/L. What is the nurse's priority?
    a. Place the patient on a cardiac monitor
    b. Check the patient's BP
    c. Teach the patient to avoid high-potassium foods
    d. Call the laboratory and request a redraw of the laboratory to verify results

14. A patient with AKI has a serum potassium level of 6.7 mEq/L (6.7 mmol/L) and the following arterial blood gas results: pH 7.28, $PaCO_2$ 30 mm Hg, PaO_2 86 mm Hg, HCO_3^- 18 mEq/L (18 mmol/L). The nurse recognizes that treatment of the acid–base problem with sodium bicarbonate would cause a decrease in which value?
    a. pH
    b. Potassium level
    c. Bicarbonate level
    d. Carbon dioxide level

15. What information is used to stage a patient with chronic kidney disease (CKD?
    a. Total daily urine output
    b. Glomerular filtration rate (GFR)
    c. Degree of altered mental status
    d. Serum creatinine and urea levels

16. The patient with CKD is receiving dialysis and the nurse observes excoriations on the patient's skin. What pathophysiologic changes in CKD occur that can contribute to this finding? **Select all that apply.**
    a. Dry skin
    b. Sensory neuropathy
    c. Vascular calcifications
    d. Calcium-phosphate skin deposits
    e. Uremic crystallization from high BUN

17. What causes the gastrointestinal (GI) manifestation of stomatitis in the patient with CKD?
    a. High serum sodium levels
    b. Irritation of the GI tract from creatinine
    c. Increased ammonia from bacterial breakdown of urea
    d. Iron salts, calcium-containing phosphate binders, and limited fluid intake

18. The patient with CKD is brought to the emergency department with Kussmaul respirations. What would cause this clinical manifestation?
    a. Uremic pleuritis is occurring.
    b. There is decreased pulmonary macrophage activity.
    c. They are caused by respiratory compensation for metabolic acidosis.
    d. Pulmonary edema from heart failure and fluid overload is occurring.

19. Which serum laboratory value indicates to the nurse that the patient's CKD is getting worse?
    a. Decreased BUN
    b. Decreased sodium
    c. Decreased creatinine
    d. Decreased calculated glomerular filtration rate (GFR)

20. What is the most serious electrolyte disorder associated with kidney disease?
    a. Hypocalcemia
    b. Hyperkalemia
    c. Hyponatremia
    d. Hypermagnesemia

21. The nurse identifies that a patient with CKD is at risk for fractures because of alterations in calcium and phosphorus metabolism. What is the pathologic process that causes an increased risk for fractures? Number the processes in order beginning with 1 as the first process and 6 as the last process.
    _____a. Bone remodeling causes weakened bone matrix
    _____b. Bone demineralization for calcium and phosphate release
    _____c. Decalcification of the bone and replacement of bone tissue with fibrous tissue
    _____d. Impaired vitamin D activation resulting in decreased GI absorption of calcium
    _____e. Increased release of parathyroid hormone in response to decreased calcium levels
    _____f. Hyperphosphatemia decreases serum calcium levels and reduces kidney's vitamin D activation

22. What is the most appropriate snack for the nurse to offer a patient with stage 4 CKD?
    a. Raisins
    b. Ice cream
    c. Dill pickles
    d. Hard candy

23. Which complication of chronic kidney disease is treated with erythropoietin?
    a. Anemia
    b. Hypertension
    c. Hyperkalemia
    d. Mineral and bone disorder

24. The patient with CKD asks why she is receiving nifedipine (Procardia) and furosemide (Lasix). What would the nurse tell the patient these drugs are being used to treat?
    a. Anemia
    b. Hypertension
    c. Hyperkalemia
    d. Mineral and bone disorder

25. Which drugs will be used to treat mineral and bone disorder associated with CKD? **Select all that apply.**
    a. Calcium acetate
    b. Cinacalcet (Sensipar)
    c. IV glucose and insulin
    d. IV 10% calcium gluconate
    e. Sevelamer carbonate (Renvela)

26. Which statement describes the care of the patient with CKD?
    a. Iron is a nutrient that is commonly supplemented for the patient on dialysis because it is dialyzable.
    b. The syndrome that includes all of the signs and symptoms seen in the various body systems in CKD is azotemia.
    c. The use of morphine is contraindicated in the patient with CKD because accumulation of its metabolites may cause seizures.
    d. The use of calcium-based phosphate binders in the patient with CKD is contraindicated when serum calcium levels are increased.

27. During the assessment of the patient with renal insufficiency, what history would the nurse ask the patient about?
    a. Angina
    b. Asthma
    c. Hypertension
    d. Rheumatoid arthritis

28. The patient with CKD is considering whether to use peritoneal dialysis (PD) or hemodialysis (HD). What are advantages of PD? **Select all that apply.**
    a. Less protein loss
    b. Rapid fluid removal
    c. Less cardiovascular stress
    d. Decreased hyperlipidemia
    e. Requires fewer dietary restrictions

29. What does the dialysate for PD routinely contain?
    a. Calcium in a lower concentration than in the blood
    b. Sodium in a higher concentration than in the blood
    c. Dextrose in a higher concentration than in the blood
    d. Electrolytes in an equal concentration to that of the blood

30. Beginning with 1 as the first phase and 3 as the last phase, number the phases of exchange in PD.
    _____ a. Drain
    _____ b. Dwell
    _____ c. Inflow

31. Which type of dialysis has fluid dwelling in the abdomen during the day and dialyzes the patient while they sleep?
    a. Long nocturnal HD
    b. Automated peritoneal dialysis (APD)
    c. Continuous veno-venous hemofiltration (CVVH)
    d. Continuous ambulatory peritoneal dialysis (CAPD)

32. What is important for the nurse to do to prevent the most common complication of PD?
    a. Infuse the dialysate slowly
    b. Use strict aseptic technique in the dialysis procedures
    c. Have the patient empty the bowel before the inflow phase
    d. Reposition the patient frequently and promote deep breathing

33. A patient on HD develops a thrombus of a subcutaneous arteriovenous graft (AVG), requiring its removal. While waiting for a replacement graft or fistula, how will the patient be dialyzed?
    a. Peritoneal dialysis
    b. Peripheral vascular access using the radial artery
    c. Long-term cuffed catheter tunneled subcutaneously to the jugular vein
    d. Peripherally inserted central catheter (PICC) line inserted into subclavian vein

34. A man with end-stage renal disease (ESRD) is scheduled for HD following healing of an arteriovenous fistula (AVF). What would the nurse explain will occur during dialysis?
    a. He will be able to visit, read, sleep, or watch TV while reclining in a chair.
    b. He will be placed on a cardiac monitor to detect any adverse effects that may occur.
    c. The dialyzer will remove and hold part of his blood for 20 to 30 minutes to remove the waste products.
    d. A large catheter with 2 lumens will be inserted into the fistula to send blood to and return it from the dialyzer.

35. How would the nurse evaluate the patency of an AVF?
    a. Palpate for pulses distal to the graft site.
    b. Auscultate for the presence of a bruit at the site.
    c. Evaluate the color and temperature of the extremity.
    d. Assess for the presence of numbness and tingling distal to the site.

36. A patient with AKI is a candidate for continuous renal replacement therapy (CRRT). What is the most common indication for using CRRT?
    a. Pericarditis
    b. Hyperkalemia
    c. Fluid overload
    d. Hypernatremia

37. A patient rapidly progressing toward ESRD asks about the possibility of a kidney transplant. When responding to the patient, what would the nurse state is a contraindication to kidney transplantation?
    a. Hepatitis C infection
    b. Coronary artery disease
    c. Refractory hypertension
    d. Extensive vascular disease

38. During the immediate postoperative care of a kidney transplant recipient, what nursing action is a priority?
    a. Regulate fluid intake hourly based on urine output.
    b. Monitor urine-tinged drainage on abdominal dressing.
    c. Medicate the patient frequently for incisional flank pain.
    d. Remove the urinary catheter to evaluate the ureteral implant.

39. A month ago, a patient received a kidney transplant. Because of the effects of immunosuppressive drugs and CKD, what complication would the nurse be assessing the patient for to decrease the risk of mortality?
    a. Cancer
    b. Infection
    c. Rejection
    d. Cardiovascular disease

CASE STUDY Kidney Transplant

(STUDIO GRAND
OUEST/iStock/
Thinkstock)

Patient Profile

D.B., a 46-year-old female, has CKD resulting from type 1 diabetes and hypertension. She was on hemodialysis for 2 years and then received a cadaveric renal transplant 1 year ago. She had 1 episode of acute rejection 3 months after transplant. Her baseline creatinine has been 1.2 to 1.3 mg/dL (106 to 115 mmol/L). She came to the clinic reporting decreased urinary output, fever, and tenderness at the transplant site. She is admitted to the hospital for testing and possible kidney biopsy.

Subjective Data
- Tells the nurse that if she loses this kidney, she does not think she can stand to go back on dialysis

Objective Data
Physical Examination
- BP: 150/90 mm Hg, HR 103 beats/min, RR 28 breaths/min and deep
- Flank area tender to palpation

Laboratory Tests
- Serum creatinine: 3.0 mg/dL (265 mmol/L)
- BUN: 70 mg/dL (25 mmol/L)
- Glucose: 404 mg/dL (22.4 mmol/L)
- K^+: 5.1 mEq/L (5.1 mmol/L)
- HCO_3^-: 18 mEq/L (18 mmol/L)

Interprofessional Care
- IV insulin
- Furosemide (Lasix)
- Nifedipine (Procardia)
- Sodium bicarbonate
- Mycophenolate mofetil (CellCept)
- Methylprednisolone (Solu-Medrol)
- Tacrolimus (Prograf)

Questions

1. The nurse is evaluating D.B.'s assessment findings. What would the nurse know is a potential complication associated with these assessment findings? **Indicate which assessment finding listed in the far-left column is associated with each complication. Note that some assessment findings may apply to more than 1 potential complication.**

Assessment Finding	Potential Complication	Appropriate Assessment Finding Associated with Each Complication
Creatinine 3.0 mg/dL	Diabetic ketoacidosis	
BUN 70 mg/dL	Cardiac dysrhythmias	
Glucose 404 mg/dL	Kidney failure	
K^+ 5.1 mEq/L		
HCO_3^- 18 mEq/L		
BP 150/90 mm Hg		
RR 28 and deep		

2. What interventions would the nurse include when planning care for D.B.? **Use an X to indicate whether the nursing action is Indicated (is appropriate or necessary), Contraindicated (could be harmful), or Non-essential (makes no difference or is unnecessary).**

Nursing Action	Indicated	Contraindicated	Non-Essential
Begin a continuous insulin infusion			
Administer 50 mL of dextrose 50%			
Have the patient use the incentive spirometer			
Offer juice and crackers			
Monitor urine output hourly			

Nursing Action	Indicated	Contraindicated	Non-Essential
Administer Kayexalate PO			
Transfuse 1 unit PRBC			
Perform continuous SpO$_2$ monitoring			
Place patient on continuous cardiac monitoring			
Place patient on droplet precautions			
Encourage patient to eat the spinach on her dinner tray			

3. The nurse performs the medication reconciliation. What is the indication or purpose for each drug that D.B. has been prescribed? **Match each prescribed drug listed in the far-left column with its intended use. Note that some drugs may have more than 1 use.**

Prescribed Drug	Intended Use	Appropriate Intended Use for Each Prescribed Drug
Insulin	Hypertension	
Sodium bicarbonate	Metabolic Acidosis	
Nifedipine	Renal Transplant	
Mycophenolate mofetil	Diabetes	
Tacrolimus		
Furosemide		
Methylprednisolone		

4. If D.B. has to resume dialysis, what information would the nurse provide so that she understands advantages and disadvantages of each type? **Use an X to indicate if the description applies to <u>Hemodialysis</u>, <u>Peritoneal Dialysis</u>, or <u>CRRT</u>.**

Description	Hemodialysis	Peritoneal Dialysis	CRRT
This type is only performed in the acute care setting			
You will need surgery to create a graft or fistula			
You will need a catheter implanted in your abdomen			
This type cleans your blood continuously over 24 hours			
You will need dialysis at least 3 times/week			
You may develop peritonitis			
You may become hypotensive			
It is preferred because you have diabetes			

5. What information would the nurse provide D.B. when doing discharge teaching? **Select all that apply.**
   A. Report fevers to your HCP immediately.
   B. Stay away from crowded spaces.
   C. Get an annual live virus influenza vaccine.
   D. You are more susceptible to developing cancer.
   E. Cardiovascular disease is the leading cause of death in patients after kidney transplant.
   F. Stop taking your immunosuppressant medications when you are ill.
   G. Corticosteroids won't have any effect on your blood glucose levels.
   H. Diabetes increases your risk of heart disease.
   I. You will need lifelong monitoring for organ rejection.

Assessment: Endocrine System

1. Identify the glands in the illustration below.

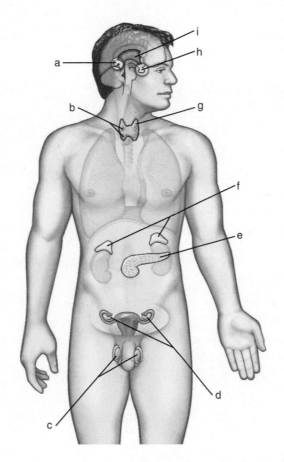

a. _____

b. _____

c. _____

d. _____

e. _____

f. _____

g. _____

h. _____

i. _____

2. Which hormones are secreted by the anterior pituitary gland? **Select all that apply.**
   a. Prolactin
   b. Melatonin
   c. Somatostatin
   d. Parathyroid hormone
   e. Growth hormone (GH)
   f. Gonadotropic hormones
   g. Antidiuretic hormone (ADH)
   h. Melanocyte-stimulating hormone
   i. Thyroid-stimulating hormone (TSH)
   j. Adrenocorticotropic hormone (ACTH)

3. From where is the hormone glucagon secreted?
   a. F cells of the islets of Langerhans
   b. β-cells of the islets of Langerhans
   c. α-cells of the islets of Langerhans
   d. Delta cells of the islets of Langerhans

4. Which endocrine gland secretes cortisol in a diurnal pattern?
   a. Ovaries
   b. Thyroid
   c. Adrenal cortex
   d. Adrenal medulla

5. Which statement about the adrenal medulla hormones is accurate?
   a. Overproduction of androgens may cause masculinization in women.
   b. Both the adrenal medulla and the thyroid gland have a negative feedback system to the hypothalamus.
   c. Cortisol levels would be altered in a person who normally works a night shift from 11:00 PM to 7:00 AM and sleeps from 8:00 AM to 3:00 PM.
   d. Catecholamines are considered hormones when they are secreted by the adrenal medulla and neurotransmitters when they are secreted by nerve cells.

6. Match each hormone with the primary factor that stimulates its secretion and the primary factor that inhibits its secretion (factors may be used more than once).

Stimulate	Inhibit	Hormone	Primary Factor
_____	_____	a. TSH or thyrotropin	1. Increased stress
_____	_____	b. Corticotropin-releasing hormone	2. Increased serum T_3
_____	_____	c. ADH	3. Decreased serum T_3
_____	_____	d. Follicle-stimulating hormone (FSH)	4. Increased serum cortisol
_____	_____	e. Calcitonin	5. Increased serum estrogen
_____	_____	f. Aldosterone	6. Decreased serum estrogen
_____	_____	g. Glucagon	7. Increased serum glucose
_____	_____	h. Parathyroid hormone (PTH)	8. Decreased serum glucose
_____	_____	i. Insulin	9. Increased serum calcium
			10. Decreased serum calcium
			11. Decreased BP
			12. Increased arterial BP
			13. Increased plasma osmolality
			14. Decreased plasma osmolality

7. What is released in the normal response to increased serum osmolality?
   a. Aldosterone from the adrenal cortex, which stimulates sodium excretion by the kidney
   b. ADH from the posterior pituitary gland, which stimulates the kidney to reabsorb water
   c. Mineralocorticoids from the adrenal gland, which stimulate the kidney to excrete potassium
   d. Calcitonin from the thyroid gland, which increases bone resorption and decreases serum calcium levels

8. What accurately demonstrates that hormones of one gland influence the function of hormones of another gland?
   a. Increased insulin levels inhibit the secretion of glucagon.
   b. Increased cortisol levels stimulate the secretion of insulin.
   c. Increased testosterone levels inhibit the release of estrogen.
   d. Increased atrial natriuretic peptide (ANP) levels inhibit the secretion of aldosterone.

9. How do hormones respond following the ingestion of a high-protein, carbohydrate-free meal?
   a. Both insulin and glucagon are inhibited because blood glucose levels are unchanged.
   b. Insulin is inhibited by low glucose levels, and glucagon is released to promote gluconeogenesis.
   c. Insulin is released to facilitate the breakdown of amino acids into glucose, and glucagon is inhibited.
   d. Glucagon is released to promote gluconeogenesis, and insulin is released to facilitate movement of amino acids into muscle cells.

10. What are 2 effects of hypokalemia on the endocrine system?
    a. Decreased insulin and aldosterone release
    b. Decreased glucagon and increased cortisol release
    c. Decreased release of ANP and increased ADH release
    d. Decreased release of parathyroid hormone and increased calcitonin release

11. Identify 1 specific finding identified by the nurse during assessment of each of the patient's functional health patterns that indicates a risk factor for endocrine problems or a patient response to an actual endocrine problem.

Functional Health Pattern	Risk Factor for or Response to Endocrine Problem
Health perception–health management	
Nutritional-metabolic	
Elimination	
Activity-exercise	
Sleep-rest	
Cognitive-perceptual	
Self-perception–self-concept	
Role-relationship	
Sexuality-reproductive	
Coping–stress tolerance	
Value-belief	

12. In a patient with an elevated serum cortisol, what would the nurse expect other laboratory findings to reveal?
    a. Hypokalemia
    b. Hyponatremia
    c. Hypoglycemia
    d. Decreased serum triglycerides

13. What manifestations of endocrine problems in the older adult are commonly attributed to the aging process?
    a. Tremors and paresthesias
    b. Fatigue and mental impairment
    c. Hyperpigmentation and oily skin
    d. Fluid retention and hypertension

14. What common nonspecific manifestations may alert the nurse to endocrine dysfunction?
    a. goiter and alopecia.
    b. exophthalmos and tremors.
    c. weight loss, fatigue, and depression.
    d. polyuria, polydipsia, and polyphagia.

15. What is a potential adverse effect of palpation of an enlarged thyroid gland?
    a. Carotid artery obstruction
    b. Damage to the cricoid cartilage
    c. Release of excessive thyroid hormone into circulation
    d. Hoarseness from pressure on the recurrent laryngeal nerve

16. Which abnormal assessment findings are related to thyroid dysfunction? **Select all that apply.**
    a. Tetanic muscle spasms with hypofunction
    b. Heat intolerance caused by hyperfunction
    c. Exophthalmos associated with excessive secretion
    d. Hyperpigmentation associated with hypofunction
    e. A goiter with either hyperfunction or hypofunction
    f. Increase in hand and foot size associated with excessive secretion

17. A patient has a low serum T_3 level. The health care provider (HCP) orders measurement of the TSH level. If the TSH level is elevated, what does this indicate?
    a. The cause of the low T_3 level is most likely primary hypothyroidism.
    b. The negative feedback system is failing to stimulate the anterior pituitary gland.
    c. The patient has an underactive thyroid gland that is not receiving TSH stimulation.
    d. A tumor on the anterior pituitary gland that is causing increased production of TSH.

18. To ensure accurate results of a fasting blood glucose analysis, how long would the nurse instruct the patient to fast?
    a. 2 hours
    b. 4 hours
    c. 8 hours
    d. 12 hours

19. A 30-year-old female patient was brought to the emergency department (ED) after a seizure at work. During the assessment, she mentions hair loss and menstrual irregularities. What diagnostic tests would be helpful to determine if endocrine problems are a cause of her problem? **Select all that apply.**
    a. Thyroglobulin
    b. Luteinizing hormone (LH)
    c. PTH
    d. FSH
    e. MRI of the head
    f. ACTH suppression

20. A patient is admitted with a new diagnosis of Cushing syndrome with elevated serum and urine cortisol levels. Which assessment findings would the nurse expect to see in this patient?
    a. Hair loss and moon face
    b. Decreased weight and hirsutism
    c. Decreased muscle mass and thick skin
    d. Elevated BP and blood glucose

21. The patient with type 1 diabetes is in the clinic to check their long-term glycemic control. Which test would be used?
    a. Water deprivation test
    b. Fasting blood glucose test
    c. Oral glucose tolerance test
    d. Glycosylated hemoglobin (A_1C)

Diabetes

1. In addition to promoting the transport of glucose from the blood into the cell, what does insulin do?
   a. Enhances the breakdown of adipose tissue for energy
   b. Stimulates hepatic glycogenolysis and gluconeogenesis
   c. Prevents the transport of triglycerides into adipose tissue
   d. Increases amino acid transport into cells and protein synthesis

2. Which tissues require insulin to enable movement of glucose into the tissue cells? **Select all that apply.**
   a. Liver
   b. Brain
   c. Adipose
   d. Blood cells
   e. Skeletal muscle

3. Cortisol, glucagon, epinephrine, and growth hormone are referred to as counterregulatory hormones. What do they do?
   a. Decrease glucose production
   b. Stimulate glucose output by the liver
   c. Increase glucose transport into the cells
   d. Independently regulate glucose level in the blood

4. What characterizes type 2 diabetes? **Select all that apply.**
   a. β-cell exhaustion
   b. Insulin resistance
   c. Genetic predisposition
   d. Altered production of adipokines
   e. Inherited defect in insulin receptors
   f. Inappropriate glucose production by the liver

5. Which laboratory results indicate the patient has prediabetes?
   a. Glucose tolerance result of 132 mg/dL (7.3 mmol/L)
   b. Glucose tolerance result of 240 mg/dL (13.3 mmol/L)
   c. Fasting blood glucose result of 80 mg/dL (4.4 mmol/L)
   d. Fasting blood glucose result of 120 mg/dL (6.7 mmol/L)

6. What information would the nurse include when teaching the patient with prediabetes about ways to prevent or delay the development of type 2 diabetes? **Select all that apply.**
   a. Exercise regularly
   b. Maintain a healthy weight
   c. Have BP checked regularly
   d. Assess for visual changes on a monthly basis
   e. Monitor for polyuria, polyphagia, and polydipsia

7. In type 1 diabetes, glucose has an osmotic effect when insulin deficiency prevents the use of glucose for energy. Which symptom is caused by the osmotic effect of glucose?
   a. Fatigue
   b. Polydipsia
   c. Polyphagia
   d. Recurrent infections

8. Which patient would the nurse plan to teach how to prevent or delay the development of diabetes?
   a. An obese 40-year-old Hispanic woman
   b. A 20-year-old man whose father has type 1 diabetes
   c. A 34-year-old woman whose parents both have type 2 diabetes
   d. A 12-year-old boy whose father has maturity-onset diabetes of the young (MODY)

9. Which treatment plan would the nurse give the highest priority to when caring for a patient with metabolic syndrome?
   a. Achieving a normal weight
   b. Performing daily aerobic exercise
   c. Eliminating red meat from the diet
   d. Monitoring the blood glucose periodically

10. During routine health screening, a patient is found to have fasting plasma glucose (FPG) of 132 mg/dL (7.33 mmol/L). At a follow-up visit, which laboratory results would a diagnosis of diabetes be made? **Select all that apply.**
    a. A1C of 7.5%
    b. Glycosuria of 3 +
    c. FPG $\geq$ 127 mg/dL (7.0 mmol/L).
    d. Random blood glucose of 126 mg/dL (7.0 mmol/L)
    e. A 2-hour oral glucose tolerance test (OGTT) of 190 mg/dL (10.5 mmol/L)

11. What would the nurse determine a patient has with a 2-hour OGTT of 152 mg/dL?
    a. Diabetes
    b. Elevated A1C
    c. Impaired fasting glucose
    d. Impaired glucose tolerance

12. Which instruction would the nurse include when teaching the patient with diabetes about insulin administration?
    a. Pull back on the plunger after inserting the needle to check for blood.
    b. Consistently use the same size of insulin syringe to avoid dosing errors.
    c. Clean the skin at the injection site with an alcohol swab before each injection.
    d. Rotate injection sites from arms to thighs to abdomen with each injection to prevent lipodystrophies.

13. A patient with type 1 diabetes uses 20 U of Novolin 70/30 (NPH/regular) in the morning and at 6:00 PM. What would the nurse emphasize when teaching the patient about this regimen?
    a. Hypoglycemia is most likely to occur before the noon meal.
    b. A set meal pattern with a bedtime snack is necessary to prevent hypoglycemia.
    c. Flexibility in food intake is possible because insulin is available 24 hours a day.
    d. Glucose checks before meals are required to determine needed changes in daily dosing.

14. Lispro insulin (Humalog) with NPH (Humulin N) insulin is ordered for a patient with newly diagnosed type 1 diabetes. When would the nurse administer lispro insulin?
    a. Only once a day
    b. 1 hour before meals
    c. 30 to 45 minutes before meals
    d. At mealtime or within 15 minutes of meals

15. A patient with diabetes is learning to mix regular insulin and NPH insulin in the same syringe. The nurse determines that additional teaching is needed when the patient does what?
    a. Withdraws the NPH dose into the syringe first
    b. Injects air equal to the NPH dose into the NPH vial first
    c. Removes any air bubbles after withdrawing the first insulin
    d. Adds air equal to the insulin dose into the regular vial and withdraws the dose

16. The following interventions are planned for a patient with diabetes. Which intervention can the nurse delegate to assistive personnel (AP)?
    a. Discuss complications of diabetes.
    b. Check that the bath water is not too hot.
    c. Check the patient's technique for drawing up insulin.
    d. Teach the patient to use a meter for self-monitoring of blood glucose.

17. The home care nurse is reviewing insulin administration with a patient. What action by the patient causes the home care nurse to intervene?
    a. The patient warms a prefilled refrigerated syringe in the hands before administration.
    b. The patient stores syringes prefilled with NPH and regular insulin needle-up in the refrigerator.
    c. The patient places the insulin bottle currently in use in a small container on the bathroom countertop.
    d. The patient mixes an evening dose of regular insulin with insulin glargine in 1 syringe for administration.

18. When teaching the patient with type 1 diabetes, what would the nurse emphasize as the major advantage of using an insulin pump?
    a. Tight glycemic control can be maintained.
    b. Errors in insulin dosing are less likely to occur.
    c. Complications of insulin therapy are prevented.
    d. Frequent blood glucose monitoring is unnecessary.

19. A patient taking insulin has recorded fasting glucose levels above 200 mg/dL (11.1 mmol/L) for the last 5 mornings. What would the nurse have the patient do first?
    a. Increase the evening insulin dose to prevent the dawn phenomenon.
    b. Use a single-dose insulin regimen with an intermediate-acting insulin.
    c. Monitor the glucose level at bedtime, between 2:00 AM and 4:00 AM, and on arising.
    d. Decrease the evening insulin dosage to prevent night hypoglycemia and the Somogyi effect.

20. Which class of oral glucose-lowering agents (OA) is most commonly used for people with type 2 diabetes because it reduces hepatic glucose production and enhances tissue uptake of glucose?
    a. Insulin
    b. Biguanide
    c. Meglitinide
    d. Sulfonylurea

21. The patient with type 2 diabetes is being prescribed acarbose (Precose) and wants to know about taking it. What would the nurse include in this patient's teaching? **Select all that apply.**
    a. Take it with the first bite of each meal.
    b. It is not used in patients with heart failure.
    c. Endogenous glucose production is decreased.
    d. Effectiveness is measured by 2-hour postprandial glucose.
    e. It delays glucose absorption from the gastrointestinal (GI) tract.

22. The patient with type 2 diabetes has had trouble controlling his-glucose with several OAs but wants to avoid the risks of insulin. Which medication will increase insulin synthesis and release from the pancreas, inhibit glucagon secretion, and slow gastric emptying?
    a. Dopamine receptor agonist, bromocriptine (Cycloset)
    b. Dipeptidyl peptidase-4 (DPP-4) inhibitor, sitagliptin (Januvia)
    c. Sodium-glucose co-transporter 2 (SGLT2) inhibitor, canagliflozin (Invokana)
    d. Glucagon-like peptide-1 receptor agonist, exenatide extended release (Bydureon)

23. The nurse is assessing a newly admitted patient with diabetes. Which observation would most concern the nurse?
    a. Bilateral numbness of both hands
    b. Rapid respirations with deep inspiration
    c. Stage 2 pressure injury on the right heel
    d. Areas of lumps and dents on the abdomen

24. What teaching would be included regarding individualized nutrition therapy for patients using conventional, fixed insulin regimens?
    a. Eat regular meals at regular times.
    b. Restrict calories to promote moderate weight loss.
    c. Eliminate sucrose and other simple sugars from the diet.
    d. Limit saturated fat intake to 30% of dietary calorie intake.

25. What goals of nutrition therapy are included for the patient with type 2 diabetes?
    a. Ideal body weight
    b. Normal-glucose and lipid levels
    c. A special diabetic diet using dietetic foods
    d. Five small meals per day with a bedtime snack

26. To prevent hyperglycemia or hypoglycemia related to exercise, what would the nurse teach the patient about exercise when using glucose-lowering agents?
    a. Plan activity and food intake related to glucose levels
    b. When glucose is greater than 250 mg/dL and ketones are present
    c. When glucose monitoring reveals that the glucose is in the normal range
    d. When glucose levels are high, because exercise always has a hypoglycemic effect

27. The nurse assesses the technique of a patient with diabetes for self-blood glucose monitoring (BGM) 3 months after initial instruction. Which error in the performance of BGM requires intervention?
    a. Doing the BGM before and after exercising
    b. Puncturing the finger on the side of the finger pad
    c. Cleaning the puncture site with alcohol before the puncture
    d. Holding the hand down for a few minutes before the puncture

28. A nurse working in an outpatient clinic plans a screening program for diabetes. What recommendations for screening would be included?
    a. OGTT for all minority populations every year
    b. FPG for all persons at age 45 years and then every 3 years
    c. Testing people under the age of 21 years for islet cell antibodies
    d. Testing for type 2 diabetes in all overweight or obese persons

29. A patient with diabetes calls the clinic because of nausea and flu-like symptoms. What is the nurse's best advice?
    a. Administer the usual insulin dosage.
    b. Hold fluid intake until the nausea subsides.
    c. Come to the clinic immediately for evaluation and treatment.
    d. Monitor glucose every 1 to 2 hours and call if it rises over 150 mg/dL (8.3 mmol/L).

30. When would the nurse observe the patient for symptoms of ketoacidosis?
    a. Illnesses causing nausea and vomiting lead to bicarbonate loss with body fluids.
    b. Glucose levels become so high that osmotic diuresis promotes fluid and electrolyte loss.
    c. An insulin deficit causes the body to metabolize large amounts of fatty acids rather than glucose for energy.
    d. The patient skips meals after taking insulin, leading to rapid metabolism of glucose and breakdown of fats for energy.

31. What assessment findings occur with diabetic ketoacidosis (DKA)? **Select all that apply.**
    a. Thirst
    b. Ketonuria
    c. Dehydration
    d. Metabolic acidosis
    e. Kussmaul respirations
    f. Sweet, fruity breath odor

32. What describes the main difference in treatment for diabetic ketoacidosis (DKA) and hyperosmolar hyperglycemic syndrome (HHS)?
    a. DKA requires administration of bicarbonate to correct acidosis.
    b. Potassium replacement is not necessary in management of HHS.
    c. HHS requires greater fluid replacement to correct the dehydration.
    d. Glucose is withheld in HHS until the blood glucose reaches a normal level.

33. The patient with diabetes has a blood glucose level of 248 mg/dL. Which assessment findings would be related to this blood glucose level? **Select all that apply.**
    a. Headache
    b. Unsteady gait
    c. Abdominal cramps
    d. Emotional changes
    e. Increase in urination
    f. Weakness and fatigue

34. A patient with diabetes is found unconscious at home, and a family member calls the clinic. After determining that a glucometer is not available, what would the nurse advise the family member to do?
    a. Have the patient drink some orange juice.
    b. Administer 10 U of regular insulin subcutaneously.
    c. Call for an ambulance to transport the patient to a medical facility.
    d. Administer glucagon 1 mg intramuscularly (IM) or subcutaneously.

35. The patient with diabetes is brought to the emergency department by his family members, who say that he has had an infection, is not acting like himself, and is more tired than usual. Number the nursing actions in order of priority for this patient, using number 1 as the first priority and number 6 as the last priority.
    _____a. Establish IV access.
    _____b. Check blood glucose.
    _____c. Ensure patent airway.
    _____d. Begin continuous regular insulin drip.
    _____e. Administer 0.9% NaCl solution at 1 L/hr.
    _____f. Establish time of last food and medication(s).

36. Two days after a self-managed hypoglycemic episode at home, the patient tells the nurse that their glucose levels since the episode have been between 80 and 90 mg/dL. How would the nurse respond?
    a. "That is a good range for your glucose levels."
    b. "You should call your HCP because you need to have your insulin increased."
    c. "That level is too low in view of your recent hypoglycemia and you should increase your food intake."
    d. "You should take only half your insulin dosage for the next few days to get your glucose level back to normal."

37. Which statement best describes atherosclerotic disease affecting the cerebrovascular, cardiovascular, and peripheral vascular systems in patients with diabetes?
    a. It can be prevented by tight glucose control.
    b. It occurs with a higher frequency and earlier onset than in the nondiabetic population.
    c. It is caused by hyperinsulinemia related to insulin resistance common in type 2 diabetes.
    d. It cannot be modified by reducing risk factors, such as smoking, obesity, and high fat intake.

38. What disorders and diseases are related to macrovascular complications of diabetes? **Select all that apply.**
    a. Chronic kidney disease
    b. Coronary artery disease
    c. Microaneurysms and destruction of retinal vessels
    d. Ulceration and amputation of the lower extremities
    e. Capillary and arteriole membrane thickening specific to diabetes

39. The patient with diabetes has been diagnosed with autonomic neuropathy. What problems would the nurse assess for in this patient? **Select all that apply.**
    a. Painless foot ulcers
    b. Erectile dysfunction
    c. Burning foot pain at night
    d. Loss of fine motor control
    e. Vomiting undigested food
    f. Painless myocardial infarction

40. Following the teaching of foot care to a patient with diabetes, the nurse determines that additional instruction is needed when the patient makes which statement?
    a. "I should wash my feet daily with soap and warm water."
    b. "I should always wear shoes to protect my feet from injury."
    c. "If my feet are cold, I should wear socks instead of using a heating pad."
    d. "I'll know if I have sores or lesions on my feet because they will be painful."

41. A 72-year-old woman is diagnosed with diabetes. What does the nurse know about managing diabetes in the older adult?
    a. It is harder to achieve strict glucose control than in younger patients.
    b. Treatment is not warranted unless the patient develops severe hyperglycemia.
    c. It does not include treatment with insulin because of limited dexterity and vision.
    d. It usually requires that a younger family member be responsible for care of the patient.

42. A patient with newly diagnosed type 2 diabetes has been given a prescription to start an oral hypoglycemic medication, but would rather control their glucose with herbal therapy. What would the nurse do?
    a. Teach the patient that herbal therapy is not safe and should not be used.
    b. Advise the patient to discuss using herbal therapy with her HCP before using it.
    c. Encourage the patient to give the prescriptive medication time to work before using herbal therapy.
    d. Teach the patient that if they take herbal therapy, they will have to monitor their glucose more often.

CASE STUDY Hypoglycemia

Patient Profile

After running in her first half-marathon, F.W., a 24-year-old woman with type 1 diabetes, was brought to the first aid tent provided for participants in a charity run. She manages her diabetes using a regimen of self-blood glucose monitoring, intensive insulin therapy, and diet.

(Minerva Studio/ iStock/Thinkstock)

Subjective Data
- Reports that she feels cold and has a headache; her fingers feel numb
- She took her usual insulin dose this morning but did not eat her entire breakfast because of a lack of time and fear of nausea when she ran
- Completed the half-marathon faster than her practice times

Objective Data
- Has slurred speech and unsteady gait
- HR: 120 beats/min
- Confused
- Finger-stick BG level: 48 mg/dL (2.7 mmol/L)

Questions

1. What is the etiology of the manifestations that F.W. exhibits? **Use an X to indicate if the assessment finding is associated with the effects of epinephrine on the <u>Sympathetic Nervous System</u> or is a result of <u>Hypoglycemia to the Brain</u>.**

Assessment Finding	Sympathetic Nervous System	Hypoglycemia to the Brain
Headache		
HR 120 beats/min		
Slurred speech		
Numbness in fingers		
Unsteady gait		
Confused		
Feels cold		

2. What other clinical manifestations of hypoglycemia would the nurse expect? **Use an X to indicate whether the assessment finding is Expected (is a sign or symptom of hypoglycemia) or Unexpected (is not a sign or symptom of hypoglycemia).**

Assessment Finding	Expected	Unexpected
Tremors		
Skin is flushed and warm		
Diaphoresis		
Lips are numb		
Abdominal cramping		
Polyuria		
Dizziness		

3. **Choose the most likely options for the information missing from the paragraph below by selecting from the lists of options provided.**

If the patient is conscious, have the patient ingest _____**1**_____ of _____**2**_____. This can be _____**3**_____ or _____**3**_____. Recheck the glucose _____**4**_____ minutes later. If still less than _____**5**_____ mg/dL, repeat the previous steps. In an acute care setting, treat hypoglycemia with 25–50 mL of _____**6**_____. If IV access is not available, administer _____**7**_____ mg of _____**8**_____ IM or SQ.

Options for 1	Options for 2	Options for 3	Options for 4
5–10 g	Fats	Diet soda	5
1–5 g	Proteins	Apple juice	10
10–15 g	Simple carbohydrates	Water	15
15–20 g	Complex carbohydrates	Soft drink	20
20–25 g	Vitamins	Black coffee	25
25–30 g	Fiber	Milk	30

Options for 5	Options for 6	Options for 7	Options for 8
25	5% dextrose	1	Epinephrine
50	10% dextrose	0.5	Cortisol
70	0.9% saline	2	Hydrocortisone
75	3% saline	3	Glucagon
100	0.45% saline	5	Dextrose
120	50% dextrose	10	Insulin

4. What statements by F.W. indicate teaching about how to prevent future episodes of hypoglycemia has been effective? **Use an X to indicate if the patient's statement indicates teaching is Effective (patient understands), Ineffective (needs clarification) or Unrelated (doesn't pertain to this topic).**

Patient Statement	Effective	Ineffective	Unrelated
"I will carry a snack with me."			
"My insulin requirements will be higher with exercise."			
"I will drink lots of water during exercise."			
"I will dress lightly during strenuous exercise."			

Patient Statement	Effective	Ineffective	Unrelated
"I will increase my calories before I exercise."			
"I should wait 60 minutes after meals before exercising."			
"Exercise doesn't affect my blood glucose levels."			

5. What would the nurse include when teaching F.W. about diabetes-related ketoacidosis (DKA)? **Select all that apply.**

_____A. DKA doesn't occur in patients with type 1 diabetes.

_____B. It is caused by too much insulin.

_____C. Illness and physiologic stress are causes.

_____D. Vomiting occurs from acidosis.

_____E. You should test your urine for ketones during illnesses.

_____F. You won't need to be hospitalized.

_____G. Closely monitor your glucose during illnesses.

_____H. Restrict fluids to minimize nausea and vomiting.

1. A patient suspected of having acromegaly has an increased plasma growth hormone (GH) level. In acromegaly, what would the nurse expect the patient's diagnostic results to show?
   a. Hyperinsulinemia
   b. Plasma glucose of less than 70 mg/dL (3.9 mmol/L)
   c. Decreased GH levels with an oral glucose challenge test
   d. Increased levels of plasma insulin-like growth factor-1 (IGF-1)

2. During assessment of the patient with acromegaly, what would the nurse expect the patient to report?
   a. Infertility
   b. Dry, irritated skin
   c. Undesirable changes in appearance
   d. An increase in height of 2 to 3 inches a year

3. A patient with acromegaly is treated with a transsphenoidal hypophysectomy. What would the nurse do postoperatively?
   a. Ensure that any clear nasal drainage is tested for glucose and protein.
   b. Maintain the patient flat in bed to prevent cerebrospinal fluid (CSF) leakage.
   c. Aid the patient with tooth brushing every 4 hours to keep the surgical area clean.
   d. Encourage deep breathing, coughing, and turning to prevent respiratory complications.

4. What assessment findings are common in a patient with a prolactinoma?
   a. Gynecomastia in men
   b. Profuse menstruation in women
   c. Excess follicle-stimulating hormone (FSH) and luteinizing hormone (LH)
   d. Signs of increased intracranial pressure, including headache, nausea, and vomiting

5. A woman with a history of breast cancer has panhypopituitarism from radiation therapy to treat a primary pituitary tumor. Which lifelong medications would the nurse teach her about taking? **Select all that apply.**
   a. Cortisol
   b. Vasopressin
   c. Sex hormones
   d. Levothyroxine (Synthroid)
   e. Growth hormone (somatropin)
   f. Dopamine agonists (bromocriptine)

6. The patient is diagnosed with syndrome of inappropriate antidiuretic hormone (SIADH). What manifestation would the nurse expect?
   a. Decreased body weight
   b. Decreased urinary output
   c. Increased plasma osmolality
   d. Increased serum sodium levels

7. When caring for a patient with SIADH, what action would the nurse include in the plan of care?
   a. Monitor neurologic status at least every 2 hours.
   b. Teach the patient receiving diuretic therapy to restrict sodium intake.
   c. Keep the head of the bed elevated to prevent antidiuretic hormone (ADH) release.
   d. Notify the health care provider (HCP) if the patient's BP decreases more than 20 mm Hg from baseline.

8. A patient with SIADH is treated with water restriction. Which findings would indicate that treatment has been effective?
   a. Increased urine output, decreased serum sodium, and increased urine specific gravity
   b. Increased urine output, increased serum sodium, and decreased urine specific gravity
   c. Decreased urine output, increased serum sodium, and decreased urine specific gravity
   d. Decreased urine output, decreased serum sodium, and increased urine specific gravity

9. The patient with diabetes insipidus presents to the emergency department (ED) with confusion and dehydration after excretion of a large volume of urine today even though several liters of fluid were consumed. What diagnostic test would be done first to help make a diagnosis?
   a. Blood glucose
   b. Serum sodium level
   c. CT scan of the head
   d. Water deprivation test

10. In a patient with central diabetes insipidus, what is the expected outcome of administering ADH during a water deprivation test?
    a. Decrease in body weight
    b. Increase in urinary output
    c. Decrease in blood pressure
    d. Increase in urine osmolality

11. A patient with diabetes insipidus is treated with nasal desmopressin acetate (DDAVP). What would indicate that the drug is not having an adequate therapeutic effect?
    a. Headache and weight gain
    b. Nasal irritation and nausea
    c. A urine specific gravity of 1.002
    d. An oral intake greater than urinary output

12. What would the nurse expect the treatment of a patient with nephrogenic diabetes insipidus to include?
    a. Fluid restriction
    b. Thiazide diuretics
    c. A high-sodium diet
    d. Metformin (Glucophage)

13. What characteristic is related to Hashimoto's thyroiditis?
    a. Enlarged thyroid gland
    b. Viral-induced hyperthyroidism
    c. Bacterial or fungal infection of thyroid gland
    d. Chronic autoimmune thyroiditis with antibody destruction of thyroid tissue

14. Which statement accurately describes Graves' disease?
    a. Exophthalmos occurs in Graves' disease.
    b. It is an uncommon form of hyperthyroidism.
    c. Manifestations of hyperthyroidism occur from tissue desensitization to the sympathetic nervous system.
    d. Diagnostic testing in the patient with Graves' disease will reveal an increased thyroid-stimulating hormone (TSH) level.

15. A patient with Graves' disease asks the nurse what caused the disorder. How would the nurse respond?
    a. "The cause of Graves' disease is not known, although it is thought to be genetic."
    b. "It is usually associated with goiter formation from an iodine deficiency over a long period."
    c. "Antibodies develop against thyroid tissue and destroy it, causing a deficiency of thyroid hormones."
    d. "In genetically susceptible persons, antibodies are formed that cause excessive thyroid hormone secretion."

16. A patient is admitted to the hospital with acute thyrotoxicosis. What would the nurse expect during physical assessment of the patient?
    a. Hoarseness and laryngeal stridor
    b. Bulging eyeballs and dysrhythmias
    c. Increased temperature and signs of heart failure
    d. Lethargy progressing suddenly to impaired consciousness

17. What medication is administered in thyrotoxicosis to block the effects of the sympathetic nervous stimulation of the thyroid hormones?
    a. Potassium iodine
    b. Propylthiouracil
    c. Propranolol (Inderal)
    d. Radioactive iodine (RAI)

18. Which characteristics most accurately describe the use of RAI? **Select all that apply.**
    a. Decreases release of thyroid hormones
    b. Often causes hypothyroidism over time
    c. Blocks peripheral conversion of T_4 to T_3
    d. Treatment of choice in nonpregnant adults
    e. Often used with iodine to produce euthyroid before surgery
    f. Decreases thyroid hormone secretion by damaging thyroid gland

19. What preoperative instruction would the nurse give to the patient scheduled for a subtotal thyroidectomy?
    a. How to support the head with the hands when turning in bed
    b. Coughing should be avoided to prevent pressure on the incision
    c. Head and neck will have to remain immobile until the incision heals
    d. Any tingling around the lips or in the fingers after surgery is expected and temporary

20. As a precaution for vocal cord paralysis from damage to the superior laryngeal nerve during thyroidectomy surgery, what equipment is most important to have in the room in case it is needed for an emergency situation?
    a. Tracheostomy tray
    b. Oxygen equipment
    c. IV calcium gluconate
    d. Paper and pencil for communication

21. When providing discharge instructions to a patient who had a subtotal thyroidectomy for hyperthyroidism, what would the nurse teach the patient?
    a. Never miss a daily dose of thyroid replacement therapy.
    b. Avoid regular exercise until thyroid function is normalized.
    c. Use warm saltwater gargles several times a day to relieve throat pain.
    d. Substantially reduce caloric intake compared to what was eaten before surgery.

22. What is a cause of primary hypothyroidism in adults?
    a. Malignant or benign thyroid nodules
    b. Surgical removal or failure of the pituitary gland
    c. Surgical removal or radiation of the thyroid gland
    d. Autoimmune-induced atrophy of the thyroid gland

23. What action would the nurse include in the plan of care for a patient experiencing fatigue from hypothyroidism?
    a. Assess for changes in orientation, cognition, and behavior.
    b. Monitor for vital signs and cardiac rhythm response to activity.
    c. Monitor bowel movement frequency, consistency, shape, volume, and color.
    d. Help in developing well-balanced meal plans consistent with energy expenditure level.

24. A patient with long-standing hypothyroidism starts replacement therapy. What is most important for the nurse to monitor for in the patient?
    a. Insomnia
    b. Weight loss
    c. Nervousness
    d. Dysrhythmias

25. A patient with hypothyroidism is treated with levothyroxine (Synthroid). What would the nurse include when teaching the patient about this medication?
    a. Explain that alternate-day dosage may be used if side effects occur.
    b. Provide written instruction for all information related to the drug therapy.
    c. Tell the patient that the drug must be taken until the hormone balance is reestablished.
    d. Assure the patient that a return to normal function will occur with replacement therapy.

26. A patient who recently had a calcium oxalate renal stone had a bone density study. What endocrine problem could cause a decrease in bone density?
    a. SIADH
    b. Hypothyroidism
    c. Cushing syndrome
    d. Hyperparathyroidism

27. What is an appropriate nursing intervention for the patient with hyperparathyroidism?
    a. Pad side rails as a seizure precaution.
    b. Increase fluid intake to 3000 to 4000 mL daily.
    c. Maintain bed rest to prevent pathologic fractures.
    d. Monitor the patient for Trousseau's and Chvostek's signs.

28. A patient has been diagnosed with hypoparathyroidism. What manifestations would the nurse expect? **Select all that apply.**
    a. Skeletal pain
    b. Dysrhythmias
    c. Dry, scaly skin
    d. Personality changes
    e. Abdominal cramping
    f. Muscle spasms and stiffness

29. When the patient with parathyroid disease has symptoms of hypocalcemia, what measure can temporarily raise serum calcium levels?
    a. Administer IV normal saline.
    b. Have patient rebreathe in a paper bag.
    c. Administer oral phosphorus supplements.
    d. Administer furosemide (Lasix) as ordered.

30. What would the nurse include in discharge instructions for a patient with hypoparathyroidism from surgical treatment of hyperparathyroidism?
    a. Milk and milk products should be increased in the diet.
    b. Parenteral replacement of parathyroid hormone will be needed for life.
    c. Calcium supplements with vitamin D can effectively maintain calcium balance.
    d. Bran and whole-grain foods should be used to prevent gastrointestinal (GI) effects of replacement therapy.

31. A patient is admitted to the hospital with a diagnosis of Cushing syndrome. What would the nurse expect when assessing the patient?
    a. Hypertension, peripheral edema, and petechiae
    b. Weight loss, buffalo hump, and moon face with acne
    c. Abdominal and buttock striae, truncal obesity, and hypotension
    d. Anorexia, signs of dehydration, and hyperpigmentation of the skin

32. A patient is scheduled for a bilateral adrenalectomy. During the postoperative period, what action would the nurse expect related to the administration of corticosteroids?
    a. Reduced to promote wound healing
    b. Withheld until symptoms of hypocortisolism appear
    c. Increased to promote an adequate response to the stress of surgery
    d. Reduced with excessive hormone release during surgical manipulation of adrenal glands

33. A patient with Addison's disease comes to the ED with reports of nausea, vomiting, diarrhea, and fever. What interprofessional care would the nurse expect?
    a. IV administration of vasopressors
    b. IV administration of hydrocortisone
    c. IV administration of D_5W with 20 mEq KCl
    d. Parenteral injections of adrenocorticotropic hormone (ACTH)

34. After providing discharge teaching to the patient with Addison's disease, which statement indicates the need for further teaching?
    a. "I should always call the doctor if I develop vomiting or diarrhea."
    b. "If my weight goes down, my dosage of steroid is probably too high."
    c. "I should double or triple my steroid dose if I undergo rigorous physical exercise."
    d. "I need to carry an emergency kit with injectable hydrocortisone in case I can't take my medication by mouth."

35. A patient who is taking corticosteroids to treat an autoimmune disorder has the following drugs ordered. Which one is used to prevent corticosteroid-induced osteoporosis?
    a. Potassium
    b. Furosemide (Lasix)
    c. Alendronate (Fosamax)
    d. Pantoprazole (Protonix)

36. A patient with mild iatrogenic Cushing syndrome is on an alternate-day regimen of corticosteroid therapy. What would the nurse explain to the patient about this regimen?
    a. It maintains normal adrenal hormone balance.
    b. It prevents ACTH release from the pituitary gland.
    c. It minimizes hypothalamic-pituitary-adrenal suppression.
    d. It provides a more effective therapeutic effect of the drug.

37. When caring for a patient with primary hyperaldosteronism, which prescription would the nurse question?
    a. Ketoconazole
    b. Furosemide (Lasix)
    c. Eplerenone (Inspra)
    d. Spironolactone (Aldactone)

38. What is the priority nursing intervention during the management of the patient with pheochromocytoma?
    a. Administering IV fluids
    b. Monitoring blood pressure
    c. Administering β-adrenergic blockers
    d. Monitoring intake and output and daily weights

CASE STUDY   Cushing Syndrome

(Thinkstock)

Patient Profile

T.H. is a 34-year-old male elementary school teacher. He seeks the advice of his HCP because of changes in his appearance over the past year.

Subjective Data
- Reports weight gain (particularly through his midsection), easy bruising, and edema of his feet, lower legs, and hands
- Reports increasing weakness and insomnia

Objective Data
- Physical assessment: BP 150/110 mm Hg; 2 + edema of lower extremities; purplish striae on abdomen; thin extremities with thin, friable skin; severe acne of the face and neck
- Blood analysis: Glucose 167 mg/dL (9.3 mmol/L); white blood cell (WBC) count 13,600/μL; lymphocytes 12%; red blood cell (RBC) count 6.0×10^6/μL; K$^+$ 3.2 mEq/L (3.2 mmol/L)

Questions
1. What hormones would the nurse attribute to T.H.'s clinical manifestations? **Use an X to indicate whether the assessment finding is caused by Glucocorticoids, Mineralocorticoids, or Androgens. Note that some assessment findings may be applicable to multiple hormones.**

Assessment Finding	Glucocorticoids	Mineralocorticoids	Androgens
Truncal obesity			
Weakness			

Assessment Finding	Glucocorticoids	Mineralocorticoids	Androgens
Purple striae			
Peripheral edema			
Insomnia			
Hyperglycemia			
Hypokalemia			
Acne			
Hypertension			

2. What diagnostic testing would identify the cause of T.H.'s Cushing syndrome? **Use an X to indicate whether the diagnostic test is Indicated (helps diagnose) or is Unrelated (does not help diagnose).**

Diagnostic Test	Indicated	Unrelated
Ultrasound of adrenal glands		
MRI of head		
24-hour urine cortisol		
Dexamethasone suppression test		
Creatinine clearance		
D-dimer		
Salivary cortisol		

3. T.H. asks the nurse what is meant by a "medical adrenalectomy." **Choose the most likely options for the information missing from the statements below by selecting from the list of options provided.**

A medical adrenalectomy uses drug therapy to stop the secretion of _____. These drugs include _____ and _____. Other medications that may be necessary to avoid adrenal insufficiency are _____ or _____. Patients who have type 2 diabetes and need help controlling hyperglycemia may be prescribed _____.

Options:	
Mifepristone	Hydrocortisone
Prednisone	Cortisol
Insulin	ADH
Ketoconazole	Demeclocycline
Fludrocortisone	Mitotane

4. T.H. has been informed of the 2 surgical options depending on the location of the tumor causing Cushing disease. What nursing interventions would the nurse plan postoperatively for each type of surgery? **Use an X to indicate if the nursing action applies mainly to the Hypophysectomy, the Adrenalectomy or Both.**

Nursing Action	Hypophysectomy	Adrenalectomy	Both
Splint the abdominal incision			
Administer hydrocortisone			
Monitor blood glucose			
Apply a "moustache" dressing			

Nursing Action	Hypophysectomy	Adrenalectomy	Both
Report BP fluctuations			
Report severe headaches			
Perform sterile dressing changes			
Elevate the HOB ≥ 30°			
Monitor electrolytes			
Assess peripheral vision			

5. T.H. is status-post a transphenoidal hypophysectomy 3 days ago. What discharge instructions would the nurse include when discharging T.H. to home? **Select all that apply.**

_____A. You can use a soft bristle toothbrush to brush your teeth.

_____B. Clear drainage from your nose is normal.

_____C. Perform saline rinses to clean your nose.

_____D. Report any vision changes to your HCP.

_____E. You will need to take levothyroxine for the remainder of your life.

_____F. It is normal to urinate frequently.

_____G. Pinch your nose when you sneeze or cough.

_____H. You may gently blow your nose.

_____I. Report any symptoms of a stiff neck.

Assessment: Reproductive System

1. Identify the structures in the illustrations below by filling in the blanks with the correct answers from the list of terms. **(Some terms will be used in both illustrations.)**

Terms

Anus
Bladder
Body of uterus
Cervix
Cowper's gland
Ductus deferens
Ejaculatory duct
Epididymis

Fallopian tube
Fundus of uterus
Glans
Ovary
Penis
Prostate gland
Rectum
Scrotum

Seminal vesicle
Testis
Ureter
Urethra
Vagina
Vaginal introitus

a. _____
b. _____
c. _____
d. _____
e. _____
f. _____
g. _____
h. _____
i. _____
j. _____
k. _____
l. _____
m. _____
n. _____

o. _____
p. _____
q. _____
r. _____
s. _____
t. _____
u. _____
v. _____
w. _____
x. _____
y. _____
z. _____
aa. _____

2. Using the list of terms, identify the structures in the illustrations below.

Terms

Alveoli	Labia majora	Perineum
Areola	Labia minora	Prepuce
Bartholin's gland	Mons pubis	Urethral meatus
Clitoris	Nipple	Vaginal introitus
Hymen	Pectoralis major muscle	Vestibule

a. _____   i. _____

b. _____   j. _____

c. _____   k. _____

d. _____   l. _____

e. _____   m. _____

f. _____   n. _____

g. _____   o. _____

h. _____

3. Number in sequence from 1 to 8 the passage of sperm through, and the formation of semen in, the structures of the male reproductive system.

_____ a. Ductus deferens   _____ e. Seminiferous tubules
_____ b. Urethra   _____ f. Cowper's glands
_____ c. Epididymis   _____ g. Seminal vesicles
_____ d. Prostate gland   _____ h. Ejaculatory duct

4. Which structure of the female breast carries milk from the alveoli to the lactiferous sinuses?
   a. Ducts   c. Nipple
   b. Areola   d. Adipose tissue

5. What describes Montgomery's tubercles in the female breast?
   a. Store milk during lactation   c. Sebaceous-like glands on areola
   b. Secrete milk during lactation   d. Erectile tissues containing pores

6. Which statement accurately describes the female reproductive system?
   a. Fertilization of an ovum by sperm occurs in the uterus.
   b. Only the ectocervix is used for obtaining Papanicolaou (Pap) tests.
   c. A middle-aged woman is considered to be in menopause when she has not had a menstrual period for 1 year.
   d. The normal process of reabsorption of immature oocytes throughout the female life span is caused by follicle-stimulating hormone (FSH) and luteinizing hormone (LH).

7. What are characteristics of LH? **Select all that apply.**
   a. Maintains implanted egg
   b. Completes follicle maturation
   c. Stimulates testosterone production
   d. Required for female sex characteristics
   e. Needed for growth of mammary glands
   f. Called interstitial cell-stimulating hormone (ICSH) in men

8. FSH is secreted by the anterior pituitary gland in both women and men. Which characteristics describe FSH? **Select all that apply.**
   a. Produced by testes
   b. Increased at onset of menopause
   c. Responsible for spermatogenesis
   d. Stimulated by high estrogen levels
   e. Needed for male sex characteristics
   f. Stimulates growth and maturity of ovarian follicles

9. A 72-year-old man asks the nurse whether it is normal for him to have erectile dysfunction at his age. What is the best response by the nurse?
   a. Most decreased sexual function in older adults is caused by psychologic stress.
   b. Physiologic changes of aging may require increased stimulation for an erection to occur.
   c. Although the penis decreases in size in older men, there should be no change in sexual function.
   d. Benign changes in the prostate gland that occur with aging can decrease the ability to attain an erection.

10. List 1 problem associated with each of these factors that may be identified during assessment of the reproductive system.

Factor	Problem Identified During Assessment
Rubella	
Mumps	
Diabetes	
Antihypertensive agents	

11. A 58-year-old man is being assessed by the nurse. Which information would identify the need for further examination for benign prostatic hyperplasia (BPH)?
    a. A mass on the scrotum or testes
    b. A slow and difficult start of a urinary stream
    c. Patient describes a single, small, painless blister
    d. A bulging inguinal ring while the patient bears down

12. When assessing an aging adult man, what would the nurse consider as a normal finding?
    a. Decreased penis size
    b. Decreased pubic hair
    c. A change in scrotal color
    d. Unilateral breast enlargement

13. When assessing an aging adult woman, what would the nurse consider as a normal finding?
    a. Rectocele
    b. Larger breasts
    c. Vaginal dryness
    d. Severe osteoporosis

14. Identify 1 specific finding identified by the nurse during assessment of each of the patient's functional health patterns that indicates a risk factor for reproductive problems or a patient response to an actual reproductive problem.

Functional Health Pattern	Risk Factor for or Patient Response to Reproductive Problem
Health perception–health management	
Nutritional-metabolic	
Elimination	
Activity-exercise	
Sleep-rest	
Cognitive-perceptual	
Self-perception–self-concept	
Role-relationship	
Sexuality-reproductive	
Coping–stress tolerance	
Value-belief	

15. A 25-year-old female patient is at the clinic and says that she has white, curd-like vaginal drainage and itching. Which problem would the nurse suspect?
   a. Cancer
   b. Candidiasis
   c. Trichomonas vaginalis
   d. Bacterial vaginosis infection

16. During examination of the female reproductive system, which finding would the nurse consider abnormal?
   a. Clear vaginal discharge
   b. Perineal episiotomy scars
   c. Nonpalpable Skene's glands
   d. Reddened base of the vulva

17. Which laboratory tests are used to diagnose *Chlamydia?* **Select all that apply.**
   a. Pap test
   b. Gram stain
   c. Rapid plasma reagin (RPR)
   d. Nucleic acid amplified test (NAAT)
   e. Venereal Disease Research Laboratory (VDRL)
   f. Fluorescent treponemal antibody absorption (FTA-Abs)

18. Why is the serum estradiol laboratory test used?
   a. To detect pregnancy
   b. To detect prostate cancer
   c. To measure ovarian function
   d. To identify secondary gonadal failure

19. After a dilation and curettage (D&C), what complication would the nurse prioritize?
   a. Infection
   b. Hemorrhage
   c. Urinary retention
   d. Perforation of the bladder

20. Which diagnostic tests of the female reproductive system are operative procedures requiring surgical anesthesia? **Select all that apply.**
   a. D&C
   b. Conization
   c. Culdoscopy
   d. Colposcopy
   e. Laparoscopy
   f. Endometrial biopsy

21. Which fertility test requires a couple to have no sexual intercourse for 2 to 3 days before the test?
   a. Urinary LH
   b. Semen analysis
   c. Endometrial biopsy
   d. Hysterosalpingogram

Breast Disorders

1. A woman at the health clinic tells the nurse that she does not do breast self-examination (BSE) because it just seems too much of a bother. What is the best response by the nurse about BSE?
   a. BSE is the most common way that breast cancer is discovered.
   b. It reduces mortality from breast cancer in women under the age of 50 years.
   c. It is useful to help women learn how their breasts normally look and feel.
   d. BSE has little value in detecting cancer and is not recommended anymore.

2. Identify the 4 screening guidelines recommended by the American Cancer Society for breast cancer.
   a.
   b.
   c.
   d.

3. When teaching a 24-year-old woman who wants to learn BSE, the nurse knows that it is important to do what?
   a. Provide time for a return demonstration.
   b. Emphasize the statistics related to breast cancer survival and mortality.
   c. Have the woman set a consistent monthly date for performing the examination.
   d. Inform the woman that professional examinations are not necessary unless she finds an abnormality.

4. Which diagnostic test is most accurate and advantageous in terms of time and expense in diagnosing breast cancer?
   a. Mammography
   b. Excisional biopsy
   c. Fine-needle aspiration
   d. Core (core needle) biopsy

5. A 44-year-old female patient has breast cancer with estrogen receptor–negative cells. Which genomic assay test can be used to provide information about the likely recurrence and need for chemotherapy?
   a. CA 27-29
   b. TNM system
   c. Oncotype DX
   d. Direct to consumer

6. While examining a patient's breasts, the nurse palpates multiple, bilateral mobile lumps. To assess the patient further, what is the most appropriate question by the nurse?
   a. "Do you have a high caffeine intake?"
   b. "When did you last have a mammogram?"
   c. "Is there a history of breast cancer in your mother or sisters?"
   d. "Do the size and tenderness of the lumps change with your menstrual cycle?"

7. A patient has fibrocystic changes in her breast. What would the nurse tell the patient is significant about this condition?
   a. Often turns to cancer over time
   b. Can be controlled with hormone therapy
   c. Makes it more difficult to examine the breasts
   d. Will eventually cause atrophy of normal breast tissue

8. Which characteristics describe an intraductal papilloma? **Select all that apply.**
   a. Associated with breast trauma
   b. Occurs in 10% of women ages 15 to 40 years
   c. Is more common in women ages 30 to 50 years
   d. Has multicolored, sticky nipple discharge
   e. Is associated with an increased cancer risk
   f. Has wartlike growth in mammary ducts near nipple

9. Which benign breast disorder occurs most often during lactation and is commonly caused by *Staphylococcus aureus*?
   a. Mastitis
   b. Ductal ectasia
   c. Fibroadenoma
   d. Senescent gynecomastia

10. Which patient has the highest risk of breast cancer?
    a. 60-year-old obese man
    b. 58-year-old woman with sedentary lifestyle
    c. 55-year-old woman with fibrocystic breast changes
    d. 65-year-old woman with a sister diagnosed with breast cancer

11. Which finding from a breast examination would most concern the nurse?
    a. A large, tender, moveable mass in the upper inner quadrant
    b. An immobile, hard, nontender lesion in the upper outer quadrant
    c. A 2- to 3-cm, firm, defined, mobile mass in the lower outer quadrant
    d. A painful, immobile mass with reddened skin in the upper outer quadrant

12. What diagnostic results have the best prognosis for a patient with breast cancer?
    a. Negative axillary lymph nodes
    b. Aneuploid DNA tumor content
    c. Cells with high S-phase fractions
    d. An estrogen receptor– and progesterone receptor–negative tumor

13. The health care provider of a patient with a positive biopsy of a 2-cm breast tumor has recommended a lumpectomy with radiation therapy or a modified radical mastectomy as treatment. The patient says that she does not know how to choose and asks the female nurse what she would do if she had to make the choice. What is the best response by the nurse?
    a. "It doesn't matter what I would do. It is a decision you have to make for yourself."
    b. "There are advantages and disadvantages of both procedures. What do you know about these procedures?"
    c. "I would choose the modified radical mastectomy because it would ensure that the entire tumor was removed."
    d. "The lumpectomy maintains a nearly normal breast, but the survival rate is not as good as it is with a mastectomy."

14. What additional treatment would be recommended for a patient undergoing either a mastectomy or a lumpectomy for breast cancer?
    a. Chemotherapy
    b. Radiation therapy
    c. Hormonal therapy
    d. Sentinel lymph node dissection (SLNB)

15. SLNB is planned for a patient undergoing a modified radical mastectomy for breast cancer. What would the nurse teach the patient and her family about the purpose of this procedure?
    a. SLNB provides metastatic lymph nodes to test for responsiveness to chemotherapy.
    b. If cancer cells are found in any sentinel nodes, a complete axillary lymph node dissection will be done.
    c. If 1 sentinel lymph node is positive for malignant cells, all the sentinel lymph nodes will be removed.
    d. A radioisotope shows which lymph nodes are most likely to have metastasis, and all those nodes are removed.

16. What describes the use of high-dose brachytherapy radiation? **Select all that apply.**
    a. May be completed in 5 days
    b. A primary treatment after mastectomy of breast
    c. Alternative to traditional radiation therapy for early-stage breast cancer
    d. Used to treat possible local residual cancer cells following a mastectomy
    e. Used to reduce tumor size and stabilize metastatic lesions for pain relief

17. A patient with a positive breast biopsy tells the nurse that she read about tamoxifen on the Internet and asks about its use. What information would the nurse include when responding?
    a. Tamoxifen is the treatment of choice if the tumor has receptors for estrogen on its cells.
    b. Tamoxifen is the primary treatment for breast cancer if axillary lymph nodes are positive for cancer.
    c. Tamoxifen is used only to prevent the development of new primary tumors in women with high risk for breast cancer.
    d. Because tamoxifen has been shown to increase the risk for uterine cancer, it is used only when other treatment has not been successful.

18. During the immediate postoperative period after a modified radical mastectomy, which exercises would the nurse initially include for the affected arm?
    a. Have the patient brush or comb her hair with the affected arm.
    b. Perform full passive range-of-motion (ROM) exercises to the affected arm.
    c. Ask the patient to flex and extend the fingers and wrist of the operative side.
    d. Have the patient crawl her fingers up the wall, raising her arm above her head.

19. Following a mastectomy, a patient develops lymphedema of the affected arm. What would the nurse teach the patient to do?
    a. Avoid skin-softening agents on the arm.
    b. Protect the arm from any type of trauma.
    c. Abduct and adduct the arm at the shoulder hourly.
    d. Keep the arm positioned so that it is in straight and dependent alignment.

20. A patient who had a mastectomy and is undergoing radiation for treatment of breast cancer is experiencing disturbed body image. What is an appropriate nursing intervention?
    a. Provide the patient with information about surgical breast reconstruction.
    b. Restrict visitors and phone calls until the patient feels better about herself.
    c. Arrange for a Reach-to-Recovery visitor or similar resource available in the community.
    d. Encourage the patient to obtain a permanent breast prosthesis as soon as she is discharged from the hospital.

21. A 56-year-old patient is undergoing a mammoplasty for breast reconstruction following a mastectomy 1 year ago. During the preoperative preparation of the patient, what is important for the nurse to do?
    a. Determine why the patient is choosing reconstruction surgery rather than the use of an external prosthesis.
    b. Ensure that the patient has realistic expectations about the outcome and complications of the surgery.
    c. Inform the patient that implants used for breast reconstruction have been shown to cause immune-related diseases.
    d. Let the patient know that, although the shape will be different from the other breast, the nipple can be reconstructed from other erectile tissue.

22. A patient undergoing a modified radical mastectomy for cancer of the breast is going to use tissue expansion and an implant for breast reconstruction. What would the nurse teach the patient about tissue expansion?
    a. Injections of sterile saline into the expander will be needed over weeks to months.
    b. The expander cannot be placed until healing from the mastectomy is complete.
    c. This method of breast reconstruction uses the patient's own tissue to replace breast tissue.
    d. The nipple from the affected breast will be saved to be grafted onto the reconstructed breast.

CASE STUDY Metastatic Breast Cancer

(RuslanGuzov/
iStock/Thinkstock)

Patient Profile

P.T. is a 57-year-old married female lawyer who is having a routine physical examination. Her HCP has found a 4 × 6-cm firm, fixed mass in the upper, outer quadrant of the right breast during a clinical breast examination.

Subjective Data

- States that she deserves to have breast cancer for being so careless about her health
- Reports that she is just so busy with work
- Menopausal
- Uses estrogen therapy to treat hot flashes
- Reports using oral contraceptives until she reached 48 years of age
- Denies family history of breast cancer

Objective Data

- Height 5 ft 5 in, weight 165 lbs (75 kg)
- Appears anxious
- Breasts are round without indentation
- Small amount of clear nipple discharge in the right breast
- Mammogram at age 50 showed fibrocystic changes

Questions

1. What could P.T. have done to screen for breast cancer at an earlier age? **Use an X to indicate if the type of screening is Recommended to screen for breast cancer or Not Recommended to screen for breast cancer.**

Screening	Recommended	Not Recommended
Perform self-breast exams monthly		
Genetic testing		
Annual clinical breast exam		
Mammogram once every 5 years, starting at age 25		
Annual Pap smear testing for HPV		
Annual mammogram starting at age 45		
Annual MRIs		

2. What risk factors or clinical manifestations does P.T. have for breast cancer? **Use an X to indicate if the assessment finding is a Risk Factor (causative factor), a Clinical Manifestation (symptom of breast cancer) or is Unrelated (not a causative factor nor a clinical manifestation).**

Assessment Finding	Risk Factor	Clinical Manifestation	Unrelated
Age			
Clear nipple discharge			
Treats hot flashes with estrogen therapy			
Fibrocystic changes			
Breasts are round			
Menopausal			
No family history			
Weight			
Contraceptive use			

3. **Choose the most likely options for the information missing from the statements below by selecting from the lists of options provided.**

_____1_____ is a non-invasive type of breast cancer that does not grow or invade normal tissue. It tends to be unilateral but can progress to invasive if left untreated. It accounts for approximately ___2___ of all non-invasive breast cancer. _____3_____ is a benign condition that is a risk factor for developing breast cancer. _____4_____ is the most common type of breast cancer and accounts for about ___5___ of all invasive breast cancers. _____6_____ begins in the lobules of the breast and accounts for ___7___ of invasive breast cancers. _____8_____ is an aggressive and fast-growing breast cancer with a high risk for metastasis. It accounts for ___9___ of all breast cancers.

Options for 1, 3, 4, 6, and 8:	Options for 2, 5, 7, and 9:
Paget's Disease	1%–3%
Inflammatory breast cancer	10%–15%
Invasive ductal carcinoma	< 1%
Invasive lobular carcinoma	50%
Ductal carcinoma in situ	80%
Lobular carcinoma in situ	20%
Phyllodes tumor	75%
Triple-negative breast cancer	25%–30%
Peau d'orange	5%–10%

4. P.T. has been diagnosed with a malignant tumor. What statements are true about breast cancer and its treatment? **Select all that apply.**

_____A. HER-2 negative tumors are more aggressive and have a poorer prognosis.

_____B. Patients with triple-negative tumors do not respond well to hormone therapy.

_____C. Surgery is the main treatment.

_____D. A double-mastectomy is recommended if BRCA1 and BRCA2 mutations are present.

_____E. Estrogen receptor-positive tumors have a greater chance to recur.

_____F. Progesterone receptor-negative tumors are more often poorly differentiated.

_____G. Tamoxifen is often prescribed to treat estrogen receptor-positive tumors.

_____H. Postmenopausal women are at greater risk of endometrial cancer if prescribed Tamoxifen.

5. P.T. opted for a right modified radical mastectomy with sentinel lymph node biopsy and tissue expander. What patient statements would indicate discharge teaching has been effective? **Use an X to indicate if teaching has been <u>Effective</u> (meets expected outcomes) or <u>Ineffective</u> (does not meet expected outcomes).**

Patient Statement	Effective	Ineffective
"I may have phantom breast pain."		
"I will not be allowed to raise my arm more than 90 degrees for 2 weeks."		
"I will not allow blood pressures to be measured on my right arm."		
"Blood can be drawn from my right arm only if blood cultures are necessary."		
"Lymphedema won't be an issue for me."		
"I may get breast implants in the future."		
"I can put ice on the breast incision to reduce swelling."		

Sexually Transmitted Infections

1. In part, what is the current incidence of sexually transmitted infections (STIs) related to?
   a. Increased social acceptance of homosexuality
   b. Increased virulence of organisms that cause STIs
   c. Use of oral agents rather than condoms as contraceptives
   d. Increased microorganism resistance to common antibiotics

2. When establishing screening programs for populations at high risk for STIs, which microorganism causes nongonococcal urethritis in men and cervicitis in women?
   a. *Treponema pallidum*
   b. *Neisseria gonorrhoeae*
   c. *Chlamydia trachomatis*
   d. Herpes simplex virus (HSV)

3. The laboratory result of a specimen from a patient is positive for fluorescent treponemal antibodies (FTA). What would the nurse expect the diagnosis to be?
   a. Syphilis
   b. Gonorrhea
   c. Genital warts
   d. Genital herpes

4. A patient with a purulent vaginal discharge is seen at an outpatient clinic. The nurse suspects a diagnosis of gonorrhea. How will this STI be treated?
   a. Oral acyclovir (Zovirax)
   b. Penicillin G Benzathine given IM
   c. Need a confirmatory test result before treatment
   d. Ceftriaxone IM with oral azithromycin (Zithromax)

5. A 22-year-old woman with multiple sexual partners seeks care after several weeks of having painful and frequent urination and vaginal discharge. Although the results of a culture of cervical secretions are not yet available, what complications would the nurse explain to the patient are being prevented by treating her as if she has gonorrhea and chlamydia?
   a. Damage to the fallopian tubes
   b. Endocarditis and aortic aneurysms
   c. Disseminated gonococcal infection
   d. Polyarthritis and generalized adenopathy

6. During evaluation and treatment of a patient with gonorrhea, what question is most important for the nurse to ask the patient?
   a. "Do you have a prior history of STIs?"
   b. "When did the symptoms begin?"
   c. "What date was your last sexual activity?"
   d. "What are the names of your recent sexual partners?"

7. Which manifestations are characteristic of the late or tertiary stage of syphilis? **Select all that apply.**
   a. Heart failure
   b. Tabes dorsalis
   c. Aortic aneurysms
   d. Mental deterioration
   e. Generalized cutaneous rash
   f. Destructive skin, bone, and soft tissue lesions

8. Which stage of syphilis is identified by the absence of clinical manifestations and a positive fluorescent treponemal antibody absorption (FTA-Abs) test?
   a. Latent
   b. Primary
   c. Secondary
   d. Late (tertiary)

9. A blood test for syphilis reveals that a patient has a positive Venereal Disease Research Laboratory (VDRL) test. How would the nurse advise the patient?
   a. A single dose of penicillin will cure the syphilis.
   b. The patient should question their partner about prior sexual contacts.
   c. Additional testing to detect specific antitreponemal antibodies is necessary.
   d. A lumbar puncture to evaluate cerebrospinal fluid (CSF) is needed to rule out active syphilis.

10. Why would the nurse encourage serologic testing for human immunodeficiency virus (HIV) in the patient with syphilis?
    a. Syphilis is harder to treat in patients with HIV infection.
    b. The presence of HIV infection increases the risk of contracting syphilis.
    c. Central nervous system (CNS) involvement is common in patients with HIV infection and syphilis.
    d. The incidence of syphilis is increased in those with high rates of indiscriminate sexual activity and drug use.

11. A female patient returns to the clinic with a recurrent urethral discharge after being treated for a chlamydial infection 2 weeks ago. Which statement by the patient indicates the most likely cause of the recurrence of her infection?
    a. "I took the doxycycline twice a day for a week."
    b. "I haven't told my boyfriend about my infection yet."
    c. "I had a couple of beers while I was taking the medication."
    d. "I've only had sexual intercourse once since I finished the medication."

12. What is the most common way to determine a diagnosis of chlamydial infection in a male patient?
    a. Cultures for chlamydial organisms are positive.
    b. The nucleic acid amplification test (NAAT) is positive.
    c. Gram stain smears and cultures are negative for gonorrhea.
    d. Signs and symptoms of epididymitis or proctitis are also present.

13. What are characteristics of HSV infection? **Select all that apply.**
    a. Treatment with acyclovir can cure genital herpes.
    b. Herpes simplex virus type 2 (HSV-2) is capable of causing only genital lesions.
    c. Recurrent symptomatic genital herpes may be precipitated by sexual activity and stress.
    d. To prevent transmission of genital herpes, condoms should be used when lesions are present.
    e. The primary symptom of genital herpes is painful vesicular lesions that rupture and ulcerate.

14. What would the nurse expect during the physical assessment of a female patient with human papilloma virus (HPV) infection?
    a. Purulent vaginal discharge
    b. Painful perineal vesicles and ulcerations
    c. A painless, indurated lesion on the vulva
    d. Multiple coalescing gray warts in the perineal area

15. What is most important for the nurse to teach the female patient with genital warts?
    a. Have an annual Papanicolaou (Pap) test.
    b. Apply topical acyclovir faithfully as directed.
    c. Have her sexual partner treated for the condition.
    d. Use a contraceptive to prevent pregnancy, which may worsen the disease.

16. During the birth of a woman's baby, which STI actively occurring at the time of delivery would indicate the need for a cesarean section?
    a. Syphilis
    b. Gonorrhea
    c. Chlamydia
    d. Genital herpes

17. Although an 18-year-old girl knows that abstinence is one way to prevent STIs, she does not consider that as an alternative. She asks the nurse at the clinic if there are other measures for preventing STIs. What would the nurse teach her?
    a. Abstinence is the only way to prevent STIs.
    b. Voiding immediately after intercourse will decrease the risk for infection.
    c. A vaccine can prevent genital warts and cervical cancer caused by some strains of HPV.
    d. Thorough hand washing after contact with genitals can prevent oral-genital spread of STIs.

18. Which STI are patients most likely to avoid obtaining and following treatment measures for their infection?
    a. Syphilis
    b. Gonorrhea
    c. HPV infection
    d. Genital herpes

CASE STUDY Gonorrhea

(Thinkstock)

Patient Profile
C.J., a 26-year-old male graduate student, had intercourse with an unfamiliar partner while he was on vacation. He returns home 3 days later and has intercourse with his fiancée, Ms. A. The next day he begins to have symptoms of an STI.

Subjective Data
- Reports pain and burning on urination
- Reports yellowish-white discharge from his penis
- Expresses concern over the possibility of having an STI and what this diagnosis would mean in his relationship with his fiancée

Objective Data
- Positive Gram stain for *N. gonorrhoeae*

Questions
1. What symptoms will Ms. A. have if she has an uncomplicated gonorrhea infection? **Use an X to indicate if the assessment finding is Indicated (a symptom of infection) or Unrelated (symptom is not related to infection).**

Assessment Finding	Indicated	Unrelated
Breast tenderness		
Vaginal discharge		
Fever		
Shortness of breath		
Bleeding after intercourse		
Dysmenorrhea		
Urinary frequency		

2. What physical examinations and laboratory procedures are required to establish a diagnosis of gonorrhea in C.J. and Ms. A.? **Use an X to indicate if the examination or procedure is Indicated (is necessary) for C.J. only, Ms. A. only, both C.J. and Ms. A. or is Unrelated (is unnecessary or makes no difference) to both C.J. and Ms. A.**

Examination or Procedure	Indicated for C.J.	Indicated for Ms. A.	Indicated for both C.J. & Ms. A.	Unrelated to both C.J. & Ms. A.
History of symptoms				
Endocervical swab				
Urethral swab				
Oropharyngeal swab				
Gram-stain				
Treponemal serologic test				
PCR testing				
NAAT				
HIV testing				

3. What would the nurse include when teaching C.J. about the diagnosis? **Select all that apply.**
    _____A. Your fiancé doesn't need to be told about your diagnosis.
    _____B. Your fiancé may be asymptomatic.
    _____C. The Public Health Department will be notified.
    _____D. Once you have had gonorrhea, you won't get it again.
    _____E. Your fiancé may experience infertility if she is not treated.
    _____F. You should abstain from sexual contact for at least 7 days.
    _____G. You should have repeat testing done in 1 month.
    _____H. You cannot transmit gonorrhea through oral sex.

4. What clinical manifestations could C.J. and Ms. A. have if they experience complications of gonorrhea? **Indicate which assessment finding listed in the far-left column is appropriate for the potential complication. Note that each assessment finding should only apply to one complication.**

Assessment Finding	Potential Complication	Appropriate Assessment Finding for Complication
Increased abdominal pain with walking	Epididymitis	
Pain with urination	Pelvic Inflammatory Disease	
Chills	Disseminated Gonococcal Infection	
Swelling of external genitalia		
Joint pain		
Scrotal pain		
Chest pain		
Skin lesions		

5. **Choose the most likely options for the information missing from the statements below by selecting from the options provided. Note that some options may not be used, but options that are used are used only once.**

Treatment for gonorrhea will be high-dose_____. Penicillin G benzathine is the antibiotic of choice to treat_____, but if penicillin is contraindicated then _____ will be used. Genital herpes would be treated with _____ or _____. Alternative treatment for chlamydia is _____.

Options:	
Doxycycline	Genital warts
Acyclovir	Human papillomavirus
Azithromycin	Syphilis
Ceftriaxone	Trichomoniasis
Metronidazole	Pubic lice (crabs)
Valacyclovir	

Female Reproductive Problems

1. A couple seeks assistance from an infertility specialist for evaluation of infertility. What does the nurse inform the couple they can expect during the initial visit?
   a. Physical and psychosocial functioning assessments
   b. Assessment of tubal patency with a hysterosalpingogram
   c. Pelvic ultrasound for the woman and semen analysis for the man
   d. Postcoital testing to evaluate sperm numbers and motility in cervical and vaginal secretions

2. A couple has not conceived using at-home basal body temperature and ovulation testing. What therapy would most likely be used next to treat this couple's infertility?
   a. Surgery to reduce endometriosis
   b. Intrauterine insemination with sperm from the husband
   c. Selective estrogen receptor modulator (clomiphene citrate [Clomid])
   d. Assisted reproductive technologies (e.g., in vitro fertilization [IVF])

3. A patient with a 10-week pregnancy is admitted to the emergency department (ED) with vaginal bleeding and abdominal cramping. What does the nurse recognize about this situation?
   a. The patient will require a blood transfusion.
   b. The patient is most likely having a spontaneous abortion.
   c. The patient must undergo an immediate dilation and curettage (D&C).
   d. Placing the patient on bed rest is usually successful in preventing further bleeding.

4. A woman has an unwanted pregnancy and is seeking an abortion. What would the nurse teach her about the effects of an abortion?
   a. D&C will be done in the hospital.
   b. She will feel much better afterward.
   c. The products of conception will pass immediately.
   d. She will need someone to support her through her loss.

5. Which is true about premenstrual syndrome (PMS)?
   a. Symptoms can be controlled with the use of progesterone.
   b. The woman has symptoms only when oral contraceptives are used.
   c. Symptoms can be correlated with altered serum levels of estrogen and progesterone.
   d. The woman has consistent syndrome complex with symptoms ending after menses begins.

6. What would the nurse teach a patient with premenstrual dysphoric disorder (PMDD) about managing the disorder?
   a. Limit diet intake of caffeine and refined sugar
   b. Use estrogen supplements during the luteal phase
   c. Supplement the diet with vitamin B_6, calcium, and magnesium
   d. Limit exercise and physical activity when symptoms are present

7. What is the rationale for the regular use of nonsteroidal antiinflammatory drugs (NSAIDs) during the first several days of the menstrual period for women who have primary dysmenorrhea?
   a. They suppress ovulation and the production of prostaglandins that occur with ovulation.
   b. They cause uterine relaxation and small vessel constriction, preventing cramping and abdominal congestion.
   c. They inhibit the production of prostaglandins believed to be responsible for menstrual pain and associated symptoms.
   d. They block the release of luteinizing hormone, preventing the increase in progesterone associated with maturation of the corpus luteum.

8. A 20-year-old woman is a college softball player who participates in strenuous practices and a heavy class schedule. She is describing an absence of menses. What could be contributing to her amenorrhea?
   a. Decreased sexual activity
   b. Excess prostaglandin production
   c. Strenuous exercise or elevated stress
   d. Endometrial cancer or uterine fibroids

9. A young woman who runs vigorously as a form of exercise has not had a menstrual period in more than 6 months. What would the nurse teach her?
   a. Normal periods will return when she stops running.
   b. Uterine balloon therapy may be necessary to promote uterine sloughing of the overgrown endometrium.
   c. Progesterone or combined oral contraceptives should be used to prevent persistent overgrowth of the endometrium.
   d. Unopposed progesterone production causes an overgrowth of the endometrium that increases her risk for endometrial cancer.

10. A 29-year-old woman is at the clinic with heavy menstrual bleeding. What assessment finding would the nurse anticipate?
    a. Pain with each menstrual period
    b. Excessive bleeding at irregular intervals
    c. Bleeding between regular menstrual cycles
    d. Increased duration or amount of menstrual bleeding

11. A patient with abdominal pain and irregular vaginal bleeding is admitted to the hospital with a suspected ectopic pregnancy. Before actual diagnosis, what is the most appropriate action by the nurse?
    a. Provide analgesics for pain relief.
    b. Monitor vital signs, pain, and bleeding frequently.
    c. Offer support for the patient's emotional response to the loss of the pregnancy.
    d. Explain the need to obtain a blood sample for β-human chorionic gonadotropin monitoring.

12. Which manifestations of menopause are related to estrogen deficiency? **Select all that apply.**
    a. Cessation of menses
    b. Breast engorgement
    c. Vasomotor instability
    d. Reduction of bone fractures
    e. Decreased cardiovascular risk

13. A 51-year-old woman is having symptoms of menopause. She has her uterus and is interested in starting hormone replacement therapy (HRT). What would the nurse include when discussing the risks and benefits of HRT?
    a. Taking only progesterone is suggested for a woman with a uterus.
    b. Taking both estrogen and progesterone may decrease her bone loss.
    c. The risk of breast cancer and cardiovascular disease is decreased with HRT.
    d. Taking estrogen and progesterone will increase the risk of endometrial cancer.

14. The patient at the urgent care facility reports that her vaginal discharge has a fishy smell. What would the nurse suspect as the cause?
    a. Cervicitis
    b. Trichomoniasis
    c. Bacterial vaginosis
    d. Vulvovaginal candidiasis

15. The patient calls the office and says that she thinks she has a "yeast infection." What signs and symptoms would the nurse expect? **Select all that apply.**
    a. Intense itching and dysuria
    b. Hemorrhagic cervix and vagina
    c. Pruritic, frothy greenish or gray discharge
    d. Thick, white, cottage cheese–like discharge
    e. Mucopurulent discharge and postcoital spotting

16. A patient is diagnosed and treated for a *Gardnerella vaginalis* infection at a clinic. For her treatment to be effective, what would the nurse tell the patient?
    a. Her sexual partner should be examined and treated.
    b. Her sexual partner must use a condom during intercourse.
    c. She can wear pads to prevent reinfection as long as she has vaginal drainage.
    d. A vaginal suppository should be used in the morning so that it will fight the infection all day.

17. A young woman is admitted to the hospital with acute pelvic inflammatory disease (PID). Which risk factor in the health history would the nurse consider as most significant?
    a. Lack of any method of birth control
    b. Sexual activity with multiple partners
    c. Use of a vaginal sponge for contraception
    d. Recent antibiotic-induced monilial vaginitis

18. What would the nurse include when teaching the patient with acute PID about self-care?
    a. Rest in a semi-Fowler's position.
    b. Perform vaginal irrigations every 4 hours.
    c. Use tampons to contain the vaginal drainage.
    d. Ambulate frequently to promote drainage of exudate.

19. A 20-year-old patient with PID is crying and tells the nurse that she is afraid she will not be able to have children as a result of the infection. What is the nurse's best response to this patient?
    a. "I would not worry about that now. Our immediate concern is to cure the infection you have."
    b. "PID increases the possibility of infertility. Would you like to talk about what it means to you?"
    c. "Sterility following PID is possible but not common, and it is too soon to know what the effects will be."
    d. "The infection can cause more serious complications, such as abscesses and shock, which you should be more concerned about."

20. The patient is suspected of having endometriosis and/or uterine leiomyoma. What best describes what is found with these conditions?
    a. Endometriosis and uterine leiomyoma increase in incidence with the onset of menopause.
    b. Lupron (GnRH analog) is used to treat endometriosis and leiomyomas to create a pseudopregnancy.
    c. Treatment of endometriosis and leiomyomas depends on the severity of symptoms and the woman's desire to maintain her fertility.
    d. The presence of ectopic uterine tissue that bleeds and causes pelvic and abdominal adhesions, cysts, and pain is known as *uterine leiomyoma*.

21. An 18-year-old patient with irregular menstrual periods, hirsutism, and obesity has been diagnosed with polycystic ovary syndrome (PCOS). What is an accurate rationale for the expected treatment?
    a. Hirsutism may be treated with leuprolide to decrease an altered body image.
    b. The medication used will cure the hormonal abnormality of excess testosterone.
    c. Untreated PCOS leads to cardiovascular disease and abnormal insulin resistance.
    d. Since weight loss will improve all the symptoms, this will be the first treatment tried.

22. A patient with a stage 0 cervical cancer identified from a Papanicolaou (Pap) test asks the nurse what this finding means. What information would the nurse include?
    a. Atypical cells characteristic of inflammation are present.
    b. Cancer cells have extended beyond the cervix to the upper vagina.
    c. Cancer cells are present and are confined to the epithelial layer of the cervix.
    d. This is a common finding on Pap testing, and she will be examined often to see if the abnormal cells spread beyond the cervix.

23. Fertility and normal reproductive function can be maintained when a cancer of the cervix is successfully treated with which therapy?
    a. External radiation therapy
    b. Internal radiation implants
    c. Conization or laser surgery
    d. Cryotherapy or subtotal hysterectomy

24. A woman who has been postmenopausal for 10 years calls the clinic because of vaginal bleeding. The nurse schedules a visit for the patient and informs her to expect to have which diagnostic procedure?
    a. An endometrial biopsy
    b. Abdominal radiography
    c. A laser treatment to the cervix
    d. Only a routine pelvic examination and Pap test

25. A patient has been diagnosed with ovarian cancer. When planning patient care, the nurse recognizes that which factor influences treatment?
    a. Results of a direct-needle biopsy of the ovary
    b. Results of a laparotomy with multiple biopsies
    c. Whether the patient desires to maintain fertility
    d. The findings of metastasis by ultrasound or CT scan

26. Which cancer is associated with intrauterine exposure to diethylstilbestrol (DES) or metastasis from another gynecological cancer?
    a. Vaginal
    b. Ovarian
    c. Cervical
    d. Endometrial

27. Which risk factors are associated with endometrial cancer? **Select all that apply.**
    a. Obesity
    b. Smoking
    c. Family history
    d. Early sexual activity
    e. Early menarche and late menopause
    f. Unopposed estrogen-only replacement therapy

28. What would the nurse expect during assessment of the patient with vulvar cancer?
    a. Soreness and itching of the vulva
    b. Labial lesions with purulent exudate
    c. Severe excoriation of the labia and perineum
    d. Painless, firm nodules embedded in the labia

29. A 44-year-old woman undergoing a total abdominal hysterectomy asks if she will need to take estrogen until she reaches the age of menopause. What is the nurse's best response?
    a. "Yes, it will help prevent the more intense symptoms caused by surgically induced menopause."
    b. "You are close enough to normal menopause that you probably won't need additional estrogen."
    c. "Because your ovaries won't be removed, they will continue to secrete estrogen until your normal menopause."
    d. "There are so many risks associated with estrogen replacement therapy that it is best to begin menopause now."

30. Any patient undergoing gynecological surgery may need assistance in coping with changes in body image. This will be most likely to occur after which surgery?
    a. Vaginectomy
    b. Hemivulvectomy
    c. Pelvic exenteration
    d. Radical hysterectomy

31. What occurs during treatment of the patient with an intrauterine radioactive implant?
    a. All care should be provided by the same nurse.
    b. The patient may ambulate in the room as desired.
    c. There can be unlimited number and duration of visitors.
    d. The patient is restricted to bed rest with turning from side to side.

32. When teaching a patient with pelvic support problems, how would the nurse tell the patient to perform Kegel exercises?
    a. Contract the muscles used to stop rectal gas expulsion.
    b. Tighten the lower abdominal muscles over the bladder area.
    c. Squeeze all of the perineal muscles as if trying to close the vagina.
    d. Lie on the floor and do leg lifts to strengthen the abdominal muscles.

33. The patient is describing a feeling of something coming down her vagina and having a backache. What is most likely the cause of this discomfort?
    a. Cystocele
    b. Dysmenorrhea
    c. Uterine prolapse
    d. Abdominal distension

34. The patient with a large rectocele is undergoing surgery. What nursing intervention would be a priority postoperatively?
    a. An ice pack to relieve swelling
    b. An enema each day to relieve constipation
    c. Administration of a stool softener each night
    d. Perineal care after each urination or defecation

35. What is an appropriate outcome for a patient who undergoes an anterior colporrhaphy?
    a. Maintain normal bowel patterns
    b. Adjust to temporary ileal conduit
    c. Urinate within 8 hours postoperatively
    d. Have healing of excoriated vaginal and vulvar tissue

36. When admitting a victim of sexual assault to the ED, what would be the nurse's first priority?
    a. Contact a rape support person for the patient.
    b. Assess the patient for urgent medical problems.
    c. Question the patient about the details of the assault.
    d. Tell the patient what procedures and treatments will be performed.

37. To prepare a woman who has been raped for physical examination, what would the nurse do first?
    a. Ensure that a signed informed consent is obtained from the patient.
    b. Provide a private place for the patient to talk about what happened to her.
    c. Instruct the patient not to wash, eat, drink, or urinate before the examination.
    d. Administer prophylaxis for sexually transmitted infections (STIs) and tetanus.

CASE STUDY   Acute Pelvic Inflammatory Disease

Patient Profile
A.R. is a 27-year-old single woman. For the past several weeks, she has had a heavy purulent vaginal discharge, lower abdominal pain, and general malaise. Concerned that her symptoms appear to be worsening, A.R. makes an appointment at the gynecologic clinic.

(Szepy/iStock/
Thinkstock)

Subjective Data
- Has an increase in lower abdominal pain during vaginal examination
- Expresses concern over worsening of her condition and the effect this will have on future childbearing ability

Objective Data
- Vital signs: Temp 101°F (38.3°C), HR 90 beats/min, RR 18 breaths/min, BP 110/58 mm Hg
- Physical assessment: heavy, purulent vaginal discharge

Questions
1. Which assessment finding would the nurse identify as a clinical manifestation of each of these female problems? **Use an X to indicate if the assessment finding is applicable to <u>Gynecological Cancer</u>, <u>Vaginitis</u>, or <u>Pelvic Inflammatory Disease (PID)</u>. Note that some assessment findings may apply to more than one category.**

Assessment Finding	Gynecological Cancer	Vaginitis	PID
Temperature 101°F (38.3°C)			
Purulent vaginal discharge			
General malaise			
Abdominal pain			
Increased pain during vaginal exam			
Young age			

2. Based on the assessment findings, what diagnostic tests should be performed to diagnose A.R.'s condition? **Use an X to indicate if the diagnostic test is <u>Indicated</u> (is appropriate or necessary) or is <u>Non-essential</u> (is unnecessary or makes no difference).**

Diagnostic Test	Indicated	Non-Essential
Pap test		
Chest x-ray		
Genetic testing		
HIV testing		
Pregnancy test		
Abdominal CT scan		
STI testing		

3. A.R. is diagnosed as having Pelvic Inflammatory Disease (PID) due to a co-infection. Cytology results from the pelvic exam also indicate she has human papillomavirus (HPV). What would the nurse tell A.R. about HPV? **Select all that apply.**

_____A. HPV is a sexually transmitted infection.

_____B. It is the leading cause of ovarian cancer.

_____C. HPV infection can increase your risk for vulvar cancer.

_____D. HPV infection is usually asymptomatic.

_____E. HPV is the most common STI in the U.S.

_____F. HPV will need to be treated with antibiotics.

_____G. HPV cannot be transmitted through oral sex.

_____H. You will need to get annual Pap tests.

4. A.R. is admitted to the hospital for treatment. What nursing interventions would the nurse include in this patient's plan of care? **Use an X to indicate if the nursing action is Indicated (is appropriate or necessary), Contraindicated (could cause harm), or is Non-essential (is unnecessary or makes no difference).**

Nursing Action	Indicated	Contraindicated	Non-Essential
Administer high-dose Cephalosporin			
Administer doxycycline			
Place A.R. on a fluid restriction			
Administer high-dose Ceftriaxone			
Place A.R. on contact precautions			
Monitor and document vaginal discharge			
Ask her about how to contact recent sexual partners			
Palpate abdomen to assess for deep pain			

5. What discharge instructions would the nurse provide A.R.? **Select all that apply.**

_____A. You should get a vaccine to protect you from future HPV strains.

_____B. Take the antibiotics until the pain and discharge stop.

_____C. Avoid sexual intercourse until the antibiotics are gone.

_____D. You should have your male partners wear a condom during sex.

_____E. Birth control pills will help prevent STIs.

_____F. PID can cause infertility.

_____G. Tell your HCP if your abdominal pain persists longer than 2 weeks.

_____H. Avoid douching.

Male Reproductive Problems

1. A patient asks the nurse what the difference is between benign prostatic hyperplasia (BPH) and prostate cancer. The best response by the nurse includes what information about BPH?
   a. BPH is a benign tumor that does not spread beyond the prostate gland.
   b. BPH is a precursor to prostate cancer but does not yet show any malignant changes.
   c. BPH is an enlargement of the gland caused by an increase in the size of existing cells.
   d. BPH is a benign enlargement of the gland caused by an increase in the number of normal cells.

2. When taking a history from a patient with BPH, what would the nurse expect the patient to report?
   a. Nocturia, dysuria, and bladder spasms
   b. Urinary frequency, hematuria, and perineal pain
   c. Urinary hesitancy, postvoid dribbling, and weak urinary stream
   d. Urinary urgency with a forceful urinary stream and cloudy urine

3. Which diagnostic study can determine the extent of urinary obstruction caused by BPH?
   a. Uroflowmetry
   b. A cystometrogram
   c. Transrectal ultrasound
   d. Postvoiding catheterization

4. What is the effect of finasteride (Proscar) in the treatment of BPH?
   a. A reduction in the size of the prostate gland
   b. Relaxation of the smooth muscle of the urethra
   c. Increased bladder tone that promotes bladder emptying
   d. Relaxation of the bladder detrusor muscle promoting urine flow

5. On admission to the ambulatory surgical center, a patient with BPH tells the nurse that he is going to have a laser treatment of his enlarged prostate. What would the nurse include when teaching the patient about this treatment?
   a. The effects of general anesthesia
   b. The possibility of short-term incontinence
   c. Home management of an indwelling catheter
   d. Monitoring for postoperative urinary retention

6. What is the most common screening intervention for detecting BPH in men over age 50 years?
   a. Prostate-specific antigen (PSA) level
   b. Urinalysis
   c. Cystoscopy
   d. Digital rectal examination

7. Which treatment for BPH uses a low-wave radiofrequency to precisely destroy prostate tissue?
   a. Laser prostatectomy
   b. Transurethral needle ablation (TUNA)
   c. Transurethral microwave thermotherapy (TUMT)
   d. Transurethral vaporization of prostate (TUVP)

8. Which characteristics describe transurethral resection of the prostate (TURP)? **Select all that apply.**
   a. Best used for a very large prostate gland
   b. Inappropriate for men with rectal problems
   c. Involves an external incision prostatectomy
   d. Uses transurethral incision into the prostate
   e. Most common surgical procedure to treat BPH
   f. Resectoscopic excision and cauterization of prostate tissue

9. Which therapies for BPH are done on an outpatient basis? **Select all that apply.**
   a. Intraprostatic urethral stents
   b. TUNA
   c. Photoselective vaporization of the prostate (PVP)
   d. Transurethral incision of prostate (TUIP)
   e. TUMT

10. Before undergoing a TURP, what would the nurse teach the patient?
    a. This surgery requires an external incision.
    b. The procedure is done under local anesthesia.
    c. Recurrent urinary tract infections are likely to occur.
    d. An indwelling catheter will be used to maintain urinary output until healing is complete.

11. Following a TURP, a patient has continuous bladder irrigation. Four hours after surgery, the catheter is draining thick, bright red clots and tissue. What would the nurse do?
    a. Release the traction on the catheter.
    b. Clamp the drainage tube and notify the patient's health care provider (HCP).
    c. Manually irrigate the catheter until the drainage is clear.
    d. Increase the rate of the irrigation and take the patient's vital signs.

12. A patient with continuous bladder irrigation after a prostatectomy tells the nurse that he has bladder spasms and leaking of urine around the catheter. What would the nurse do first?
    a. Slow the rate of the irrigation.
    b. Assess the patency of the catheter.
    c. Encourage the patient to try to urinate around the catheter.
    d. Administer a belladonna and opium (B&O) suppository as prescribed.

13. The nurse provides discharge teaching to a patient after a TURP. Which statement indicates that the patient understands the instructions?
    a. "I should use daily enemas to avoid straining until healing is complete."
    b. "I will avoid heavy lifting, climbing, and driving until my follow-up visit."
    c. "At least I don't have to worry about developing cancer of the prostate now."
    d. "Every day I should drink 10 to 12 glasses of liquids, such as coffee, tea, or soft drinks."

14. A 55-year-old man with a history of prostate cancer in his family asks the nurse what he can do to decrease his risk of prostate cancer. What would the nurse teach him about risks of prostate cancer?
    a. Nothing can decrease the risk because prostate cancer is primarily a disease of aging.
    b. Treatment of any enlargement of the prostate gland will help prevent prostate cancer.
    c. Substituting fresh fruits and vegetables for high-fat foods in the diet may lower the risk of prostate cancer.
    d. Using a natural herb, such as saw palmetto, has been found to be an effective protection against prostate cancer.

15. When caring for a patient after a radical prostatectomy with a perineal approach, what is the priority nursing intervention to prevent complications?
    a. Use chemotherapy to prevent metastasis.
    b. Administer sildenafil (Viagra) as needed for erectile dysfunction (ED).
    c. Provide wound care after each bowel movement to prevent infection.
    d. Insert a smaller indwelling urinary catheter to prevent urinary retention.

16. What accurately describes prostate cancer detection and/or treatment? **Select all that apply.**
    a. The symptoms of lumbosacral pain and lower urinary tract symptoms may be present.
    b. Orchiectomy is a treatment option for all patients with prostatic cancer except those with stage IV tumors.
    c. Palpation of the prostate reveals hard and asymmetric enlargement with areas of induration or nodules.
    d. The preferred hormonal therapy for treatment of prostate cancer includes estrogen and androgen receptor blockers.
    e. Early detection of prostate cancer is increased with annual rectal examinations and serum prostatic acid phosphatase (PAP) measurements.
    f. An annual prostate examination is recommended starting at age 45 years for black men with a first-degree relative with prostate cancer at an early age.

17. What differentiates chronic bacterial prostatitis from acute prostatitis?
    a. Postejaculatory pain
    b. Frequency, urgency, and dysuria
    c. Symptoms of a urinary tract infection (UTI)
    d. Most common reason for recurrent UTIs in adult men

18. What describes hypospadias?
    a. Scrotal lymphedema
    b. Undescended testicle
    c. Ventral urinary mcatus
    d. Inflammation of the prepuce

19. What explanation would the nurse give to the wife of the patient who asks what her husband's diagnosis of paraphimosis means?
    a. Painful, prolonged erection
    b. Inflammation of the epididymis
    c. Painful downward curvature of an erect penis
    d. Retracted tight foreskin preventing return over the glans

20. With which problem of the scrotum and testes is the cremasteric reflex absent?
    a. Hydrocele
    b. Varicocele
    c. Spermatocele
    d. Testicular torsion

21. What serum tumor markers may be elevated in testicular cancer and used to monitor the response to therapy?
    a. Tumor necrosis factor (TNF) and C-reactive protein (CRP)
    b. α-fetoprotein (AFP) and human chorionic gonadotropin (hCG)
    c. PSA and PAP
    d. Carcinoembryonic antigen (CEA), antinuclear antibody (ANA) and human epidermal growth factor receptor 2 (HER-2)

22. After having a vasectomy, what would the nurse teach the patient?
    a. The amount of ejaculate will be noticeably decreased.
    b. He may have difficulty maintaining an erection for several months.
    c. The testes will gradually decrease production of sperm and testosterone.
    d. An alternative form of contraception must be used until semen examination shows no sperm.

23. A patient is seeking medical intervention for erectile dysfunction (ED). Why should he be thoroughly evaluated?
    a. It is important to determine if ED is reversible before treatment is started.
    b. Psychologic counseling can reverse the problem in 80% to 90% of the cases.
    c. Most treatments for ED are contraindicated in patients with systemic diseases.
    d. New invasive and experimental techniques currently used have unknown risks.

24. A 66-year-old male patient is experiencing ED. He and his partner have used tadalafil (Cialis), but because he had priapism, they decided to change treatment to an intraurethral device. How would the nurse explain how this device works?
    a. The device relaxes smooth muscle in the penis.
    b. Blood is drawn into corporeal bodies and held with a ring.
    c. The device is implanted into corporeal bodies to firm the penis.
    d. The device directly applies drugs that increase blood flow in the penis.

25. A 47-year-old patient who has hypogonadism has decided to try the testosterone gel, Testim. What would the nurse teach the patient and his partner about this gel?
    a. Wash the hands with soap and water after applying it.
    b. His partner should apply it to help him feel better about using it.
    c. Do not wear clothing over the area until it has been absorbed.
    d. The gel may be taken buccally if it is not effective on the abdomen.

26. A couple has not been able to become pregnant. When considering the most common cause of male infertility, which intervention will the nurse to teach the couple about?
    a. Antibiotics
    b. Semen analysis
    c. Avoidance of scrotal heat
    d. Surgery to correct the problem

CASE STUDY   Testicular Cancer

Patient Profile
C.E., a 19-year-old, noticed scrotal swelling and discovered a firm lump on his left testicle while in the shower last evening. After a medical examination, he was admitted to the hospital for a left orchiectomy and lymph node dissection.

(Siri Stafford/
DigitalVision/
Thinkstock)

Subjective Data
- Has a history of an undescended left testicle, which was surgically corrected at age 2 years
- Expresses concern about surgery and how it will affect him
- Asks about his prognosis and chances for recovery after the surgery
- Denies back pain

Objective Data
- Firm, nontender nodule on left testicle
- Local lymph node enlargement
- Appears anxious with assessment and diagnostic studies
- Chest x-ray is clear
- Biopsy revealed seminoma germ cell tumor

Questions
1. What would the nurse tell C.E. about the development and risk factors regarding testicular cancer? **Select all that apply.**
    _____A. It is a common type of cancer in men, especially between 15–34 years of age.
    _____B. Testicular cancer is more common in males with a family history.
    _____C. This type of cancer is common in males who have had cryptorchidism.
    _____D. Orchitis is not a predisposing factor.
    _____E. Maternal exposure to exogenous estrogen is a predisposing factor.
    _____F. All forms of testicular cancers are aggressive.
    _____G. Acute pain is usually the first symptom in the majority of patients.
    _____H. Most testicular cancers arise from embryonic germ cells.

2. What diagnostic studies would the nurse tell C.E. may be performed? **Use an X to indicate whether the diagnostic test is Indicated or Unrelated.**

Diagnostic Test	Indicated	Unrelated
Palpating scrotal contents		
PSA level		
α-fetoprotein (AFP) marker		

Diagnostic Test	Indicated	Unrelated
LDL level		
hCG level		
CT scans of the abdomen and pelvis		
Liver function tests		

3. What statements made by C.E. indicate to the nurse that he understands the treatments and is coping with this diagnosis? **Use an X to indicate if the teaching is <u>Effective</u> (meets expected outcomes), <u>Ineffective</u> (does not meet expected outcomes), or <u>Unrelated</u> (is not related to the expected outcomes).**

Patient Statement	Effective	Ineffective	Unrelated
"I know this type of cancer has a poor survival rate."			
"I will need to store semen before treatments begin."			
"An orchiectomy will not be necessary."			
"This type of tumor is sensitive to radiation therapy."			
"Ejaculatory dysfunction may occur from the lymph node dissection."			
"The therapies will cause gynecomastia."			
"I may have lung damage from chemotherapy treatment."			

4. C.E. undergoes chemotherapy using bleomycin prior to having an orchiectomy to shrink the tumor. What nursing actions are appropriate after surgery? **Use an X to indicate if the nursing action is <u>Indicated</u> (is appropriate or necessary), <u>Contraindicated</u> (could be harmful) or <u>Non-essential</u> (makes no difference or is unnecessary).**

Nursing Action	Indicated	Contraindicated	Non-Essential
Apply 2 L/min via nasal cannula for SpO$_2$ < 94%			
Apply SCDs while on bedrest			
Wait 2 days before ambulating			
Obtain coagulation studies			
Have the patient wear a jock strap			
Apply ice to the scrotum			
Obtain a 12-lead ECG postoperatively			

5. What instructions would the nurse provide C.E. upon discharge home after surgery? **Select all that apply.**
_____A. Avoid bicycle riding until approved by your HCP.
_____B. Report any shortness of breath to your HCP.
_____C. Wear scrotal support for the first 48 hours.
_____D. After 72 hours, apply heat to the incision.
_____E. You can soak in a bathtub after 48 hours.
_____F. Avoid driving if taking Tylenol or ibuprofen for pain.
_____G. Take ibuprofen with food.
_____H. Report malodorous drainage to your HCP.

Assessment: Nervous System

1. Using the following list of terms, identify the structures of the neuron in the illustration below.

Terms

Axon	Neuron cell body	Synaptic knobs
Myelin sheath	Schwann cell	Mitochondrion
Nucleus	Dendrites	Nucleolus
Collateral axon	Node of Ranvier	Telodendria (presynaptic terminal)

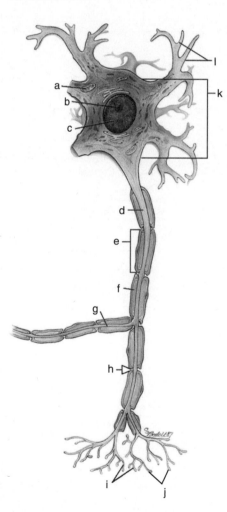

a. _____

b. _____

c. _____

d. _____

e. _____

f. _____

g. _____

h. _____

i. _____

j. _____

k. _____

l. _____

2. Using the following list of terms, identify the structures in the illustration below.

Terms

Medulla   Occipital lobe   Broca's motor speech
Cerebellum   Temporal lobe   Superior temporal gyrus
Frontal lobe   Precentral gyrus   Wernicke's receptive speech
Parietal lobe   Postcentral gyrus

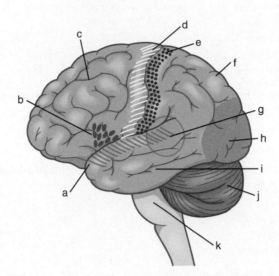

a. _____   g. _____

b. _____   h. _____

c. _____   i. _____

d. _____   j. _____

e. _____   k. _____

f. _____

3. Which structure protects the central nervous system (CNS)?
   a. Synaptic cleft
   b. Limbic system
   c. Myelin sheath
   d. Cerebrospinal fluid (CSF)

4. Which type of macroglial cells myelinate peripheral nerve fibers?
   a. Neurons
   b. Astrocytes
   c. Schwann cells
   d. Ependymal cells

5. What happens at the synapse?
   a. The synapse physically joins 2 neurons.
   b. The nerve impulse is transmitted only from 1 neuron to another neuron.
   c. The presynaptic terminal submits a nerve impulse through the synaptic cleft to the receptor site on the postsynaptic cell.
   d. When a presynaptic cell releases excitatory neurotransmitters, the postsynaptic cell depolarizes enough to generate an action potential.

6. What is the purpose of the dendrite?
   a. Provides gap in peripheral nerve axons
   b. Carries impulses to the nerve cell body
   c. Carries impulses from the nerve cell body
   d. Helps repair damage to peripheral axons

7. A patient has a lesion involving the fasciculus gracilis and fasciculus cuneatus of the spinal cord. The nurse would expect the patient to experience what loss?
   a. Pain and temperature sensations
   b. Touch, deep pressure, vibration, and position sense
   c. Subconscious information about body position and muscle tension
   d. Voluntary muscle control from the cerebral cortex to the peripheral nerves

8. What is the effect when a lesion occurs in a lower motor neuron compared to in an upper motor neuron?
   a. Causes hyporeflexia and flaccidity
   b. Affects motor control of the lower body
   c. Arises in structures above the spinal cord
   d. Interferes with reflex arcs in the spinal cord

9. The patient is admitted to the emergency department having difficulty with respiratory, vasomotor, and cardiac function. A problem with which part of the brain may be causing these manifestations?
   a. Medulla
   b. Cerebellum
   c. Parietal lobe
   d. Wernicke's area

10. A 28-year-old female patient has been diagnosed with occipital lobe damage after a car accident. The nurse would expect the patient to need help with which task?
    a. Being able to feel heat
    b. Processing visual images
    c. Identifying smells appropriately
    d. Being able to say what she means

11. Which area of the brain regulates functions of the endocrine system and autonomic nervous system (ANS)?
    a. Basal ganglia
    b. Temporal lobe
    c. Hypothalamus
    d. Reticular activating system

12. What are the functions of the thalamus?
    a. Registers auditory input
    b. Integrates past experiences
    c. Relays sensory and motor input to and from the cerebrum
    d. Controls and facilitates learned and automatic movements

13. How do spinal nerves of the peripheral nervous system (PNS) differ from cranial nerves (CNs)?
    a. Only spinal nerves occur in pairs.
    b. CNs affect only the sensory and motor functions of the head and neck.
    c. Cell bodies of all CNs are located in the brain, whereas cell bodies of spinal nerves are located in the spinal cord.
    d. All spinal nerves contain both afferent sensory and efferent motor fibers, whereas CNs contain one or the other or both.

14. When the patient has a rapidly growing brain tumor, what part of the brain slows expansion of cerebral brain tissue into the adjacent hemisphere?
    a. Ventricles
    b. Falx cerebri
    c. Arachnoid layer
    d. Tentorium cerebella

15. After talking with the health care provider (HCP), the patient asks what the blood–brain barrier does. What description would the nurse give the patient?
    a. Protects the brain from external trauma
    b. Protects against harmful blood-borne agents
    c. Provides for flexibility while protecting the spinal cord
    d. Forms the outer layer of protective membranes around the brain and spinal cord

16. During neurologic assessment of the older adult, what would the nurse determine is an effect of aging on the neurologic system?
    a. Absent deep tendon reflexes
    b. Below-average intelligence score
    c. Decreased sensation of touch and temperature
    d. Decreased frequency of spontaneous awakening

17. What factors are priorities when taking the history of a patient with a neurologic problem? **Select all that apply.**
    a. Avoid suggesting symptoms.
    b. Include the CN assessment as the first assessment.
    c. Mental status must be accurately assessed to ensure that the reported history is factual.
    d. Do a focused assessment of the neurologic system, as other body systems will not be affected.
    e. The mode of onset and course of illness are especially important aspects of the nursing history.

18. Identify 1 specific finding from the nurse's assessment of each of the patient's functional health patterns that indicates a risk factor for neurologic problems or a patient response to an actual neurologic problem.

Functional Health Pattern	Risk Factor for or Patient Response to Neurologic Problem
Health perception–health management	
Nutritional-metabolic	
Elimination	
Activity-exercise	
Sleep-rest	
Cognitive-perceptual	
Self-perception–self-concept	
Role-relationship	
Sexuality-reproductive	
Coping–stress tolerance	
Value-belief	

19. Which CNs are involved with oblique eye movements? **Select all that apply.**
    a. Optic (CN II)
    b. Trochlear (CN IV)
    c. Trigeminal (CN V)
    d. Abducens (CN VI)
    e. Oculomotor (CN III)

20. Which CN responds to the corneal reflex test?
    a. Optic (CN II)
    b. Vagus (CN X)
    c. Trigeminal (CN V)
    d. Spinal accessory (CN XI)

21. What methods are used to assess the facial (CN VII) nerve? **Select all that apply.**
    a. Gag reflex
    b. Visual fields
    c. Corneal (blink) reflex test
    d. Light touch to the face
    e. Smile, frown, and close eyes
    f. Salt and sugar discrimination

22. Which CN is being tested with tongue protrusion?
    a. Vagus (CN X)
    b. Olfactory (CN I)
    c. Hypoglossal (CN XII)
    d. Glossopharyngeal (CN IX)

23. During the neurologic assessment, the patient is unable to hear a ticking watch. What neurologic problem would the nurse identify as the cause?
    a. The patient is distracted.
    b. The patient is hard of hearing.
    c. The vagus (CN X) nerve is malfunctioning.
    d. The cochlear branch of the acoustic (CN VIII) nerve is damaged.

24. During an assessment of the motor system, the nurse finds that the patient has a staggering gait and an abnormal arm swing. What would the nurse do with this information?
    a. Assist the patient to cope with the disability.
    b. Plan a rehabilitation program for the patient.
    c. Protect the patient from injury caused by falls.
    d. Help establish a diagnosis of cerebellar dysfunction.

25. The nurse would use the heel-to-shin test to assess for what abnormality?
    a. Hypertonia
    b. Lack of coordination
    c. Extension of the toes
    d. Loss of proprioception

26. What method is used to assess for extinction?
    a. Cotton wisp
    b. Sharp and dull end of a pin
    c. Tuning fork to bony prominences
    d. Simultaneously touching both sides of the body

27. When the patient stands with their feet close together and eyes closed and they sway or fall, what would the nurse document?
    a. Pronator drift
    b. Absent patellar reflex
    c. Positive Romberg test
    d. Absence of 2-point discrimination

28. What is the normal response to striking the triceps tendon with a reflex hammer?
    a. Forearm pronation
    b. Extension of the arm
    c. Flexion of the arm at the elbow
    d. Flexion and supination of the elbow

29. The patellar tendon is struck and the leg extends with contraction of the quadriceps. What grade, out of 5, would the nurse give this response?
    a. 1
    b. 2
    c. 3
    d. 4

30. What would the nurse do to prepare a patient for a lumbar puncture?
    a. Sedate the patient with medication before the test.
    b. Withhold beverages containing caffeine for 8 hours.
    c. Assess the patient for a stroke before the procedure for baseline data.
    d. Position the patient in a lateral recumbent position with the hips, knees, and neck flexed.

31. What would the nurse assess the patient for following a lumbar puncture?
    a. Headache
    b. Lower limb paralysis
    c. Allergic reactions to the dye
    d. Hemorrhage from the puncture site

32. The patient has just had a myelogram. What would the nurse include in the plan of care?
    a. Restrict fluids until the patient is ambulatory.
    b. Keep the patient positioned flat in bed for several hours.
    c. Position the patient with the head of the bed elevated 30 degrees.
    d. Provide mild analgesics for pain associated with the insertion of needles.

33. What neurologic diagnostic test has the highest risk of complications and requires the nurse to frequently monitoring of neurologic and vital signs following the procedure?
    a. Electromyelogram
    b. Cerebral angiography
    c. Electroencephalogram
    d. Transcranial Doppler sonography

34. When evaluating the results of a CSF analysis, what would the nurse identify as an abnormal finding?
    a. pH of 7.35
    b. Clear, colorless appearance
    c. Glucose level of 30 mg/dL (1.7 mmol/L)
    d. White blood cell (WBC) count of 5 cells/μL (5×10^6 cells/L)

Acute Intracranial Problems

1. Which components can change to adapt to small increases in intracranial pressure (ICP)? **Select all that apply.**
   a. Blood
   b. Skull bone
   c. Brain tissue
   d. Scalp tissue
   e. Cerebrospinal fluid (CSF)

2. The cerebral perfusion pressure (CPP) is the pressure needed to ensure blood flow to the brain. Normal CPP is 60 to 100 mm Hg. Calculate the CPP for a patient whose BP is 106/52 mm Hg and ICP is 14 mm Hg.

   _____ mm Hg

3. Calculate the CPP for a patient with an ICP of 34 mm Hg and a systemic BP of 108/64 mm Hg.

   _____ mm Hg

4. Which factors decrease cerebral blood flow? **Select all that apply.**
   a. Increased ICP
   b. Partial pressure of oxygen in arterial blood (PaO_2) of 45 mm Hg
   c. Partial pressure of carbon dioxide in arterial blood ($PaCO_2$) of 30 mm Hg
   d. Arterial blood pH of 7.3
   e. Decreased mean arterial pressure (MAP)

5. What are causes of vasogenic cerebral edema? **Select all that apply.**
   a. Hydrocephalus
   b. Ingested toxins
   c. Destructive lesions or trauma
   d. Local disruption of cell membranes
   e. Fluid flowing from intravascular to extravascular space

6. Which events cause an increase in ICP? **Select all that apply.**
   a. Vasodilation
   b. Necrotic cerebral tissue
   c. Blood vessel compression
   d. Edema from initial brain insult
   e. Brainstem compression and herniation

7. What is an early sign of increased ICP?
   a. Cushing's triad
   b. Unexpected vomiting
   c. Decreasing level of consciousness (LOC)
   d. Dilated pupil with sluggish response to light

8. Which vital sign changes indicate the presence of Cushing's triad?
   a. Increased pulse, irregular respiration, increased BP
   b. Decreased pulse, increased respiration, decreased systolic BP
   c. Decreased pulse, irregular respiration, widened pulse pressure
   d. Increased pulse, decreased respiration, widened pulse pressure

9. Increased ICP in the left cerebral cortex caused by intracranial bleeding causes displacement of brain tissue to the right hemisphere beneath the falx cerebri. The nurse knows that this is referred to as what?
   a. Uncal herniation
   b. Tentorial herniation
   c. Cingulate herniation
   d. Temporal lobe herniation

10. A patient has ICP monitoring with an intraventricular catheter. What nursing intervention is a priority?
    a. Aseptic technique to prevent infection
    b. Constant monitoring of ICP waveforms
    c. Removal of CSF to maintain normal ICP
    d. Sampling CSF to determine abnormalities

11. When using intraventricular ICP monitoring, what would cause inaccurate readings?
    a. The P2 wave is higher than the P1 wave.
    b. CSF is leaking around the monitoring device.
    c. The stopcock of the drainage device is open to drain the CSF fluid.
    d. The transducer of the ventriculostomy monitor is at the tragus of the ear.

12. The patient with increased ICP is being monitored with a brain tissue oxygenation catheter. What range for the pressure of oxygen in brain tissue ($PbtO_2$) will maintain cerebral oxygen supply and demand?
    a. 55% to 75%
    b. 20 to 40 mm Hg
    c. 70 to 150 mm Hg
    d. 80 to 100 mm Hg

13. Which drug helps decrease ICP by expanding plasma and has an osmotic effect to move fluid?
    a. Dexamethasone
    b. Oxygen administration
    c. Pentobarbital (Nembutal)
    d. Mannitol (Osmitrol) (25%)

14. How are the metabolic and nutrition needs of the patient with increased ICP best met?
    a. Enteral feedings that are low in sodium
    b. Simple glucose available in D_5W IV solutions
    c. Fluid restriction that promotes a moderate dehydration
    d. Balanced, essential nutrition in a form that the patient can tolerate

15. Why would the nurse use the Glasgow Coma Scale (GCS)?
    a. To quickly assess the LOC
    b. To assess the patient's ability to communicate
    c. To assess the patient's ability to respond to commands
    d. To assess the patient's coordination with motor responses

16. A patient with an intracranial problem does not open his eyes to any stimulus, has no verbal response except moaning and muttering when stimulated, and flexes his arm in response to painful stimuli. What would the nurse document as the patient's GCS score?
    a. 6
    b. 7
    c. 9
    d. 11

17. When assessing the body functions of a patient with increased ICP, what would the nurse assess first?
    a. Corneal reflex testing
    b. Pupillary reaction to light
    c. Extremity strength testing
    d. Circulatory and respiratory status

18. How would the nurse assess cranial nerve (CN) III for an early sign of pressure on the brainstem?
    a. Assess for nystagmus
    b. Test the corneal reflex
    c. Test pupillary reaction to light
    d. Check the oculocephalic (doll's eyes) reflex

19. What is an appropriate nursing intervention for a patient with cerebral edema and increased ICP?
    a. Avoid positioning the patient with neck and hip flexion.
    b. Maintain hyperventilation to a $PaCO_2$ of 15 to 20 mm Hg.
    c. Cluster nursing activities to provide periods of uninterrupted rest.
    d. Routinely suction to prevent accumulation of respiratory secretions.

20. An unconscious patient with increased ICP is on ventilatory support. Which arterial blood gas (ABG) measurement would the nurse report to the health care provider (HCP)?
    a. pH of 7.43
    b. Partial pressure of oxygen in arterial blood (SaO_2) of 94%
    c. PaO_2 of 70 mm Hg
    d. $PaCO_2$ of 35 mm Hg

21. What assessment findings would lead the nurse to suspect a patient with a head injury has developed increased ICP? **Select all that apply.**
    a. Fever
    b. Oriented to name only
    c. Narrowing pulse pressure
    d. Right pupil dilated greater than left pupil
    e. Decorticate posturing to painful stimulus

22. While the nurse performs range of motion (ROM) for an unconscious patient with increased ICP, the patient has severe decerebrate posturing reflexes. What would the nurse do first?
    a. Use restraints to protect the patient from injury while posturing.
    b. Perform the exercises less often because posturing indicates increased ICP.
    c. Administer CNS depressants to lightly sedate the patient.
    d. Continue the exercises because they are necessary to maintain musculoskeletal function.

23. What manifestations would the nurse expect in a patient diagnosed with a cerebral concussion?
    a. Deafness, loss of taste, and CSF otorrhea
    b. CSF otorrhea, vertigo, and Battle's sign with a dural tear
    c. Boggy temporal muscle because of extravasation of blood
    d. Headache, retrograde amnesia, and transient reduction in LOC

24. The patient comes to the emergency department (ED) with cortical blindness and visual field defects. Which type of head injury would the nurse suspect?
    a. Cerebral contusion
    b. Orbital skull fracture
    c. Posterior fossa fracture
    d. Frontal lobe skull fracture

25. The patient has a depressed skull fracture and scalp lacerations with communication to the intracranial cavity. Which type of injury would the nurse document?
    a. Linear skull fracture
    b. Depressed skull fracture
    c. Compound skull fracture
    d. Comminuted skull fracture

26. A patient with a head injury has bloody drainage from the ear. What would the nurse do to determine if CSF is present in the drainage?
    a. Examine the tympanic membrane for a tear.
    b. Test the fluid for a halo sign on a white dressing.
    c. Test the fluid with a glucose-identifying strip or stick.
    d. Collect 5 mL of fluid in a test tube and send it to the laboratory for analysis.

27. What clinical manifestation would cause the nurse to suspect an epidural hematoma ?
    a. Failure to regain consciousness following a head injury.
    b. A rapid deterioration of neurologic function within 24 to 48 hours following a head injury.
    c. Nonspecific, nonlocalizing progression of alteration in LOC occurring over weeks or months.
    d. Unconsciousness at the time of a head injury with a brief period of consciousness followed by a decrease in LOC.

28. Skull x-rays and a CT scan show a depressed parietal fracture with a subdural hematoma in a patient admitted to the ED following an automobile accident. What treatment would the nurse anticipate when planning care?
    a. The patient will receive life support measures until the condition stabilizes.
    b. Immediate burr holes will be made to rapidly decompress the intracranial cavity.
    c. The patient will be treated conservatively with close monitoring for changes in neurologic status.
    d. The patient will be taken to surgery for a craniotomy for evacuation of blood and decompression of the cranium.

29. A patient is admitted to the ED following a head injury. Using 1 for the top priority action and 6 for the last priority action, number the nurse's actions when providing care to the patient.
    a. _____ Confirm patent airway.
    b. _____ Anticipate cerebral surgery.
    c. _____ Maintain cervical spine precautions.
    d. _____ Monitor for changes in neurologic status.
    e. _____ Determine the presence of increased ICP.
    f. _____ Establish IV access with a large-bore catheter.

30. A 54-year-old man is recovering from a skull fracture with a subacute subdural hematoma that caused unconsciousness. He has return of motor control and orientation, but appears apathetic and has reduced awareness of his environment. When planning discharge, what would the nurse explain to the patient's family?
    a. The patient will likely have long-term emotional and mental changes and need professional help.
    b. Continuous improvement in the patient's condition should occur until he has returned to pretrauma status.
    c. The patient's complete recovery may take years, and the family should plan for his long-term dependent care.
    d. Role changes in family members will be necessary because the patient will be dependent on his family for care and support.

31. The patient is suspected of having a new brain tumor. Which diagnostic test would they undergo to detect a small tumor?
    a. CT scan
    b. Angiography
    c. Electroencephalography (EEG)
    d. Positron emission tomography (PET) scan

32. Assisting the family to understand what is happening to the patient is an especially important role of the nurse when the patient has a tumor in which part of the brain?
    a. Ventricles
    b. Frontal lobe
    c. Parietal lobe
    d. Occipital lobe

33. Which cranial surgery would require the patient to learn how to protect the surgical area from trauma?
    a. Burr holes
    b. Craniotomy
    c. Cranioplasty
    d. Craniectomy

34. What is the best explanation of stereotactic radiosurgery?
    a. Radioactive seeds are implanted in the brain.
    b. Very precisely focused radiation destroys tumor cells.
    c. Tubes are placed to redirect CSF from one area to another.
    d. The cranium is opened with removal of a bone flap to open the dura.

35. For the patient undergoing a craniotomy, when would the nurse provide information about the use of wigs and hairpieces or other methods to disguise hair loss?
    a. During preoperative teaching
    b. If the patient asks about their use
    c. In the immediate postoperative period
    d. When the patient expresses negative feelings about his or her appearance

36. What would best indicate successful achievement of outcomes for the patient with cranial surgery?
    a. Ability to return home in 6 days
    b. Ability to meet all self-care needs
    c. Acceptance of residual neurologic deficits
    d. Absence of signs and symptoms of increased ICP

37. During physical examination of a patient with headache and fever, what findings would lead the nurse to suspect a brain abscess?
    a. Seizures
    b. Nuchal rigidity
    c. Focal symptoms
    d. Signs of increased ICP

38. Which descriptions are characteristic of encephalitis? **Select all that apply.**
    a. Increased CSF production
    b. Most often caused by bacteria
    c. Is an inflammation of the brain
    d. Almost always has a viral cause
    e. May be transmitted by insect vectors
    f. Involves inflammation of tissues surrounding the brain and spinal cord

39. A patient is admitted to the hospital with possible bacterial meningitis. During the initial assessment, the nurse questions the patient about a recent history of what?
    a. Mosquito or tick bites
    b. Chickenpox or measles
    c. Cold sores or fever blisters
    d. An upper respiratory infection

40. What are manifestations of bacterial meningitis?
    a. Papilledema and psychomotor seizures
    b. High fever, nuchal rigidity, and severe headache
    c. Behavioral changes with memory loss and lethargy
    d. Jerky eye movements, loss of corneal reflex, and hemiparesis

41. Vigorous control of fever in the patient with meningitis is needed to prevent complications of increased cerebral edema, seizure frequency, neurologic damage, and fluid loss. What nursing care would be included?
    a. Administer analgesics as ordered.
    b. Monitor LOC related to increased brain metabolism.
    c. Rapidly decrease temperature with a cooling blanket.
    d. Assess for peripheral edema from rapid fluid infusion.

CASE STUDY   Head Injury

(Riddfranz/
iStock/Thinkstock)

Patient Profile
J.K., a 25-year-old unrestrained driver, suffered a compound fracture of the skull and facial fractures in a motor vehicle accident. On admission to the hospital, he was immediately taken to surgery for evacuation of a right subdural hematoma in the temporal region and repair of facial fractures. On the fourth postoperative day, the nurse discovers the following assessment findings.

Subjective Data
• Increasingly difficult to arouse

Objective Data
• GCS score decreased from 10 to 5
• Signs of nuchal rigidity
• Vital signs: temp 102.2°F (39°C), BP 110/60 (77) mm Hg, HR 114 beats/min
• ICP ranges 20–30 mm Hg
• External ventricular drain (EVD) closed to drain

Questions
1. Based on the nursing assessment, what interventions would the nurse include in J.K.'s plan of care? **Use an X to indicate if the nursing action is Indicated (appropriate or necessary), Contraindicated (could be harmful), or Non-essential (makes no difference or is unnecessary).**

Nursing Action	Indicated	Contraindicated	Non-Essential
Administer mannitol			
Keep the HOB flat			

Nursing Action	Indicated	Contraindicated	Non-Essential
Administer a beta-blocker			
Assess pupils			
Use EVD to drain CSF			
Auscultate bowel sounds			
Apply antibiotic ointment to cranial staples			

2. The nurse suspects diabetes insipidus (DI) and is collecting data to report to the HCP. **Highlight the information in the nurse's note below that indicates the possibility of DI**.

NURSE'S NOTE:

Patient is obtunded, decorticate posturing with noxious stimulation. PERRLA 4 mm. Lung sounds clear. Hypoactive bowel sounds. Vital signs: ICP 28 mm Hg, temperature 38.7°C, HR 120 beats/min, BP 95/55 mm Hg, RR 25 breaths/min, SpO$_2$ 93% on 6 L/min simple face mask. CSF drained from EVD is clear. Urine output clear, 400 mL/hr. Specific gravity 1.0. Labs: Hct. 50%, sodium 155 mg/dL, creatinine 1.1 mg/dL, urine osmolality 50 mOsm/kg.

3. The nurse has assigned the following clinical problems for J.K. **Indicate which nursing action listed in the far-left column is appropriate for each clinical problem. Note that some nursing actions may apply to more than one problem.**

Nursing Action	Clinical Problem	Appropriate Nursing Action for Each Clinical Problem
Administer antibiotics	Risk for Injury	
Pad side rails	Increased Intracranial Pressure	
Keep HOB 30-45°	Altered Temperature	
Administer phenytoin		
Obtain CSF culture		
Drain 10 mL/hr from EVD		
Perform aseptic dressing changes		
3% saline infusion		
Lock all bed controls when EVD is open to drain		

4. J.K. has been diagnosed with meningitis. What does the nurse know about this type of infection? **Select all that apply**.
_____A. Nuchal rigidity is a key sign.
_____B. Seizures occur in about 50% of these patients.
_____C. Meningitis may cause an increase in ICP.
_____D. Meningitis likely caused the change in J.K.'s GCS.
_____E. Unequal pupils are unexpected.
_____F. J.K. may have headaches for months.
_____G. Meningitis may cause photophobia.
_____H. Respiratory isolation is not necessary for bacterial meningitis.
_____I. A cooling blanket may be necessary to reduce fever.

5. What assessment findings indicate treatment has been effective? **Use an X to indicate if the assessment findings indicate whether treatment has been <u>Effective</u> (helped to meet expected outcomes), <u>Ineffective</u> (did not help to meet expected outcomes), or <u>Unrelated</u> (not related to expected outcomes).**

Assessment Finding	Effective	Ineffective	Unrelated
ICP is 22 mm Hg			
Urine specific gravity 1.025			
HR 100 beats/min			
BP 125/75 (92) mm Hg			
Peripheral pulses 3+			
Temperature 38°C			
Patient withdraws to painful stimulus			
Pupils are unequal			

Stroke

1. In promoting health maintenance for prevention of strokes, the nurse understands that the highest risk for the most common type of stroke is present in which people?
   a. Blacks
   b. Women who smoke
   c. Persons with hypertension and diabetes
   d. Those who are obese with high dietary fat intake

2. Why does a thrombus that develops in a cerebral artery not always cause a loss of neurologic function?
   a. The body can dissolve atherosclerotic plaques as they form.
   b. Some tissues of the brain do not require constant blood supply to prevent damage.
   c. Circulation via the Circle of Willis may provide blood supply to the affected area of the brain.
   d. Neurologic deficits occur only when major arteries are occluded by thrombus formation around atherosclerotic plaque.

3. A patient comes to the emergency department (ED) with numbness of the face and an inability to speak. While the patient awaits examination, the symptoms disappear and the patient requests discharge. Why should the nurse emphasize that it is important for the patient to be treated before leaving?
   a. The patient has probably had an asymptomatic lacunar stroke.
   b. The symptoms are likely to return and progress to worsening neurologic deficit in the next 24 hours.
   c. Neurologic deficits that are transient occur most often as a result of small hemorrhages that clot off.
   d. The patient has probably had a transient ischemic attack (TIA), which is a sign of progressive cerebrovascular disease.

4. Which statements describe characteristics of a stroke caused by an intracerebral hemorrhage? **Select all that apply.**
   a. Carries a poor prognosis
   b. Caused by rupture of a vessel
   c. Strong association with hypertension
   d. Commonly occurs during or after sleep
   e. Creates a mass that compresses the brain

5. Which type of stroke is associated with endocardial disorders, has a rapid onset, and is likely to occur during activity?
   a. Embolic
   b. Thrombotic
   c. Intracerebral hemorrhage
   d. Subarachnoid hemorrhage

6. What primarily determines the neurologic functions that are affected by a stroke?
   a. The amount of tissue area involved
   b. The rapidity of the onset of symptoms
   c. The brain area perfused by the affected artery
   d. The presence or absence of collateral circulation

7. Indicate whether the following manifestations of a stroke are more likely to occur with right-brain stroke (R) or left-brain stroke (L).
   a. _____ Aphasia
   b. _____ Impaired judgment
   c. _____ Quick, impulsive behavior
   d. _____ Inability to remember words
   e. _____ Left homonymous hemianopsia
   f. _____ Neglect of the left side of the body
   g. _____ Hemiplegia of the right side of the body

8. The patient has a lack of comprehension of both verbal and written language. Which type of communication problem does this patient have?
   a. Dysarthria
   b. Fluent dysphasia
   c. Receptive aphasia
   d. Expressive aphasia

9. A patient is admitted to the hospital with a left hemiplegia. To determine the size and location and to ascertain whether a stroke is ischemic or hemorrhagic, what diagnostic test does the nurse anticipate the health care provider (HCP) will order?
   a. Lumbar puncture
   b. Cerebral angiography
   c. MRI
   d. CT scan with contrast

10. A carotid endarterectomy is being considered as treatment for a patient who has had several TIAs. What should the nurse explain to the patient about this surgery?
    a. It involves intracranial surgery to join a superficial extracranial artery to an intracranial artery.
    b. It is used to restore blood circulation to the brain following an obstruction of a cerebral artery.
    c. It is used to open a stenosis in a carotid artery with a balloon and stent to restore cerebral circulation.
    d. It involves removing an atherosclerotic plaque in the carotid artery to prevent an impending stroke.

11. The incidence of ischemic stroke in patients with TIAs and other risk factors is reduced with the administration of which medication?
    a. Nimodipine
    b. Furosemide (Lasix)
    c. Warfarin (Coumadin)
    d. Daily low-dose aspirin

12. What is the priority intervention in the ED for the patient with a stroke?
    a. IV fluid replacement
    b. Giving osmotic diuretics to reduce cerebral edema
    c. Starting hypothermia to decrease the oxygen needs of the brain
    d. Maintaining respiratory function with a patent airway and oxygen administration

13. A ruptured cerebral aneurysm has been diagnosed in a patient with manifestations of a stroke. Which treatment option would the nurse anticipate?
    a. Hyperventilation therapy
    b. Surgical clipping of the aneurysm
    c. Administration of hyperosmotic agents
    d. Administration of thrombolytic therapy

14. During the acute phase of a stroke, the nurse assesses the patient's vital signs and neurologic status at least every 4 hours. What would the nurse observe as the body attempts to increase cerebral blood flow?
    a. Hypertension
    b. Fluid overload
    c. Cardiac dysrhythmias
    d. S_3 and S_4 heart sounds

15. What should be included during the secondary assessment of the patient with a stroke? **Select all that apply.**
    a. Gaze
    b. Sensation
    c. Facial palsy
    d. Proprioception
    e. Current medications
    f. Distal motor function

16. What nursing intervention is indicated for the patient with hemiplegia?
    a. The use of a footboard to prevent plantar flexion
    b. Immobilization of the affected arm against the chest with a sling
    c. Positioning the patient in bed with each joint lower than the joint proximal to it
    d. Having the patient perform passive range of motion of the affected limb with the unaffected limb

17. A newly admitted patient diagnosed with a right-sided brain stroke has homonymous hemianopsia. What would the nurse do when caring for this patient?
    a. Place objects on the right side within the patient's field of vision.
    b. Approach the patient from the left side to encourage the patient to turn the head.
    c. Place objects on the patient's left side to assess the patient's ability to compensate.
    d. Patch the affected eye to encourage the patient to turn the head to scan the environment.

18. Four days following a stroke, a patient is to start oral fluids and feedings. What would the nurse do first before feeding the patient?
    a. Check the patient's gag reflex.
    b. Order a soft diet for the patient.
    c. Raise the head of the bed to a sitting position.
    d. Assess the patient's ability to swallow tiny amounts of crushed ice.

19. What is an appropriate food for a patient who has mild dysphagia from a stroke?
    a. Fruit juices
    b. Pureed meat
    c. Scrambled eggs
    d. Fortified milkshakes

20. A patient's wife asks the nurse why her husband, who is diagnosed with a hemorrhagic stroke, did not receive the clot-busting medication (tissue plasminogen activator [t-PA]). What is the best response by the nurse to the patient's wife?
    a. "He didn't arrive within the time frame for that therapy."
    b. "Not everyone is eligible for this drug. Has he had surgery lately?"
    c. "You should discuss the treatment of your husband with his doctor."
    d. "The medication you are talking about dissolves clots and could cause more bleeding in your husband's brain."

21. The rehabilitation nurse assesses the patient, caregiver, and family before planning the rehabilitation program for this patient. What must be included in this assessment? **Select all that apply.**
    a. Cognitive status of the family
    b. Patient resources and support
    c. Physical status of all body systems
    d. Rehabilitation potential of the patient
    e. Body strength remaining after the stroke
    f. Patient and caregiver expectations of the rehabilitation

22. What is an appropriate nursing intervention to promote communication during rehabilitation of the patient with aphasia?
    a. Allow time for the patient to complete their thoughts.
    b. Use gestures, pictures, and music to stimulate patient responses.
    c. Structure statements so that the patient does not have to respond verbally.
    d. Use flashcards with simple words and pictures to promote recall of language.

23. A patient with a right hemisphere stroke has unilateral neglect. During the patient's rehabilitation, what is an important nursing intervention?
    a. Avoid positioning the patient on the affected side.
    b. Place all objects for care on the patient's unaffected side.
    c. Teach the patient to care consciously for the affected side.
    d. Protect the affected side from injury with pillows and supports.

24. A patient with a stroke has right-sided hemiplegia. What does the nurse teach the family to prepare them to cope with the behavior changes seen with this type of stroke?
    a. Ignore undesirable behaviors manifested by the patient.
    b. Provide directions to the patient verbally in small steps.
    c. Distract the patient from inappropriate emotional responses.
    d. Supervise all activities before allowing the patient to do them independently.

25. What can the nurse do to best assist the patient and family in coping with the long-term effects of a stroke?
    a. Informing family members that the patient will need assistance with almost all activities of daily living (ADLs)
    b. Explaining that the patient's prestroke behavior will return as improvement progresses
    c. Encouraging the patient and family members to seek assistance from family therapy or stroke support groups
    d. Helping the patient and family understand the significance of residual stroke damage to promote problem solving and planning

26. Which intervention can the nurse delegate to the licensed practical nurse (LPN/VN) when caring for a patient following an acute stroke?
    a. Assess the patient's neurologic status.
    b. Assess the patient's gag reflex before beginning feeding.
    c. Administer ordered antihypertensives and platelet inhibitors.
    d. Teach the patient's caregivers strategies to minimize unilateral neglect.

CASE STUDY   Stroke

(leungchopan/
iStock/Thinkstock)

Patient Profile
R.C., a 38-year-old married woman, was admitted to the hospital unconscious after her family could not rouse her in the morning. She is accompanied by her husband and 3 daughters, ages 10, 13, and 15 years.

Subjective Data
• No history of hypertension or other health problems
• Reported a headache the day before she became unconsciousness

Objective Data
• Diagnostic tests show a subarachnoid hemorrhage
• Vital signs: BP 150/82 mm Hg, RR 16 breaths/min, HR 56 beats/min, Temp 101°F (38.3°C)
• Glasgow Coma Scale score: 5

Questions
1. Select the anticipated health care provider orders from each category. Each category must have at least 1 option selected.

Category	Orders
Imaging	☐ PET scan
	☐ Echocardiogram
	☐ CT scan
	☐ Chest x-ray
Monitoring	☐ Continuous EEG monitoring
	☐ Neurologic assessment every hour
	☐ Continuous pulse oximetry
	☐ Intracranial pressure (ICP) monitoring
Medications	☐ Nimodipine
	☐ Aspirin
	☐ Atropine
	☐ Metoprolol
	☐ Mannitol

2. For each potential nursing intervention, use an X to specify whether the intervention is **Indicated** (appropriate or necessary), **Contraindicated** (could be harmful), or **Non-Essential** (makes no difference or is unnecessary) for the care of R.C.

Potential Intervention	Indicated	Contraindicated	Non-Essential
Raise the HOB to 30 degrees			
Orient the patient to place and time			
Perform a 12-lead ECG			
Use the Trendelenburg position to treat hypotension			
Prepare to administer t-PA			
Insert an oropharyngeal airway			
Prepare the patient for surgery			

3. Below is the nurse's note upon admission to the ICU. **Highlight the information that requires follow-up by the nurse**.

The patient is unresponsive with a GCS of 3. Her vital signs are: HR 48 beats/min, BP 160/70 mm Hg, RR 10 and irregular, Temp 101°F (38.3°C), O_2 saturation 95% on 100% NRB. Pupils are equal 3 mm bilaterally but sluggish to light. She has an 18G right antecubital IV infusing 0.9% NSS at 50 mL/hr. She does not have an indwelling urinary catheter; bladder scan shows 650 mL. Her skin is hot, dry and intact. Cardiac monitor shows sinus bradycardia. Peripheral pulses +3 × 4. Capillary refill < 3 sec. Breath sounds clear in all fields.

4. R.C.'s husband asks the nurse if this could have been prevented. Which risk factors or signs would the nurse identify as possible contributing factors? **Select all that apply**.

_____A. Family history of AVMs
_____B. Smokes cigarettes socially
_____C. Has a glass of wine with dinner once/week
_____D. Sleeps 5 hours per night
_____E. Runs 2 miles 3x/week
_____F. Takes oral contraceptives on and off for 20 years
_____G. Has had frequent headaches during the last month
_____H. Takes "baby" aspirin daily

5. R.C. remains unresponsive. She is intubated and placed on mechanical ventilation. **For each nursing intervention, use an X to specify whether the intervention is Indicated (appropriate or necessary), Contraindicated (could be harmful), or Non-Essential (makes no difference or is unnecessary) in R.C.'s plan of care.**

Nursing Intervention	Indicated	Contraindicated	Non-Essential
Use a specialized air mattress			
Apply SCDs to bilateral lower extremities			
Massage lower legs twice a day			
Place on contact precautions			
Suction the endotracheal tube every 2 hours			
Perform mouth care once daily			
Turn every 2 hours			
Administer enteral nutrition through a gastrostomy tube			
Start an additional IV for extra access			
Initiate fall precautions			

63

Chronic Neurologic Problems

1. Which type of headache would the nurse suspect when the headaches are unilateral and throbbing, preceded by a premonitory symptom of photophobia, and associated with a family history?
   a. Cluster
   b. Migraine
   c. Frontal-type
   d. Tension-type

2. A patient is diagnosed with cluster headaches. Which characteristics would the nurse associate with this type of headache? **Select all that apply.**
   a. Family history
   b. Alcohol is the only dietary trigger
   c. Severe, sharp, penetrating head pain
   d. Abrupt onset lasting 5 to 180 minutes
   e. Bilateral pressure or tightness sensation
   f. May be accompanied by unilateral ptosis or lacrimation

3. What is the most important method of diagnosing functional headaches?
   a. CT scan
   b. Electromyography (EMG)
   c. Cerebral blood flow studies
   d. Thorough history of the headache

4. Which drug therapy for acute migraine and cluster headaches appears to alter the pathophysiologic process for these headaches?
   a. Tricyclic antidepressants, such as amitriptyline
   b. Nonsteroidal antiinflammatory drugs (NSAIDs)
   c. β-adrenergic blockers, such as propranolol (Inderal)
   d. Specific serotonin receptor agonists, such as sumatriptan (Imitrex)

5. What intervention would the nurse implement for the patient with anxiety caused by a lack of knowledge about the cause and treatment of headache?
   a. Help the patient examine lifestyle patterns and precipitating factors.
   b. Administer medications as ordered to relieve pain and promote relaxation.
   c. Provide a quiet, dimly lit environment to reduce stimuli that increase muscle tension and anxiety.
   d. Support the patient's use of counseling or psychotherapy to enhance conflict resolution and stress reduction.

6. The nurse is preparing to admit a newly diagnosed patient with tonic-clonic seizures. What would the nurse delegate to assistive personnel (AP)?
   a. Complete the admission assessment.
   b. Assess the details of the seizure event.
   c. Obtain the suction equipment from the supply cabinet.
   d. Place a padded tongue blade on the wall above the patient's bed.

7. How do generalized seizures differ from focal seizures?
   a. Focal seizures are confined to one side of the brain and remain focal in nature.
   b. Generalized seizures result in loss of consciousness, whereas focal seizures do not.
   c. Generalized seizures result in temporary residual deficits during the postictal phase.
   d. Generalized seizures have bilateral synchronous epileptic discharges affecting the whole brain at onset of the seizure.

8. Which type of seizure occurs in children and consists of a staring spell that lasts for a few seconds?
   a. Atonic
   b. Typical absence
   c. Atypical absence
   d. Focal impaired awareness

9. The patient is diagnosed with focal impaired awareness seizures. Which characteristics are related to this type of seizures? **Select all that apply.**
   a. Formerly known as "grand mal seizure"
   b. Often accompanied by incontinence or tongue or cheek biting
   c. Psychomotor seizures with repetitive behaviors and lip smacking
   d. Altered memory, sexual sensations, and distortions of visual or auditory sensations
   e. Loss of consciousness and stiffening of the body with subsequent jerking of extremities
   f. Often involves behavioral, emotional, and cognitive functions with altered consciousness

10. Which condition could cause a patient to die?
    a. Status epilepticus
    b. Myoclonic seizures
    c. Subclinical seizures
    d. Psychogenic seizures

11. A patient admitted to the hospital following a generalized tonic-clonic seizure asks the nurse what caused the seizure. How would the nurse respond?
    a. "So many factors can cause epilepsy that it is impossible to say what caused your seizure."
    b. "Epilepsy is an inherited disorder. Does anyone else in your family have a seizure disorder?"
    c. "In seizures, some type of trigger causes sudden, abnormal bursts of electrical brain activity."
    d. "Scar tissue in the brain alters the chemical balance, creating uncontrolled electrical discharges."

12. A patient with seizure disorder is being evaluated for surgical treatment of the seizures. What would the nurse recognize as one of the requirements for surgical treatment?
    a. Identification of scar tissue that is able to be removed
    b. An adequate trial of drug therapy that had unsatisfactory results
    c. Development of toxic syndromes from long-term use of antiseizure drugs
    d. The presence of symptoms of cerebral degeneration from repeated seizures

13. The patient is taking antiseizure drugs. Which method would the nurse teach the patient is most commonly used to assess compliance and monitor for drug toxicity?
    a. A daily seizure log
    b. Urine testing for drug levels
    c. Blood testing for drug levels
    d. Monthly electroencephalography (EEG)

14. When teaching a patient with seizure disorder about the medication regimen, what is most important for the nurse to emphasize?
    a. The patient should increase the dosage of the medication if stress is increased.
    b. Most over-the-counter and prescription drugs are safe to take with antiseizure drugs.
    c. Stopping the medication abruptly may increase the intensity and frequency of seizures.
    d. If gingival hypertrophy occurs, notify the health care provider (HCP) so the drug may be changed.

15. The nurse finds a patient in bed having a generalized tonic-clonic seizure. As the patient is seizing, what actions would the nurse take? **Select all that apply.**
    a. Loosen restrictive clothing.
    b. Turn the patient to the side.
    c. Protect the patient's head from injury.
    d. Place a padded tongue blade between the patient's teeth.
    e. Restrain the patient's extremities to prevent soft tissue and bone injury.

16. Following a generalized tonic-clonic seizure, the patient is tired and sleepy. What action would the nurse take?
    a. Suction the patient before allowing him to rest.
    b. Allow the patient to sleep as long as he feels sleepy.
    c. Stimulate the patient to increase his level of consciousness.
    d. Check the patient's level of consciousness every 15 minutes for an hour.

17. During the diagnosis and long-term management of seizure disorder, what would the nurse recognize as one of the major needs of the patient?
    a. Managing the complicated drug regimen of seizure control
    b. Coping with the effects of negative social attitudes toward epilepsy
    c. Adjusting to the restricted lifestyle required by a diagnosis of epilepsy
    d. Learning to minimize the effect of the condition to obtain employment

18. A patient, at the clinic for a routine health examination, mentions that she is exhausted because her legs bother her so much at night that she cannot sleep. What knowledge about restless legs syndrome would the nurse use to base questions about the patient's symptoms?
    a. The condition can be readily diagnosed with EMG.
    b. Other more serious nervous system dysfunctions may be present.
    c. Dopaminergic agents are often effective in managing the symptoms.
    d. Symptoms can be controlled by vigorous exercise of the legs during the day.

19. Which chronic neurologic disorder involves a deficiency of the neurotransmitters acetylcholine and γ-aminobutyric acid (GABA) in the basal ganglia and extrapyramidal system?
    a. Myasthenia gravis
    b. Parkinson's disease
    c. Huntington's disease
    d. Amyotrophic lateral sclerosis (ALS)

20. A 38-year-old woman has newly diagnosed multiple sclerosis (MS) and asks the nurse what is going to happen to her. How would the nurse respond?
    a. "You will have either periods of attacks and remissions or progression of nerve damage over time."
    b. "You need to plan for a continuous loss of movement, sensory functions, and mental capabilities."
    c. "You will most likely have a steady course of chronic progressive nerve damage that will change your personality."
    d. "It is common for people with MS to have an acute attack of weakness and then not to have any other symptoms for years."

21. What would the nurse expect when assessing a patient admitted to the hospital with an acute exacerbation of MS?
    a. Tremors, dysphasia, and ptosis
    b. Bowel and bladder incontinence and loss of memory
    c. Motor impairment, visual disturbances, and paresthesias
    d. Excessive involuntary movements, hearing loss, and ataxia

22. How does the health care provider primarily diagnose MS?
    a. Spinal x-ray results
    b. T-cell analysis of the blood
    c. Analysis of cerebrospinal fluid
    d. History and clinical manifestations

23. Ocrelizumab is being considered as treatment for a patient with progressive-relapsing MS. What would the nurse explain is a disadvantage of this drug compared with other drugs used for MS?
    a. It must be given subcutaneously every day.
    b. It has an increased risk of infection and breast cancer.
    c. It is a muscle relaxant that increases the risk for drowsiness.
    d. It is an anticholinergic agent that causes urinary incontinence.

24. A patient with MS is having difficulty with hygienic care due to muscle spasticity and neuromuscular deficits. When providing care for the patient, what is most important for the nurse to do?
    a. Teach the family members how to care adequately for the patient's needs.
    b. Encourage the patient to maintain social interactions to prevent social isolation.
    c. Promote the use of assistive devices so that the patient can take part in self-care activities.
    d. Perform all activities of daily living (ADLs) for the patient to conserve the patient's energy.

25. A patient with newly diagnosed MS has been hospitalized for evaluation and initial treatment of the disease. Following discharge teaching, which patient statement indicates that additional instruction is needed?
    a. "It is important for me to avoid exposure to people with upper respiratory infections."
    b. "When I begin to feel better, I will stop taking the prednisone to prevent side effects."
    c. "I plan to use vitamin supplements and a diet high in fiber to help manage my condition."
    d. "I must plan with my family how we are going to manage my care if I become more incapacitated."

26. The classic manifestations associated with Parkinson's disease are tremor, rigidity, akinesia, and postural instability. What is a consequence of rigidity?
    a. Shuffling gait
    b. Impaired handwriting
    c. Lack of postural stability
    d. Muscle soreness and pain

27. A patient with a tremor is being evaluated for Parkinson's disease. What would the nurse tell the patient can confirm the diagnosis of Parkinson's disease?
    a. CT and MRI scans.
    b. Relief of symptoms with administration of dopaminergic agents.
    c. The presence of tremors that increase during voluntary movement.
    d. Cerebral angiogram that reveals the presence of cerebral atherosclerosis.

28. Which assessment finding is most indicative of Parkinson's disease?
    a. Large, embellished handwriting
    b. Weakness of one leg resulting in a limping walk
    c. Difficulty rising from a chair and beginning to walk
    d. Onset of muscle spasms occurring with voluntary movement

29. A patient with Parkinson's disease is started on levodopa. What would the nurse teach the patient about this drug?
    a. It stimulates dopamine receptors in the basal ganglia.
    b. It promotes the release of dopamine from brain neurons.
    c. It is a precursor of dopamine that is converted to dopamine in the brain.
    d. It prevents the excessive breakdown of dopamine in the peripheral tissues.

30. To reduce the risk of falls in the patient with Parkinson's disease, what would the nurse teach the patient to do?
    a. Use an elevated toilet seat.
    b. Use a wheelchair for mobility.
    c. Use a walker or cane for support.
    d. Consciously think about stepping over an imaginary object.

31. A patient with myasthenia gravis is admitted to the hospital with respiratory insufficiency and severe weakness. What would the nurse recognize will confirm a diagnosis of myasthenia gravis?
    a. History and physical examination reveal weakness.
    b. Serum acetylcholine receptor antibodies are present.
    c. The patient's respiratory function is impaired because of muscle weakness.
    d. EMG reveals an increased response with repeated stimulation of muscles.

32. When caring for a patient in myasthenic crisis, what would be the nurse's first priority?
    a. Maintaining mobility
    b. Adequate nutrition
    c. Maintaining respiratory function
    d. Maintaining verbal communication

33. When providing care for a patient with ALS, what would the nurse recognize as one of the most distressing problems experienced by the patient?
    a. Painful spasticity of the face and extremities
    b. Retention of cognitive function with total degeneration of motor function
    c. Uncontrollable writhing and twisting movements of the face, limbs, and body
    d. Knowledge that there is a 50% chance the disease has been passed to any offspring

34. When providing care for patients with chronic, progressive neurologic disease, what would the nurse identify as the main goal of treatment?
    a. Meet the patient's personal care needs.
    b. Return the patient to normal neurologic function.
    c. Maximize neurologic functioning for as long as possible.
    d. Prevent the future development of additional chronic diseases.

CASE STUDY   Multiple Sclerosis

(Julialine/iStock/
Thinkstock)

Patient Profile

D.S., a 32-year-old white woman of European descent, born and raised in Minneapolis, is diagnosed with MS after an episode of numbness and tingling on the left side of her body that started several months ago. Two years ago, she had an episode of viral neuritis in the right eye.

Subjective Data
- Reports difficulty seeing out of the right eye
- Denies dry eyes or mouth, ruling out Sjögren's disease
- Reports numbness and tingling on the left side that worsens in hot weather
- Tires easily
- Used all sick days at work; concerned about loss of her job and her ability to care for her 3-year-old son
- History of high cholesterol
- Smokes cigarettes and drinks alcohol at parties

Objective Data
- Cries softly during the interview
- Appears tense and anxious
- Results of visual evoked potential: prolonged in right eye
- MRI of the brain shows several plaques in white matter; ruling out fibromyalgia and stroke
- No rash and negative test for Lyme disease
- No cobalamin deficiency
- Deficient Vitamin D levels

Questions

1. What risk factors does D.S. have for multiple sclerosis? **Use an X to indicate whether the assessment finding is <u>Expected</u> (associated with MS) or <u>Unrelated</u> (not associated with MS).**

Assessment Finding	Expected	Unrelated
32 years of age		
History of high cholesterol		
European descent		
Born and raised in Minneapolis		
Social smoking		
Vitamin D deficiency		
Viral neuritis 2 years ago		
Social drinking		

2. **Choose the most likely options for the information missing from the table below by selecting from the lists of options provided.**

Multiple sclerosis (MS) is a chronic, progressive and degenerative disorder of the _____**1**_____ system. People diagnosed at __**2**__ years of age or older often have more progressive disease. The primary problem is a(n) _____**3**_____ process driven by activated ____**4**____. Nerve impulses are disrupted by ___**5**___ scar tissue. Eventually, ____**6**____, ____**6**____, and _____**6**_____ matter are affected.

Options for 1:	Options for 2:	Options for 3:
Central nervous	30	Inflammatory
Respiratory	45	Malignant
Autonomic nervous	50	Extrapyramidal
Musculoskeletal	65	Autoimmune
Sympathetic nervous	80	Dopaminergic

Options for 4:	Options for 5:	Options for 6:
B cells	Neuron	White
Red blood cells	Myelin	Black
White blood cells	Astrocytes	Axonal
T cells	Oligodendrocytes	Grey
Cancer cells	Glial	Brown

3. What orders from the health care provider would the nurse expect? **Select the anticipated health care provider orders from each of the following categories. Each category must have at least 1 option selected.**

Category	Orders
Diagnostic	☐ PET scan
	☐ Liver function tests
	☐ Lumbar puncture
	☐ CT scan
	☐ EEG
Nursing Care	☐ Neutropenic precautions
	☐ Neurologic assessment every hour
	☐ Routine vision assessment
	☐ Out of bed with assistance
	☐ Bladder ultrasound if unable to void
Ancillary Care	☐ Respiratory therapy
	☐ Speech therapy
	☐ Palliative care
	☐ Physical therapy
	☐ Pastoral care
Medications	☐ Cladribine
	☐ Oxybutinin
	☐ Alemtuzumab
	☐ Cefazolin
	☐ Mannitol
	☐ Hydrocortisone

4. Drug therapy may treat symptoms and slow progression of MS. **Choose the most likely options for the information missing from the table below by selecting from the lists of options provided.**

Drug	Mechanism of Action	Nursing Considerations
β-Interferon	Suppresses the immune system	1
2	Immunomodulatory agent	Liver toxicity
Cladribine	3	Increases risk of breast cancer
Fingolimod	Prevents lymphocytes from reaching CNS	4
5	Reduces inflammation at site of demyelination	Delays wound healing

Options for 1 and 4:	Options for 2 and 5:	Options for 3:
Causes hyperglycemia	Fluticasone	Prevents glial scar tissue formation
May cause suicidal ideation	Dimethyl fumarate	Slows attack on myelin by lymphocytes
May cause kidney injury	Teriflunomide	Monoclonal antibodies that suppress immunologic activity
Susceptible to fatal brain infection	Prednisone	Blocks passage through the blood brain barrier
May cause hemorrhagic stroke	Natalizumab	Prevents demyelination

5. What instructions would the nurse include when doing discharge teaching with D.S.? **Select all that apply.**
_____A. You can reduce your risk of getting the flu by getting a live virus influenza vaccine.
_____B. You need to rest when you feel tired.
_____C. Avoid working or recreation outside on hot days.
_____D. Schedule annual eye examinations with your eye doctor.
_____E. Adhering to the medications will prevent MS from getting worse.
_____F. You should limit yourself to drinking 1 cup of coffee per day.
_____G. There isn't anything to help with urinary incontinence.
_____H. Acute exacerbations will occur, but shouldn't interfere with your ADLs.

Dementia and Delirium

1. What manifestations of cognitive impairment are primarily characteristic of delirium? **Select all that apply.**
   a. Reduced awareness
   b. Impaired judgments
   c. Words difficult to find
   d. Sleep/wake cycle reversed
   e. Distorted thinking and perception
   f. Insidious onset with prolonged duration

2. Which statement most accurately describes dementia?
   a. Overproduction of β-amyloid protein causes all dementias.
   b. Dementia from neurodegenerative causes can be prevented.
   c. Dementia caused by hepatic or renal encephalopathy cannot be reversed.
   d. Vascular dementia can be diagnosed by brain lesions found on neuroimaging.

3. A patient with Alzheimer's disease (AD) dementia has manifestations of depression. The nurse knows that treating the patient with antidepressants will most likely do what?
   a. Improve cognitive function
   b. Not alter the course of either condition
   c. Cause interactions with the drugs used to treat the dementia
   d. Be contraindicated because of the central nervous system (CNS)–depressant effect of antidepressants

4. For what purpose would the nurse use the Mini-Mental State Examination to evaluate a patient with cognitive impairment?
   a. It is a useful tool to determine the cause of dementia.
   b. It is the best tool to evaluate mood and thought processes.
   c. It can help to document the degree of cognitive impairment in delirium and dementia.
   d. It is only useful for the initial evaluation of mental status, other tools are used to evaluate changes in cognition over time.

5. After obtaining a health history of a patient with dementia, the nurse determines that the condition is potentially reversible when finding out what about the patient?
   a. Has long-standing abuse of alcohol
   b. Has a history of Parkinson's disease
   c. Recently developed symptoms of hypothyroidism
   d. Was infected with human immunodeficiency virus (HIV) 15 years ago

6. The husband of a patient is reporting that his wife's memory has been deteriorating lately. When asked for examples of her memory loss, the husband says that she is forgetting the neighbors' names and forgot their granddaughter's birthday. What kind of memory loss is this?
   a. Delirium
   b. Memory loss in AD
   c. Normal forgetfulness
   d. Memory loss in mild cognitive impairment

7. The wife of a patient who has deterioration in memory asks the nurse whether her husband has AD. The nurse explains that a diagnosis of AD is usually made when what happens?
   a. A urine test shows high levels of isoprostanes.
   b. All other possible causes of dementia have been eliminated.
   c. Blood analysis reveals increased amounts of β-amyloid protein.
   d. A CT scan of the brain shows brain atrophy.

8. A newly admitted patient has moderate AD. What will the patient need help with that the nurse includes when planning care?
   a. Eating
   b. Walking
   c. Dressing
   d. Self-care activities

9. What is one focus of interprofessional care of patients with AD?
   a. Replacement of deficient acetylcholine in the brain
   b. Drug therapy for cognitive problems and undesirable behaviors
   c. The use of memory-enhancing techniques to delay disease progression
   d. Prevention of other chronic diseases that hasten the progression of AD

10. The nurse is reviewing the medication record of a patient with AD. What benzodiazepine medication is being used to help manage the patient's behavior?
    a. Sertraline (Zoloft)
    b. Donepezil (Aricept)
    c. Lorazepam (Ativan)
    d. Risperidone (Risperdal)

11. What *N*-methyl-D-aspartate (NMDA) receptor antagonist is often used for a patient with AD who has decreased memory and cognition?
    a. Zolpidem (Ambien)
    b. Olanzapine (Zyprexa)
    c. Rivastigmine (Exelon)
    d. Memantine (Namenda)

12. A patient with AD in a long-term care facility is wandering the halls very agitated, asking for her "mommy" and crying. What is the best response by the nurse?
    a. Ask the patient, "Why are you behaving this way?"
    b. Tell the patient, "Let's go get a snack in the kitchen."
    c. Ask the patient, "Wouldn't you like to lie down now?"
    d. Tell the patient, "Just take some deep breaths and calm down."

13. The sister of a patient with AD asks the nurse whether preventing the disease is possible. When responding, the nurse explains that there is no known way to prevent AD, but there are ways to keep the brain healthy. What is recommended to keep the brain healthy? **Select all that apply.**
    a. Avoid trauma to the brain.
    b. Recognize and treat depression early.
    c. Avoid social gatherings to avoid infections.
    d. Do not overtax the brain by trying to learn new skills.
    e. Daily wine intake will increase circulation to the brain.
    f. Exercise regularly to decrease the risk for cognitive decline.

14. The son of a patient with early onset AD asks if he will get AD. What would the nurse tell him about the genetics of AD?
    a. The risk for it is higher for the children of parents of early onset AD.
    b. Women get AD more often than men do, so his chances of getting AD are slim.
    c. The blood test for the *ApoE* gene to identify this type of AD can predict who will develop it.
    d. This type of AD is not as complex as regular AD, so he does not need to worry about getting AD.

15. The nurse is planning care to address confusion in a patient with moderate AD. What is an appropriate nursing intervention to include?
    a. Post clocks and calendars in the patient's environment.
    b. Establish and consistently follow a daily schedule with the patient.
    c. Monitor the patient's activities to maintain a safe patient environment.
    d. Stimulate thought processes by asking the patient questions about recent activities.

16. The family caregiver for a patient with AD expresses an inability to make decisions, concentrate, or sleep. What does the nurse determine about the caregiver?
    a. The caregiver is also developing signs of AD.
    b. The caregiver has symptoms of caregiver role strain.
    c. The caregiver needs a period of respite from caring for the patient.
    d. The caregiver should ask other family members to help with the patient's care.

17. The partner of a man with moderate AD is experiencing social isolation. What is a nursing intervention that would be appropriate to provide respite care and allow the partner to have satisfactory contact with significant others?
    a. Help the partner arrange for adult day care for the patient.
    b. Encourage placing the patient permanently in the Alzheimer's unit of a long-term care facility.
    c. Refer the partner to a home health agency to arrange daily home nursing visits to help with the patient's care.
    d. Arrange for hospitalization of the patient for 3 or 4 days so the partner can visit out-of-town friends and relatives.

18. For a patient with moderate cognitive impairment, the health care provider (HCP) is trying to distinguish between a diagnosis of dementia and dementia with Lewy bodies (DLB). What observations by the nurse support a diagnosis of DLB? **Select all that apply.**
    a. Tremors
    b. Fluctuating cognitive ability
    c. Disturbed behavior, sleep, and personality
    d. Symptoms of pneumonia, including congested lung sounds
    e. Bradykinesia, rigidity, and postural instability without tremor

19. Which activities could the registered nurse (RN), in charge at a long-term care facility, delegate to assistive personnel (AP)? **Select all that apply.**
    a. Help the patient with eating.
    b. Provide personal hygiene and skin care.
    c. Check the environment for safety hazards.
    d. Help the patient to the bathroom at regular intervals.
    e. Monitor for skin breakdown and swallowing difficulties.

20. A 72-year-old woman is hospitalized in the intensive care unit (ICU) with pneumonia resulting from chronic obstructive pulmonary disease (COPD). She has a fever, productive cough, and adventitious breath sounds throughout her lungs. In the past 24 hours, her fluid intake was 1000 mL and her urine output was 700 mL. She was diagnosed with early stage AD 6 months ago but has been able to maintain her activities of daily living (ADLs) with supervision. Identify 6 risk factors that place her at risk for developing delirium.
    a.
    b.
    c.
    d.
    e.
    f.

21. A 68-year-old man is admitted to the ED with multiple blunt trauma wounds following a one-vehicle car accident. He is restless; disoriented to person, place, and time; and agitated. He resists attempts at examination and calls out the name "Janice." Why would the nurse suspect delirium rather than dementia in this patient?
    a. The fact that he should not have been allowed to drive if he had dementia
    b. His hyperactive behavior, which distinguishes his condition from the hypoactive behavior of dementia
    c. Emergency personnel reported he was noncommunicative when they arrived at the accident scene
    d. The report of his family that, although he has heart disease and is "very hard of hearing," this behavior is unlike him

22. What would be included in the management of a patient with delirium?
    a. The use of restraints to protect the patient from injury
    b. The use of short-acting benzodiazepines to sedate the patient
    c. Identification and treatment of underlying causes when possible
    d. Administration of high doses of an antipsychotic drug, such as haloperidol (Haldol)

23. When caring for a patient in the severe stage of AD, what diversion or distraction activities would the nurse use?
    a. Watching TV
    b. Books to read
    c. Playing games
    d. Mobiles or dangling ribbons

24. An 81-yr-old patient who has been in the intensive care unit (ICU) for a week is now stable and transfer to the progressive care unit is planned. On rounds, the nurse notices that the patient has new onset confusion. What would the nurse plan to do?
    a. Give PRN lorazepam (Ativan) and cancel the transfer.
    b. Inform the receiving nurse and then transfer the patient.
    c. Notify the health care provider and postpone the transfer.
    d. Obtain an order for restraints as needed and transfer the patient.

CASE STUDY   Alzheimer's Disease

Patient Profile

G.D. is a 71-year-old man whose wife noticed that he has become increasingly forgetful over the past 3 years. Recently he was diagnosed with AD.

(lekcej/iStock/Thinkstock)

Subjective Data
- Wanders out of the house at night
- Reports that he "has trouble balancing the checkbook"
- Can dress, bathe, and feed himself
- Has trouble figuring out how to use his electric razor
- His wife is distressed about his cognitive decline
- His wife says she is depressed and cannot watch him at night and get rest herself

Objective Data
- CT scan: evidence of previous stroke

Questions

1. The nurse expects several diagnostic tests to be performed to evaluate G.D.'s disease and explains these to his wife. **Complete the statements below by choosing the most likely options for the missing information from the lists of options provided.**

   A _____ may show brain _____ in later stages of the disease. A _____ uses glucose tracers to determine brain metabolism and can detect _____. Serum levels may be evaluated for the _____ vitamins.

Options:	
V/Q scan	amyloid
Neurofibrillary tangles	atrophy
EEG	A & E
CT scan	C & D
Gamma-knife	B-complex

2. Neuropsychologic testing, which includes the Mini-Cog and the Mini-Mental State Examination (MMSE), are performed to assess G.D. **Use an X to indicate if the task or question is part of the <u>Mini-Cog</u> or part of the <u>MMSE</u>.**

Task or Question	Mini-Cog	MMSE
Repeat the 3 words previously stated at the end of the examination		
Ask the patient to name an object		
Read this and do what it says		
"What is today's date?"		
Draw a clock and put the clock hands on 11:10		

3. The nurse explains to G.D.'s wife that there are 3 stages of AD. **Use an X to indicate if the assessment finding is associated with the <u>Mild</u> stage, <u>Moderate</u> stage, or <u>Severe</u> stage of Alzheimer's disease (AD).**

Assessment Finding	Mild	Moderate	Severe
Wanders out of the house at night			
Has trouble speaking			
Occasionally misplaces eyeglasses			
Puts the car keys in the refrigerator			
Has trouble recognizing his children			
Becomes agitated easily			
Has trouble finding the right word			

4. What medications may be recommended to slow the progression or treat effects of the disease? **Choose the most likely options for the information missing from the table below by selecting from the lists of options provided.**

Drug	Drug Class	AD Problem it Treats
Memantine	Cholinesterase inhibitor	5
1	Atypical antidepressant	Depression
2	Benzodiazepine	Agitation
Zolpidem	Benzodiazepine Receptor Agonist	6
Fluoxetine	3	7
Aripiprazole	Antipsychotic	8
Donepezil	4	Decreased cognition

Options for 1 and 2:	Options for 3 and 4:	Options for 5, 6, 7, and 8:
Midazolam	SSRI	Forgetfulness
Lithium	Non-SSRI	Depression
Clonazepam	Anticholinergic	Manic phase
Duloxetine	Cholinesterase inhibitor	Insomnia
Trazodone	Mood stabilizer	Disinhibition

5. What would the nurse include when teaching G.D. and his wife about managing Alzheimer's disease? **Select all that apply**.

_____A. You should select a durable power of attorney for healthcare.

_____B. Use distraction to cope with behavior problems.

_____C. G.D. should wear a MedicAlert bracelet.

_____D. Avoid interactions with friends or family to avoid embarrassment.

_____E. G.D. can drive until he is physically unable to do so.

_____F. Join community support groups.

_____G. Take actions like removing throw rugs to ensure safety in the home.

_____H. Correct mistakes G.D. makes.

Spinal Cord and Peripheral Nerve Problems

1. What group would the nurse target when planning community education about preventing spinal cord injuries (SCIs)?
   a. Older men
   b. Teenage girls
   c. Elementary school-age children
   d. Adolescent and young adult men

2. A 70-year-old patient is admitted after falling off his roof. He has an SCI at the level of C7. What assessment findings would indicate the presence of spinal shock?
   a. Paraplegia with a flaccid paralysis
   b. Tetraplegia with total sensory loss
   c. Total hemiplegia with sensory and motor loss
   d. Spastic tetraplegia with loss of pressure sensation

3. Which syndrome of incomplete SCI is described as cord damage common in the cervical region that results in greater weakness in upper extremities than lower?
   a. Central cord syndrome
   b. Anterior cord syndrome
   c. Posterior cord syndrome
   d. Cauda equina and conus medullaris syndromes

4. The patient is diagnosed with Brown-Séquard syndrome after a knife wound to the spine. Which description accurately describes this syndrome?
   a. Damage to the most distal cord and nerve roots, resulting in flaccid paralysis of the lower limbs and areflexic bowel and bladder
   b. Spinal cord damage resulting in ipsilateral motor paralysis and contralateral loss of pain and sensation below the level of the injury
   c. Rare cord damage resulting in loss of proprioception below the lesion level with retention of motor control and temperature and pain sensation
   d. Often caused by flexion injury with acute compression of cord resulting in complete motor paralysis and loss of pain and temperature sensation below the level of injury

5. What causes an initial incomplete SCI to result in complete cord damage?
   a. Edematous compression of the cord above the level of the injury
   b. Continued trauma to the cord resulting from damage to stabilizing ligaments
   c. Infarction and necrosis of the cord caused by edema, hemorrhage, and metabolites
   d. Mechanical transection of the cord by sharp vertebral bone fragments after the initial injury

6. A patient with SCI has spinal shock. The nurse plans care for the patient based on what knowledge?
   a. Rehabilitation measures cannot be started until spinal shock has resolved.
   b. The patient needs continuous monitoring for hypotension, tachycardia, and hypoxemia.
   c. Resolution of spinal shock is manifested by spasticity, reflex return, and neurogenic bladder.
   d. Patient will have complete loss of motor and sensory functions below the level of the injury, but autonomic functions are not affected.

7. Two days after SCI, a patient asks about the extent of impairment that will result from the injury. What is the nurse's best response?
   a. "You will have more normal function when spinal shock resolves and the reflex arc returns."
   b. "The extent of your injury cannot be determined until the secondary injury to the cord is resolved."
   c. "When your condition is more stable, MRI will be done to reveal the extent of the cord damage."
   d. "Because rehabilitation can affect the return of function, it will be years before we can tell what the complete effect will be."

8. The patient has loss of function below C4 due to injuries sustained in a traffic collision. Which effect most influences how the nurse prioritizes care?
   a. Respiratory diaphragmatic breathing
   b. Loss of all respiratory muscle function
   c. Decreased response of the sympathetic nervous system
   d. Gastrointestinal (GI) hypomotility with paralytic ileus and gastric distention

9. A patient is admitted to the emergency department (ED) with SCI at the level of T2. Which assessment finding would most concern the nurse?
   a. Arterial oxygen saturation by pulse oximetry (SpO_2) of 92%
   b. Heart rate of 42 bpm
   c. BP of 88/60 mm Hg
   d. Loss of motor and sensory function in arms and legs

10. The patient's SCI is at T4. What is the highest-level goal of rehabilitation that is realistic for this patient?
    a. Indoor mobility in manual wheelchair
    b. Ambulate with crutches and leg braces
    c. Be independent in self-care and wheelchair use
    d. Completely independent ambulation with short leg braces and canes

11. What is an indication for early surgical therapy of the patient with SCI?
    a. There is incomplete cord lesion involvement.
    b. The ligaments that support the spine are torn.
    c. A high cervical injury causes loss of respiratory function.
    d. Evidence of continued compression of the cord is apparent.

12. A patient is admitted to the ED with a possible cervical SCI following an automobile accident. During admission, what is the highest priority?
    a. Maintaining a patent airway
    b. Assessing the patient for head and other injuries
    c. Maintaining immobilization of the cervical spine
    d. Assessing the patient's motor and sensory function

13. Before surgical stabilization of a cervical SCI, what method of patient immobilization would the nurse expect?
    a. Kinetic beds
    b. Hard cervical collar
    c. Skeletal traction with skull tongs
    d. Sternal-occipital-mandibular immobilizer brace

14. The health care provider (HCP) has prescribed IV norepinephrine (Levophed) for a patient in the ED with SCI. What finding indicates the drug is having the desired effect?
    a. Heart rate of 68 bpm
    b. Respiratory rate of 24 breaths/min
    c. Temperature of 96.8°F (36.0°C)
    d. BP of 106/82 mm Hg

15. During assessment of a patient with SCI, the nurse determines that the patient has a poor cough with diaphragmatic breathing. Based on this finding, what would be the nurse's first action?
    a. Begin frequent turning and repositioning.
    b. Use tracheal suctioning to remove secretions.
    c. Assess lung sounds and respiratory rate and depth.
    d. Prepare the patient for endotracheal intubation and mechanical ventilation.

16. Following a T2 spinal cord injury, the patient develops paralytic ileus. What would the nurse expect will be necessary?
    a. IV fluids
    b. Enteral nutrition
    c. Parenteral nutrition
    d. Nasogastric suctioning

17. How is urinary function best maintained during the acute phase of SCI?
    a. An indwelling catheter
    b. Intermittent catheterization
    c. Insertion of a suprapubic catheter
    d. Use of incontinent pads to protect the skin

18. A week after SCI at T2, a patient has movement in his leg and tells the nurse that he is recovering some function. What is the nurse's best response?
    a. "It is really still too soon to know if you will have a return of function."
    b. "That could be a really positive finding. Can you show me the movement?"
    c. "That's wonderful. We will start exercising your legs more frequently now."
    d. "I'm sorry, but the movement is only a reflex and does not indicate normal function."

19. A patient with SCI suddenly develops a throbbing headache, flushed skin, and diaphoresis above the level of injury. The nurse checks the patient's vital signs and finds a systolic blood pressure of 210 mm Hg and a heart rate of 40 beats/min. Beginning with number 1 as the first priority, number the following nursing actions in order of highest priority to lowest.
    a. _____ Administer ordered as needed nitroglycerin.
    b. _____ Check for bladder distention.
    c. _____ Document the occurrence, treatment, and response.
    d. _____ Call the HCP.
    e. _____ Raise the head of bed (HOB) to 45 degrees or above.
    f. _____ Loosen tight clothing on the patient.

20. A patient with paraplegia has developed an irritable bladder with reflex emptying. Along with the use of medications, what would be most helpful for the nurse to teach the patient?
    a. Hygiene care for an indwelling urinary catheter
    b. How to perform intermittent self-catheterization
    c. To empty the bladder with manual pelvic pressure in coordination with reflex voiding patterns
    d. That a urinary diversion, such as an ileal conduit, is the easiest way to handle urinary elimination

21. When counseling patients with SCI about sexual function, what would the nurse teach a male patient with a complete lower motor neuron lesion?
    a. He may have uncontrolled reflex erections, but orgasm and ejaculation are usually not possible.
    b. He is most likely to have reflex erections and may have orgasm if S2-S4 nerve pathways are intact.
    c. He has a lesion with the greatest possibility of successful psychogenic erection with ejaculation and orgasm.
    d. He will probably be unable to have either psychogenic or reflex erections and no ejaculation or orgasm.

22. During the patient's process of grieving for the losses resulting from SCI, what would the nurse do?
    a. Help the patient understand that working through the grief will be a lifelong process.
    b. Assist the patient to move through all stages of the mourning and grief process to acceptance.
    c. Let the patient know that anger directed at the staff or the family is not a positive coping mechanism.
    d. Facilitate the grieving process so that it is completed by the time the patient is discharged from rehabilitation.

23. A patient with a metastatic tumor of the spinal cord is scheduled for a laminectomy to remove the tumor. What would the nurse consider when planning postoperative patient care?
    a. Most cord tumors cause autodestruction of the cord as in traumatic injuries.
    b. Metastatic tumors are commonly extradural lesions that are treated palliatively.
    c. Radiation therapy is routinely given after surgery for all malignant spinal cord tumors.
    d. Because complete removal of intramedullary tumors is not possible, the surgery is considered palliative.

24. When planning care for the patient with trigeminal neuralgia, which patient outcome would the nurse set as the highest priority?
    a. Relief of pain
    b. Protecting the cornea
    c. Maintaining optimal nutrition
    d. Maintaining a positive body image

25. Surgical intervention is being considered for a patient with trigeminal neuralgia. Which procedure has the least residual effects with a positive outcome?
    a. Glycerol rhizotomy
    b. Gamma knife radiosurgery
    c. Microvascular decompression
    d. Percutaneous radiofrequency rhizotomy

26. What would the nurse do when providing care for a patient experiencing an acute attack of trigeminal neuralgia?
    a. Carry out all hygiene and oral care for the patient.
    b. Use conversation to distract the patient from pain.
    c. Maintain a quiet, comfortable, draft-free environment.
    d. Have the patient examine the mouth after each meal for residual food.

27. A patient is diagnosed with Bell's palsy. What information would the nurse teach the patient about Bell's palsy? **Select all that apply.**
    a. Bell's palsy affects the motor branches of the facial nerve.
    b. Antiseizure drugs are the drugs of choice for treatment of Bell's palsy.
    c. Nutrition and avoiding hot foods or beverages are special needs of this patient.
    d. Herpes simplex virus 1 is strongly associated with the development of Bell's palsy.
    e. Moist heat, gentle massage, electrical nerve stimulation, and exercises are used to treat Bell's palsy.
    f. An inability to close the eyelid, with an upward movement of the eyeball when closure is attempted, is evident.

28. A patient is admitted to the hospital with Guillain-Barré syndrome. She had weakness in her feet and ankles that has progressed to weakness with numbness and tingling in both legs. During the acute phase of the illness, what information about Guillain-Barré syndrome would the nurse apply?
    a. The most important aspect of care is to monitor the patient's respiratory rate and depth and vital capacity.
    b. Early treatment with corticosteroids can suppress the immune response and prevent ascending nerve damage.
    c. The most serious complication of this condition is ascending demyelination of the peripheral nerves and the cranial nerves.
    d. Although voluntary motor neurons are damaged by the inflammatory response, the autonomic nervous system is unaffected by the disease.

29. A patient with Guillain-Barré syndrome asks whether he is going to die as the paralysis spreads toward his chest. What information would the nurse use to answer this question?
    a. Patients who need ventilatory support almost always die.
    b. Death occurs when nerve damage affects the brain and meninges.
    c. Most patients with Guillain-Barré syndrome do not die, but recover.
    d. If death is prevented, residual paralysis and sensory impairment are usually permanent.

30. The patient is diagnosed with chronic inflammatory demyelinating polyneuropathy (CIDP) after nerve conduction velocity test. How will this patient with CIDP be treated differently than a patient with Guillain-Barré syndrome?
    a. Rehabilitation
    b. Corticosteroids
    c. Plasmapheresis
    d. IV immunoglobulin

31. Which condition is transmitted through wound contamination, causes painful tonic spasms or seizures, and can be prevented by immunization?
    a. Tetanus
    b. Botulism
    c. Neurosyphilis
    d. Systemic inflammatory response syndrome

CASE STUDY Spinal Cord Injury

Patient Profile

S.M. is an 18-year-old high school student who sustained a C7 spinal cord injury when she dove into a lake while swimming with her friends. S.M. is admitted directly to the intensive care unit (ICU).

(monkeybusiness
images/iStock/
Thinkstock)

Subjective Data
- Has patchy sensation in her upper extremities

Objective Data
- Very weak biceps and triceps strength bilaterally
- Moderate strength in both lower extremities
- Bladder control present
- X-rays show no fracture dislocation of the spine
- Hard cervical collar in place
- On bed rest

Interprofessional Care
- Diagnosed as central cord syndrome

Questions

1. What interventions would the nurse include when planning care for S.M. during the acute phase of care? **Use an X to indicate if the nursing action is <u>Indicated</u> (is necessary or appropriate), <u>Contraindicated</u> (could be harmful), or is <u>Non-Essential</u> (makes no difference or is unnecessary).**

Nursing Action	Indicated	Contraindicated	Non-Essential
Maintain MAP > 85 mm Hg			
Encourage use of incentive spirometer			
Raise HOB to 45°			
Perform ROM exercises			
Maintain SpO$_2$ > 92%			
Monitor EtCO$_2$			
Turn patient every 2 hours			
Administer a PPI			

2. The following medications have been ordered to treat S.M. **Choose the most likely options for the information missing from the table below by selecting from the lists of options provided.**

Drug	Drug Class	Rationale for its Use	Nursing Consideration
Enoxaparin	3	5	Hemorrhage
1	H$_2$ antagonist	Prevent gastric ulcer	Acute kidney injury
Norepinephrine	Cardiac stimulant	6	8
Atropine	4	7	Tachycardia
2	Corticosteroid	Reduces swelling	9

Options for 1 and 2:	Options for 3 and 4:	Options for 5, 6, and 7:	Options for 8 and 9:
Famotidine	Proton pump inhibitor	Treat bradycardia	Extravasation
Omeprazole	Beta-blocker	Treat chest pain	Liver toxicity
Sucralfate	Cardiac glycoside	Prevent dysrhythmias	Hypotension
Methylprednisolone	Anticoagulant	Prevent VTE	Hyperglycemia
Nitroglycerin	Anticholinergic	Treat hypertension	Hypokalemia
Esmolol	Nitrate	Treat hypotension	Cyanide poisoning

3. What would the nurse include in the plan of care to prevent or treat autonomic dysreflexia? **Select all that apply.**

_____A. Straight catheterize to treat urinary retention.

_____B. Keep the HOB flat to treat a severe headache.

_____C. Administer stool softeners or laxatives.

_____D. Maintain neck alignment.

_____E. Raise HOB to lower blood pressure.

_____F. Encourage patient to report changes in vision.

_____G. Logroll the patient when turning.

_____H. Treat headaches with acetaminophen.

4. How would the nurse provide psychological care to S.M.? **Use an X to indicate if the statements made by the nurse are Therapeutic or Nontherapeutic.**

Nurse's Statements	Therapeutic	Nontherapeutic
"You only have an incomplete spinal cord injury, so you have a good chance for a full recovery."		
"Tell me how you are feeling."		
"You shouldn't be angry, unfortunately these accidents happen."		
"I understand how you feel."		
"You may experience depression, but there is professional help if you need it."		
"Rehabilitation can help you function at your highest potential."		
"You must eventually accept what has happened to you."		

5. S.M. will be discharged with a halo vest. What statements indicate patient teaching has been effective? **Use an X to indicate whether the statement indicates if teaching has been Effective (patient understands), Ineffective (needs clarification), or Unrelated (isn't related to this topic).**

Patient Statement	Effective	Ineffective	Unrelated
"I can wear a T-shirt under the vest."			
"I can wear high heels when going out on a date."			
"The sheepskin pad cannot be washed."			
"I will need to perform pin site care using hydrogen peroxide."			
"I need to avoid wearing tight clothing."			
"I need to report fevers to my HCP."			
"Severe headaches mean the pins are too tight."			

Assessment: Musculoskeletal System

1. Using the terms listed, identify the structures of an adult long bone in the illustration below.

   Terms

   Articular cartilage   Epiphysis   Spongy bone
   Compact bone   Medullary cavity   Yellow marrow#
   Diaphysis   Periosteum
   Epiphyseal line   Red marrow cavities

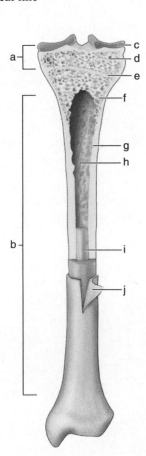

   a. _____

   b. _____

   c. _____

   d. _____

   e. _____

   f. _____

   g. _____

   h. _____

   i. _____

   j. _____

2. Using the terms listed, identify the cortical bone structures in the illustration below.

Terms
Blood vessels
Canaliculi
Osteon (Haversian system)
Periosteum

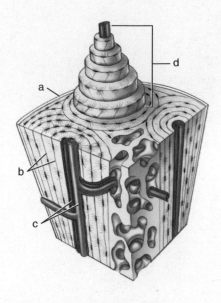

a. _____

b. _____

c. _____

d. _____

3. Using the terms listed, identify the structures of a diarthrodial (synovial) joint in the illustration below. **(Terms may be used more than once.)**

Terms

Articular cartilage	Joint capsule	Synovial membrane
Blood vessel	Joint cavity with synovial fluid	Tendon sheath
Bone	Nerve	
Bursa	Periosteum	

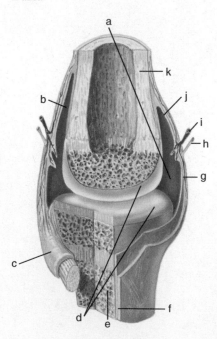

a. _____

b. _____

c. _____

d. _____

e. _____

f. _____

g. _____

h. _____

i. _____

j. _____

k. _____

4. Which type of cell is responsible for the formation of bone?
   a. Osteocyte
   b. Osteoclast
   c. Osteoblast
   d. Sarcomere

5. The patient is told by the health care provider (HCP) that the size of the patient's muscle has decreased. How would the nurse document this?
   a. Hyaline
   b. Atrophy
   c. Isometric
   d. Hypertrophy

6. An older patient is describing increased stiffness in the shoulders, back, and hips. The loss of elasticity in what tissue contributes to this?
   a. Actin
   b. Fascia
   c. Myosin
   d. Ligament

7. What is the best description of the periosteum?
   a. Lining of a joint capsule
   b. A characteristic of skeletal muscle
   c. Most common type of cartilage tissue
   d. Fibrous connective tissue covering bone

8. What is the function of a tendon?
   a. Attaches muscle to bone
   b. Connects bone to bone at the joint
   c. Connects cartilage to muscle in joints
   d. Attaches synovium to the joint capsule

9. The nurse performing range of motion (ROM) with a patient puts each joint through its full movement. Which joints are capable of abduction and adduction? **Select all that apply.**
   a. Hip
   b. Knee
   c. Wrist
   d. Elbow
   e. Thumb
   f. Shoulder

10. While having his height measured during a routine health examination, a 79-year-old man asks the nurse why he is "shrinking." How would the nurse explain the decreased height that occurs with aging?
    a. Decreased muscle mass results in a stooped posture.
    b. Loss of cartilage in the knees and hip joints causes a loss of height.
    c. Long bones become less dense and shorten as bone tissue compacts.
    d. Vertebrae become more compressed with thinning of intervertebral discs.

11. A 78-year-old woman has physiologic changes in her joints related to aging. What is an appropriate nursing intervention related to common changes of aging in the musculoskeletal system?
    a. Encourage adequate rest to eliminate fatigue.
    b. Provide all care for the patient to ensure that care is completed.
    c. Encourage eating enough calories to avoid the risk for impaired skin integrity.
    d. Have the patient exercise to maintain muscle strength and avoid the risk for falls.

12. When obtaining information about the patient's use of medications, the nurse is concerned that both bone and muscle function may be impaired when the patient reports taking what type of drug?
    a. Corticosteroids
    b. Oral hypoglycemic agents
    c. Potassium-depleting diuretics
    d. Nonsteroidal antiinflammatory drugs (NSAIDs)

13. Identify 1 specific finding noted by the nurse during assessment of each of the patient's functional health patterns that indicates a risk factor for musculoskeletal problems or a patient response to an actual musculoskeletal problem.

Functional Health Pattern	Risk Factor for or Response to Musculoskeletal Problem
Health perception–health management	
Nutritional-metabolic	
Elimination	
Activity-exercise	
Sleep-rest	
Cognitive-perceptual	
Self-perception–self-concept	
Role-relationship	
Sexuality-reproductive	
Coping–stress tolerance	
Value-belief	

14. During muscle strength testing, the patient has active movement against gravity and some resistance to pressure. What score would the nurse document? _____

15. When observing the patient, the nurse notes the presence of a limping gait. How would the nurse further evaluate the patient?
    a. Palpate the hips for crepitation.
    b. Measure the length of the limbs.
    c. Evaluate the degree of leg movement.
    d. Compare the muscle mass of 1 leg with the other.

16. A patient with severe joint immobility is receiving physical and exercise therapy. To evaluate the effect of the treatment, the nurse may assess joint range of motion using what equipment?
    a. Ergometer
    b. Myometer
    c. Goniometer
    d. Peak flow meter

17. An adolescent patient referred to the office by the school nurse is found to have a lateral curvature of the spine. How would the nurse document this condition?
    a. Lordosis
    b. Scoliosis
    c. Ankylosis
    d. Kyphosis

18. In report, the nurse is told that the patient has a contracture of the right arm. What would the nurse expect to find when assessing the patient?
    a. A fluid-filled cyst
    b. Generalized muscle pain
    c. Shortening of a muscle or ligament
    d. Grating sensation between bones with movement

19. The patient is diagnosed with torticollis. What care whould the nurse need to provide the patient?
    a. An immobilizer to hold the bones in place
    b. Exercises to increase the strength of the muscles
    c. A pillow to use to support the knees while sleeping
    d. Enough pillows to support the patient's head comfortably

20. The patient describes having burning, sharp pain on the sole of the foot, especially in the morning. What common musculoskeletal problem does this describe?
    a. Pes planus
    b. Tenosynovitis
    c. Plantar fasciitis
    d. Muscle atrophy

21. When assessing the patient, the nurse notices that the patient has foot drop and the foot slaps down on the floor as the patient walks. How would the nurse document this gait?
    a. Ataxic gait
    b. Spastic gait
    c. Antalgic gait
    d. Steppage gait

22. What is the most common diagnostic test used to assess musculoskeletal disorders?
    a. Myelogram
    b. Arthroscopy
    c. Standard x-ray
    d. MRI

23. What test provides fast, precise measurement of the bone mass of the spine, femur, forearm, and total body to evaluate osteoporosis?
    a. Bone scan
    b. Diskogram
    c. Quantitative ultrasound (QUS)
    d. Dual-energy x-ray absorptiometry (DEXA)

24. Which serologic studies would be done to evaluate rheumatoid arthritis? **Select all that apply.**
    a. Uric acid
    b. Anti-DNA antibody
    c. Rheumatoid factor (RF)
    d. Antinuclear antibody (ANA)
    e. C-reactive protein (CRP)
    f. Anticyclic citrullinated peptide (anti-CCP)

Musculoskeletal Trauma and Orthopedic Surgery

1. A 72-year-old man tells the nurse that he cannot perform most of the physical activities he could do 5 years ago because of overall joint aches and pains. What can the nurse do to help the patient prevent further deconditioning and decrease the risk for developing musculoskeletal problems?
   a. Limit weight-bearing exercise to prevent stress on fragile bones and possible hip fractures.
   b. Tell the patient to avoid using canes and walkers because they increase dependence on ambulation aids.
   c. Teach the patient to increase his activity by climbing stairs in buildings and other environments with steps.
   d. Discuss the use of stretching and strengthening exercises to decrease aches and pain so that exercise can be maintained.

2. The patient asks, "What does the doctor mean when he says that I have an avulsion fracture in my leg? I thought I had a sprain!" How would the nurse respond?
   a. "It is a fracture with more than 2 fragments."
   b. "It means that a ligament pulled a bone fragment loose."
   c. "The line of the fracture is twisted along the shaft of the bone."
   d. "The line of the fracture is at right angles to the longitudinal axis of the bone."

3. The patient with osteoporosis had a spontaneous hip fracture. How would the nurse document this type of fracture?
   a. Open fracture
   b. Oblique fracture
   c. Pathologic fracture
   d. Greenstick fracture

4. What kind of injury would the nurse assess for in a patient who works on a computer 8 hours each day?
   a. Meniscus injury
   b. Rotator cuff injury
   c. Radial-ulnar fracture
   d. Carpal tunnel syndrome

5. An athlete comes to the clinic with bursitis. What would the nurse expect is the cause of the patient's pain?
   a. Tearing of a ligament
   b. Stretching of muscle and fascia sheath
   c. Inflammation of synovial membrane sac at friction sites
   d. Incomplete separation of articular surfaces of joint caused by ligament injury

6. Application of RICE (rest, ice, compression, elevation) is indicated for initial management of which type of injury?
   a. Muscle spasms
   b. Sprains and strains
   c. Repetitive strain injury
   d. Dislocations and subluxations

7. During the first 48 hours after an acute soft tissue injury of the ankle, what would be included in the management? **Select all that apply.**
   a. Use of elastic wrap
   b. Initial immobilization and rest
   c. Elevation of ankle above the heart
   d. Alternating the use of heat and cold
   e. Administration of antiinflammatory drugs

8. At 3 weeks to 6 months of fracture healing, there is clinical union which is the first stage of healing that is sufficient to prevent movement of the fracture site when the bones are gently stressed. How is this stage of fracture healing documented?
   a. Ossification
   b. Remodeling
   c. Consolidation
   d. Callus formation

9. The x-ray shows that the patient's fracture is at the remodeling stage. What characteristics of the fracture healing process occur at this stage? **Select all that apply.**
   a. Radiologic union
   b. Absorption of excess bone cells
   c. Return to preinjury strength and shape
   d. Semisolid blood clot at the ends of fragments
   e. Deposition and absorption of bone in response to stress
   f. Unorganized network of bone woven around fracture parts

10. A patient is brought to the emergency department (ED) with an injured lower left leg after falling while rock climbing. The nurse identifies the presence of a fracture based on what cardinal sign?
    a. Muscle spasms
    b. Obvious deformity
    c. Edema and swelling
    d. Pain and tenderness

11. A patient with a fractured femur develops the complication of malunion. The nurse plans care recognizing what has happened to the patient?
    a. The fracture heals in an unsatisfactory position.
    b. The fracture fails to heal properly despite treatment.
    c. Fracture healing progresses more slowly than expected.
    d. Loss of bone substances occurs as a result of immobilization.

12. What is a disadvantage of open reduction and internal fixation (ORIF) of a fracture compared to closed reduction?
    a. Infection
    b. Skin irritation
    c. Nerve impairment
    d. Complications of immobility

13. A young patient with a fractured femur has a hip spica cast applied. What is the most important action by the nurse while the cast is drying?
    a. Elevate the legs above the level of the heart for 24 hours.
    b. Turn the patient to both sides and prone to supine every 2 hours.
    c. Cover the cast with a light blanket to avoid chilling from evaporation.
    d. Assess the patient frequently for abdominal pain, nausea, and vomiting.

14. A patient is admitted with an open fracture of the tibia after a bicycle accident. What information would the nurse obtain when assessing the patient?
    a. Any previous injuries to the leg
    b. The status of tetanus immunization
    c. The use of antibiotics in the last month
    d. Whether the injury was exposed to dirt or gravel

15. A patient who fell in the bathroom of the hospital room reports pain in the upper right arm and elbow. Which action would the nurse take first in managing a possible fracture before splinting the injury?
    a. Elevate the arm
    b. Apply ice to the site
    c. Notify the health care provider
    d. Perform a neurovascular check below the injury

16. How would the nurse assess the neurologic status of the patient with a fractured humerus?
    a. Have the patient evert, invert, dorsiflex, and plantar flex the foot.
    b. Assess the location, quality, and intensity of pain below the site of the injury.
    c. Have the patient abduct the fingers, oppose the thumb and fingers, and flex and extend the wrist.
    d. Assess the color, temperature, capillary refill, peripheral pulses, and edema in the extremity.

17. A patient is discharged from the outpatient clinic after application of a synthetic fiberglass long arm cast for a fractured ulna. Before discharge, what instruction would the nurse provide to the patient?
    a. Never get the cast wet
    b. Move the shoulder and fingers frequently
    c. Place tape petals around the edges of the cast when it is dry
    d. Use a sling to support the arm at waist level for the first 48 hours

18. A patient with a fractured tibia accompanied by extensive soft tissue damage initially has a splint applied and held in place with an elastic bandage. What early sign would alert the nurse that the patient is developing compartment syndrome?
    a. Paralysis of the toes
    b. Absence of peripheral pulses
    c. Distal pain unrelieved by opioid analgesics
    d. Skin over the injury site is blanched when the bandage is removed

19. If surgery is needed, which procedure would the nurse first prepare the patient for to treat compartment syndrome?
    a. Fasciotomy
    b. Amputation
    c. Internal fixation
    d. Release of tendons

20. Which type of fracture can cause radial nerve and brachial artery damage and is reduced with a hanging arm cast?
    a. Fractured tibia
    b. Colles' fracture
    c. Fractured humerus
    d. Femoral shaft fracture

21. A woman with osteoporosis slipped on the ice and reports pain in her wrist. If there is a fracture, what type is expected?
    a. Dislocation
    b. Open fracture
    c. Colles' fracture
    d. Incomplete fracture

22. What emergency considerations are part of the management of facial fractures? **Select all that apply.**
    a. Airway patency
    b. Oral examination
    c. Cervical spine injury
    d. Cranial nerve assessment
    e. Immobilization of the jaw

23. In a patient with a stable vertebral fracture, what would the nurse teach the patient?
    a. Remain on bed rest until the pain is gone.
    b. Logroll to keep the spine straight when turning.
    c. How to use bone cement to correct the problem.
    d. Take as much analgesic as needed to relieve the pain.

24. When is a fat embolism most likely to occur?
    a. 24 to 48 hours after a fractured tibia
    b. 36 to 72 hours after a skull fracture
    c. 4 to 5 days after a fractured femur
    d. 5 to 6 days after a pelvic fracture

25. In a patient with a fracture, what assessment findings distinguish a fat embolism from a pulmonary embolism?
    a. Tachycardia and dyspnea
    b. A sudden onset of chest pain
    c. Petechiae around the neck and upper chest
    d. Electrocardiographic (ECG) changes and decreased partial pressure of oxygen in arterial blood (PaO_2)

26. Which kind of hip fracture is usually repaired with a prosthesis?
    a. Intracapsular
    b. Extracapsular
    c. Subtrochanteric
    d. Intertrochanteric

27. An older adult woman is admitted to the ED after falling at home. What data collected during the patient assessment causes the nurse to caution her to not put weight on the leg?
    a. Inability to move the toes and ankle
    b. Edema of the thigh extending to the knee
    c. Internal rotation of the leg with groin pain
    d. Shortening and external rotation of the leg

28. A patient with an extracapsular hip fracture is admitted to the orthopedic unit and placed in Buck's traction. How would the nurse explain the purpose of the traction to the patient?
    a. Pulls bone fragments back into alignment
    b. Immobilizes the leg until healing is complete
    c. Reduces pain and muscle spasms before surgery
    d. Prevents damage to the blood vessels at the fracture site

29. A patient with a fractured right hip has an anterior ORIF of the fracture. What would the nurse plan to do postoperatively?
    a. Get the patient up to the chair on the first postoperative day.
    b. Ambulate the patient with partial weight bearing by discharge.
    c. Keep the leg abductor pillow on the patient even when bathing.
    d. Position the patient only on the back and the nonoperative side.

30. What would the nurse include in discharge instructions for the patient after a hip prosthesis with a posterior approach?
    a. Restrict walking for 2 to 3 months.
    b. Take a bath rather than a shower to prevent falling.
    c. Keep the leg internally rotated while sitting and standing.
    d. Have a family member help the patient put on shoes and socks.

31. When preparing a patient for discharge after intermaxillary fixation of a mandibular fracture, which statement indicates that patient teaching has been successful?
    a. "I can keep my mouth moist by sucking on hard candy."
    b. "I should cut the wires with scissors if I begin to vomit."
    c. "I may use a bulk-forming laxative if my liquid diet causes constipation."
    d. "I should use a moist swab to clean my mouth every time I eat something."

32. Twenty-four hours after a below-the-knee amputation, a patient uses the call system to tell the nurse that his dressing (a compression bandage) has fallen off. What would be the nurse's first action?
    a. Apply ice to the site.
    b. Cover the incision with dry gauze.
    c. Reapply the compression dressing.
    d. Elevate the extremity on 2 pillows.

33. A patient reports pain in the foot of a leg that was recently amputated. What would the nurse recognize about this pain?
    a. It is caused by swelling at the incision.
    b. It would be treated with ordered analgesics.
    c. It will become worse with the use of a prosthesis.
    d. It can be managed with diversion because it is psychologic.

34. An immediate postoperative prosthetic fitting during surgery is used for a patient with a traumatic below-the-knee amputation. During the immediate postoperative period, what is a priority nursing intervention?
    a. Monitor the patient's vital signs.
    b. Assess the incision for hemorrhage.
    c. Elevate the residual limb on pillows.
    d. Have the patient flex and extend the knee every hour.

35. What is the reason a nurse would position a patient prone several times a day after an above-the-knee amputation with a delayed prosthetic fitting?
    a. To prevent flexion contractures
    b. To assess the posterior skin flap
    c. To reduce edema in the residual limb
    d. To relieve pressure on the incision site

36. A patient who had a below-the-knee amputation is to be fitted with a temporary prosthesis. What is most important to teach the patient?
    a. Inspect the residual limb daily for irritation.
    b. Apply an elastic shrinker before applying the prosthesis.
    c. Perform range-of-motion (ROM) exercises to the affected leg 4 times a day.
    d. Apply alcohol to the residual limb every morning and evening to toughen the skin.

37. Which joint surgery is used to arthroscopically remove devitalized tissue in joints?
    a. Osteotomy
    b. Arthrodesis
    c. Debridement
    d. Synovectomy

38. How would the nurse describe an arthroplasty?
    a. Surgical fusion of a joint to relieve pain
    b. Correction of bone deformity by removal of a wedge or slice of bone
    c. Reconstruction or replacement of a joint to relieve pain and correct deformity
    d. Used in rheumatoid arthritis to remove the tissue involved in joint destruction

39. A patient had a right total hip arthroplasty with a cemented prosthesis for treatment of severe osteoarthritis of the hip. What activity would the nurse include on the patient's first postoperative day?
    a. Transfer from the bed to the chair twice a day only
    b. Only turning from the back to both sides every 2 hours
    c. Crutch walking with non–weight bearing on the operative leg
    d. Ambulation with a walker and limited weight bearing on the right leg

40. When positioning the patient after a total hip arthroplasty with a posterior approach, in what position would the affected extremity be maintained?
    a. Adduction and flexion
    b. Abduction and extension
    c. Abduction and internal rotation
    d. Adduction and external rotation

41. After a total knee arthroplasty, a patient has a continuous passive motion (CPM) machine for the affected joint. What would the nurse explain to the patient is the purpose of this device?
    a. To relieve edema and pain at the incision site
    b. To promote early joint mobility and increase knee flexion
    c. To prevent venous stasis and the formation of a deep venous thrombosis
    d. To improve arterial circulation to the affected extremity to promote healing

42. A patient with severe ulnar deviation of the hands undergoes an arthroplasty with reconstruction and replacement of finger joints. Postoperatively, what is most important for the nurse to do?
    a. Position the fingers lower than the elbow at all times.
    b. Perform neurovascular assessments of the fingers every 2 to 4 hours.
    c. Encourage the patient to gently flex, extend, abduct, and adduct the fingers every 4 hours.
    d. Remind the patient that function of the hands is more important than cosmetic appearance.

43. After change-of-shift handoff, which patient would the nurse assess first?
    a. A 58-year-old male reporting phantom pain and requesting an analgesic
    b. A 72-year-old male being transferred to a skilled nursing unit after repair of a hip fracture
    c. A 25-year-old female in left leg skeletal traction asking for the weights to be lifted for a few minutes
    d. A 68-year-old male with a new lower leg cast reporting the cast is too tight and he cannot feel his toes

CASE STUDY Fracture

Patient Profile

H.A., a 30-year-old telephone lineman, is seen in the emergency department after falling from a pole. His right lower extremity was splinted with a cardboard splint and a large, bulky dressing applied.

(g-stockstudio/
iStock/Thinkstock)

Subjective Data
- Reports severe pain in the right leg
- Expresses concern about notifying his wife about the accident and his whereabouts
- Asks how long he will be off work

Objective Data
- Open oblique fracture of the anterolateral aspect of the tibia
- Obvious deformity, marked swelling, and bruising in region of injury
- To be treated with closed reduction and a cast

Questions

1. When performing a physical assessment of H.A., what assessment findings are expected from this type of injury? **Use an X to indicate if the assessment finding is <u>Expected</u> (normal), <u>Unexpected</u> (indicates a complication) or <u>Unrelated</u> (is not relevant).**

Assessment Finding	Expected	Unexpected	Unrelated
"My right leg feels like pins and needles."			
Right dorsalis pedis pulse 2+			
RLE edema present			
RLE pale and cool			
"I feel a significant amount of tightness in my right leg."			
Moves toes and ankle on RLE			
Reports burning with urination			
Petichiae on the chest			

2. What interventions would the nurse include in H.A.'s plan of care? **Use an X to indicate whether the nursing action is <u>Indicated</u> (is appropriate or necessary), <u>Contraindicated</u> (may be harmful), or <u>Non-essential</u> (makes no difference or is unnecessary).**

Nursing Action	Indicated	Contraindicated	Non-Essential
Apply sequential compression device to RLE			
Apply ice to RLE			
Do not allow weight bearing on the RLE			
Perform ROM exercises with RLE			
Immobilize RLE			
Perform a 12-lead ECG			
Obtain a CBC			
Administer a 1 L bolus of 0.9% saline solution			

3. What patient care can be delegated to assistive personnel (AP)? **Use an X to indicate if the patient care task can be <u>Delegated</u> (the assistive personnel can perform the task) or Cannot be Delegated (the assistive personnel cannot perform the task).**

Patient Care	Delegated	Cannot be Delegated
Elevate the casted RLE on 2 pillows		
Document the skin color and temperature of the RLE		
Teach the patient how to use crutches		
Offer the patient a urinal to void		
Obtain the patient's vital signs		
Give the patient an oral opioid for pain		
Transport the patient to x-ray		

4. What instructions would the nurse include when discharging H.A. from the ED? **Select all that apply.**

_____A. Never put anything down the cast.

_____B. You can take a shower and get the cast wet.

_____C. Do not put any weight on the RLE until approved by your HCP.

_____D. Keep your RLE elevated above your heart as much as possible in the next 72 hours.

_____E. You can drive while taking the opioid pain medication.

_____F. If taking the opioid pain medication, take a stool softener.

_____G. Report any discoloration of your toes on the RLE.

_____H. Foul odor from the cast is expected.

5. **Choose the most likely options for the information missing from the statements below by selecting from the options provided.**

Several problems can be associated with musculoskeletal injuries. _____**1**_____ occur when muscle fibers and ligaments shorten. A decrease in muscle mass is called _____**2**_____ which can be reduced through the use of _____**3**_____. _____**4**_____ may help prevent footdrop which occurs when the _____**5**_____ shortens. _____**6**_____ may reduce _____**7**_____ which are caused by involuntary muscle contractions.

Options for 1, 2, and 7:	Options for 3 and 4:	Options for 5:
Atrophy	ROM exercises	Anterior cruciate ligament
Footdrop	Isometric exercises	Tibialis anterior tendon
Contractures	Crutch walking	Medial collateral ligament
Muscle spasms	High-top tennis shoes	Achilles tendon
Compartment syndrome	Isotonic exercises	Patellar ligament

Options for 6:
NSAIDs
Cryotherapy
Potassium
Thermotherapy
Opioids

1. A patient with chronic osteomyelitis has been hospitalized for a surgical debridement procedure. What would the nurse explain to the patient is the reason for the surgical treatment?
   a. Removal of the infection prevents the need for bone and skin grafting.
   b. Formation of scar tissue has led to a protected area of bacterial growth.
   c. The process of depositing new bone blocks the vascular supply to the bone.
   d. Antibiotics are not effective against microorganisms that cause chronic osteomyelitis.

2. A patient with osteomyelitis is at risk for injury. What is an appropriate nursing intervention?
   a. Use careful and appropriate disposal of soiled dressings.
   b. Gently handle the involved extremity during movement.
   c. Measure the circumference of the affected extremity daily.
   d. Range-of-motion (ROM) exercise every 4 hours to the involved extremity.

3. A patient who had an open fracture of the humerus 2 weeks ago is having increased pain at the fracture site. To determine if the patient has developed osteomyelitis at the site, what diagnostic test would the nurse expect?
   a. X-rays
   b. CT scan
   c. Bone biopsy
   d. White blood cell (WBC) count and erythrocyte sedimentation rate (ESR)

4. After 7 days of IV antibiotic therapy, a patient with acute osteomyelitis of the tibia is preparing for discharge from the hospital. The nurse determines that additional instruction is needed when the patient makes which statement?
   a. "I will need to continue antibiotic therapy for 4 to 6 weeks."
   b. "I will notify the health care provider if the pain in my leg becomes worse."
   c. "I shouldn't bear weight on my affected leg until healing is complete."
   d. "I do not need to do anything special while taking the antibiotic therapy."

5. During a follow-up visit to a patient with acute osteomyelitis treated with IV antibiotics, the home health nurse is told by the patient's wife that she can hardly get the patient to eat because his mouth is so sore. What would the nurse expect when assessing the patient's mouth?
   a. A dry, cracked tongue with a central furrow
   b. White, curdlike membranous lesions of the mucosa
   c. Ulcers of the mouth and lips surrounded by a reddened base
   d. Single or clustered vesicles on the tongue and buccal mucosa

6. Which type of bone tumor is a benign overgrowth of bone and cartilage that may transform into a malignant form?
   a. Enchondroma
   b. Osteoclastoma
   c. Ewing's sarcoma
   d. Osteochondroma

7. Which statement describes osteosarcoma?
   a. High rate of local recurrence
   b. Very malignant and metastasizes early
   c. Arises in cancellous ends of long bones
   d. Develops in the medullary cavity of long bones

8. A 24-year-old patient with a 12-year history of Becker muscular dystrophy is hospitalized with heart failure. What intervention would be included in the plan of care?
   a. Feed and bathe the patient to avoid exhausting the muscle.
   b. Reposition frequently to avoid skin and respiratory complications.
   c. Provide hand weights for the patient to exercise the upper extremities.
   d. Use orthopedic braces to promote ambulation and prevent muscle wasting.

9. What does radicular pain that radiates down the buttock and below the knee, along the distribution of the sciatic nerve, generally indicate?
   a. Cervical disc herniation
   b. Acute lumbosacral strain
   c. Degenerative disc disease
   d. Herniated lumbar disc disease

10. What would the nurse teach the patient recovering from an episode of acute low back pain?
    a. Perform daily exercise as a lifelong routine.
    b. Sit in a chair with the hips higher than the knees.
    c. Avoid occupations in which the use of the body is required.
    d. Sleep on the abdomen or on the back with the legs extended.

11. A laminectomy and spinal fusion were done on a patient with a herniated lumbar intervertebral disc. During the postoperative period, which assessment finding most concerns the nurse?
    a. Paralytic ileus
    b. Urinary incontinence
    c. Greater pain at the graft site than at the lumbar incision site
    d. Leg and arm movement and sensation unchanged from preoperative status

12. What would the nurse do first before repositioning the patient on the side after a lumbar laminectomy?
    a. Raise the head of the bed 30 degrees.
    b. Have the patient flex the knees and hips.
    c. Place a pillow between the patient's legs.
    d. Have the patient grasp the side rail on the opposite side of the bed.

13. The HCP diagnoses a patient with a plantar wart. What would the nurse expect to find when assessing the patient?
    a. Painful papillomatous growth on the sole of the foot
    b. Thickening of skin on the weight-bearing part of the foot
    c. Local thickening of skin caused by pressure on bony prominences
    d. Tumor on nerve tissue between the third and fourth metatarsal heads

14. The patient has lateral angulation of the large toe toward the second toe. What will be included in the treatment?
    a. Metatarsal arch support
    b. Trimming with a scalpel after softening
    c. Surgery to remove the bursal sac and bony enlargement
    d. Intraarticular corticosteroids and passive manual stretching

15. In promoting healthy feet, which factor is associated with most foot problems?
    a. Poor foot hygiene
    b. Congenital deformities
    c. Improperly fitting shoes
    d. Peripheral vascular disease

16. What are characteristics of Paget's disease? **Select all that apply.**
    a. Results from vitamin D deficiency
    b. Loss of total bone mass and substance
    c. Abnormal remodeling and resorption of bone
    d. Most common in bones of spine, hips, and wrists
    e. Generalized bone decalcification with bone deformity
    f. Replacement of normal marrow with vascular connective tissue

17. Which female patients are at risk for developing osteoporosis? **Select all that apply.**
    a. 60-year-old white aerobics instructor
    b. 55-year-old Asian American cigarette smoker
    c. 62-year-old black who takes estrogen therapy
    d. 68-year-old white who is underweight and inactive
    e. 58-year-old Native American who started menopause prematurely

18. Identify ways to prevent osteoporosis in postmenopausal women? **Select all that apply.**
    a. Eating more beef
    b. Eating 8 ounces of yogurt daily
    c. Performing weight-bearing exercise
    d. Spending 15 minutes in the sun each day
    e. Taking postmenopausal estrogen replacement

19. A patient is started on alendronate (Fosamax) once weekly for the treatment of osteoporosis. Which patient statement indicates that further instruction about the drug is needed?
    a. "I should take the drug with a meal to prevent stomach irritation."
    b. "This drug will prevent further bone loss and increase my bone density."
    c. "I need to sit or stand upright for at least 30 minutes after taking the drug."
    d. "I will still need to take my calcium supplements while taking this new drug."

CASE STUDY Herniated Intervertebral Disc

(STEFANOLUNARDI/
iStock/Thinkstock)

Patient Profile
G.B. is a 38-year-old truck driver who slipped on a wet floor at work and landed on his buttocks.

Subjective Data
- Had immediate severe lower back pain with pain radiating into his right buttock
- Had worsening of pain in 3 days with pain radiating down his leg and into his foot
- Reported tingling of his toes
- Rested at home for 2 weeks without relief
- Smokes a pack of cigarettes a day
- History of a fractured femur in his youth

Objective Data
- Height: 5 ft 8 in
- Weight: 213 lbs (96.6 kg)
- BP 148/78 mm Hg, HR 98 beats/min, RR 24 breaths/min, Temperature 98.9°F (37.2°C)

Questions
1. What risk factors for low back pain does G.B. have? **Use an X to indicate whether the assessment finding is a Risk Factor (associated with low back pain) or Unrelated (is not associated with low back pain).**

Assessment Finding	Risk Factor	Unrelated
Height 5 ft 8 in		
BP 148/78 mm Hg		
Weight 213 lbs (96.6 kg)		
Occupation		
History of a fractured femur		
Smokes cigarettes		
Age		

2. What diagnostic tests would the nurse expect to identify the cause of G.B.'s back pain? **Use an X to indicate whether the diagnostic test is <u>Indicated</u> (necessary to help diagnose) or <u>Unrelated</u> (is unnecessary or makes no difference).**

Diagnostic Test	Indicated	Unrelated
MRI		
ABG		
Leg raise test		
PET scan		
CBC		
Epidural venogram		
Lumbar puncture		

3. The HCP diagnoses a herniated disc at L4-5. What clinical manifestations would most concern the nurse? **Highlight the findings in the Nurse's Note below that are clinical manifestations of cauda equina syndrome.**

NURSE'S NOTE:

Pt. is AOx4, responds appropriately to questions. Reports low back pain 5 out of 10 that radiates into his right buttock. He reports tingling in his right toes. He feels the urge to urinate, but is unable. Bladder scan reveals 650 mL. His right inner thigh and buttock feel numb. 3/5 dorsiflexion/plantar flexion in his RLE, 5/5 in his LLE. He has increased pain when RLE is raised. He denies shortness of breath. Lungs CTA. Peripheral pulses 3+ in all extremities. Skin warm and dry throughout.

4. G.B. is status-post a microsurgical discectomy at L4-5. What interventions would the nurse include in G.B.'s plan of care? **Use an X to indicate whether the nursing action is <u>Indicated</u> (is necessary or appropriate), <u>Contraindicated</u> (could be harmful), or is <u>Non-essential</u> (makes no difference or is unnecessary).**

Nursing Action	Indicated	Contraindicated	Non-Essential
Assess dressing			
Report complaints of a headache to the HCP			
Keep the HOB supine at all times			
Collaborate with occupational therapy			
Report lower extremity weakness present preoperatively to the HCP			
Have the patient turn himself independently			
Raise the HOB > 30° if patient reports a headache			
Encourage the use of an incentive spirometer			
Place pillows under knees and thighs to support lower back			

5. G.B. is being discharged home. What instructions would the nurse include when teaching him about self-care at home? **Select all that apply.**

_____A. You can lift weight not exceeding 25 lbs.

_____B. You will need physical therapy.

_____C. Don't stand for long periods of time.

_____D. Sleep on a soft mattress.

_____E. Try not to sleep on your stomach.

_____ F. Report any sensation or motor changes in your lower extremities to your HCP.

_____G. You can go back to work in 2 weeks.

_____H. You should perform daily twisting and stretching exercises.

Arthritis and Connective Tissue Diseases

1. A 60-year-old woman has pain when moving her fingers and asks the nurse if this is just a result of aging. How would the nurse respond?
   a. "Joint pain with functional limitation is a normal change that affects all people to some extent."
   b. "Joint pain that develops with age is usually related to previous trauma or infection of the joints."
   c. "This is a symptom of a systemic arthritis that eventually affects all joints as the disease progresses."
   d. "Changes in the cartilage and bones of joints may cause symptoms of pain and loss of function in some people as they age."

2. Number in order from 1, being the first process, to 6, being the last process, the pathophysiologic processes that occur in osteoarthritis (OA).
   _____a. Erosion of articular surfaces
   _____b. Incongruity in joint surfaces
   _____c. Reduction in motion
   _____d. Joint cartilage becomes yellow and granular
   _____e. Osteophytes form at joint edges
   _____f. Cartilage becomes softer and less elastic

3. What is most likely to cause the pain experienced in the later stages of OA?
   a. Crepitation
   b. Bouchard's nodes
   c. Heberden's nodes
   d. Bone surfaces rubbing together

4. What would the nurse teach the patient with OA to preserve function and the ability to perform activities of daily living (ADLs)?
   a. Avoid exercise that involves the affected joints.
   b. Plan and organize task performance to be less stressful to joints.
   c. Maintain normal activities during an acute episode to prevent loss of function.
   d. Use mild analgesics to control symptoms when performing tasks that cause pain.

5. A patient with OA asks the nurse if he could try glucosamine and chondroitin for symptom management. How would the nurse respond?
   a. "Results of research have been mixed and most medical groups do not recommend their use."
   b. "Most patients find these supplements helpful for relieving arthritis pain and improving mobility."
   c. "These supplements are a fad that have not been shown to reduce pain or increase joint mobility."
   d. "High dosages of these supplements are needed for the patient to receive any benefit in treating OA."

6. A patient taking ibuprofen for treatment of OA has good pain relief but reports increased dyspepsia and nausea. What would the nurse discuss with the patient's health care provider (HCP) about these side effects?
   a. Adding misoprostol to the patient's drug regimen
   b. Substituting naproxen (Naprosyn) for the ibuprofen
   c. Returning to the use of acetaminophen at a dose of 5 g/day instead of 4 g/day
   d. Administering the ibuprofen with antacids to decrease the gastrointestinal (GI) irritation

7. Which description is most characteristic of osteoarthritis (OA) when compared to rheumatoid arthritis (RA)?
   a. Not systemic or symmetric
   b. Rheumatoid factor (RF) positive
   c. Most commonly occurs in women
   d. Morning joint stiffness lasts 1 to several hours

8. What best describes the manifestations of OA?
   a. Smaller joints are typically affected first.
   b. There is joint stiffness after periods of inactivity.
   c. Joint stiffness is accompanied by fatigue, anorexia, and weight loss.
   d. Pain and immobility may be aggravated by falling barometric pressure.

9. What would the nurse check when assessing the patient with early to moderate RA?
   a. Hepatomegaly
   b. Heberden's nodes
   c. Spindle-shaped fingers
   d. Crepitus on joint movement

10. What laboratory results would the nurse expect in the patient with RA?
    a. Polycythemia
    b. Increased immunoglobulin G (IgG)
    c. Decreased white blood cell (WBC) count
    d. Antibodies to citrullinated peptide (anti-CCP)

11. Which extraarticular manifestation of RA is most likely to be seen in the patient with rheumatoid nodules?
    a. Lyme disease
    b. Felty syndrome
    c. Sjögren's syndrome
    d. Spondyloarthropathies

12. Which drug used in the management of RA prevents binding of tumor necrosis factor and inhibits the inflammatory response?
    a. Anakinra (Kineret)
    b. Etanercept (Enbrel)
    c. Leflunomide (Arava)
    d. Azathioprine (Imuran)

13. A patient who has had RA for some time has not had success with previous medications. Although there is an increased risk for tuberculosis, which tumor necrosis factor (TNF) inhibitor may be used with methotrexate to treat symptoms?
    a. Parenteral gold
    b. Certolizumab (Cimzia)
    c. Tocilizumab (Actemra)
    d. Hydroxychloroquine (Plaquenil)

14. A 70-year-old patient is being evaluated for symptoms of RA. What would the nurse recognize as the major problem in the management of RA in the older adult?
    a. RA is usually more severe in older adults.
    b. Older patients are not as likely to comply with treatment regimens.
    c. Drug interactions and toxicity are more likely to occur with multidrug therapy.
    d. Laboratory and other diagnostic tests are not effective in identifying RA in older adults.

15. After teaching a patient with RA about the prescribed therapeutic regimen, which patient statement indicates that further instruction is needed?
    a. "It is important for me to perform my prescribed exercises every day."
    b. "I should do most of my daily chores in the morning when my energy level is highest."
    c. "An ice pack to a joint for 10 minutes may help relieve pain when I have an acute flare."
    d. "I can use assistive devices, like padded utensils and elevated toilet seats, to protect my joints."

16. A patient recovering from an acute exacerbation of RA tells the nurse that she is too tired to bathe. What would the nurse do?
    a. Give the patient a bed bath to conserve her energy.
    b. Allow the patient a rest period before showering with the nurse's help.
    c. Tell the patient that she can skip bathing if she will walk in the hall later.
    d. Teach the patient that it is important for her to maintain self-care activities.

17. After teaching a patient with RA to use heat and cold therapy to relieve symptoms, which patient statement indicates to the nurse that teaching has been effective?
    a. "Heat treatments cannot be used if muscle spasms are present."
    b. "Cold applications can be applied for 25 to 30 minutes to relieve joint stiffness."
    c. "I can use heat applications for 25 minutes to relieve the symptoms of an acute flare."
    d. "When my joints are painful, using a bag of frozen corns for 10 to 15 minutes may relieve the pain."

18. Which exercise would the nurse teach the patient with RA is the most effective method of aerobic exercise?
    a. Ballet dancing
    b. Casual walking
    c. Aquatic exercises
    d. Low-impact aerobic exercises

19. A patient is seen at the outpatient clinic for a sudden onset of inflammation and severe pain in the great toe. What establishes a definitive diagnosis of gouty arthritis?
    a. A family history of gout
    b. Elevated urine uric acid levels
    c. Elevated serum uric acid levels
    d. Presence of monosodium urate crystals in synovial fluid

20. During treatment of the patient with an acute attack of gout, which drug would the nurse expect to administer first?
    a. Aspirin
    b. Colchicine
    c. Probenecid
    d. Allopurinol

21. A patient with gout is treated with drug therapy to prevent future attacks. What would the nurse teach the patient?
    a. Have periodic testing of serum uric acid levels.
    b. Avoid all foods high in purine, such as organ meats.
    c. Increase the dose of medication with the onset of an acute attack.
    d. Perform active range of motion (ROM) of all joints that are affected by gout.

22. What characteristics are common in spondyloarthropathies associated with human leukocyte antigen (HLA)–B27?
    a. Presence of RF
    b. Symmetric polyarticular arthritis
    c. Absence of extraarticular disease
    d. Sacroiliac and peripheral joint involvement

23. What would the nurse teach the patient with ankylosing spondylitis?
    a. Wear roomy shoes with good orthotic support.
    b. Sleep on the side with the knees and hips flexed.
    c. Keep the spine slightly flexed while sitting, standing, or walking.
    d. Perform back, neck, and chest stretches and deep-breathing exercises.

24. Which statements describe reactive arthritis? **Select all that apply.**
    a. Methotrexate is an initial treatment of choice
    b. Symptoms include urethritis and conjunctivitis
    c. Diagnosed by finding of hypersensitive tender points
    d. Increased risk in persons with decreased host resistance
    e. Infection of a joint often caused by hematogeneous route
    f. Self-limiting arthritis following genitourinary or GI tract infections

25. What characterizes the pathophysiology of systemic lupus erythematosus (SLE)?
    a. Destruction of nucleic acids and other self-proteins by autoantibodies
    b. Overproduction of collagen that disrupts the functioning of internal organs
    c. Formation of abnormal IgG that attaches to cellular antigens, activating complement
    d. Increased activity of T suppressor cells with B-cell hypoactivity, resulting in an immunodeficiency

26. What is an ominous sign of advanced SLE?
    a. Proteinuria from early glomerulonephritis
    b. Anemia from antibodies against blood cells
    c. Dysrhythmias from fibrosis of the atrioventricular node
    d. Cognitive dysfunction from immune complex deposit in the brain

27. A patient with newly diagnosed SLE asks the nurse how the disease will affect her life. What is the nurse's best response?
    a. "You can plan to have a near-normal life, since SLE rarely causes death."
    b. "It is hard to say because the disease is so variable in its severity and progression."
    c. "Life span is shortened in people with SLE, but the disease can be controlled with long-term corticosteroid use."
    d. "Most people with SLE have alternating periods of remissions and exacerbations that rapidly progress to permanent organ damage."

28. During an acute exacerbation, a patient with SLE is treated with corticosteroids. The nurse would expect tapering of the corticosteroids to begin when which serum laboratory results are evident?
    a. Decreased anti-DNA
    b. Increased complement
    c. Increased red blood cells (RBCs)
    d. Decreased erythrocyte sedimentation rate (ESR)

29. What would the nurse include in the teaching plan for the patient with SLE?
    a. Ways to avoid exposure to sunlight
    b. Ways to increase dietary protein and carbohydrate intake
    c. The need for genetic counseling before planning a family
    d. The use of nonpharmacologic pain interventions instead of analgesics

30. What would the nurse expect when assessing the patient with scleroderma?
    a. Thickening of the skin of the fingers and hands
    b. Cool, cyanotic fingers with thinning skin over the joints
    c. Swan neck deformity or ulnar drift deformity of the hands
    d. Low back pain, stiffness, and limitation of spine movement

31. When caring for the patient with CREST syndrome (calcinosis, Raynaud's phenomenon, esophageal dysfunction, sclerodactyly, and telangiectasia) associated with scleroderma, what would the nurse teach the patient to do?
    a. Maintain a fluid intake of at least 3000 mL/day.
    b. Avoid exposure to the sun or other ultraviolet light.
    c. Monitor and keep a log of daily BP.
    d. Protect the hands and feet from cold exposure and injury.

32. During the acute phase of dermatomyositis, what is an appropriate patient outcome?
    a. Relates improvement in pain
    b. Does not experience aspiration
    c. Performs active ROM 4 times daily
    d. Maintains absolute rest of affected joints

33. During assessment of the patient diagnosed with fibromyalgia, what would the nurse expect the patient to report in addition to widespread pain?
    a. Generalized muscle twitching and spasms
    b. Nonrestorative sleep with resulting fatigue
    c. Profound and progressive muscle weakness that limits ADLs
    d. Widespread musculoskeletal pain that is accompanied by inflammation and fever

34. What is 1 criterion identified by the American College of Rheumatology for a diagnosis of fibromyalgia?
    a. Fiber atrophy found on muscle biopsy
    b. Elimination of all other causes of musculoskeletal pain
    c. The elicitation of pain on palpation of at least 11 of 18 identified tender points
    d. The presence of manifestations of systemic exertion intolerance disease (SEID)

35. What would the nurse teach the patient with fibromyalgia?
    a. Rest the muscles as much as possible to avoid triggering pain.
    b. Plan night-time sleep and naps to obtain 12 to 14 hours of sleep a day.
    c. Try using food supplements, such as glucosamine and chondroitin, for pain relief.
    d. Use techniques, such as meditation and cognitive behavioral therapy, to manage stress.

36. A patient with debilitating fatigue has been diagnosed with SEID. Which criteria are considered the 3 major symptoms and the 1 additional manifestation that must be present to make this diagnosis? **Select all that apply.**
    a. Unrefreshing sleep
    b. Unexplained muscle pain
    c. Cognitive impairment ("brain fog")
    d. Profound fatigue lasting for 6 months
    e. Tender cervical or axillary lymph nodes
    f. Headaches of a new type, pattern, or severity
    g. Total exhaustion after minor physical or mental exertion

CASE STUDY Rheumatoid Arthritis

(Yann Poirier/
iStock/Thinkstock)

Patient Profile
N.M. is a 36-year-old overweight woman who thinks she has arthritis. When her symptoms began to interfere with her daily activities, she sought medical help.

Subjective Data
* Reports painful, stiff hands and feet
* Feels tired all of the time
* Reports an intermittent low-grade fever
* Takes naproxen (Aleve) 220 mg twice daily
* Wears a copper bracelet on the advice of a neighbor

Objective Data
* Hands show mild ulnar drift and puffiness
* Temp: 100°F (37.8°C)

Questions
1. The nurse determines that N.M. has either rheumatoid arthritis or osteoarthritis. What clinical manifestations are associated with each of these 2 types of arthritis? **Use an X to indicate if the assessment finding is associated with <u>Rheumatoid Arthritis</u>, <u>Osteoarthritis</u>, or <u>Both</u>.**

Assessment Finding	Rheumatoid Arthritis	Osteoarthritis	Both
Age			
Fatigue			
Low-grade fever			
Painful, stiff hands and feet			
Mild ulnar drift			
Puffy hands			
Overweight			

2. What diagnostic studies would confirm the diagnosis of RA? **Use an X to indicate if the diagnostic study is <u>Indicated</u> (helps diagnose RA) or is <u>Unrelated</u> (will not help diagnose RA).**

Diagnostic Study	Indicated	Unrelated
Rheumatoid factor		
Joint ultrasound		
Electrolyte panel		
C-reactive protein		

Diagnostic Study	Indicated	Unrelated
V/Q scan		
Antinuclear antibody (ANA) titer		
Bone scan		

3. What interventions would the nurse include when caring for N.M. in the acute care setting? **Use an X to indicate if the nursing action is Indicated (is necessary or appropriate), Contraindicated (may be harmful), or Non-Essential (is unnecessary or makes no difference).**

Nursing Action	Indicated	Contraindicated	Non-Essential
Obtain a physical therapy consult			
Restrict purines in her diet			
Administer antibiotics as ordered			
Assess labs for evidence of leukocytosis			
Assist with ROM exercises			
Check urine for hematuria			
Use assistive devices as necessary			
Administer calcium channel blockers as ordered			

4. N.M. will be started on drug therapy to treat RA. The following drugs are possible options for her treatment. **Choose the most likely options for the information missing from the table below by selecting from the lists of options provided. Note that options will only be used once.**

Drug	Mechanism of Action	Nursing Consideration
1	Inhibits DNA/RNA synthesis	Report severe fatigue
Hydroxychloroquine	May suppress antigen formation	2
3	Analgesic	Avoid sun and UV light exposure
Rituximab	4	Monitor for bleeding
Sulfasalazine	Blocks prostaglandin synthesis	5
6	Binds to TNF	Increased risk for tuberculosis
Prednisone	Inhibits synthesis of inflammatory mediators	7
Capsaicin	8	Risk for topical burn

Options for 1, 3, and 6	Options for 4 and 8	Options for 2, 5, and 7
Methotrexate	Sulfonamide	Report vision changes
Abatacept	Depletes substance P	Don't use with heating pads
Diclofenac	Cox-2 inhibitor	Avoid pregnancy
Tofacitinib	Immunomodulatory agent	Limit potassium intake
Acetaminophen	NSAID	Avoid overusing affected joint
Adalimumab	Monoclonal antibody	Monitor for change in level of consciousness
Anakinra	Antimetabolite	May cause orange-yellow urine or skin
Mycophenolate	Interleukin-1 receptor antagonist	Taper dose to withdrawal from drug

5. The HCP prescribes methotrexate to treat N.M.'s RA. What would the nurse teach N.M. about this drug? **Select all that apply.**

_____A. It has a lower risk for toxicity than other drugs.
_____B. It won't increase your risk of infection.
_____C. You should see therapeutic effects with 4–6 weeks.
_____D. It may be necessary to add another drug.
_____E. We need to do a pregnancy test before starting the drug.
_____F. The drug must be stopped 6 months before you become pregnant.
_____G. This medication is a chemotherapeutic agent used to treat cancer.
_____H. Rare side effects include kidney failure.
_____I. This drug may cause you to lose your hair.

CHAPTER 1

1. a, b, d, f, g, i
2. a, b, d. Certification usually requires an examination to verify a certain knowledge base and clinical experience in the specialty area to develop the expertise. Certification is a voluntary process that gives recognition of one's expertise.
3. b. Standards of Practice describe a competent level of nursing based on the nursing process. Standards of Professional Performance describe behavioral competencies expected of a nurse. Quality and Safety Education for Nurses defines specific competencies nurses need to possess to practice safely and effectively. The state Nurse Practice Act defines nursing scope of practice in addition to delegating patient care.
4. QSEN's 6 competencies are: (1) patient-centered care, (2) teamwork and collaboration, (3) safety, (4) quality improvement, (5) informatics, and (6) evidence-based practice.
5. Numbered in order:
   6 Share the results of the EBP change
   1 Ask a clinical question
   3 Critically analyze the evidence
   2 Find and collect the evidence
   5 Evaluate patient outcomes
   4 Implementing the evidence in practice
6. b. The *C* part of the PICOT format stands for Comparison. "Restraint" is the Intervention. "During a seizure" is the Time period. "Adult seizure patients" is the Patient/population. "Protecting them from injury" is the Outcome.
7. d. Evidence-based clinical practice guidelines are developed from summaries of research results and reflect the best-known state of practice at the time. Use of these guidelines leads to more positive outcomes of care and would be best to use in planning care or programs.
8. c. An electronic health record (EHR) is being used to place patient care orders, review and update patient's health records, and document care provided. The cost is not reduced; more people have access to the records, but this is being monitored to protect patient privacy; all health systems are currently not able to communicate via EHRs.
9. a. 2; b. 3; c. 4; d. 1; e. 2; f. 5; g. 3; h. 2; i. 5; j. 4
10. a, c, d. Clinical problems are based on a single clinical finding, such as pain or anxiety, or result from a complex decision about a particular focus, such as impaired nutrition or musculoskeletal problem. Sepsis, COPD, and myocardial infarction are medical diagnoses.
11. Many answers may be correct. Examples include the following:
    a. Turn the patient every 2 hours using the following schedule: L side to back to R side to L side to back. Inspect and document all at-risk areas for blanching and erythema during each position change.
    b. Provide 8 oz. of fluids every 2 hours (even hours) while the patient is awake (the patient prefers cold liquids). Assist the patient in choosing 5 fresh fruits or vegetables from the menu each day.

12. d. The mistake was made during assessment when the nurse did not ask why the patient had not taken her medication regularly and the etiology for the clinical problem was not validated.
13. b, d, f, g, h. Right task, right person, right circumstance, right supervision and evaluation, right directions and communication.
14. a, c, d, f, g. These actions or interventions require judgment and clinical decision making; therefore they should be performed by a registered nurse (RN).
15. 3 A plan that directs an entire health care team
    1 Used as guides for routine nursing care
    1, 2 Used in nursing education to teach the nursing process and care planning
    3 A description of patient care required at specific times during treatment
    1 Should be personalized and specific to each patient
    2 A visual diagram representing relationships between patient problems, interventions, and data
    3 Used for high-volume and highly predictable case types
16. c, e. Hands are to be washed with soap and water or gel before and after each patient. Quickly communicating test results to the right staff person increases effectiveness of patient care by the health care team. Restraints are not suggested as part of the National Patient Safety Goals (NPSG), although evaluating fall risk and taking action to reduce fall risk are included. All medications may not be administered if there is interaction between them. The health care provider (HCP) would be notified before administering any questionable medications. The "time-out" is not for the nurse's fatigue but to ensure that the correct patient procedure and site are verified before surgical procedures. To prevent health care–related pressure ulcers, NPSG suggest assessing patients at risk initially on admission and on a regular basis throughout their care. To improve the accuracy of patient identification, it is suggested that 2 identifiers are used whenever a patient is identified, including for but not limited to medication administration.
17. a, b, c, e. Clinical outcomes, patient satisfaction, use of evidence-based practice, and occurrence of serious reportable events are all care and performance initiatives that influence payment for health care services by third-party payers. Adoption of information technology no longer affects payment for care, although requirements for the Affordable Care Act are changing in this area.
18. c. Accountable Care Organizations (ACO) are the groups that coordinate care to ensure the right care is given at the right time. National Quality Forum (NQF) reduces the occurrence of serious reportable events by providing a list of effective *Safe Practices* to be used in health care settings. Preferred provider organizations (PPOs) and health maintenance organizations (HMOs) provide health care services with charges established with predetermined reimbursement rates or capitation fees in advance of the medical, hospital, and other health care services delivered.

CHAPTER 2

1. b. The determinants of health are factors that influence the health of individuals and groups. The major determinant of health is behavior. Although the other factors could influence this patient's health, the smoking behavior is the *most* important causative factor in this situation.

2. a. Rural setting; b. Low income; c. Gender; d. Age. Low health literacy also leads to health disparities.

3. a, b, e, f. Health literacy is the patient's ability to obtain, process, and understand basic health information needed to make appropriate decisions. Age, language, and education influence the patient's ability to read, understand, and analyze information to make health care decisions. Place may be associated with limited health literacy because rural populations tend to be older and have lower literacy rates. The accepted health behaviors are affected by the areas in which people grow up, work, and live. Although gender, race, ethnicity, and sexual preferences are not associated with health literacy, they may lead to health disparity.

4. a, b, c. Values, culture, and ethnicity provide the nurse with information to help plan care for the patient that ensures that cultural histories, experiences, and traditions are valued. Stereotyping, acculturation, and ethnocentrism all presuppose information about the individual because of their culture or ethnicity without assessing the individual.

5. d. Culture is dynamic and ever changing, may not be shared by all members of the same cultural group, is adapted to specific conditions such as environmental factors, and is learned through oral and written histories as well as socialization.

6. a. Cultural skill is the ability to complete a cultural assessment by collecting cultural data.

7. Examples may include, but are not limited to, any instances *given in the Table below*:

Cultural Factor	Effect on Nursing Care	Health Care Team
Time orientation	Patients may be late for appointments, skip appointments entirely, or delay seeing a HCP because social events are more important to them.	HCPs may be late to work or in providing time-sensitive care.
Economic factors	Lack of health insurance, limited financial resources, or undocumented immigrant status may deter patients from using the health care system.	The health care worker may not be able to afford new uniform items or transportation to work.
Nutrition	Ethnic foods may be high in sodium and fat or low in calcium and protein. If dietary changes required by health problems are not made within the context of the patient's normal diet, chances are high that the patient will not make the changes.	Ethnic foods may not be available in the cafeteria, so the HCP must bring food for meals.
Personal space	Personal space zones are a variable and subjective cultural trait.	A patient may move closer to the nurse, causing a feeling of discomfort for the nurse, or if the nurse increases the personal space, the patient may be offended.
Beliefs and practices	Religious beliefs or practices, faith in folk medicine, or negative experiences with culturally insensitive health care may delay or prevent patients from seeking health care.	Health care workers may need to practice certain behaviors while at work (i.e., fasting during Ramadan, not caring for patients having abortions, not eating milk and meat together).

8. As a follower of Islam, eating pork is prohibited (this is also true for strict followers of Judaism). Hinduism prohibits eating meat because it harms a living creature. Judaism prohibits eating shellfish as well as predatory fowl. Seventh Day Adventism encourages a vegetarian diet.

9.

Social Determinant of Health	Health Disparity
Neighborhood	Poor living conditions or overcrowding can negatively impact health as well as living in high crime areas or in poverty. Rural residents have higher obesity and cancer rates.
Economic stability	Those with lower incomes cannot afford health care, food or safe housing. They may work in hazardous jobs or occupations. They die at younger ages.
Education	Impacts health literacy. Those with lower education levels are 3 times likelier to die before age 65.
Health care	Those who are uninsured, underinsured or lack financial resources forgo health care visits, screenings, and treatments. They may encounter bias and discrimination in the health care setting.
Community context	Positive relationships improve health. People who are bullied may not get the support they need.

10. a. A *curandera* is a folk healer who in some parts of Mexico and Central and South American countries is used because they speak their native language and is less expensive than traditional health care providers. *Parteras* are midwives that some Latino women may request.

11. b. In some cultural groups, especially Asian, Hispanic, and Native American, there is an emphasis on interdependence

rather than independence. The nurse should be aware that in some cultures, decisions for the patient may be made by other family members or may be made collectively by the patient and their family. All the other options reflect an insensitive assumption that the patient should make an autonomous decision.

12. a. Community context; b. Economic stability; c. Neighborhood; d. Health care; e. Education

13. d. Antihypertensives are not responded to as well by blacks as they are by European Americans. There is no difference in the effect of analgesics, anticoagulants, or benzodiazepines.

14. a, b, e. Muslim-Arab women exhibit modesty when avoiding eye contact with men other than their husbands and when in public situations. Many Native Americans are comfortable with silence and interpret silence as essential for thinking and carefully considering a response. In traditional Asian cultures, the speaker may stop talking and leave a period of silence for the listener to think about what was said before continuing.

15. a, d. To communicate with a patient who does not speak the dominant language, the nurse should obtain an interpreter. But if one is not available, use of pantomime with specific words and a website or phrase book with both the nurse's and patient's language may be helpful. The patient may think you are angry if you speak in a loud voice. Only use family members if there are no other choices.

16. a, c. Using cultural competency guidelines guides the nurse in practice. Using standardized evidence-based care guidelines guides care based on the patient's outcomes. Using a family member as the interpreter is not recommended because of the possibility of misunderstanding as well as potential privacy issues. Completing the health history rapidly may not allow patients from other cultures than the nurse to explain themselves well enough. Racial cultural differences cannot be assumed. The individual patient must be assessed to determine the differences to be included in the care.

CHAPTER 3

1.

Subjective	Objective
Short of breath, pain in chest upon breathing, coughing makes head hurt, aches all over	Respiratory rate of 28 breaths/minute, coughing up yellow sputum, skin hot and moist, temperature 102.2°F (39°C), increased white blood cell (WBC) count

2. d. The focused assessment is used to evaluate the status of previously identified problems and monitor for signs of new problems. In this case, the chest must be assessed related to the shortness of breath, chest pain with breathing, increased respiratory rate, yellow sputum, increased temperature, and elevated WBC count. If the patient's headache and achiness are not reduced after the cough and temperature have been treated, further nursing and medical assessments will be done.

3. Examples: many answers could be correct. It is helpful to preface the question with the reason it is being asked.

a. "Many patients taking drugs for hypertension have problems with sexual function. Have you experienced any problems?"

b. "Alcohol may interact dangerously with drugs you receive, or it may cause withdrawal problems in the hospital. Can you describe your recent alcohol intake?"

c. "It is important to contact and treat others who may have the same infection you do. Would you tell me with whom you have been sexually intimate in the last 6 weeks?"

d. "Today medications are so expensive that some people must choose between eating and taking their medications. Are you able to get and take all of the medications prescribed for you?"

4. d. Data are required regarding the immediate problem, but gathering additional information can be delayed. The patient should not receive pain medication before pertinent information related to allergies or the nature of the problem is obtained. Questions that require brief answers do not elicit adequate information for a health profile.

5. c. When a patient describes a feeling, the nurse should ask about the factors surrounding the situation to clarify the etiology of the problem. An incorrect clinical problem may be assigned if the statement is taken literally and its meaning is not explored with the patient. A sense of "being tired and unable to function" does not necessarily indicate a need for rest or sleep, and there is no way to know that treatment will relieve the problem.

6. There may be many correct answers. Examples include the following:
   a. "Can you tell me how you are feeling?"
   b. "Describe your relationship with your spouse."
   c. "Can you describe your experience with this illness?"
   d. "What is your usual activity during the day?"

7. c, d, e. Severity, palliative, and radiation are not addressed. The timing, quality, and precipitating factors are described.

8. a. 1; b. 10; c. 10; d. 8; e. 4; f. 4, 12; g. 2, 3; h. 3; i. 3; j. 6; k. 7; l. 5; m. 3, 9; n. 2; o. 4; p. 12; q. 11; r. 2; s. 10; t. 13

9. d. Abnormal lung sounds are usually associated with chronic bronchitis, and their absence is a negative finding. Chest pain is a positive finding, and radiation is not expected for all chest pain. Elevated BP in hypertension is a positive finding, and pupils that are equal and react to light and accommodation are normal findings.

10. a. 2; b. 4; c. 3; d. 2; e. 1; f. 4; g. 1; h. 2

11. d. The usual sequence of physical assessment techniques is inspection, palpation, percussion, and auscultation. However, because palpation and percussion can alter bowel sounds, in abdominal assessment the sequence should be inspection, auscultation, percussion, and palpation.

12. b. A nurse should use the same efficient sequence in each examination to avoid forgetting a procedure, a step in the sequence, or a body part. However, a specific method is not required. Patient safety, comfort, and privacy are considerations but are not the priorities. The nursing history data should be collected in an interview to avoid prolonging the examination.

13. b, c, e. Older adults may have decreased vision and hearing, so providing a quiet environment free from distractions will make the assessment easier than having the distraction of the TV.

14. b, c. These are situations in which an initial and thorough baseline assessment must be completed. Options a and e

would require focused assessments; option d would require an emergency assessment.

15. a, b, e. The watch is used to assess pulses, the stethoscope is used to hear pulses and heart sounds, and the BP cuff is used to assess BP. The ophthalmoscope is used to assess the retina, and the percussion hammer is used to assess reflexes.

16. c. Subjective data or symptoms are obtained by interview during the nursing history. These data can be described only by the patient or caregiver. Objective data or signs are data that are obtained on physical examination. Comprehensive data are obtained from a detailed health history and physical examination of 1 or more body systems.

17. a, d, e. The general survey is considered a scanning procedure that includes mental state, behavior, speech, body movements, body features, obvious physical signs, and nutritional status. The physical examination includes auscultation and percussion of lung sounds and bowel sounds, palpation of body temperature and pulses, auscultation of pulses and heart sounds, and inspection of mobility. If there are obvious physical signs or abnormal sounds, a focused assessment will be done to assess the specific problems.

CHAPTER 4

1. a. Health promotion. b. Management of illness.
   c. Appropriate choice and use of treatment options.
   d. Disease prevention.
2. Stated in your own words, the answer should be something like this: Use every opportunity (interaction [e.g., administering medications]) to assess patients for educational needs, to provide the teaching needed, and to reinforce the teaching that has already occurred. The time for patient teaching is limited, and every opportunity must be used efficiently.
3. a, b, e. Learning is acquiring a skill or knowledge and may occur from experience rather than teaching. Planned teaching using a variety of methods may increase learning, and teaching that is planned helps make learning more efficient. Teaching may occur as an incidental experience without prior planning. One hopes that the learner's behavior will change as a result of teaching. However, it is the choice of the learner to either change behavior or not.
4. a. 1, 2; b. 1, 2, 4, 6; c. 2, 4; d. 5; e. 2, 6; f. 2, 4, 5; g. 3
5. c. This patient is in the precontemplation stage of behavior change; he is not considering a change, nor is he ready to learn. During this stage, the best intervention by the nurse is to describe the benefits of change and the risks of not changing. The consequences of not changing should not be presented as threats but rather as a disadvantage of the current behavior. Describing what is involved in behavior change and setting priorities are recommended for later stages of change.
6. a. Example: A sudden episode (acute) in which the heart muscle (myocardium) is damaged from a lack of blood supply (infarction) b. Example: The IV injection of a dye to visually record (-gram) the kidneys (pylon-) c. Example: Damage (-pathy) to the retina (retino-) of the eye as a complication of diabetes
7. b. An empathetic approach to teaching requires that the nurse provide positive feedback and try to understand the

patient's world. The other options are important but are not directly related to empathy.

8.

Barrier	Strategy
Lack of time	Set learning priorities with the patient and use every encounter. Let the patient know how much time you have for each session.
Your feeling as a teacher	Prepare ahead of time. Use available written materials. Respect the patient's response to the health problem.
Nurse-patient differences	Expectations of teaching may be different for the patient, caregiver, and nurse. The patient may not be ready to learn or understand the urgency of the teaching and the early discharge.

9. c. Because the patient's father died of a myocardial infarction at a young age, the nurse needs to assess how his anxiety may affect his ability to learn about his treatment and follow-up care. There is no information about the learner characteristics or sociocultural characteristics, although these areas would also need to be assessed.

10. b. To promote self-efficacy it is important that the person is successful in new endeavors to strengthen the belief in their ability to manage a situation. To avoid early failure, the nurse should work with the patient to present simple concepts related to knowledge and skills that the person already has. Motivation and relevancy are important factors in adult learning but are more often a result of self-efficacy, not a method of promoting it.

11.

Patient Characteristic	Teaching Intervention
Impaired hearing	Use supplementary illustrations and written materials. Provide audiotapes or audiovisual presentations with headphones that block environmental noise and promote auditory function.
Patient refuses to see a need for a change in health behaviors	Support the patient during this time and do not argue about the need for a change in health behaviors. Wait until the patient is ready to learn before beginning teaching.
Drowsiness caused by use of sedatives	Evaluate the medication schedule and change it, if possible, to increase alertness. If sedation is the objective of the medication, consider teaching family members or other caregivers.
Presence of pain	Provide only brief explanations and wait until the pain has been controlled to present more detailed instruction.
Uncertain of reading ability	Be sure that educational materials are written at fifth-grade or lower reading level. Use audiovisual materials with simple, layperson language.

Patient Characteristic	Teaching Intervention
Visual learning style	Provide a variety of written educational materials. Refer the patient to appropriate Internet resources for information.
Primary language is not English	Use interpreters and translation software programs. Obtain patient teaching materials in the patient's primary language.

12. c. Adjusting to rather than opposing the patient's resistance, as well as expressing empathy and reinforcing the positive outcome of attending therapy previously, will encourage her to continue therapy. The other options are argumentative and confrontational, focus on the negative rather than the patient's strengths, and do not help the patient recognize the "gap" between where she is and where she hopes to be.

13. Example: By the time of discharge the patient will identify foods that are high in potassium from a given list of common foods.

14. a, c, d, f. DVDs, discussion, printed materials, and Web-based programs can be left with the patient, then discussed or "taught back" later to be sure that all goals are met. Role play and lecture-discussion may take more time than is available to meet the goals.

15. c. If audiovisual and written materials do not help the patient meet the learning goals, they are a waste of time and expense. The nurse should ensure that these materials are accurate and appropriate for each patient. Audiovisual materials are often supplementary materials that are used either before or after other presentation of information and do not have to include all the information the patient needs to learn to be of value. Patients with auditory and visual limitations may find these materials useful because they can adjust the volume and size of the images.

16. a, e. When using the Internet as a teaching strategy, the nurse will assist the patient or caregiver in accessing trustworthy sites. The nurse personally cannot evaluate all sites that a patient or caregiver uses. The Internet is a valuable source of health information, but it is also unregulated and much information is unreliable or inaccurate. As a result, both nurses and patients should learn to evaluate sources and identify accurate information. Reliable sources include universities, government health agencies, and reputable health care organizations.

17.

Learning Goal	Evaluation Technique
The patient will demonstrate to the nurse the preparation and administration of a subcutaneous insulin injection to himself with correct technique before discharge.	Direct observation

Learning Goal	Evaluation Technique
Before discharge, the patient will identify 5 serious side effects of Coumadin that should be reported to the HCP.	Ask a direct question or use a written measurement tool (ask the patient to write down the serious side effects that must be reported to the doctor)
The patient's wife will select the foods highest in potassium for each meal from the hospital menu with 80% accuracy.	Direct observation with observation of verbal and nonverbal cues
The patient will verbalize "no shortness of breath" when ambulating unassisted with the walker each of 3 times a day.	Direct observation with observation of verbal and nonverbal cues
The patient's caregiver will state that they are ready to change the patient's dressing today.	Talk with a member of the patient's family and then observe the dressing change to validate the caregiver's self-evaluation

18. b. A statement that documents what the patient does as a result of teaching indicates whether the learning objective has been met and provides the best documentation of patient instruction. "Understand" is not a measurable behavior and does not validate that learning has occurred.

19. d, f. Baby boomers grew up sitting quietly in rows at school with the teacher lecturing or watching a movie and then discussing the information. They are used to learning with these methods, although some individuals may be comfortable with the other methods as well.

20. a, b, c, e. With the stressors the daughter is experiencing, the best strategies to help her cope are to keep a journal; get regular exercise; join a support group to share feelings and learn she is not alone; and use humor for both herself and her father. A weight loss diet could increase stress at this time. Reading more books could distract her but also take her away from her father's needs, so this is not the best strategy.

CHAPTER 5

1. b, c, e, f. The diabetes and residual right-sided weakness from the cerebrovascular accident (CVA) contribute to the residual disability and permanent impairments. Diabetes requires long-term management, and both problems contribute to nonreversible pathologic changes.

2.

Chronic Condition	Task
Diabetes	Prevent and manage crisis, carry out prescribed regimen, control symptoms, adjust to changes in the course of the disease

Chronic Condition	Task
Visual impairment	Prevent social isolation, try to normalize interactions with others
Heart disease	Carry out prescribed regimen, control symptoms, prevent and manage a crisis
Hearing impairment	Prevent social isolation, try to normalize interactions with others
Alzheimer's disease	Prevent and manage crisis, reorder time, control symptoms, adjust to changes in the course of the disease, try to normalize interactions with others, prevent social isolation
Arthritis	Control symptoms, carry out prescribed regimen, reorder time, adjust to changes in the course of the disease, prevent social isolation
Orthopedic impairment	Reorder time, prevent and manage crisis, prevent social isolation

3. a. secondary; b. primary
4. c. Heart disease is the leading cause of death in the United States.
5. d. The trajectory defines a life-threatening situation as a crisis. Increasing disability is described as downward. A gradual return to an acceptable way of life is a comeback.
6. a, b, d, e. Ageism is a negative attitude based on age.
7. There may be other correct responses, but examples include the following:
   a. Decreased intestinal villi, decreased digestive enzyme production and secretion, decreased dentine and gingival retraction, decreased taste of salt and sugar
   b. Decreased force of cardiac contraction, decreased cardiac muscle mass, increased fat and collagen
   c. Decreased skeletal muscle mass; decreased joint flexion; stiffening of tendons and ligaments; decreased cortical and trabecular bone; changes in eyes and ears that impair vision, hearing, and balance; slowed response/reaction timed.
   d. Decreased bladder smooth muscle and elastic tissue, decreased sphincter control
   e. Decreased ciliary action, decreased respiratory muscle strength, decreased elastic recoil, decreased cough force
   f. Decreased muscle and subcutaneous fat, collagen stiffening, decreased sebaceous gland activity, decreased sensory receptors, decreased tissue fluid, increased capillary fragility
   g. Decreased vessel elastin and smooth muscle, increased arterial rigidity
   h. Decreased blood flow to colon, decreased intestinal motility, decreased sensation to defecate, decreased muscle mass
8. d. Age-associated memory impairment is characterized by a memory lapse or benign forgetfulness that is different from a decline in cognitive functioning. Forgetting a name, date, or recent event is not serious, but the other examples indicate abnormal functioning.

9.

S	Sadness (mood)
C	Cholesterol (high)
A	Albumin (low)
L	Loss (or gain of weight)
E	Eating problems
S	Shopping (and food preparation problems)

10. d. Older adults with an ethnic identity often have disproportionately low incomes and may not be able to afford Medicare deductibles or medications to treat health problems. Although they often live in older urban neighborhoods with extended families, they are not isolated. Ethnic diets have adequate nutrition, but health could be impaired if money is not available for food.
11. c. This statement shows that this patient does not understand the importance of having the test every week and that the test results will determine ongoing dosing. The other statements indicate that the patient is thinking about ways to get into town weekly.
12. Any 3 of the following are criteria for frailty: unplanned weight loss ($\geq$ 10 lb in a year), self-reported exhaustion, weakness (measured by grip strength), slow walking speed, and low level of physical activity.
13. a. Psychologic abuse, psychologic neglect, physical neglect, and perhaps violation of personal rights b. Perform a very careful medical history and screening for mistreatment; interview the mother alone; use an assessment tool designed specifically for elder mistreatment; specifically assess for depression, dehydration, malnutrition, pressure ulcers, and poor personal hygiene; evaluate explanations about physical findings that are not consistent with what is seen or contradictory statements made by the daughter and the mother c. Caregiver role strain, spiritual distress, or dysfunctional family processes d. Community caregiver support group; and to help care for her mother, formal support system for respite care, adult day care, Programs for All-Inclusive Care for the Elderly (PACE)
14. Factors that precipitate placement are rapid patient deterioration, caregiver stress and burnout, and change in or loss of family support system. Possible factors that hasten placement decisions are progressive dementia, urinary incontinence, or a major health event.
15. d. During an initial contact with an older adult, the nurse should perform a comprehensive nursing assessment that includes a health history using physical, psychologic, functional, developmental, socioeconomic, and cultural assessments. If available, a comprehensive interprofessional geriatric assessment may then be done to maintain and enhance the functional abilities of the older adult. The older adult and caregiver should be interviewed separately, and the older adult should identify their own needs, if possible.
16. a. The results of mental status evaluation often determine whether the patient can manage independent living, a major issue in older adulthood. Other elements of comprehensive assessment could determine eligibility for special problems, determination of frailty, and total service and placement needs.
17. c. Exercise for all older adults is important to prevent deconditioning and subsequent functional decline from many

different causes. Walkers and canes may improve mobility but can also decrease mobility if they are too difficult for the patient to use. Nutrition is important for muscles, but muscle strength is primarily dependent on use. Risk appraisals are usually performed for specific health problems.

18. Any of the following 9 nursing interventions listed in Table 5.12: (1) assess cognitive function, (2) try to reduce medication use that is not essential, (3) assess ability to self-administer medication, (4) assess alcohol and illicit drug use, (5) encourage the use of written or electronic medication-reminder systems, (6) encourage the use of 1 pharmacy, (7) work with HCPs and pharmacists to set up routine drug profiles on each older adult patient, (8) advocate for low-income prescription support services, (9) obtain and maintain a complete medication record.

19. a, b, c. These actions are alternatives to restraints that may help reduce falls and keep the patient safe. A jacket vest and a seat belt are forms of restraint and require an order and frequent reassessment and order renewal.

20. a, b, c, d, e. Any of these actions will promote health.

21. b, e. Long-term acute care provides acute care for an average length of >25 days. Programs for All-Inclusive Care for the Elderly (PACE) provide skilled nursing home level care for adults age 55 years and older if they have Medicaid or Medicare. Being dual-eligible will provide the care at no cost. Acute rehabilitation is a postacute level of care with therapies for returning the patient to the patient's best level of functioning. Intermediate care facilities provide convalescent care. Transitional subacute care facilities are used for 5 to 21 days.

CHAPTER 6

1. b. Some persons may have genitalia or chromosomal make up that cannot be categorized as male or female which is called intersex.

2. a. 2; b. 1; c. 3

3. a. Gender dysphoria is a diagnostic classification that describes the distress that occurs when there is conflict between a person's gender identity and their sex assigned at birth.

4. a. 7; b. 4; c. 2; d. 3; e. 6; f. 5; g. 1

5. B., D., G., I., J. Poverty rates are higher in LGBTQ+ persons compared to cisgender persons. Depression is a significant issue for LGBTQ+ persons. More than 50% of transgender and non-binary youth have considered suicide compared to 40% of LGBTQ+ youth. Lesbian and bisexual women have a higher rate of obesity than heterosexual women. Gay and bisexual men have a higher rate of HPV infections than lesbian and bisexual women.

6. b. The best method to use when establishing a patient's identity is to ask what they would like to be called, either their preferred name and/or pronoun. Don't make assumptions based on first names or appearance. Some individuals do not use their name listed on legal documents.

7. c. Estradiol is a hormone used to develop feminine characteristics, like growing breasts.

8. A history of cardiovascular disease could contraindicate the use of testosterone. A cardiology consult should be obtained prior to its use in higher risk patients.

9. c. A polyamorous relationship is having more than 1 romantic relationship at the same time.

10. a. 4; b. 3; c. 5; d. 1; e. 2

11. b. Facial feminization surgery involves brow lifts, hairline adjustment, nose reshaping, cheek implants, blepharoplasty, mandibular angle reduction, chin width reduction, lip reshaping, and tracheal shave (thyroid chondroplasty). Maintaining a patent airway should be the nurse's top priority.

Case Study

1. 1 = angiotensin converting enzyme (ACE) inhibitor; 2 = 0.5 mg IV every 1 hour PRN; 3 = ondansetron; 4 = androgen inhibitor; 5 = 15 mg IV every 6 hr; 6 = promethazine

2. 1 = Estradiol; 2 = breast growth and skin softening; 3 = breast cancer and venous thromboembolic event (VTE)

3. NPH insulin IV = **Contraindicated** as it is only administered subcutaneously. Morphine sulfate = **Indicated** to treat the patient's pain. The normal saline bolus = **Non-essential** as there isn't an indication for its use. Elevating the HOB to 30 degrees = **Indicated** to decrease facial edema and maintain a patent airway. Inserting an oropharyngeal airway (OPA) = **Contraindicated** as it could stimulate the gag reflex in an awake or semi-conscious patient increasing their risk of aspiration. Inserting an additional IV = **Non-essential** as there isn't an indication for an extra IV, such as a blood transfusion or administering incompatible medications. Applying ice packs to eyes and cheeks = **Indicated** to help decrease surgical-related facial edema. Administering 6 L/min of oxygen = **Indicated** because the patient's O$_2$ saturation is 93%, there is inspiratory stridor, and the RR is 28 breaths/min. Teaching the patient about pursed-lip breathing = **Non-essential** as this type of breathing technique helps expel carbon dioxide, which is applicable to patients who retain carbon dioxide, like those who have COPD or during an asthma attack.

4. Reporting a pain level of 3 = **Effective** as the patient previously reported pain at 7. Temperature of 99°F (37.2°C) = **Unrelated** because it is expected to have a low-grade fever after surgery and there weren't any therapies implemented to decrease the temperature. Oxygen saturation of 94% = **Ineffective** because a 6 L/min simple face mask should significantly increase the oxygen saturation level and not just increase the saturation by 1%. Heart rate = **Effective** as it decreased from 120 beats/min to 100 beats/min which may indicate the patient is more comfortable and less anxious. The FSBS of 220 mg/dL = **Unrelated** as there wasn't a previous reading and nothing was prescribed to treat it. A&O x3 = **Unrelated** as this is a natural progression when recovering from anesthesia. Clear breath sounds = **Effective** as there were coarse breath sounds during the initial assessment.

5. B; D; F; G. Ice packs to decrease edema are only effective for approximately 3 days after surgery. The HOB should be elevated at a minimum of 30 degrees or higher to help decrease edema and promote a patent airway. This patient has been prescribed spironolactone which is a potassium-sparing diuretic. The patient should be instructed to decrease their dietary intake of dietary potassium to reduce the risk of hyperkalemia. Green leafy vegetables, like spinach, are high in potassium. Palpitations could indicate a cardiac dysrhythmia which may occur if potassium levels are too high or too low.

CHAPTER 7

1. b. When individuals do not become stressed with a situation or an event, it is because the event is not perceived by them as a demand that is being made on them or as a threat to their well-being. Perceptions of stressors have great variability and, for whatever reasons, this patient does not perceive this diagnosis as stressful.

2. b. The student's stress related to difficulty studying for the important examination, and the emotional and spiritual stress from the mother's diagnosis will affect the student's body by weakening the immune system and making the student more likely to catch a cold or other illness. Failure of the examination and driving skill are not effects of stress on the student's body. To prevent illness, the student will want to plan a healthy diet and sleep pattern before the examination.

3. Resilience, hardiness, attitude, and optimism. Other factors that could have been selected are age, health status, personality characteristics, prior experience with stress, nutritional status, sleep status, and genetic background. These are all factors that are internal to the individual and may affect the response to stress.

4.

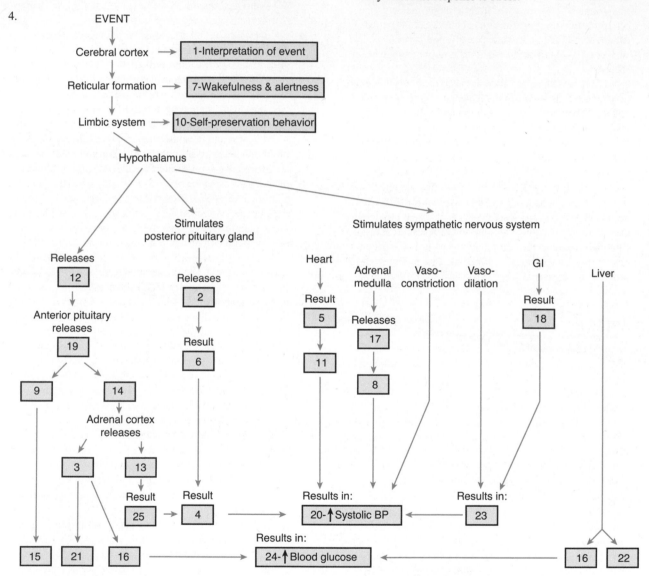

Word and phrase list

1. Interpretation of event
2. ↑ antidiuretic hormone (ADH)
3. Cortisol
4. ↑ Blood volume
5. ↑ Heart rate and stroke volume
6. ↑ Water retention
7. Wakefulness and alertness
8. ↑ Sympathetic response
9. β-Endorphin
10. Self-preservation behaviors
11. ↑ Cardiac output
12. Corticotropin-releasing hormone
13. Aldosterone
14. ACTH (adrenocorticotropic hormone)
15. Blunted pain perception
16. ↑ Gluconeogenesis
17. Epinephrine and norepinephrine
18. ↓ Digestion
19. ↑ Proopiomelanocortin (POMC)
20. ↑ Systolic BP
21. ↓ Inflammatory response
22. Glycogenolysis
23. ↑ Blood to vital organs and large muscles
24. ↑ Blood glucose
25. ↑ Na and H_2O reabsorption

5. **Objective manifestations**
   a. Increased heart rate
   b. Increased BP
   c. Cool, clammy skin
   d. Decreased bowel sounds
   e. Hyperglycemia
   f. Decreased lymphocytes
   g. Decreased neutrophils
   h. Decreased urinary output
   Subjective findings
   a. Anxiety, fear
   b. Decreased perception of pain
   c. Verbalization of stress
   d. Wakefulness, restlessness

6. b. One of the many physiologic changes that occur as a result of prolonged, increased stress is immunosuppression, which may exacerbate or increase the risk of progression of immune-based diseases, including asthma. The other options are not valid explanations for the worsening asthma.

7. a. N; b. N; c. P; d. P; e. P

8. a, d, e. The other answers are problem-focused coping mechanisms.

9. b. Because it is almost impossible to maintain muscle tension while breathing slowly and deeply, relaxation breathing is a component of all relaxation therapies. With fibromyalgia, exercise would not relax this patient. Progressive muscle relaxation first requires relaxed breathing, and although soft music can decrease stress, it should be used with other therapies.

10. a. Peptic ulcer disease is 1 of several disorders with a known stress component. Although many patients have stress related to a health problem, stress-relieving interventions are always indicated for patients with diseases in which stress contributes to the problem.

11. a, c, e. Humor, journaling, and relaxation activities are realistic strategies that can be used during hospitalization by a patient with an acute episode of a chronic disease. Exercise or a cleansing diet would not be appropriate for an exacerbation of Crohn's disease.

Case Study

1. **Physiologic**: pain, anemia, inflammatory disease; **Psychologic**: no insurance, duration and chronicity of the disease, frequent hospital admissions; **Effects**: weight loss and depression

2. A., B., D., E., F. Having a good support system (boyfriend and sister) and pets are thought to positively affect adaptation to stress. Increased weight, hemoglobin and hematocrit levels, strength. Decreased body temperature and number of stools

3. **Indicated**: treating pain, promoting restful sleep, teaching relaxation breathing, and consulting with a social worker will help M.J.'s adaptation to stress. **Contraindicated**: avoiding meditation and restricting visitors will not be helpful as meditation and interaction with a good support system are beneficial. **Non-essential**: physical therapy is not essential for this patient.

4. **Effective** assessment findings include: gaining weight, walking the dogs 2x/day, and decreased number of stools per day all indicate the patient is responding positively to therapies and showing physiologic as well as psychologic improvement. **Ineffective**: refusing to share her illness with her sister and crying twice per week both indicate that she is not coping as well as expected. **Unrelated**: platelet

count doesn't indicate an improvement of her condition like increased hemoglobin and hematocrit levels would.

5. **1**=difficulty coping (Refer to Appendix B for a list of clinical problems and their definitions); **2**=art therapy and journaling, respectively. (Refer to Table 7.3) **3**=emotion-focused coping; **4**=yoga, Qigong, Tai Chi. (Refer to Table 7.5)

CHAPTER 8

1. c. During sleep, individuals are not consciously aware of the environment. Lack of sleep does not cause medical and psychiatric disorders, although people with these diagnoses may have fragmented sleep. Most adults need 7 to 8 hours of sleep per day. An estimated 50 to 70 million people in the United States have a sleep disorder.

2. b, c, e, f. Manifestations of insomnia include difficulty falling asleep, frequent awakenings, prolonged nighttime awakening, awakening too early and not being able to fall back to sleep, feeling unrefreshed on awakening, and having daytime sleepiness and difficulty concentrating.

3. d. Sleep terrors, sleepwalking, and nightmares are parasomnias that are unusual and often undesirable behaviors that occur while falling asleep, transitioning between sleep stages, or arousing from sleep. Cataplexy is brief and sudden loss of skeletal muscle tone and is experienced with narcolepsy episodes. Hypopnea is slow, shallow respirations, and sleep apnea is the cessation of spontaneous respirations for longer than 10 seconds.

4. c. The suprachiasmatic nucleus in the hypothalamus is the master clock and controls the cyclic changes of wake and sleep through a complex arrangement of nerve pathways with the brainstem, hypothalamus, and thalamus. Melatonin is an endogenous hormone that increases sleep efficiency and is released in the evening related to darkness. The light-dark cycles influence our circadian rhythms and neuropeptides influence wake behavior. These all play a role in the sleep/wake cycle and are components of the nervous system but are regulated by the suprachiasmatic nucleus in the hypothalamus.

5. a. 4; b. 3; c. 2, 3; d. 4; e. 4; f. 1; g. 2; h. 1; i. 2; j. 3

6. Any 3 of these can contribute to insomnia:
   • consumption of stimulants (caffeine, nicotine, methamphetamine) close to bedtime;
   • side effect of medications (antidepressants, antihypertensives, corticosteroids, psychostimulants, analgesics);
   • drinking alcohol, or using over-the-counter (OTC) medications as a sleep aid;
   • long naps in the afternoon;
   • sleeping in late;
   • exercise near bedtime;
   • jet lag;
   • nightmares;
   • stressful life event;
   • medical conditions or psychiatric illnesses;
   • irregular sleep/wake schedules;
   • worry about getting enough sleep.

7. a, b, e, f, g, h, i, k

8. d. Cognitive-behavioral therapies for insomnia (CBT-I) are effective therapies for insomnia and should be tried first. These include relaxation techniques, guided imagery, education about good sleep hygiene, and regular exercise several hours before bedtime. The other therapies are used

to treat insomnia, with benzodiazepine-receptor agents being the first choice for drug therapy. Many patients will try OTC medications, such as diphenhydramine, but tolerance develops rapidly. Complementary and alternative therapies, such as melatonin have been found to be useful to help individuals with jet lag.

9. b. Alcohol should not be consumed within 6 hours of bedtime. It is not recommended that a person lie in bed awake. A light snack with milk and cheese, which contain tryptophan, may help the person relax. Exercise is good but not within 6 hours of bedtime.

10. c. A&W root beer has no caffeine, so this would be the best beverage in the afternoon. Cola has 22 mg of caffeine; Green tea has 28 mg; decaffeinated coffee has 2 mg (see Table 8.6).

11. a. Reducing the light and noise levels in the ICU can help promote opportunities for sleep. Having the TV on at all times will only add to the noise level. The alarms should not be silenced except for short periods to address why they were alarming. Silencing alarms to prevent them from making noise puts the patient at risk because the nurse may not be alerted to patient changes on the monitor or problems with the infusion device. Analgesics given for actual pain may help a patient sleep or rest, but they may also alter sleep.

12. b. Modafinil (Provigil) is a first-line nonamphetamine wake-promotion drug used to treat narcolepsy. Solriamfetol (Sunosi) and pitolisant (Wakix) are newer wake-promoting drugs that exert effects at the histamine receptor. Amitriptyline is a tricyclic antidepressant used to treat narcolepsy with cataplexy.

13. Any of these responses would be appropriate:
    - Start to get in harmony with the Moscow time zone several days before you travel.
    - Melatonin and exposure to daylight help synchronize the body's clock to environmental time.
    - Resynchronization of the body's clock will occur at a rate of 1 hr/day if the patient travels eastward and 1.5 hr/day when traveling westward.

14. a. 3; b. 6; c. 5; d. 4; e. 2; f. 1; g. 7. Risk factors for obstructive sleep apnea include obesity, a neck circumference of 16 inches or larger, male sex, postmenopause in women, and age > 65 years. Airflow obstruction occurs because of narrowing of the air passages with relaxation of muscle tone during sleep and/or when the tongue and soft palate fall backward and partially or completely obstruct the pharynx. With apnea lasting 10 to 90 seconds, hypoxemia and hypercapnia occur, which cause a startle response with a brief arousal, so the tongue and soft palate move forward and the airway opens. This cycle occurs 180 (30 per hour x 6 hours) to 400 (50 per hour x 8 hours) times during 6 to 8 hours of sleep.

15. c. Continuous positive airway pressure (CPAP) is the treatment of choice for more serious sleep apnea. CPAP is not well tolerated, and compliance is low. Compliance may be improved by involving the patient in the selection of the device and mask, showing the CPAP before therapy begins, and teaching troubleshooting to reduce anxiety. An oral appliance is used to prevent airway occlusion from the relaxed mandible and tongue. Bilevel positive airway pressure (BiPAP) is the therapy that delivers a high inspiratory pressure and a low expiratory pressure to prevent airway collapse.

16. d. The most common complications in the immediate postoperative period are airway obstruction and hemorrhage. The patient may experience a sore throat,

foul-smelling breath, and snoring during the recovery, but these will resolve. Infection is a potential complication of any surgery but is not common with this procedure. Loss of voice and electrolyte imbalance generally are not complications of this procedure.

17. d. Assess the patient to determine what the problem is and then offer sleep hygiene instruction and collaborate with the HCP to improve the patient's sleep behavior. Disturbed sleep is not a normal result of aging, and people need about the same amount of sleep throughout their life span. OTC and prescription sleep aids must be used very cautiously in older adults, and patient response must be monitored closely.

18. Any 3 of these would be correct:
    - nurse is too sleepy to be fully awake at work;
    - nurse is too alert to sleep soundly the next day;
    - increased morbidity and mortality related to cardiovascular problems;
    - mood disorders are higher;
    - fatigue could result in errors and accidents, as perceptual skills, judgment, and decision-making abilities may be diminished;
    - reduced ability to cope and handle stress, which may result in physical, mental and emotional exhaustion.

19. a, b, c, d, e. All these measures can be used to help a nurse who works rotating shifts to get adequate sleep.

Case Study

1. A., B., C., D., E., I. W.D.'s risk factors for chronic insomnia include his age, Parkinson's disease, uses a variety of OTC sleep aids, and drinks a few glasses of wine at night. He is likely waking up to urinate during the night because he takes a diuretic before bedtime. He also complains of a persistent cough that wakes him up at night, which is likely caused by the ACE inhibitor. Heart failure is not a contributing factor for W.D.'s insomnia as he is taking medications to manage the disease and he denies shortness of breath. Diabetes is not a contributing factor. Osteoarthritis causes pain in the morning which isn't disturbing his sleep.

2. Assessment findings that require follow-up by the nurse:
    - Alcohol intake before bed (contributing to insomnia)
    - Lives alone and is anxious about discharge (safety concern and may be contributing to insomnia)
    - The patient takes furosemide before bed (contributing to insomnia)
    - W.D. has a persistent cough (a side effect of ACE inhibitors contributing to insomnia)
    - BP 150/80 mm Hg (hypertension)
    - Temperature 35.9°C (hypothermia)
    - Hip dressing is 50% saturated (may be expected or unexpected, notify HCP and continue to assess for signs of active bleeding)

3. **Indicated**: administer the anti-hypertensive medication (BP is 150/80 mm Hg), turn the TV off before bedtime (patient has a history of chronic insomnia and this would promote an environment conducive to sleep), place the patient in a private room (patient has a history of chronic insomnia and this promotes an environment conducive to sleep), schedule physical therapy in the early afternoon (this is recommended to avoid strenuous exercise within 6 hours of bedtime); **Contraindicated**: position the patient on his right side (the patient should not lay on the operative hip

due to possible dislocation), prepare to administer a blood transfusion (EBL was 75 mL which is considered a small amount of blood loss. The patient doesn't have any signs of hemorrhage or hypovolemia), allow the patient to nap during the day (this could negatively impact his ability to sleep during the nighttime), administer the furosemide at 9 PM (having to urinate throughout the night will interrupt the patient's sleep); **Non-essential**: initiate oxygen therapy (95% on room air is acceptable), administer opioid pain medication (3 out of 10 is acceptable on postop day 0)

4. **Effective teaching:**
   - "I will contact my HCP to ask about changing captopril to a different medication." (this may improve the persistent cough)
   - "I will stop using the Internet several hours before bedtime." (blue light emitted from a computer or smartphone is thought to interrupt melatonin production and interfere with falling asleep)
   - "I can drink 7-Up with dinner." (7-Up isn't caffeinated)
   - "I will get up and read a book if I cannot fall asleep within 20 minutes after going to bed." (this is recommended)

   Ineffective teaching: (needs clarification)
   - "I will continue to take furosemide at bedtime." (this will cause nocturia and interrupt his sleep)
   - "I will avoid drinking a cup of coffee in the morning." (drinking coffee in the morning is acceptable, but he should avoid caffeine 4-6 hours before bedtime)

5. **1**=captopril; **2**=5-10 mg PO every 4 hr PRN; **3**=carbidopa-levodopa; **4**=heart failure; **5**=beta blocker; **6**=5 mg PO twice daily; **7**=cardiac glycoside; **8**=heart failure

CHAPTER 9

1. c. Because the patient's self-report is the most valid means of pain assessment, patients who have decreased cognitive function, such as those who are comatose, have dementia, are mentally disabled or have expressive aphasia, may not be able to report pain. In these cases, nonverbal information and behaviors are necessary considerations in pain assessment.

2. c. Unnecessary suffering, impaired recovery from acute illness, increased morbidity from respiratory dysfunction, increased heart rate and cardiac workload, and other physical dysfunction can occur. Giving the smallest prescribed analgesic dose when given a choice is not consistent with current pain management guidelines and leads to undertreatment of pain and inadequate pain control. Without reassessing the pain within 30 minutes of the IV analgesic, the nurse is unsure how well the previous dose of medication worked for the patient to determine the current dose needed. Respiratory and sedation effects of the analgesic must be assessed before fearing overdosage. "Start low and go slow" applies to pain therapy in older adults, but age is not a factor for this patient.

3. a. Physiologic: the genetic, anatomic, and physical determinants of pain b. Affective: the emotional response to pain c. Cognitive: the beliefs, attitudes, memories, and meaning attributed to pain d. Behavioral: observable actions that express or control pain, or changed behavior e. Sociocultural: age and gender influences, family and caregiver influence, and culture that influences the pain experience

4. c. Although a peripheral nerve is 1 cell that carries an impulse directly from the periphery to the dorsal horn of the spinal cord with no synapses, transmission of the impulse can be interrupted by drugs known as "membrane stabilizers" or "sodium-channel inhibitors", such as local anesthetics and some antiseizure drugs. The nerve fiber produces neurotransmitters at the dorsal root of the spinal cord, not during transmission of the action potential.

5. a. The anterior and posterior right neck, shoulder, and posterior flank are common areas of referred pain from the liver. Examination of the liver should be considered when pain occurs without other findings in these areas. Other common referred areas are midscapular and left arm for cardiac pain, inner legs for bladder pain, shoulders for gallbladder pain, and hip for gynecologic or back pain.

6. b. It is known that the brain is necessary for pain perception but because it is not clearly understood where in the brain pain is perceived, pain may be perceived even in a comatose patient who may not respond behaviorally to noxious stimuli. Any noxious stimulus should be treated as potentially painful.

7. a. 3; b. 4; c. 2; d. 1

8. a. 2, 7, 9; b. 2, 7; c. 2, 6; d. 1, 3; e. 1, 5; f. 2, 8; g. 1, 4

9. c. Several antidepressants affect the modulatory systems by inhibiting the reuptake of serotonin and norepinephrine in descending modulatory fibers, thereby increasing their availability to inhibit transmission of pain impulses. Although chronic pain is often accompanied by anxiety and depression, the antidepressants that affect the physiologic process of pain modulation are used for pain control whether depression is present or not.

10. a. Trigeminal neuralgia is neuropathic pain from damage to peripheral or cranial nerves that is not well controlled by opioid analgesics alone and often includes the adjuvant use of tricyclic antidepressants, antiseizure drugs, or γ-aminobutyric acid (GABA) receptor agonists to help inhibit pain transmission. Salicylates and nonsteroidal antiinflammatory drugs (NSAIDs) are not effective for the intensity of neuropathic pain.

11.

Element of Pain Assessment	Assessment Finding
Onset	About 4 hours ago
Duration and pattern of pain	Continuously for about 4 hours. Similar episodes in the past month but lasted only 2 hours.
Location	Right upper quadrant
Intensity	Severe, 10 on a scale of 0 to 10, "This is the worst pain I can imagine."
Quality	Severe cramping, radiates to back
Associated symptoms	Nausea
Management strategies	Pain better walking bent forward, more intense lying in bed

12. a. Follow the principles of pain assessment. b. Use a holistic approach to pain management. c. Every patient

deserves adequate pain management. d. Base the treatment plan on the patient's goals. e. Use both drug and nondrug therapies. f. When appropriate, use a multimodal approach to analgesic therapy. g. Address pain using an interprofessional approach. h. Evaluate the effectiveness of all therapies to ensure that they are meeting the patient's goals. i. Prevent or manage medication side effects. j. Incorporate patient and caregiver teaching throughout assessment and treatment.

13. a. Analgesics should be scheduled around the clock for patients with constant pain to prevent pain from escalating and becoming difficult to relieve. If pain control is not adequate, the analgesic dose may be increased or an adjunctive drug may be added to the treatment plan.

14. a. As cancer pain increases, stronger drugs are added to the regimen. This patient is using an NSAID and an antidepressant. A stronger preparation would be an opioid, but because an NSAID is already being used, a combination NSAID/opioid is not indicated. An appropriate stronger drug would be an oral opioid, in this case oral oxycodone, and this still leaves stronger drugs for expected increasing pain.

15. c. Although tolerance to many of the side effects of opioids (pruritus, dizziness, nausea, sedation, respiratory depression) develops within days, tolerance to opioid-induced constipation does not occur. A bowel regimen that includes a gentle-stimulant laxative and a stool softener should be started at the beginning of opioid therapy and continued for as long as the drug is taken.

16. d. Use of a basal dose may increase the risk of serious respiratory events in opioid-naive patients and those at risk for respiratory difficulties (older age, existing pulmonary disease, etc.). Overdose is not expected, as the dosages are calculated and the patient-controlled analgesia (PCA) pump is programmed to prevent this. Nausea and itching are common side effects but not related to a basal dose of analgesic. A lack of pain control would not be expected with or without a basal dose. The nurse should be assessing the patient and notify the HCP if a lack of pain control occurs but, again, this is not related to receiving a basal dose of analgesic via PCA pump.

17. b, d, e, f. Corticosteroids, local anesthetics, antiseizure medications, and NSAIDs are effective in the transduction stage of pain. Distraction is effective in the perception stage. Epidural opioids are effective in the transmission stage.

18. a, b, c, d, e, f. The major complications of epidural analgesia are catheter displacement and migration, accidental infusions of neurotoxic agents, and infection. These actions will help reduce those risks.

19. b. When a patient wants to be stoic about pain, it is important that they understand that pain itself can have harmful physiologic effects and that failure to report pain and participate in its control can result in severe unrelieved pain. No evidence that indicates fear of taking the medication is present in this situation.

20. a. Fentanyl is frequently used for chronic pain in patients who are not opiate-naive. Hydrocodone is used for acute and short-term pain, not chronic pain. Intranasal butorphanol is used for acute headaches and recurrent, not chronic, pain. Sustained-release morphine given buccally will have the same absorption as morphine, so it would not be expected to be more effective than oral morphine. The route used will depend on the swallowing ability of the patient.

21. b. If the nurse knows enough acupressure to suggest its use, it is appropriate to use with the patient's permission; otherwise massage, heat or cold, distraction, or meditation may help. The as needed analgesic prescribed for postoperative pain is not usually appropriate for a headache, nor would biofeedback training be appropriate for this situation. Simply reassuring the patient that the headache will go away is not helpful. The HCP could be called for an analgesic for his headache.

Case Study

1. **Affective**: worried about worsening of disease, afraid of addiction; **Behavioral**: rigid posture, slow gait, stays in bed with severe pain; **Cognitive**: empties his mind to block pain

2. Findings that indicate poor pain management include: being preoccupied as evidenced by having to repeat questions. The patient is fidgety and grimaces when he moves. HR 98 beats/min (approaching tachycardia); BP 155/82 mm Hg (no history of HTN, but this BP is elevated); requests to use the urinal instead of ambulating to the bathroom; didn't drive himself because he cannot concentrate.

3. Assessment findings **associated** with withdrawal syndrome are: diaphoresis, chills, rhinorrhea, and insomnia. Assessment findings that are **unrelated** are: oliguria, bradycardia (tachycardia is a manifestation), constipation (diarrhea is a manifestation), and hypoxemia.

4. **1**=drowsiness; **2**=methadone; **3**=SNRI; **4**=diclofenac; **5**=cox-II inhibitor; **6**=cardiovascular thrombotic events; **7**=dexamethasone; **8**=hyperglycemia

5. A., C., D., H. Percocet is an opioid which has acetaminophen in it; therefore, it should not be doubled because of the risk of opioid overdose as well as acetaminophen toxicity. The patient shouldn't learn to tolerate severe pain. Instead, the patient should contact the HCP for evaluation of the cause as well as management options. Being pain free is an unrealistic goal when considering the cause of the pain and progression of the disease. Because Percocet has acetaminophen in it, additional acetaminophen isn't advisable due to the risk of liver toxicity. The patient shouldn't drive while taking opioids as it is considered driving under the influence.

CHAPTER 10

1. a, c, d, f, g, i. Table 9.1 lists the goals of palliative care. Overall, goals of palliative care are to prevent and relieve suffering and to improve the quality of life for the patient.

2. a. The family may not understand what hospice care is and may need information. Some cultures and ethnic groups may underuse hospice care because of a lack of awareness of the services offered, a desire to continue with potentially curative therapies, and concerns about a lack of minority hospice workers.

3. a. Patient must desire services and agree in writing that only hospice care can be used to treat the terminal illness (palliative care). b. Patient must meet eligibility, which is <6 months to live, certified initially by 2 HCPs.

4. **Respiratory**
   a. Cheyne-Stokes respiration
   b. Death rattle (mouth breathing and inability to clear secretions)
   c. Increased, then slowing, respiratory rate
   (Also: irregular breathing, terminal gasping)
   Skin
   a. Mottling on hands, feet, and legs that progresses to the torso
   b. Cold, clammy skin
   c. Cyanosis of nose, nail beds, and knees
   (Also: waxlike skin when very near death)
   Gastrointestinal
   a. Slowing of the gastrointestinal tract with accumulation of gas and abdominal distention
   b. Loss of sphincter control with incontinence
   c. Bowel movement before imminent death or at time of death
   Musculoskeletal
   a. Loss of muscle tone with sagging jaw
   b. Difficulty speaking
   c. Difficulty swallowing
   (Also: loss of ability to move or maintain body position, loss of gag reflex)

5. b. Hearing is often the last sense to disappear with declining consciousness, and conversations can distress patients even when they appear unresponsive. Conversation around unresponsive patients should never be other than that which one would maintain if the patients were alert.

6. a. Coma or unresponsiveness b. Absent brainstem reflexes c. Apnea

7. b. Kübler-Ross describes bargaining as being demonstrated by "if-then" grief behavior. Kübler-Ross's stage of depression is seen when the person says, "Yes me, and I am sad." Prolonged grief disorder is seen when there is a dysfunctional reaction to loss, and the individual is unable to move forward after the death of a loved one. In the Grief Wheel model, the new normal stage is when the grief is resolved but the normal state, because of the loss, is different from before.

8. a. Spiritual distress may surface when a person is faced with a terminal illness. It is characterized by verbalization of inner conflicts about beliefs and questioning the meaning of one's own existence. People in spiritual distress may be able to resolve the problem and die peacefully with effective grief work, but referral to spiritual leaders should be the patient's choice.

9. a. Natural death acts are the legal documents in each state that have the state's requirements related to an individual's choice of health care. Allow natural death is a new term being used for the Do Not Resuscitate order. Advance care planning is the process of having patients and their families think through their values and goals for treatment and document those wishes as advance directives.

10. b. Palliative care is aimed at symptom management rather than curative treatment for diseases that no longer respond to treatment and is focused on caring interventions rather than curative treatments. "Palliative care" and "hospice" are often used interchangeably.

11. d. There currently are no clinical practice guidelines to relieve the shortness of breath and air hunger that often occur at the end of life. The principle of beneficence would encourage any of the options to be tried, based on knowing that whatever gives the patient the most relief should be used.

12. d. End-of-life care assists patients with dying and focuses on physical and psychosocial needs for the patient and family. Physical care is very important for physical comfort. Assessment should be limited to essential data related to the patient's symptoms. Analgesics should be given for pain, but patients who are sedated cannot take part in the grieving process.

13. a, b, c, d, e, f. Teaching, along with support and encouragement, can decrease some of the anxiety. Teaching about pain relief, the dying process, and the care provided will help the patient and family know what to expect. The nurse who is the target of anger needs to not react to this anger on a personal level. Allowing the patient to make decisions will help decrease feelings of powerlessness and hopelessness.

14. d. Using the open-ended statement to seek information related to the patient's and family's perspective and expectations will best guide the plan of care for this patient. This will open the discussion about palliative or hospice care and preferences for end-of-life care.

Case Study

1. **Difficulty coping**: Children are withdrawn spending most of their time out of the house; S.J. and her husband haven't talked to their children about her dying; **Caregiver Role Strain**: Husband tries to do as much work at home to help care for S.J.; husband doesn't know how to help S.J. anymore; husband feels guilty because he wishes it was all over; **Grief**: Children are withdrawn spending most of their time out of the house; her children don't care about her; husband feels guilty because he wishes it was all over

2. **Essential**: Reasons for not discussing her impending death with their children (children need to know and be allowed to express their feelings of grief); assessment of spiritual needs; S.J.'s dying preferences (palliative care preferences); assessment of her functional status (regarding ADLs); assessment of how S.J. and her husband are coping; **Non-essential**: funeral plans (unless patient wants to discuss them); determine if S.J. is competent to make decisions (no evidence provided; if patient was not able to make her own decisions, refer to legal documents like an advance directive)

3. **Indicated**: Auscultate her lungs (patient is short of breath); apply SCDs (if confined to bed due to pain); turning schedule (patient is confined to bed and at risk of pressure ulcers); consult palliative care team (to discuss plans for end of life); **Contraindicated**: avoiding opioids (opioids are a staple when treating symptoms at the end of life unless the patient refuses their use); recommend a chiropractor (patient has metastasis to vertebrae which are likely brittle and susceptible to pathologic fractures); **Non-essential**: NG feeding tube (may be necessary to provide nutrition, but goals at the end of life are different than those for patients who are not terminal; the patient would have to desire a feeding tube); neutropenic precautions (there is no evidence that the patient is neutropenic and at risk of infection; her temperature is normal and there isn't a WBC result); obtain an arterial blood gas (an SpO$_2$ reading should be sufficient; aggressive measures and treatments

are unlikely when the patient decides to enter hospice care as the focus is symptom management)

4. A., D., E., F., G., H. Even if patients seem withdrawn at the end of life, hearing is still intact. Usually patients at the end of life are not hungry or thirsty. If a patient at the end of life experiences dyspnea, opioid medication administration is recommended to improve comfort.

5. **1**=8; **2**=Psychologic and psychiatric aspects; **3**=symptom management; **4**=4; **5**=patient must agree in writing and 2 physicians determine the patient is terminal

CHAPTER 11

1. d. Substance use disorder (SUD) negatively affects psychologic, physiologic, and/or social functioning of an individual. The compulsive need for pleasure is psychologic dependence. Behavior to maintain addiction is addictive behavior. Absence of a substance causing withdrawal symptoms is physical dependence.

2. b. Tolerance is described. Relapse is when the person returns to substance use after a period of abstinence. Abstinence is avoidance of substance use. Withdrawal is the response that occurs after abrupt cessation of a substance.

3. a. Ask; b. Advise; c. Assess; d. Assist; e. Arrange

4. d. The Joint Commission mandates that every health care professional, including nurses, identify tobacco users and provide them with information about ways to stop smoking. The advice and motivation of health care professionals can be very helpful to the individual. Nurses should encourage and provide information to patients and work with HCPs to identify ways to assist patients with quitting.

5. **Nicotine**
   a. Chronic obstructive pulmonary disease (COPD)
   b. Cancers: lung, mouth, larynx, esophagus, stomach, bladder, pancreas and others
   Others: coronary artery disease, peripheral artery disease, hypertension, hip fractures (see Fig. 10.1)
   Alcohol
   a. Dementia
   b. Cirrhosis
   Others: labile moods, depressed immune function, anemia, coronary artery disease (CAD), hypertension, gastroesophageal reflux disease (GERD) (see Table 10.7)
   Cocaine and amphetamines
   a. Dysrhythmias, myocardial ischemia and infarction
   b. Psychosis
   Others: septal necrosis, seizures, stroke (see Table 10.2)
   Opioids
   a. Gastric ulcer
   b. Glomerulonephritis
   Other: sexual dysfunction (see Table 10.2)
   Cannabis
   a. Bronchitis, chronic cough
   b. Memory impairment
   Other: anxiety, schizophrenia, depression (see Table 10.2)

6. b, f. Cocaine and amphetamines cause nasal damage when snorted as well as tachycardia and hypertension. Drowsiness is seen with sedative-hypnotics and opioids. Stimulants cause dilated, not constricted, pupils. Sexual dysfunction is associated with opioids. There is anorexia with cocaine, not increased appetite.

7. a. Opioids produce these physiologic responses. Although alcohol intake can cause euphoria, drowsiness, and slurred speech, a person with alcohol use disorder (AUD) develops tolerance and does not usually have these manifestations. Effects of chronic alcohol use include impairment of all body systems (see Table 10.7). Cannabis produces euphoria, sedation, and hallucinations. Depressants may cause slurred speech and drowsiness but not euphoria or decreased respirations unless there is an overdose.

8. a, d. Seizures, tremors, and anxiety may be experienced with sedative-hypnotic withdrawal. Violence and suicidal thoughts are more likely to occur in patients withdrawing from stimulants. Sweating, nausea, and cramps are seen with opioid withdrawal. Hallucinogens are least likely to have withdrawal symptoms.

9. d. While the addiction is treated, the carcinogens and gases associated with tobacco smoke are eliminated. Nicotine replacements do not create an aversion to nicotine. Nicotine has not been determined to be carcinogenic. The replacements reduce cravings and withdrawal symptoms by supplying smaller amounts of nicotine. They do not prevent weight gain.

10. a. 2; b. 3; c. 4; d. 1; e. 2; f. 4; g. 3

11. a. Headache is a common symptom of caffeine withdrawal and often occurs in heavy caffeine users who are NPO for diagnostic tests and surgery. Nervousness and mild tremors are more likely to be caused by the intake of caffeine. Shortness of breath is not directly related to caffeine intake or withdrawal.

12. b, c, f. Manifestations of alcohol withdrawal include seizures, disorientation, and visual, tactile, or auditory hallucinations. Apathy and depression occur in withdrawal from stimulants. Cardiovascular collapse is seen in sedative-hypnotic withdrawal.

13. c. Open-ended questions indicating that substance use is normal or at least understandable are helpful in eliciting information from patients who are reluctant to disclose substance use.

14. b. Smoking is a leading cause of preventable death, and most smokers start smoking at a young age. If smoking in preadolescents and adolescents could be prevented, it is unlikely that these individuals would start smoking at a later age. Health problems associated with smoking and future use of other addictive substances would be significantly reduced. Alcohol and other addictions are not leading causes of death in the United States.

15. a. Naloxone is given when opioids are the cause of central nervous system (CNS) depression. b. Flumazenil is given when benzodiazepines are the cause of CNS depression.

16. a. The knowledge of when the patient last had alcohol intake will help the nurse anticipate the onset of withdrawal symptoms. In patients with alcohol tolerance, the amount of alcohol and the blood alcohol concentration do not reflect impairment as consistently as in the nondrinker. The type of alcohol ingested is not important because in the body it is all alcohol.

17. c. An extreme autonomic nervous system response may be life threatening and requires immediate intervention. A quiet room is recommended, but it should be well lighted to prevent misinterpretation of the environment and visual hallucinations. Cessation of alcohol intake causes low blood alcohol levels, leading to withdrawal symptoms, and fluids should be given carefully to prevent dysrhythmias. Patients should not be restrained if possible because injury and exhaustion can occur as patients struggle against restraint.

18. d. Alcohol-induced CNS depression can lead to respiratory and circulatory failure in an alcoholic patient. Vital signs are monitored closely because of the increased risk of infection from malnutrition. Emergency magnesium would not be expected, although an emergency dose of thiamine may have been given before surgery. Pain medication requirements may be increased if the patient is cross-tolerant to opiates.

19. a. Patients with hypoglycemia may receive glucose-containing IV solutions. IV thiamine may be given before or with IV glucose solutions to prevent Wernicke-Korsakoff syndrome, which can cause seizures and brain damage. Benzodiazepines may be used for sedation and to minimize withdrawal symptoms but would not be given before thiamine, and haloperidol could be used if hallucinations occur. Naloxone is used for opioid overdose.

20. d. The "5 *R's*" are used for individuals who are unwilling to quit tobacco use. The "5 *A's*" are used for individuals who want to quit tobacco use. Although cost, cough, cleanliness, and the use of Chantix as well as deduce, describe, decide, and deadline may be ways to assist this patient, these are not recommendations or clinical practice guidelines.

21. d. Older adult patients have the highest use of OTC and prescription drugs, and simultaneous use of these drugs with alcohol is a major problem. Illegal drug use is minimal in older patients except in long-term addicts.

Case Study

1. **Myocardial infarction:** nausea, dizziness, pale and diaphoresis, chest pain; **Stroke:** migraine-like headache, hypertensive BP, dizziness; **Psychosis:** nervous and irritable, paranoia

2. **Indicated:** obtain 12-lead ECG (the patient complains of chest pain and "feels like he is having a heart attack"), obtain a blood alcohol level (has been drinking alcohol), initiate seizure precautions (stimulant toxicity can cause seizures), administer nitroglycerin 0.4 mg SL (to treat chest pain); **Contraindicated:** administer D_5W 500 mL bolus (this solution is not to be used as a bolus as it physiologically acts as a hypotonic solution, plus there isn't an indication to administer a bolus), insert an oropharyngeal airway to keep airway patent (no indication that the patient has an obstructed airway as he is awake and talking; this would be appropriate if his LOC deteriorates and he obstructs his airway; if an OPA was inserted while the patient is conscious, it would stimulate the gag reflex and possibly cause vomiting placing the patient at risk of aspiration pneumonia); **Non-essential:** administer acetaminophen 650 mg PO (no indication for its use), apply sequential compression device (unnecessary unless the patient is placed on prolonged bedrest or has an increased risk of blood clot formation)

3. B., C., E., F., G. Having ever been arrested, having ever coerced someone to do drugs, or having ever been injured or injuring someone as a result of drug use are not questions included in the DAST-10.

4. Appropriate teaching statements are: experiencing severe mood swings, sleeping when desired, taking a multivitamin, and may need hospitalization if withdrawal symptoms are severe. There are no recommendations to lessen withdrawal symptoms by consuming 1 drink per day. Withdrawing from either cocaine or alcohol will cause cravings for hours or days. There are no antidotes to treat cocaine or alcohol withdrawal.

CHAPTER 12

1.

Clinical Manifestation	Chemical Mediators	Physiologic Change
Fever	Cytokines released from monocytes/macrophages (i.e. IL-1, IL-6, TNF) which promote prostaglandin E_2 (PGE_2) synthesis and secretion	Increases the hypothalamic thermostatic set point and stimulates autonomic nervous system resulting in shivering, muscle contraction and peripheral vasoconstriction.
Redness	Histamines and prostaglandins	Vasodilation and increased capillary permeability
Edema	Prostaglandins	Vasodilators contributing to increased blood flow
Leukocytosis	Release of chemotactic factors at site of injury	Increased release of neutrophils and monocytes from bone marrow

2. d. A *shift to the left* is the term used to describe the presence of immature, banded neutrophils in the blood in response to an increased demand for neutrophils during tissue injury. Monocytes are increased in leukocytosis but are mature cells.

3. c. Chemotaxis involves the release of chemicals at the site of tissue injury that attract neutrophils and monocytes to the site of injury. When monocytes move from the blood into tissue, they are transformed into macrophages. The complement system is a pathway of chemical processes that results in cellular lysis, vasodilation, and increased capillary permeability causing the slowing of blood flow at the area. Prostaglandins slow blood flow to allow for clot formation at the injury.

4. d. The processes that are stimulated by the activation of the complement system include enhanced phagocytosis, increased vascular permeability, chemotaxis, and cellular lysis. Prostaglandins and leukotrienes are released by damaged cells, and body temperature is increased by the action of prostaglandins and interleukins. All chemical mediators of inflammation increase the inflammatory response and, as a result, increase pain.

5. c. The nurse will encourage Rest and Immobility to prevent further injury. Ice or cold Compresses will be applied to decrease swelling with vasoconstriction. Compression will help reduce edema and stop bleeding if it is occurring. Elevation will help decrease edema and pain. The other options are not correct.

6. b. The injurious agent of chronic inflammation persists or repeatedly injures tissue. It lasts for weeks, months, or years. Infective endocarditis is a subacute inflammation that lasts for weeks or months. Neutrophils are the predominant cell type in acute inflammation. Lymphocytes and macrophages are the predominant cell types at chronic inflammation sites.

7. a. Labile cells of the skin, lymphoid organs, bone marrow, and mucous membranes divide constantly and regenerate rapidly following injury. Stable cells, such as those in bone, liver, pancreas, and kidney, regenerate slowly only if they are injured. Axons in the CNS are generally less successful at regeneration than peripheral axons. There may be a certain amount of recovery after injury involving the neurons. Cardiac muscle is not expected to regenerate but will scar when damaged.

8. a. 2; b. 1; c. 10; d. 4; e. 8; f. 6; g. 7; h. 9; i. 3; j. 5

9. c. The process of healing by secondary intention is essentially the same as primary healing. With the greater defect and gaping wound edges of an open wound, healing and granulation take place from the edges inward and from the bottom of the wound up, resulting in more granulation tissue and a much larger scar. Secondary healing may require surgical debridement for healing to occur. In primary healing, the edges of the wound are aligned and may be sutured. Tertiary healing involves delayed suturing of 2 layers of granulation tissue together and may require debridement of necrotic tissue.

10. b. Adhesion is a band of scar tissue that forms between organs. It may occur in the abdominal cavity and cause intestinal obstruction. Infection could be seen with undernutrition or necrotic tissue but would not cause these symptoms. Contractures shorten the muscle or scar tissue but would not contribute to abdominal symptoms. Evisceration of an abdominal wound would occur sooner after surgery when the wound edges separate and the intestines protrude through the wound.

11. d. A fistula is an abnormal passage between organs or between a hollow organ and skin that will leak fluid or pus until it is healed. In this situation, there may be a fistula between the vagina and rectum. The student nurse did not describe dehiscence, hemorrhage, or keloid scar formation.

12. c. Vitamin C aids healing with capillary synthesis and collagen production by fibroblasts. Fats provide synthesis of fatty acids and triglycerides used for cellular membranes. Protein corrects negative nitrogen balance from increased metabolism and contributes to synthesis of immune factors, blood cells, fibroblasts, and collagen. Vitamin A aids in epithelialization, increasing collagen synthesis, and tensile strength of the healing wound.

13. d. The B-complex vitamins are necessary coenzymes for many metabolic reactions, including protein, fat, and carbohydrate metabolism. Carbohydrates provide metabolic energy for inflammation and are protein sparing. Fluid is needed to replace that used in exudates as well as the extra fluid used for the increased metabolic rate required for healing.

14. c. The stage 2 pressure injury is a shallow, partial thickness wound with a red-pink wound bed, without slough. Adherent gray necrotic tissue describes eschar tissue, which cannot be staged. Clean, moist granulating tissue occurs over time as the wound heals. Creamy exudate occurs when the wound is contaminated or infected, regardless of the stage of the pressure injury.

15. a. A clean wound would be treated with a hydrocolloid or hydrogel dressing because they provide a moist environment to encourage granulation. Transparent film would be likely to result in further tissue loss. There would not be enough drainage for an absorptive dressing unless this pressure injury became infected. An eschar wound may be treated with autolytic debridement and then negative pressure wound therapy, depending on the depth and healing of the wound.

16. c. For the negative pressure therapy to work, a vacuum is created between the device and the wound so that the excess fluid, bacteria, and debris are removed from the wound. The wound is cleaned weekly or when the dressing is replaced. A hyperbaric oxygen therapy chamber is not used with a negative pressure device. Nutrition must be maintained, as protein and electrolytes may be removed from the wound.

17. d. Hand washing is the most important factor in preventing infection transmission and is recommended before and after the use of gloves by the Centers for Disease Control and Prevention for all types of isolation precautions in health care facilities.

18. c. The immobility, mental deterioration, and possible neurologic disorder of the comatose patient present the greatest risk for tissue damage related to pressure. His Braden score is 9, which puts him at very high risk. Although obesity, hyperglycemia, advanced age, mental deterioration, malnutrition, and incontinence contribute to development of pressure injuries, the risk is not as high for any of the other patients.

19. b. Relief of pressure on tissues is critical to prevention and treatment of pressure injuries. Although pressure-reduction devices may relieve some pressure and lift sheets and trapeze bars prevent skin shear, they are no substitute for frequent repositioning individualized for the patient. Massage is contraindicated if there is the presence of acute inflammation or possibly damaged blood vessels or fragile skin.

20. d. Stage 4 pressure injuries are full-thickness tissue loss with muscle, tendon, or bone exposed. Stage 1 pressure injuries are intact skin with nonblanchable localized redness. Stage 2 pressure injuries have a shallow open area with a red-pink wound bed. Stage 3 pressure injuries exhibit full-thickness tissue loss without bone, tendon, or muscle exposure with possible tunneling into the tissue.

21. c. Stage 3 is full-thickness tissue loss; subcutaneous fat may be visible. Bone, tendon, and muscle are exposed in a stage 4 pressure injury. Abrasion, blister, and shallow crater are seen in stage 2 pressure injuries. Persistent redness or discoloration of darker skin tones describes a stage 1 pressure injury.

22. c, e. Measuring the size of the wound and repositioning do not require judgment, patient teaching, or evaluation of care. The other interventions listed relate to assessment, judgment, and teaching, all of which are responsibilities of the RN. However, the LPN can reinforce teaching by the RN. The assistive personnel (AP) may also be able to help with repositioning, if delegated by the RN.

Case Study

1. **1**=neurovascular complications and sepsis; **2**=leukocytosis, fever, and diminished left dorsalis pedis pulse; **3**=cleansing the wound using 0.9% NSS, elevating LLE above the level of the heart to decrease swelling, and increasing fluid intake to replace fluid loss from perspiration and exudate formation. Contraindicated interventions would be using alcohol to clean the wound because it can damage tissue, applying ice packs to LLE because it causes vasoconstriction and may compromise circulation to the extremity which affects wound healing, and applying SCDs bilaterally. Applying a SCD to RLE is acceptable, but not to the LLE because it could reduce circulation to the extremity as well as contribute to spread of the infection.

2. **C. Correct Wound Care Dressing for its Use**
   1. Alginates — Wounds with heavy exudate
   2. Hydrocolloids — Wounds with light drainage
   3. Antimicrobials — Prophylactic in non-healing wounds
   4. Hydrogels — Necrotic wounds
   5. Transparent films — Dry, uninfected wounds
   6. Nonadherent — Used for minor wounds
   7. Foams — Used to prevent pressure injuries
   8. Gauze — Used on almost any wound

3. Pulse=110 beats/min (tachycardia); BP is hypotensive; Temp is febrile and capillary refill is delayed. Patient is lethargic which may indicate decreased perfusion to the brain.

4. **Indicated**: administer acetaminophen 650 mg PO (treats fever); check FSBG before meals and at bedtime (patient has type I diabetes which warrants frequent glucose monitoring); assess the patient's hemoglobin A1C (diabetes is likely a contributing factor for this patient's cellulitis and ankle wound and an A1C can evaluate a 3-month history of glucose control); **Contraindicated**: cleanse the ankle wound with hydrogen peroxide (hydrogen peroxide is caustic to tissue and should not be used); administer D_5W at 125 mL/hr (patient is hyperglycemic, therefore additional dextrose is contraindicated); **Non-essential**: teach the patient to use an incentive spirometer (isn't essential as there isn't evidence to warrant its use); weigh the patient daily (there is no reason or benefit to weighing the patient daily)

5. B., C., D., E. Antibiotics should be taken as directed until they are gone to treat the infection as well as decrease the risk of developing a resistance. Fevers indicate the infection is not resolving and should be reported to the HCP for evaluation. Elevating the LLE will help reduce the swelling. If the patient continues to have pain when weight-bearing, she can use crutches until she can weight-bear pain free, but she shouldn't become dependent on their use. The patient should wait until her HCP tells her she can increase her activity which will be when her infection completely resolves. Alternating between acetaminophen and ibuprofen is acceptable, but more explicit instructions about dose and frequency need to be included. Hot tubs and taking baths are contraindicated until the wound has completely healed. Soaking in water will soften (macerate) the wound and could introduce bacteria. Showers will be fine, but the wound may need to be covered.

CHAPTER 13

1. c. The phenotype is the observable characteristics of the individual. An allele is 1 of 2 or more alternative forms of a gene on a particular locus. Genomics is the study of all of a person's genes (the genome), including interactions of these genes with each other and the person's environment. Chromosomes are compact structures containing DNA and proteins that are present in nearly all cells of the body.

2. a. Genotype is the genetic identity of an individual. A gene is the basic unit of heredity at a specific locus on a chromosome. Transmission of a disease from parent to child is termed *hereditary*. The pedigree is the family tree that contains the genetic characteristics and disorders of that particular family.

3. c, e. The age when the disease was diagnosed as well as the age and cause of death of 3 generations of the biologic relatives will be most helpful for making lifestyle changes, if necessary, and family planning. Cholecystitis and kidney stones are not known to be genetically linked. Prostate cancer is 2 times more likely if a close relative (e.g., father, brother) has it.

4. An error during meiosis causes an abnormal number of chromosomes. In Down syndrome, there are 3 copies of chromosome 21. There can also be a copy of a chromosome missing. Translocation occurs when genetic material is exchanged between 2 chromosomes in a cell, such as in chronic myelocytic leukemia.

5. a. 50%
   b. 50%

6. a, b, e. Genetic testing may raise psychologic and emotional issues if someone is identified with a positive result or as a carrier of a disease. A woman with a positive *BRCA1* or *BRCA2* genetic test may have a bilateral mastectomy to prevent breast cancer. Privacy issues also arise with genetic testing. Genetic testing can be used to provide the risk of a genetic condition in an offspring only if both parents are tested. Newborn screening for phenylketonuria is done in all states. It may also be completed for congenital hypothyroidism and cystic fibrosis.

7. 25%. With autosomal recessive diseases, the pedigree will show 25% having the disease, 25% not having the disease, and 50% being carriers whether the offspring are male or female.

8. a. When both parents are tested, genetic testing can provide information about the couple's risk of having a child with a genetic condition by identifying changes in the genes tested. Not all diseases are genetically identified or familial disorders. Genetic testing kits are available, but a genetic counselor will help them understand the purpose of the testing, the pros and cons of having testing, and the emotional and medical impact of the test results.

9. a. Because Huntington's disease is an autosomal dominant disease, and her father has it, she has a 50% chance of getting it. A positive result of genetic testing will mean that she will get the disease. There are no carriers of Huntington's disease, and changing her lifestyle will not affect the disease diagnosis.

10. d. Multifactorial conditions are caused by a combination of genetic and environmental factors. In diabetes, several genes have been identified that increase the likelihood of getting diabetes. Single gene disorders result from a single

gene mutation (e.g., sickle cell disease). Chromosome disorders are caused by structural changes within chromosomes or an excess or deficiency of the genes in that locus. People are born with these disorders. Acquired genetic disorders occur when there is an error in replication or damage to DNA from toxins at some time in the person's life.

11. a. Trastuzumab is effective only for women whose breast cancer tumors have genes that overproduce the protein HER-2. Testing for *BRCA* genes is used to identify women at risk for developing breast cancer. The stage of cancer is not relevant to whether this drug should be used.

12. a. Pharmacogenomic testing for genes *VKORC1* and cytochrome P4502C9 *(CYP2C9)* can assist the HCP in prescribing the appropriate dosage of warfarin. Giving bivalirudin IV would be done only in the hospital. Clopidogrel and aspirin will not give the level of anticoagulant effect that warfarin does, as they are only platelet inhibitors and do not block clotting factors. Enoxaparin injections can be given at home, but the patient is less likely to continue the therapy because of the injections and the added expense of the medication.

13. b. Yearly colonoscopies are done to monitor the polyp growth and remove polyps. A colectomy may be considered to prevent cancer. Changing the diet will not affect the growth of polyps that develop in the colon and potentially become cancerous. Gene therapy is still considered experimental therapy. If he has children, they will need to have genetic testing.

14. c. Gene therapy is an investigational technique used to treat the underlying cause of a disease. Gene therapy may be used to supply a missing gene, avoid the missing gene's role, or enhance treatment of a disease. A new gene inserted into the body usually does not function without using a carrier molecule called a *vector* to deliver it to the target cells. It will replace a mutated gene with a healthy copy of a gene.

15. b. The hematopoietic stem cells are adult stem cells. The red blood cells are returned to the donor so that they do not become anemic. Although bone marrow aspirations and transplants may be done for recipients, peripheral blood stem cells, stimulated by filgrastim, are now usually obtained from the blood via apheresis and large-bore IV needles.

Case Study

1. **1**=X-linked recessive; **2**=Usually males; **3**=Hemophilia and Wiskott-Aldrich syndrome; **4**=Daughters of affected males

2. B, F, G, H. BRCA is an inherited mutation of a protective gene. If D.L. has a daughter, she has a 50% chance to inherit the BRCA mutation.

3. **Effective**: "I will consult an oncologist about the chances of developing ovarian cancer." and "I will have my eggs harvested and consider preimplantation genetic diagnosis before getting pregnant." D.L. has the BRCA gene mutation which increases her risk of developing ovarian cancer. It may be possible to have her eggs harvested and fertilized, then have the fertilized embryos tested for genetic disorders before being implanted in utero. **Ineffective**: "I will not have any children since they will develop Duchenne muscular dystrophy." and "I will have bilateral mastectomies since I will develop breast

cancer." There is a 50% chance that her sons will develop Duchenne MD and her daughters will be carriers. It isn't guaranteed that she will develop breast cancer, but the BRCA gene mutation increases her risk. **Unrelated**: "I will eat healthy and exercise to reduce my risks of developing cancer."

4. **1**=warfarin; **2**=nucleoside reverse transcriptase inhibitor; **3**=HER-2; **4**=non-small cell lung cancer; **5**=trastuzumab; **6**=kinase inhibitor; **7**=CYP2C19; **8**=CAD

CHAPTER 14

1. b. Natural active acquired immunity is a result of exposure to the antigen via infection and the longest lasting type of immunity. Innate immunity is present at birth and its primary role is first-line defense against any pathogens. Artificial active acquired immunity is from immunization and also lasts a long time. Artificial passive acquired immunity is from gamma globulin injection and is immediate but short lived.

2. a, c. Artificial passive acquired immunity is received from the injection of gamma globulin, provides immediate immunity, and may last for several weeks or months. Immunization with an antigen and the need for boosters contribute to artificial active acquired immunity. Maternal immunoglobulins in the neonate provide temporary natural passive acquired immunity.

3. b. Both B and T lymphocytes must be sensitized by a processed antigen to activate the immune response. Processing involves the taking up of an antigen by macrophages, expression of the antigen on the macrophage cell membrane, and presentation to the lymphocytes. Antigens do not need to be proteins, and a few antigens may combine with larger molecules that are antigenic.

4. d. T cytotoxic cells directly attack antigens on the cell membrane of foreign pathogens and release cytolytic substances that destroy pathogens. Dendritic cells primarily capture antigens at sites of contact with the external environment and then transport the antigen to a T cell with specificity for the antigen. Natural killer cells are involved in cell-mediated immunity but are not considered T lymphocytes. T helper cells are involved in the regulation of cell-mediated immunity and humoral antibody response.

5. c. Interferon is antiviral by reacting with viruses and inducing the formation of an antiviral protein that mediates antiviral action of interferon by altering the cell's protein synthesis and preventing viral replication. It also may activate macrophages, neutrophils, and natural killer cells.

6. b. B lymphocytes differentiating into plasma cells and producing immunoglobulins (or antibodies) is the essential component in humoral immunity. Tumor surveillance and the production of cytokines are functions of T lymphocytes in cellular immunity. B lymphocytes do not directly attack antigens.

7. b. B lymphocytes activated in the bone marrow by the presentation of an antigen differentiate into many plasma cells that secrete immunoglobulins and only a few memory cells that retain recognition of the antigen as foreign. Helper cells are T lymphocytes and natural killer cells are large, granular lymphocytes that are neither B nor T lymphocytes. The spleen filters foreign substances from

the blood. T lymphocytes differentiate in the thymus. The bursa of Fabricius is found in birds, not humans.

8. d. IgM immunoglobulin is predominant in the primary immune response and produces antibodies against ABO blood antigens. IgA lines mucous membranes and protects body surfaces. IgD, on lymphocyte surface, assists in the differentiation of B lymphocytes. IgG crosses the placenta and is responsible for the secondary immune response.

9. a, d. IgA is passed to the neonate in the colostrum and breast milk; and IgG crosses the placenta for fetal protection.

10. a, b. Immunoglobulin E (IgE) causes allergic reactions and assists in parasitic infections. IgD assists in B-lymphocyte differentiation and is present on the lymphocyte surface. IgG is predominant in the secondary immune response. IgA protects body surfaces and mucous membranes.

11. a, c, d, e. Functions of cell-mediated immunity include fungal infections, rejection of foreign tissue, contact hypersensitivity reactions, immunity against pathogens that survive inside cells, and destruction of cancer cells and tuberculosis. Transfusion reactions are from humoral immunity.

12. d. Aging has a pronounced effect on the thymus, which decreases in size and activity, leading to a decline in T cells and cell-mediated immunity and increased T-cell differentiation and memory T cells. A decrease in T cells is responsible for decreased tumor surveillance, resulting in an increase in cancer. B cell activity also declines with advancing age, but the bone marrow is relatively unaffected by increasing age. Circulating autoantibodies increase and are a factor in autoimmune diseases.

13. c. When sensitized T lymphocytes attack antigens or release cytokines that attract macrophages and cause tissue damage, a type IV or delayed hypersensitivity reaction is occurring with transplant rejections as well as contact dermatitis, some drug sensitivity reactions, and hypersensitivity reactions to bacterial fungal and viral infections. Type I reactions occur when antigens link with specific IgE antibodies bound to mast cells of basophils and release chemical mediators. Type II reactions occur when cellular lysis or phagocytosis occurs through complement activation after antigen-antibody binding on cell surfaces. Type III reactions occur when the antigens combined with IgG and IgM are too small to be removed by the mononuclear phagocytic system and are deposited in tissue and cause complement activation.

14. a, b, c, d, e, g. These are the atopic or anaphylactic responses that can be seen with a type I or IgE-mediated hypersensitivity reaction to specific allergens. Contact dermatitis is seen with a type IV or delayed hypersensitivity reaction. Transfusion reactions and Goodpasture syndrome are seen with a type II or cytotoxic hypersensitivity reaction.

15. c. With rheumatoid arthritis and acute glomerulonephritis, type III or immune-complex reaction is seen when the antigens combined with IgG and IgM are too small to be removed by the mononuclear phagocytic system and are deposited in tissue, which activates the complement system and lead to inflammation and destruction of the involved tissue.

16. d. The best drugs for allergic rhinitis are antihistamines. However, of those listed, minor sympathomimetic/decongestant drugs are used primarily for allergic rhinitis.

Nasal corticosteroids may be used for seasonal allergic rhinitis; oral corticosteroids are used briefly if the patient does not get relief from other drugs. Immunotherapy is used when the allergen cannot be avoided and after it is found that drug therapy is not effective. Antipruritic drugs are topical and used to relieve itching.

17. a, f. Wheezing and a feeling of impending doom can both occur with anaphylaxis. Other common physiologic systemic anaphylactic responses are hypotension; dilated pupils; rapid, weak pulse; and edema and itching at the injection site. An arm rash would be more likely with a simple allergic reaction.

18. a. 3; b. 1; c. 5; d. 4; e. 2; f. 6. Airway is always first. Anticipation of intubation with severe respiratory distress is needed. Knowing that the patient has a bee sting, the stinger will be removed if present. Then an IV is started and preparation to administer epinephrine is done. Having diphenhydramine and nebulized albuterol as well as methylprednisolone IV available is important, as they may be needed. Oxygen will be used for dyspnea. For hypotension, the patient will be placed recumbent with elevated legs, and IV saline will be used.

19. c. Allergic individuals have elevated levels of IgE, which react with allergens to produce symptoms. Immunotherapy involves injecting allergen extracts that will stimulate increased IgG, which combines more readily with allergens without releasing histamine. The goal is to keep blocking the level of IgE by keeping the level of IgG high. Allergen-specific T suppressor cells develop with immunotherapy.

20. d. This describes a type IV allergic contact dermatitis that is caused by chemicals used in the manufacturing process of latex gloves. A type I allergic reaction that is a response to the natural rubber latex proteins occurs within minutes of contact with the proteins and may manifest with reactions ranging from skin redness to full-blown anaphylactic shock. Powder-free gloves will avoid respiratory exposure to latex proteins, but nonlatex gloves are more helpful. Avoidance of oil-based hand creams when wearing gloves can also help prevent latex allergic reactions.

21. b. Multiple chemical sensitivities are commonly seen with scented products, paint fumes, petroleum products, smoke, pesticides, plastics, and synthetic products. Symptoms vary but include headache, sore throat, breathing problems, nausea, fatigue, congestion, dizziness, muscle pain, skin rash, gastrointestinal (GI) problems, confusion, difficulty concentrating, memory problems, and mood changes. His symptoms do not indicate posttraumatic stress disorder. A mask may help when he paints, but it would be better to avoid painting. Psychotherapy is currently recommended.

22. c, d. Autoimmune causative factors are genetic susceptibility and initiation of autoreactivity by a trigger that may include specific viruses or medications. Females and older patients are more likely to develop autoimmune diseases.

23. c. Plasmapheresis is the removal of plasma from the blood and in autoimmune disorders is used to remove pathogenic substances found in plasma, such as autoantibodies, antigen-antibody complexes, and inflammatory mediators. Circulating blood cells are not affected by plasmapheresis, nor are blood cells added.

24. d. A crossmatch mixes recipient serum with donor lymphocytes. A positive crossmatch shows that the recipient has cytotoxic antibodies to the donor and this

organ cannot be transplanted without hyperacute rejection occurring. A negative crossmatch indicates that it is safe to do the transplant. The other options are not correct.

25. c. Drug-induced immunosuppression with antineoplastic agents and corticosteroids is the most common cause of secondary immunodeficiency. Chronic stress and human immunodeficiency virus (HIV) may cause secondary immunodeficiency, but they are not the most common causes. Primary immunodeficiency is caused by common variable hypogammaglobulinemia.

26. d, e, f. Acute transplant rejection occurs when the recipient's T cytotoxic lymphocytes attack the foreign organ. Long-term immunosuppressants help combat it, and it is usually reversible with additional immunosuppression. Treatment of chronic rejection is supportive and irreversible with infiltration of the organ with B and T lymphocytes. Hyperacute rejection occurs when the recipient has antibodies against the donor's human leukocyte antigen (HLA), is most common with kidney transplants, and results in the organ having to be removed.

27. b. Chronic rejection of a kidney transplant manifests as fibrosis and glomerulopathy (seen with proteinuria, edema, and renal failure), occurs over months or years, and is irreversible. Acute rejection occurs in the first 6 months after transplant. *Delayed rejection* is not a term used with transplantation. Hyperacute rejection occurs minutes to hours after transplantation and is rare.

28. d. Standard immunotherapy involves the use of 3 different immunosuppressants that act in different ways: a calcineurin inhibitor (tacrolimus, cyclosporine), a corticosteroid, and the antimetabolite mycophenolate mofetil. Although cyclosporine is still used, tacrolimus is the most frequently prescribed calcineurin inhibitor. Polyclonal antibodies are used for induction immunosuppression and acute rejection. Azathioprine (Imuran) is similar to mycophenolate mofetil, and they cannot be taken together.

29. c. Graft-versus-host disease (GVHD) is occurring as the graft is rejecting the host tissue, which usually manifests in a pruritic or painful skin rash; in the GI tract with diarrhea, severe abdominal pain, GI bleeding, and malabsorption; or in the liver with mild jaundice, elevated liver enzymes, or coma. GVHD is more effectively prevented with immunosuppressive agents than treated.

Case Study

1. **Essential**: history of past and present allergies, auscultating lung sounds (to assess for wheezing which indicates reactive airway disease like asthma), crackles (indicates fluid or pulmonary edema) or rhonchi (coarse breath sounds indicate secretions), family history of allergies, and presence of pets in the home (may trigger allergies). **Unrelated**: any GU problems, neurologic problems, or the presence of peripheral edema.

2. **Bronchospasm**: epinephrine (bronchodilator and stops effects of allergen), nebulized albuterol (short-acting bronchodilator); **Hypotension**: normal saline bolus (increases blood volume), epinephrine (vasoconstricts blood vessels), supine with raised legs (to improve venous return to the heart); **Hypoxemia**: high-flow oxygen, epinephrine (bronchodilator), nebulized albuterol (short-acting bronchodilator)

3. B, C, D, G. A tourniquet would be applied above, not below, the intradermal site if the patient experiences a severe reaction. Skin testing is not routinely performed to test for allergic rhinitis since empiric allergy medications is the treatment of choice. When using the scratch or intradermal skin testing methods, reactions will occur within 5-10 minutes. Patch testing requires the patient to wear the patch for 48-72 hours to assess for reactions. False-negative and false-positive test results can occur; therefore, negative or positive results are not conclusive.

4. **Effective** methods to treat allergies to household dust include using a steam vacuum to clean floors, air filters in furnaces and AC units, use a HEPA filter air purifier. **Ineffective** methods include using a duster wand to dust (use a damp duster to trap or collect dust), opening windows allows dust to enter the home. Using AC would be recommended. **Unrelated** recommendations include hypoallergenic jewelry (hypoallergenic bed coverings are recommended).

5. 1=corticosteroid; 2=pseudoephedrine; 3=use with caution in HTN; 4=monitor LFTs (liver function tests); 5=ipratropium bromide; 6=antihistamine (2nd generation); 7=diphenhydramine; 8=report palpitations (Refer to Table 29.2)

CHAPTER 15

1. a, b, c, e. Global travel and bioterrorism have increased the spread of infectious agents. Infectious agents, such as the human immunodeficiency virus (HIV) and hantavirus, have evolved to affect humans through closer association with animals as human populations push into wild animal habitats. The transfer of infectious agents from animals to humans has also resulted in West Nile virus, COVID-19, and avian flu. Bacterial infections have also become untreatable as the result of genetic and biochemical changes stimulated by unnecessary or inadequate exposure to antibiotics. The increased number of immunosuppressed and chronically ill people also increase the emergence of untreatable infections. Transmission of infectious agents from humans to animals does not increase this number.

2. The 4 common antibiotic-resistant organisms are *Enterococcus faecalis*, *Enterococcus faecium*, *Klebsiella pneumoniae*, and *Streptococcus pneumoniae*.

3. d, e. The occupational Safety and Health Administration (OSHA) requires hand washing and the use of alcohol-based sanitizers and personal protective equipment (e.g., gloves) to prevent health care–associated infections (HAIs). Although the other interventions will not hurt a patient and they are good practice, they will not prevent HAIs.

4. b. Contact precautions are used with standard precautions when microorganisms can be transmitted by direct patient contact. Droplet precautions are used to minimize contact with pathogens that are spread through the air at close contact and that affect the respiratory system. *Isolation precautions* is a general term. Airborne precautions are used if the organism can cause infection over long distances when suspended in the air.

5. a. With influenza, a surgical mask will be worn when the nurse is 3 feet or closer to the patient to avoid droplet transmission. The gown and gloves will be used as with standard precautions when working closely with the patient

and there is a risk of contamination. Shoe covers are used in surgery. Particulate respirators are used for airborne precautions (e.g., tuberculosis [TB]).

6. b. Infection in older adults often has atypical presentations, with cognitive and behavioral changes occurring before fever, pain, or altered laboratory values. Fatigue and ICU psychosis could be occurring, but these are not as dangerous for the patient as infection can be. Cognitive and behavioral changes are not typical manifestations of medication allergy.

7. d. One of the most important factors in the development of antibiotic-resistant strains of organisms has been inappropriate use of antibiotics. Following directions regarding timing and completion of antibiotics will prevent antibiotic-resistant bacteria from developing. Antibiotics are not effective against viruses that cause colds and flu. Not completing the antibiotic regimen may allow the hardiest bacteria to survive and multiply and the potential development of an antibiotic-resistant infection.

8. c. SARS-CoV-2 (a.k.a. COVID-19) is an RNA virus that primarily enters the upper respiratory tract binding with angiotensin-converting enzyme 2 (ACE2) which allows the virus to enter the cells. Research suggests that the virus can enter through the eyes and the GI tract but the respiratory tract is the most common mode of entry.

9. a, c, d, e. Surgical masks aren't recommended for health care providers caring for COVID-19 positive patients or suspected positive patients as this disease is considered to be more airborne than droplet. Hair covers are optional but not necessary PPE.

10. d. Macrolides have both bactericidal and bacteriostatic properties. Tetracyclines and sulfonamides are bacteriostatic while cephalosporins are bactericidal.

11. c. Prior to starting antibiotic therapy, the nurse should ask the patient about any allergies, collect blood cultures, review all medications the patient is taking, perform baseline and infection-specific assessments, and review baseline lab results, such as liver function tests and renal function tests.

12. c, d, f. Antibiotics shouldn't be used to treat flu or colds. They should be taken until they are gone, not just when the fever or other symptoms go away. They should not be saved for future use. These actions can cause antibiotic-resistance to occur.

13. b. The only antiviral approved to treat COVID-19 is remdesivir. Acyclovir is approved to treat cytomegalovirus, herpes simplex virus and varicella-zoster virus. Valacyclovir is approved to treat herpes simplex virus and varicella-zoster virus. Oseltamivir is approved to treat influenza.

14. a. women; b. vascular access; c. first 2 to 4 weeks of infection; d. HIV-infected mothers using no therapy; e. needle-stick exposure to HIV-infected blood

15. a. 3; b. 5; c. 1; d. 6; e. 2; f. 7; g. 4

16.

Drug	Mechanism of Action
Attachment inhibitors	Interrupts the ability of HIV to attach to the CD4 cell (step 1 from Question 9)
Entry inhibitors	Inhibit entry into cell (steps 1 and 2 from Question 9)

Drug	Mechanism of Action
Reverse transcriptase inhibitors	Block development of HIV DNA chain and inhibit the action of reverse transcriptase enzyme (steps 3 and 4 from Question 9)
Integrase inhibitors	Bind with integrase enzyme and prevent HIV from incorporating its genetic material into the host cell (step 5 from Question 9)
Protease inhibitors	Prevent protease enzyme from cutting of the long strands of viral RNA needed for viable virions (step 7 from Question 9)

17. a. Activated $CD4^+$ T cells are the target cells for HIV virus and are destroyed after replication of HIV. $CD4^+$ T cells normally are a major component of the immune system and when infected and destroyed, the immune system is ineffective against HIV and other agents. The virus does not affect natural killer cells, and B lymphocytes are functional early in the disease, as evidenced by positive antibody titers against HIV. Monocytes and tissue macrophages ingest infected cells and may become sites of HIV replication and spread the virus, but this does not make the immune response ineffective.

18. d. The symptoms of acute HIV infection occur 2 to 4 weeks after initial infection, when the $CD4^+$ T cell counts fall temporarily but quickly return to baseline levels. Symptoms include a mononucleosis-like syndrome of fever, swollen lymph nodes, sore throat, headache, malaise, nausea, muscle and joint pain, diarrhea, and/or a diffuse rash. Some people develop neurologic complications. Burkitt's lymphoma and *Pneumocystis jiroveci* pneumonia (PCP) are 2 of the opportunistic diseases that can occur in acquired immunodeficiency syndrome (AIDS). Persistent fevers and drenching night sweats occur in the symptomatic infection stage.

19. d. Cytomegalovirus retinitis could be an opportunistic viral infection that occurs when AIDS is diagnosed. Flu-like symptoms occur in the acute HIV infection stage. $CD4^+$ T cells drop to 200 to 500/μL, and oral hairy leukoplakia is seen in the symptomatic infection stage of HIV.

20. d. Organisms that are nonvirulent or that cause limited or localized diseases in an immunocompetent person can cause severe, debilitating, and life-threatening infections and cancers in persons with impaired immune function. The other options are not correct.

21. c. *P. jiroveci* infection is characterized by pneumonia with a dry, nonproductive cough, hypoxemia, and other symptoms. *Cryptococcus* infection may cause fungal meningitis. Non-Hodgkin's lymphoma is diagnosed by lymph node biopsy. Cytomegalovirus infection is characterized by viral retinitis, stomatitis, esophagitis, gastritis, or colitis.

22. a. Vascular lesions of skin, mucous membranes, and viscera are seen in Kaposi sarcoma. *Candida albicans* is a common yeast infection of the mouth, esophagus, gastrointestinal (GI) tract, or vagina. Herpes simplex type 1 infection has oral and mucocutaneous vesicular and ulcerative lesions. Varicella-zoster virus infection or shingles is a maculopapular, pruritic rash along dermatomal planes.

23. b. Because there is a median delay of several weeks after infection before antibodies can be detected, testing

during this "window" may result in false-negative results. Risky behaviors that may expose a person to HIV should be discussed and possible scheduling for repeat testing done. Positive results on initial testing will be verified by additional testing. Identification of sexual partners and prevention practices are important but do not relate immediately to the testing situation.

24. c. The "rapid" test is highly reliable and results are available in about 20 minutes. However, if results are positive from any testing, blood will be drawn for HIV viral load testing and another visit will be necessary to obtain the results of the additional testing and plan for care. CD4$^+$ T cell counts are not used for screening but rather are used to monitor the progression of HIV infection, and new assay tests measure resistance of the virus to antiviral drugs.

25. b. The major advantage of combination antiretroviral therapy (ART) is the inhibition of viral replication in several ways as well as decreasing the likelihood of drug resistance, the major factor that limits the ability of ART drugs to inhibit virus replication when they are used alone. The drugs selected should be ones with which the patient has not been previously treated and that are not cross-resistant with antiretroviral agents previously used by the patient.

26. c. Guidelines for initiating ART are being updated continuously because of the development of alternative drugs and problems with long-term side effects and compliance with regimens. Whenever treatment is started, an important consideration is the patient's readiness to initiate ART because adherence to drug regimens is a critical component of the therapy and preventing drug resistance.

27. b. The goal of antiretroviral therapy is to decrease the HIV viral load. In addition, the goal is to keep the CD4 + cell count from declining. The other options show understanding.

28. d. Pneumococcal pneumonia, influenza, and hepatitis A and B vaccines should be given as early as possible in HIV infection while there is still immunologic function. Isoniazid is used for 9 to 12 months only if a patient has reactive purified protein derivative (PPD) > 5 mm, has had high-risk exposure, or has prior untreated positive PPD. Zoster virus vaccination is not recommended for patients with HIV. Trimethoprim/sulfamethoxazole is initiated when CD4$^+$ T cell count is < 200/μL or when there is a history of PCP.

29. d. After a patient has positive HIV antibody testing and is in acute disease, the overriding goal is to keep the viral load as low as possible and to maintain a functioning immune system. The nurse should provide teaching regarding ways to enhance immune function (e.g., nutrition, vaccinations, rest and exercise, stress reduction) to prevent the onset of opportunistic diseases in addition to teaching about the spectrum of the infection, options for care, signs and symptoms to watch for, ways to prevent HIV spread, and ways to adhere to treatment regimens when ART drugs are initiated. The asymptomatic stage is too early for the other options.

30. Sexual Intercourse
    - Masturbation
    - Abstain from sexual intercourse
    - Abstain from sexual activity with multiple partners
    - Noncontact sexual activities (outercourse)
    - Use of male or female condoms during sexual activity Drug use
    - Abstain from drug use
    - Do not share equipment
    - Use needle and syringe exchange programs if available
    - Use professionals or self-help programs (e.g., Narcotics Anonymous)
    - Do not have unsafe sexual intercourse while under the influence of drugs
    - Perinatal transmission
    - Use family planning to avoid pregnancy if children not desired
    - Use antiretroviral therapy to reduce the risk of transmission

31. a. All the nursing interventions are appropriate for a patient with confusion, but the priority is the safety of the patient when cognitive and behavioral problems impair the ability to maintain a safe environment.

Case Study

1. **Anticipated**: CBC with differential (would identify anemia, leukopenia, thrombocytopenia), CD4$^+$ cell count (destroyed by HIV, assesses immune system), viral load count (determines amount of HIV in the blood), hepatitis B and C serology (often a co-infection with HIV); **Non-essential**: echocardiogram, ABG, spiral CT scan (these diagnostics may be useful in AIDS but not in early HIV infection)

2. **Indicated**: provide resources for emotional support, evaluate suicide risk, contact tracing (sex partners should be tested), treatment options; **Contraindicated**: discuss clinical manifestations of AIDS (this is an early phase of the infection and the patient is likely shocked and processing the news; it is too soon to talk about advanced disease.), discuss end of life planning (this would indicate to the patient that it is a terminal disease and may affect the patient's outlook and psyche about treatment); **Non-essential**: discuss completing an Advance Directive (this is important to discuss later at a future visit, but early counseling should focus on risk reduction and treatment), provide ideas about how to tell his coworkers (it isn't necessary for the patient to divulge this information to his coworkers unless there is a high risk exposure)

3. **1**=pneumococcal, influenza, hepatitis B; **2**=using a condom, adhering to ART; **3**=reduces viral load; **4**=phenotype, genotype

4. A., B., E., G., H. Many ART medications can cause side effects. These should be reported to the HCP so ART medications can be changed if necessary. The patient should get into a routine of taking these medications at scheduled times each day to promote adherence. Undetectable viral loads do not mean HIV is gone and medications can be discontinued. The patient must continue ART medications to maintain a low or undetectable viral load.

5. *Pneumocystis jiroveci*: any respiratory difficulty including the use of accessory muscles, night sweats, fever; **Kaposi sarcoma**: swollen lymph nodes (lymphedema); hyperpigmented lesions; *Cryptococcus neoformans*: fever; seizures; memory impairment

CHAPTER 16

1. a. Lung cancer is the leading cause of cancer deaths in the United States for both women and men. Smoking cessation is one of the most important cancer prevention behaviors. About ½ of cancer-related deaths in the United States are related to tobacco use, unhealthy diet, physical inactivity, and obesity. Cancer of the breast and prostate are the second leading causes of cancer deaths, and colon cancer is the third.

2. d. Malignant cells proliferate indiscriminately and continuously and lose the characteristic of contact inhibition, growing on top of and in between normal cells. Cancer cells usually do not proliferate at a faster rate than normal cells, nor can cell cycles be skipped in proliferation. However, malignant proliferation is continuous, unlike normal cells.

3. a. Cancer cells become more fetal and embryonic (undifferentiated) in appearance and function and some produce new proteins, such as carcinoembryonic antigen (CEA) and α-fetoprotein (AFP), on cell membranes that reflect a return to more immature functioning. The other options are unrelated to CEA and AFP.

4. d. The major difference between malignant and benign cells is the ability of malignant tumor cells to invade and metastasize. Benign tumors can cause death by expansion into normal tissues and organs. Benign tumors are more often encapsulated and often grow at the same rate as malignant tumors.

5. d. Alkylating agents are used to treat Hodgkin's lymphoma and are carcinogens associated with initiation of acute myelogenous leukemia. Working with radiation would lead to a higher incidence of bone cancer. Epstein-Barr virus is seen in vitro with Burkitt's lymphoma. Intense tanning or exposure to ultraviolet radiation is associated with skin cancers.

6. a. Mutations in the *p53* tumor suppressor gene have been found in many cancers, including bladder, breast, colorectal, esophageal, liver, lung, and ovarian cancers. *APC* gene mutations increase a person's risk for familiar adenomatous polyposis, which is a precursor for colorectal cancer. *BRCA1* and *BRCA2* mutations increase the risk for breast and ovarian cancer.

7. a, c, d. Promoting factors, such as obesity and tobacco smoke promote cancer in the promotion stage of cancer development. Eliminating risk factors can reduce the chance of cancer development as the activity of promoters is reversible in this stage. Increased growth, invasion, and metastasis are seen in the progressive stage.

8. b. Carcinoma in situ has the histologic features of cancer except invasion. Evasion of the immune system by cancer cells by various methods is immunologic escape. Oncogenic factors can cause cellular alterations associated with cancer. Tumor cell surface antigens that stimulate an immune response are tumor-associated antigens.

9. a. Oncogenes are the mutation of protooncogenes, which then induce tumors. Oncogenic viruses cause genetic alterations and mutations that allow the cell to express the abilities and properties it had in fetal development and may lead to cancer. A retrogene is a gene that has the protein coding of the original gene in retrosequence. Oncofetal antigens are antigens that are found on the surface and inside the cancer cells. They are an expression of the cells usually associated with embryonic or fetal periods of life and may be used as tumor markers to monitor treatment. Tumor angiogenesis factor is the substance within tumors that promotes blood vessel development.

10. d. Meningeal sarcoma is from the embryonal mesoderm, is in the meninges, and is malignant. A meningioma has the same tissue of origin and anatomic site, but it is benign. Meningitis is inflammation or infection of the meninges. Meningocele is a hernia cyst filled with cerebrospinal fluid.

11. c. The breast cancer origination gives it the anatomic classification of a carcinoma. Grade II has moderate abnormal cells with moderate differentiation. $T_1N_1M_0$ represents a small tumor with only minimal regional spread to the lymph nodes and no metastasis. Sarcomas originate from embryonal mesoderm or connective tissue, muscle, bone, and fat. Leukemias and lymphomas originate from the hematopoietic system. The other histologic grading and TNM classifications do not represent this patient's tumor.

12. b. Healthy men and women should have a colonoscopy every 10 years, an annual fecal occult blood test, or a barium enema every 5 years (see Chapter 42). These frequencies may change depending on the results. Annual prostate-specific antigen (PSA) and digital rectal examinations screen for prostate problems, although the decision to test is made by the patient with his HCP.

13. b. Biopsy with pathologic evaluation is the only definitive method of determining malignancy. The other tests may be used in diagnosing the presence and extent of cancer.

14. a. A simple mastectomy can be done to prevent breast cancer in this woman with high risk. Mastectomy can also be used to control, cure, or provide palliative care for breasts with cancerous tumors. A mastectomy would not be used for biopsy or otherwise to establish a diagnosis of cancer.

15. a. 4; b. 1; c. 3; d. 2; e. 3; f. 2; g. 1; h. 2. Mammoplasty is done for rehabilitation postmastectomy. A bowel resection and debulking procedure to enhance radiation therapy are done to cure or control cancer. Laminectomy for spinal cord compression and colostomy to bypass bowel obstruction are done for palliation. Supportive care includes insertion of a feeding tube, placement of a central venous catheter, and surgical fixation of bones at risk for pathologic fracture.

16. a. Neuroblastomas are cured with chemotherapy. A positive response of cancer cells to chemotherapy is most likely in solid or hematopoietic tumors that arise from tissue that has a rapid rate of cellular proliferation and new tumors with cells that are rapidly dividing. A state of optimum health and a positive attitude of the patient will also promote the success of chemotherapy.

17. a. Nitrosoureas are cell cycle phase–nonspecific, break the DNA helix, and cross the blood-brain barrier. Antimetabolites are cell cycle phase–specific drugs that mimic essential cellular metabolites to interfere with DNA synthesis. Mitotic inhibitors are cell cycle phase–specific drugs that arrest mitosis. Antitumor antibiotics are cell cycle phase–nonspecific but bind with DNA to block RNA production.

18. b. One of the major concerns with the IV administration of vesicant chemotherapy agents is infiltration or extravasation of drugs into tissue surrounding the infusion site. When infiltrated into the skin, vesicants cause pain,

severe local tissue breakdown, and necrosis. Specific measures to ensure adequate dilution, patency, and early detection of extravasation and treatment are important. The other options are not related to the administration of vesicants.

19. a. Intravesical regional chemotherapy is administered into the bladder via a urinary catheter. Leukemia is treated with IV chemotherapy. Osteogenic sarcoma is treated with intraarterial chemotherapy via vessels supplying the tumor. Metastasis to the brain is treated with intraventricular or intrathecal chemotherapy via an Ommaya reservoir or lumbar punctures.

20. d. Intraperitoneal regional chemotherapy administration is used to treat metastasis from a primary colorectal cancer. Intrathecal administration is used with the spinal cord or the brain. Intraarterial administration is used to deliver chemotherapy to tumors via specific vessels. IV administration is used for systemic administration.

21. c. Patients should always be taught what to expect during a course of chemotherapy, including side effects and expected outcome. Side effects of chemotherapy are serious, but it is important that patients be informed about what measures can be taken to help them cope with the side effects of therapy. Hair loss related to chemotherapy is usually reversible and wigs, scarves, or turbans can be used during and following chemotherapy until the hair grows back.

22. c. Tissue that is actively proliferating, such as gastrointestinal (GI) mucosa (esophageal and oropharyngeal mucosa) and bone marrow, exhibits early acute responses to radiation therapy in the area. Radiation ionization breaks chemical bonds in DNA, which makes cells incapable of surviving mitosis. This loss of proliferative ability yields cellular death at the time of division for both normal cells and cancer cells, but cancer cells are more likely to be dividing because of the loss of control of cellular division. Cartilage, bone, kidney, and nervous tissues that proliferate slowly manifest subacute or late responses.

23. d. Avoiding sources of excessive heat and cold will prevent damage to the skin. Only an electric razor is used if shaving is necessary in the treatment field. The area should be exposed to air if possible. Gentle cleansing, thorough rinsing, and patting the treatment area dry are recommended.

24. b. Brachytherapy is the implantation or insertion of radioactive materials directly into the tumor or in proximity to the tumor and may be curative. The patient is a source of radiation. In addition to implementing the principles of time, distance, and shielding, caregivers should wear film badges to monitor the amount of radiation exposure. Computerized dosimetry and simulation are used in external radiation therapy.

25. a. Walking programs, or activity the patient enjoys, scheduled during the time of day when the patient feels better are a way for patients to keep active without overtaxing themselves, stimulate appetite, enhance functional capacity, and help combat the depression caused by inactivity. Ignoring the fatigue or overstressing the body can make symptoms worse. The patient should rest before activity and as necessary.

26. b. Alkylating chemotherapeutic agents and high-dose radiation are most likely to cause secondary malignancies as a late effect of treatment, especially leukemia, angiosarcoma, and skin cancer. The other conditions are not known to be late effects of radiation or chemotherapy.

27. c. Immunotherapy uses normal components of the immune system and is used therapeutically to boost or manipulate the immune system to create an environment not conducive for cancer cell growth or that attacks cancer cells directly. Immunotherapies may cause flu-like symptoms. The other options are not correct.

28. c. The nadir is the point of the lowest blood counts after chemotherapy is started, and it is the time when the patient is most at risk for infection. Because infection is the most common cause of morbidity and death in cancer patients, identification of risk and interventions to protect the patient are of the highest priority. The other problems will be treated, but they are not the priority.

29. d. An allogeneic hematopoietic stem cell transplantation (HSCT) is one in which peripheral stems cells or bone marrow from a human leukocyte antigen (HLA)-matched donor is infused into a patient who has received high doses of chemotherapy, with or without radiation, to eradicate cancerous cells. In an autologous HSCT, the patient's own stem cells are removed before therapy to destroy the bone marrow, and they may be treated to remove cancer cells. The marrow or stem cells may be infused shortly after conditioning treatment or frozen and stored for later use. There is a risk of graft-versus-host disease in allogeneic transplants. With either source, the new bone marrow will take several weeks to produce new blood cells and protective isolation is necessary during this time.

30. a. Hyperkalemia and hyperuricemia are characteristic of tumor lysis syndrome, which is the result of rapid destruction of large numbers of tumor cells. Signs include hyperuricemia that causes acute kidney injury, hyperkalemia, hyperphosphatemia, and hypocalcemia. To prevent renal failure and other problems, the primary treatment includes increasing urine production using hydration therapy and decreasing uric acid concentrations using allopurinol (Zyloprim). Electrocardiogram (ECG) monitoring is important with hyperkalemia, but the priority is to increase urine output. Administering a bisphosphonate is for hypercalcemia.

31. d. The priority in pain management is to obtain a comprehensive history of the patient's pain. This will determine the medications most useful for this patient's pain to enable giving the dose that relieves the pain with the fewest side effects. Teaching the patient about the lack of tolerance and addiction associated with effective cancer pain management will also be important for this patient's pain management. Vital signs and behavior are not reliable indicators with the chronic pain of cancer. A pain diary identifies pain management.

32. a, b, d, e. Feeling in control, having a strong support system, and the potential of cure or control of the cancer will have a positive effect on coping with the diagnosis. The other options will make coping more difficult for the patient. (See Table 15.21.)

Case Study

1. **Significant**: WBC count: 3200/μL; Temp: 99.7°F (37.4°C); Neutrophils: 500/μL; **Unrelated**: Reports no appetite (GI); Decreased skin turgor (indicates dehydration); Nausea and vomiting (related to chemotherapy); Expresses no hope (may be depressed).

2. A., B., D., F., H. Having a strong support system, being able to openly express concerns and feelings, and managing stress through meditation are important to having a positive hopeful attitude about treatment.

3. Nursing interventions appropriate for **hyperthermia**: acetaminophen acts as an antipyretic and administer fluid bolus to keep the patient hydrated because fever can cause dehydration; **impaired immunity**: monitor for signs of infection by checking temperature every 4 hours and instituting neutropenic precautions to protect the patient from infection; **impaired gastrointestinal function (nausea and vomiting)**: administer antiemetics to control nausea and vomiting and administer fluid bolus to keep the patient hydrated because nausea and vomiting can cause dehydration; **nutritionally compromised**: encourage small frequent meals, keep a food diary to track calories and fluids, perform frequent oral care (due to nausea and vomiting and promote palatable taste for food), and monitor weight to assess for weight gain or loss.

4. **1**=Epoetin alfa; **2**=hypertension and thrombosis; **3**=Pegfilgrastim; **4**=bone pain and N/V; **5**=thrombocytopenia; **6**=tachycardia and shortness of breath

5. **Effective** teaching to prevent infection include the following statements: "I will perform frequent hand washing with antibacterial soap." "I need to report fevers to my HCP." and "I will use an electric razor to shave." (blade razors can cause open wounds) **Ineffective**: "I can walk barefoot around the house, as long as I wear shoes outside." (shoes should be worn in the house as well as outside to protect feet from injury) "I will use a clean technique when changing the PICC dressing." (PICC dressings should be changed using aseptic technique) **Unrelated**: "I will refer to online cancer resources to learn coping strategies." (this isn't germane to infection prevention)

CHAPTER 17

1. 1000
2. 54 to 45 L: 90 kg × 60% = 54, 90 kg × 50% = 45
3. a, d, e. With fluid volume deficit, the osmoreceptors stimulate thirst. Hyperosmolar extracellular fluid (ECF) draws fluid out of the cells. The sodium-potassium pump maintains the fluid balance between the intracellular fluid (ICF) and ECF. Third spacing is when fluid moves into spaces that normally have little or no fluid. A cell surrounded by hypoosmolar fluid will swell and burst as water moves into the cell.
4. a. 7; b. 6; c. 4; d. 3; e. 5; f. 1; g. 2

5. $2 \times 147 + \dfrac{6}{2.8} + \dfrac{126}{18} = 303.14$. The patient's plasma osmolality is increased.

6. c, e. At the arterial end of the capillary, capillary hydrostatic pressure exceeds plasma oncotic pressure and fluid moves into the interstitial space. At the capillary level, hydrostatic pressure is the major force causing fluid to shift from vascular to the interstitial space. The other options would not cause edema.

7.

Event or Factor	Direction of Fluid Shift	Mechanism of Fluid Movement Involved
Burns	1	b
Dehydration	2	c
Fluid overload	3, 4	d
Hyponatremia	4	a
Low serum albumin	1	e
Administration of 10% glucose	1	a
Application of elastic bandages	4	c

8. a. Serum osmolality increases as a large amount of sodium is absorbed. b. Intake of these foods stimulates antidiuretic hormone (ADH) release from the posterior pituitary, which increases water reabsorption from the kidney, lowering the sodium concentration but increasing vascular volume and hydrostatic pressure, perhaps causing fluid shift into interstitial spaces.

9. d. Aldosterone is secreted by the adrenal cortex in response to a decrease in plasma volume (loss of water) and resulting decreased renal perfusion; decreased serum sodium, increased serum potassium, or adrenocorticotropic hormone (ACTH).

10. b. A decrease in renin and aldosterone and an increase in ADH and atrial natriuretic peptide (ANP) lead to decreased sodium reabsorption and increased water retention by the kidney, both of which lead to hyponatremia. Loss of subcutaneous tissue and thinning dermis of aging lead to increased moisture lost through the skin. Plasma oncotic pressure is often decreased because of lack of protein intake.

11. a, b, c, d, e. All of these are important in assessing fluid balance in a postoperative patient. Daily weight along with these assessments will provide data about potential fluid volume abnormalities.

12. d. A major cause of hypernatremia is a water deficit, which can occur in those with a decreased sensitivity to thirst, the major protection against hyperosmolality. All other conditions lead to hyponatremia.

13. d. As water shifts into and out of cells in response to the osmolality of the blood, the cells that are most sensitive to shrinking or swelling are those of the brain, resulting in neurologic symptoms.

14. a. 4; b. 6; c. 1; d. 1, 4, 6, 7; e. 2; f. 4, 8, 9; g. 2, 3; h. 4, 6, 8, 10; i. 6, 8; j. 1, 4; k. 5; l. 1, 4; m. 3, 6, 7, 9; n. 1, 2, 4, 5, 6

15. b, c. Because of the osmotic pressure of sodium, water will be excreted with the sodium lost with the diuretic. A change in the relative concentration of sodium will not be seen, but an isotonic fluid loss will occur. Diuretics can also cause a loss of calcium in the urine.

16. c. Potassium maintains normal cardiac rhythm, transmission and conduction of nerve impulses, and contraction of muscles. Cardiac cells have the most clinically significant changes with potassium imbalances because of changes in cardiac conduction. Although paralysis may occur with severe potassium imbalances, cardiac changes are seen earlier and much more commonly.

17. b. In metabolic acidosis, hydrogen ions in the blood are taken into the cell in exchange for potassium ions as a means of buffering excess acids. This results in an increase in serum potassium until the kidneys have time to excrete the excess potassium.

18. d. Chvostek's sign is a contraction of facial muscles in response to a tap over the facial nerve. This indicates the neuromuscular irritability of low calcium levels. IV calcium is the treatment used to prevent laryngeal spasms and respiratory arrest. Calcitonin and loop diuretics are treatments for hypercalcemia. Oral vitamin D supplements are part of the treatment for hypocalcemia but not for impending tetany.

19. c. Kidneys are the major route of phosphate excretion, a function that is impaired in renal failure. A reciprocal relationship exists between phosphorus and calcium, and high serum phosphate levels of kidney failure cause low calcium concentration in the serum.

20. c. 7.35 to 7.45; 20 to 1. The other answers are incorrect.

21. a, b, c. CO_2 elimination by the lungs, neutralized HCl, and H_2CO_3 formation are all part of the carbonic acid-bicarbonate buffer system. Shifts of H^+ in and out of the cell are characteristics of the cellular buffer system. Free basic radical dissociation is characteristic of the protein buffer system.

22. a, b, d. Base neutralization to a weak base, water, and salt and elimination of sodium biphosphate by the kidneys are characteristic of the phosphate buffer system. Free acid radical dissociation is characteristic of the protein buffer system. Chloride shifting in and out of red blood cells is characteristic of the hemoglobin buffer system.

23. c. The amount of CO_2 in the blood directly relates to carbonic acid concentration and subsequently hydrogen ion concentration. The CO_2 combines with water in the blood to form carbonic acid and in cases in which CO_2 is retained in the blood, acidosis occurs.

24. a. 3; b. 4; c. 2; d. 1. Respiratory acid-base imbalances are associated with excesses or deficits of carbonic acid. Metabolic acid-base imbalances are associated with excesses or deficits of bicarbonate.

25. d. Decreased respiratory rate and kidney excretion of HCO_3^- compensates for metabolic alkalosis. Shifting of bicarbonate for Cl^- may buffer acute respiratory alkalosis. The kidney conserves bicarbonate and excretes hydrogen to compensate for respiratory acidosis. Kussmaul respirations occur with metabolic acidosis to compensate.

26. a. 1; b. 1; c. 1; d. 3; e. 2; f. 2; g. 4; h. 3; i. 4

27. b. Anion Gap $= Na^+ - (HCO_3^- + Cl^-)$. Calculate the anion gap by subtracting the serum bicarbonate and chloride levels from the serum sodium level. It should normally be 8 to 12 mmol/L. The anion gap is increased in metabolic acidosis associated with acid gain (e.g., diabetic ketoacidosis) but is normal in metabolic acidosis caused by bicarbonate loss (e.g., diarrhea).

28. a. *Interpretation*: respiratory alkalosis with hypoxemia
    1. pH, $PaCO_2$, and PaO_2 are abnormal.
    2. pH > 7.45 shows alkalosis.
    3. $PaCO_2$ is < 35 mm Hg, indicating respiratory alkalosis. Respiratory alkalosis matches the pH.
    4. HCO_3^- is within 22 to 26 mEq/L which is normal.
    5. No compensation is occurring. Although uncommon, if the HCO_3^- were decreased, compensation would be present.

    6. The PaO_2 is < 80 mm Hg, indicating hypoxemia, which is a common cause of respiratory alkalosis.

  b. *Interpretation*: partially compensated metabolic acidosis
1. pH, $PaCO_2$ and HCO_3^- are abnormal.
2. pH < 7.35 shows acidosis.
3. $PaCO_2$ is < 35 mm Hg, indicating respiratory alkalosis. The $PaCO_2$ is in the opposite direction of the pH.
4. $HCO3-$ is < 22 mEq, indicating metabolic acidosis, which matches the pH.
5. The low $PaCO_2$ indicate the lungs are trying to compensate for the metabolic acidosis.
6. The PaO_2 is within normal limits.

  c. *Interpretation*: respiratory acidosis with hypoxemia
1. pH, $PaCO_2$ and PaO_2 are abnormal.
2. pH < 7.35 shows acidosis.
3. $PaCO_2$ is > 45 mm Hg, matching the pH and indicating respiratory acidosis.
4. HCO_3- is normal.
5. Compensation is not evident until the kidneys have time to retain bicarbonate.
6. PaO_2 is < 80 mm Hg, indicating hypoxemia, which may occur with chronic obstructive pulmonary disease (COPD).

  d. *Interpretation*: partially compensated metabolic alkalosis
1. pH, $PaCO_2$ and HCO_3- are abnormal.
2. pH > 7.45 shows alkalosis.
3. $PaCO_2$ is > 45 mm Hg, indicating respiratory acidosis, and is opposite of the pH.
4. HCO_3- is > 26 mEq, indicating metabolic alkalosis, which matches the pH.
5. The $PaCO_2$ in the opposite direction of the alkalotic pH shows that the lungs are trying to compensate for the alkalosis.
6. The PaO_2 is within normal limits.

  e. *Interpretation*: compensated or chronic metabolic alkalosis indicated by the high $PaCO_2$ and a pH within normal range
1. $PaCO_2$ and HCO_3- are abnormal.
2. pH is within normal range but toward alkalosis.
3. $PaCO_2$ is > 45 mm Hg, indicating respiratory acidosis.
4. HCO_3- is > 26 mEq, indicating metabolic alkalosis. Because the body will not overcompensate, the metabolic alkalosis is a closer match with the pH.
5. The high $PaCO_2$ indicates the ability of the lungs to compensate for the metabolic alkalosis.
6. The PaO_2 is within normal limits.

  f. *Interpretation*: compensated respiratory acidosis as reflected by high HCO_3- and pH in normal range
1. $PaCO_2$ and HCO_3- are abnormal.
2. pH is within normal range but toward acidosis.
3. $PaCO_2$ is > 45 mm Hg, indicating respiratory acidosis.
4. HCO_3- is > 26 mEq, indicating metabolic alkalosis.
5. Because the body will not overcompensate, the respiratory acidosis is a closer match with the pH. The high HCO_3- indicates the ability of the kidneys to compensate for the respiratory acidosis.
6. PaO_2 is within normal limits.

29. a. Fluids such as 5% dextrose in water (D_5W) allow water to move from the ECF to the ICF. Although D_5W is physiologically isotonic, the dextrose is rapidly metabolized, leaving free water to shift into cells.

30. c. An isotonic solution does not change the osmolality of the blood and does not cause fluid shifts between the ECF and ICF. In the case of ECF loss, an isotonic solution, such as lactated Ringer's solution, is ideal because it stays in the extracellular compartment. A hypertonic solution would pull fluid from the cells into the ECF, resulting in cellular fluid loss and possible vascular overload.

31. d. The greatest risk with central venous access device (CVAD) is systemic infection. Dressings that are loose should be changed at once to reduce this risk.

32. a. 3; b. 7; c. 4; d. 8; e. 2; f. 5; g. 6; h. 1. The first nursing action after a CVAD is inserted and before it is used is to ensure proper placement with a chest x-ray. Assessments, flushing, dressing changes, and cap changes are completed according to facility policies, but hand hygiene must be completed before manipulating the CVAD to prevent infection. Strict sterile technique is used with dressing and cap changes as well as having the patient turn their face away from the insertion site to avoid contamination.

33. a. Catheters tunneled to the distal end of the superior vena cava or the right atrium are vascular access devices inserted into central veins, which decrease the incidence of extravasation, provide for rapid dilution of chemotherapy, and reduce the need for venipunctures. Most right atrial catheters, except for a Groshong catheter, must be flushed with heparin to prevent clotting in the tubing. Regional chemotherapy administration delivers the drug directly to the tumor and is the only administration route that can decrease the systemic effects of the drugs.

34. b. With a low magnesium level there is an increased risk for hypokalemia and hypocalcemia as well as altered sodium-potassium pump and altered carbohydrate and protein metabolism. Hypokalemia could lead to dysrhythmias and severe muscle weakness. The sodium and phosphate levels are also not within normal limits. However, the implications are not as life-threatening. The calcium level is normal.

Case Study

1. Abnormal laboratory results include: K^+: 2.5 mEq/L (2.5 mmol/L), Cl^-: 85 mEq/L (85 mmol/L), HCO_3^-: 40 mEq/L (40 mmol/L), BUN: 42 mg/dL (15 mmol/L), Hct: 52%, Abnormal ABG results: pH: 7.52, $PaCO_2$: 55 mm Hg, HCO_3^-: 34 mEq/L (34 mmol/L)

2. **Electrolyte imbalance**: confusion (hypochloremia and hyperkalemia), generalized weakness (hypokalemia), weak peripheral pulses (hypokalemia), pH 7.52 (hypokalemia), HCO_3^- 34 mEq/L (hypokalemia), shallow respirations (hypokalemia); **Metabolic alkalosis**: confusion, sinus tachycardia, pH 7.52, HCO_3^- 34 mEq/L, shallow respirations (compensatory to retain CO_2); **Fluid imbalance**: sinus tachycardia, decreased skin turgor, dry mucous membranes, Hct 52% (dehydration causes thicker blood), weak peripheral pulses, hypotension

3. **Indicated**: continuous cardiac monitoring (hypokalemia can cause dysrhythmias), auscultate breath sounds (fluid overload can occur during fluid resuscitation causing crackles in the lungs), monitor urine output (will indicate fluid resuscitation to treat dehydration is adequate), place patient on falls precautions (patient is confused and weak increasing risk for falls); **Contraindicated**: 3% saline infusion (patient has normal sodium lab result, is dehydrated and needs fluid resuscitation with isotonic IV fluids; 3% saline is hypertonic which will cause more dehydration and is not an acceptable fluid for fluid resuscitation), apply oxygen 4 L/min (isn't warranted with a PaO_2 of 88 mm Hg); **Non-essential**: passive ROM isn't essential as the primary problems of metabolic alkalosis and dehydration need to be addressed first. Active ROM is preferred.

4. A., C., D., H. Increased sodium intake is contraindicated in the patient due to her history of heart failure. Palpitations could indicate electrolyte imbalances, like hypo- or hyperkalemia, and should be reported to the HCP. The patient takes diuretics to treat heart failure; therefore, diuresis is expected. Weighing herself daily is recommended to monitor for fluid retention that may be caused by heart failure.

5. **1**=colloid; **2**=oncotic pressure; **3**=albumin; **4**=5% and 25% respectively; **5**=factor VIII

CHAPTER 18

1. d, e. Hysterectomy and herniorrhaphy are done to eliminate and repair pathologic conditions. Gastroscopy is for the purpose of diagnosis. Rhinoplasty is done for a cosmetic improvement. A tracheotomy is palliative.

2. a. Ambulatory surgery is usually less expensive and more convenient, generally involving fewer diagnostic studies, fewer preoperative and postoperative medications, and less susceptibility to health care–associated infections (HAIs). However, the nurse is still responsible for assessing, supporting, and teaching the patient who is undergoing surgery, regardless of where the surgery is performed.

3. a. Excessive anxiety and stress can affect surgical recovery and the nurse's role in psychologically preparing the patient for surgery is to assess for potential stressors that could negatively affect surgery. Specific fears should be identified and addressed by the nurse by listening and explaining planned postoperative care. Ignoring her behavior, falsely reassuring the patient, and telling her not to be anxious are not therapeutic.

4. a, b, d, f. Garlic, fish oil, vitamin E, and ginkgo biloba may increase bleeding for the surgical patient. Valerian may cause excess sedation. Astragalus may increase BP before and during surgery.

5. c. Risk factors for latex allergies include a history of hay fever and allergies to foods, such as avocados, kiwi, bananas, potatoes, peaches, and apricots. When a patient identifies such allergies, the patient should be further questioned about exposure to latex and specific reactions to allergens. A history of any allergic responsiveness increases the risk for hypersensitivity reactions to drugs used during anesthesia, but the hay fever and fruit allergies are specifically related to latex allergy. After the nurse identifies the allergic reaction, the anesthesia care provider (ACP) should be notified, the allergy alert wristband should be applied, and the note in the record will include the allergies and reactions as well as the nursing actions related to the allergies.

6. d. Blood urea nitrogen (BUN), serum creatinine, and electrolytes are used to assess renal function and should be evaluated before surgery. Other studies are often evaluated in the presence of heart or respiratory disease, or bleeding tendencies.

7. a. Obesity, as well as spinal, chest, and airway deformities, may compromise respiratory function during and after surgery. Dehydration may require preoperative fluid therapy. An enlarged liver may indicate hepatic dysfunction that will increase perioperative risk related to glucose control, coagulation, and drug interactions. Weak peripheral pulses may reflect circulatory problems that could affect healing.

8. a, b, e. Procedural information includes what will be done for surgical preparation, including what to bring and what to wear to the surgery center, length and type of food and fluid restrictions, physical preparation required, pain control, need for coughing and deep breathing (if appropriate), and procedures done before and during surgery (such as vital signs, IV lines, and how anesthesia is administered). Characteristics of monitoring equipment is process information. Odors and sensations experienced are sensory information (see Table 17.6).

9. a. The HCP is ultimately responsible for obtaining informed consent. However, the nurse may be responsible for obtaining and witnessing the patient's signature on the consent form. The nurse must be a patient advocate during the signing of the consent form, verifying that consent is voluntary and that the patient understands the implications of consent, but the primary legal action by the nurse is witnessing the patient's signature.

10. a. The nurse should notify the surgeon because the patient needs further explanation of the planned surgery. b. Clear understanding of the information

11. a. The preoperative fasting recommendations of the American Society of Anesthesiology indicate that clear liquids may be taken up to 2 hours before surgery for healthy patients undergoing elective procedures. There is evidence that longer fasting is not necessary (see Table 17.7).

12. b. The rationale for use of preoperative checklists is to ensure that the many preparations and precautions performed before surgery have been completed and documented. Patient identification, administration of preoperative medications, voiding, and instructions to the family may be documented on the checklist, which ensures that no details are omitted.

13. c. One of the major reasons that older adults need increased time preoperatively is the presence of impaired vision and hearing that slows understanding of preoperative instructions and preparation for surgery. Thought processes and cognitive abilities may also be impaired in some older adults. The older adult's decreased adaptation to stress because of physiologic changes may increase surgical risks, and overwhelming surgery-related losses may result in difficulty coping that is not directly related to time needed for preoperative preparation. The involvement of caregivers in preoperative activities may be appropriate for patients of all ages.

14. d. The elevated white blood count (WBC) count may indicate an infection. The surgeon will probably postpone the surgery until the cause of the elevated WBC count has been found. The other values are within normal limits.

15. a, b, c, d, e. All of these are actions that are needed to ensure that the patient is ready for surgery. In addition, the nurse should verify that the identification band and allergy band (if applicable) are on; the patient is not wearing any cosmetics; nail polish has been removed; valuables have been removed and secured; and prosthetics, such as eyeglasses, have been removed and secured.

Case Study

1. C., D., E., G., I. The patient should be instructed to be NPO after midnight. He may have clear liquids 2 hours before the procedure. The patient needs a responsible adult to accompany him home. They can take public transportation or ride share, but the patient cannot use either forms of transportation by himself. He also cannot drive himself home after receiving sedation. The patient should leave all valuables at home for safe keeping, but should bring a form of ID and health insurance information. Ibuprofen can cause bleeding and should be avoided prior to surgery.

2. **Anxiety**: "Wife will not be able to manage without him" (indicates he is worried about his diagnosis and prognosis); never been hospitalized (being new to the health care system can cause anxiety because of not knowing what to expect); fears diagnosis (he is worried about having lung cancer); has 2 children with cystic fibrosis (both children have chronic diseases which need frequent care; the patient is worried about not being able to care for them or possibly dying and leaving them without a father); mass in upper lobe of right lung (may be lung cancer which causes anxiety). **Risk for impaired respiratory function**: 28 pack-years smoking history (can lead to lung cancer and other chronic diseases like COPD which may cause respiratory distress); mild obesity (habitus may interfere with deep breathing and cause respiratory impairment); hematocrit 31% (anemia that may cause hypoxemia or an increased RR as a compensatory response); **Substance Use**: 28 pack-years smoker

3. 1=informed; 2=surgeon; 3=risks, alternatives, benefits; 4=notify the surgeon

4. Preoperative teaching that is **Indicated**: taking deep breaths and coughing after the procedure to promote adequate oxygenation and prevent atelectasis; the patient will be monitored for at least an hour after the procedure to allow the sedation to wear off, treat side effects, and to monitor the patient's respiratory status; SOB is expected after a bronchoscopy but should resolve before the patient is discharged home; **Contraindicated**: the patient is not a candidate for a blood transfusion (the hematocrit would usually need to be less than 25% and the patient would need to be symptomatic such as having tachycardia or hypotension; there is minimal blood loss during a bronchoscopy); the patient may have pain or discomfort after the procedure (it is unrealistic to expect to be pain free); **Non-essential**: the patient may need to be NPO for a specified time after the procedure, but eating and drinking is not a requirement to be discharged.

5. 1=0.2 mg IV; 2=benzodiazepine; 3=decrease respiratory secretions; 4=cefazolin; 5=anticholinergic; 6=ondansetron; 7=sedation; 8=50 mcg IV

CHAPTER 19

1. Although all of the factors listed are important to the safety and well-being of the patient, the first consideration in the physical environment of the surgical suite is prevention of transmission of infection to the patient.

2. b. Persons in street clothes or attire other than surgical scrub clothing can interact with personnel of the surgical suite in unrestricted areas, such as the holding area, nursing station, control desk, or locker rooms. Only authorized personnel wearing surgical attire and hair covering are allowed in semirestricted areas, such as corridors, and masks must be worn in restricted areas, such as operating rooms, sterile core, and scrub sink areas.

3. a, c, e. The scrub nurse is involved in sterile activities, including preparing instrument table and passing instruments to the surgeon, and remains in the sterile area of the operating room (OR). The circulating nurse documents intraoperative care, checks mechanical and electrical equipment, and monitors blood and other fluid loss and urine output.

4. a. The protection of the patient from injury in the OR environment is maintained by the circulating nurse, who ensures functioning equipment; prevents falls and injury during transport, transfer, and positioning; monitors asepsis; and provides supportive care for the anesthetized patient.

5. d. The Universal Protocol supported by The Joint Commission (TJC) is used to prevent wrong site, wrong procedure, and wrong surgery in view of a high rate of these problems nationally. It involves pausing just before the procedure starts to verify patient identity, surgical site, and surgical procedure.

6. a. The mask covering the face is not considered sterile and if in contact with sterile gloved hands, it contaminates the gloves. The gown at chest level and to 2 inches above the elbows is considered sterile, as is the drape placed at the surgical area.

7. c. Musculoskeletal deformities can be a risk factor for positioning injuries and require special padding and support on the operating table. Skin lesions and break in sterile technique are risk factors for infection and electrical or mechanical equipment failure may lead to other types of injury.

8. d. Methohexital (Brevital) is a rapid-acting, short-lasting barbiturate used to induce general anesthesia. Nitrous oxide is a weak gaseous anesthetic. Propofol (Diprivan) is a nonbarbiturate hypnotic that has a rapid onset and may be used for induction. Isoflurane (Forane) is a volatile liquid inhalation agent.

9. b. The volatile liquid inhalation agents have very little residual analgesia and patients experience early onset of pain when the agents are discontinued. These agents are associated with a low incidence of nausea and vomiting. Prolonged respiratory depression is not common because of their rapid elimination. Hypothermia is not related to use of these agents, but they may precipitate malignant hyperthermia in conjunction with neuromuscular blocking agents.

10. a. Midazolam is a rapid, short-acting, sedative-hypnotic benzodiazepine that is used to prevent recall of events under anesthesia because of its amnestic properties.

11.

Drug	Use	Nursing Interventions
Ketamine (Ketalar)	Dissociative anesthetic, analgesic and amnesic	Monitor for cardiopulmonary effects, agitation or hallucinations, early pain, and nausea and vomiting
Fentanyl (Sublimaze)	Induce and maintain anesthesia with analgesia	Monitor for and treat cardiopulmonary depression, nausea, vomiting, and pruritus
Desflurane (Suprane)	Induce and maintain anesthesia	Promote early analgesia—assess for cardiopulmonary depression, nausea and vomiting, respiratory irritation
Succinylcholine (Anectine)	Produce musculoskeletal paralysis	Monitor respiratory muscle movement, airway patency, and temperature
Dexmedetomidine (Precedex)	Induce and maintain sedation in nonintubated patients before and/or during surgical procedures	Monitor heart rate and rhythm and BP

12. d. Monitored anesthesia care (MAC) refers to sedation that is similar to general anesthesia using sedative, anxiolytic, and/or analgesic medications. It can be administered by an ACP. The patient must be assessed and the physiologic problems that may develop must be managed because of the high risk of complications resulting in clinical emergencies.

13. a. 3; b. 5; c. 1; d. 4; e. 2

14. d. Moderate sedation uses sedative, anxiolytic, and/or analgesic medications. Inhalation agents are not used. It is not expected to induce levels of sedation that would impair a patient's ability to protect the airway.

15. b. During epidural and spinal anesthesia, a sympathetic nervous system blockade may occur that results in hypotension, bradycardia, and nausea and vomiting. A spinal headache may occur after (not during) spinal anesthesia and loss of consciousness and seizures are indicative of IV absorption overdose. Upward extension of the effect of the anesthesia results in inadequate respiratory excursion and apnea.

16. a. Because ketamine is a phenyl cyclohexyl piperidine (PCP) derivative, the drug may cause hallucinations and nightmares, limiting its usefulness. Concurrent use of midazolam (Versed) can reduce or eliminate the hallucinations. Nausea and urinary retention are not common effects of ketamine. The patient who has received ketamine may appear catatonic, is amnesic, and has profound analgesia.

17. b. Although malignant hyperthermia (MH) can result in cardiac arrest and death, if the patient is known or suspected to be at risk for the disorder, appropriate precautions taken by the ACP can provide for safe anesthesia for the patient. Because preventive measures are possible if the risk is known, it is critical that preoperative assessment include a careful family history of surgical events. The definitive treatment of MH is prompt administration of dantrolene (Dantrium). The cooling blanket would have no effect.

18. c. MH occurs in susceptible people when they are exposed to certain anesthetic agents. Succinylcholine (Anectine),

especially when given with volatile inhalation agents, is the primary trigger. Other factors include stress, trauma, and heat.

Case Study

1. **Essential**: vital signs; history of COPD and heart failure; type of surgery; allergies; NPO status; baseline comfort; **Non-essential**: height; plans for discharge home; and retired occupation.

2. **Indicated**: performs a *Time Out*; positions the patient; attaches monitoring equipment; **Contraindicated**: having the patient stand to transfer to the OR table (risk for falls and injury as the patient had a benzodiazepine which causes drowsiness and possible hypotension); cut off the ID bracelet (places the patient at risk for wrong procedure and wrong medications); the surgical consent form should be signed before entering the OR and before any medications causing sedation are given; **Non-essential**: updating the family upon arrival to the OR (the family should be kept informed but this should happen further into the operation as the family is likely to have seen the patient before being transferred to the OR)

3. B., E., G., H., J. There are a variety of prep solutions, many contain alcohol but alcohol by itself isn't an appropriate prep solution. Hair should be clipped, not shaved due to skin irritation and sores that occur with shaving. The prep solution should be contained to the surgical area and not allowed to pool as it can burn the skin. The surgical area should be prepped from clean (surgical site) to dirty (distal to surgical site). Draping should occur after skin prep exposing only the surgical site.

4. Clinical problem: **Risk for injury**: allow skin prep fumes to dispel (can be flammable and cause a fire in the OR); checking electrical equipment before using it on the patient; correctly placing the grounding pad. **Hypothermia**: using Bair hugger (a forced-air warming device); only exposing surgical site (reduces patient exposure to the environment); **Risk for infection**: antibiotic administered minutes before incision is made (given prophylactically for most surgeries); confirms CHG bath is done before surgery (to reduce microorganism exposure); circulating nurse monitors aseptic technique by all providers.

5. **Expected**: temperature 36.4°C (is low but acceptable); RR of 18 is within normal range; a spinal anesthetic causes absence of sensation and movement of the lower extremities; oxygen saturation of 97% is acceptable; **Requires Follow-Up**: BP is hypotensive and needs to be addressed; patient is bradycardic with HR of 52 (which may be contributing to hypotension) which is low unless this HR is his baseline; tingling in arms and hands and having difficulty breathing are unexpected and could indicate the spinal has migrated into the epidural space causing systemic manifestations.

CHAPTER 20

1. a. Although some surgical procedures and drug administration require more intensive postanesthesia care, how fast and through which levels of care patients are moved depend on the condition of the patient. A physiologically unstable outpatient may stay an extended time in Phase I, whereas a patient requiring hospitalization but who is stable and recovering may well be transferred quickly to an inpatient unit.

2. c. Physiologic status of the patient is always prioritized with regard to airway, breathing, and circulation, and respiratory adequacy is the first assessment priority of the patient on admission to the postanesthesia care unit (PACU) from the operating room. Following assessment of respiratory function, cardiovascular, neurologic, and renal function should be assessed as well as the surgical site.

3. c. The admission of the patient to the PACU is a joint effort between the anesthesia care provider (ACP), who is responsible for supervising the postanesthesia recovery of the patient, and the PACU nurse, who provides care during anesthesia recovery. The ACP gives a verbal report that presents the details of the surgical and anesthetic course, preoperative conditions influencing the surgical and anesthetic outcome, and PACU treatment plans to ensure patient safety and continuity of care.

4. b. Even before patients awaken from anesthesia, their sense of hearing returns and all activities should be explained by the nurse from the time of admission to the PACU to assist in orientation and decrease confusion.

5. b. Electrocardiogram (ECG) monitoring is performed on patients to assess initial cardiovascular problems during anesthesia recovery. Fluid and electrolyte status is an indication of renal function. Determinations of arterial blood gases and direct arterial BP monitoring are used only in special cardiovascular or respiratory problems.

6. a. Hypoxemia occurs with atelectasis and aspiration as well as pulmonary edema, pulmonary embolism, and bronchospasm. Hypercapnia is caused by decreased removal of CO_2 from the respiratory system that could occur with airway obstruction or hypoventilation. Hypoventilation may occur with depression of central respiratory drive, poor respiratory muscle tone caused by disease or anesthesia, mechanical restriction, or pain. Airway obstruction could occur with the tongue blocking the airway, restrained thick secretions, laryngospasm, or laryngeal edema.

7. d. An unconscious or semiconscious patient should be placed in a lateral position to protect the airway from obstruction by the tongue. Deep breathing and elevation of the head of the bed are implemented to facilitate gas exchange when the patient is responsive. Oxygen administration is often used, but the patient must first have a patent airway.

8. c. Incisional pain is often the greatest deterrent to patient participation in effective ventilation and ambulation. Adequate and regular analgesic medications should be provided to encourage these activities. Controlled breathing may help the patient manage pain but does not promote coughing and deep breathing. Explanations and use of an incentive spirometer help gain patient participation but are more effective if pain is controlled.

9. c. Hypotension with normal pulse and skin assessment is typical of residual vasodilating effects of anesthesia and requires continued observation. An oxygen saturation of 88% indicates hypoxemia, whereas a narrowing pulse pressure accompanies hypoperfusion. A urinary output > 30 mL/hr is desirable and indicates normal renal function.

10. a. The most common cause of emergence delirium is hypoxemia, and initial assessment should evaluate

respiratory function. When hypoxemia is ruled out, other causes, such as a distended bladder, pain, and fluid and electrolyte disturbances, should be considered. Delayed awakening may result from neurologic injury. Dysrhythmias most often result from specific respiratory, electrolyte, or cardiac problems.

11. a. During hypothermia, oxygen demand is increased and metabolic processes slow down. Oxygen therapy is used to treat the increased demand for oxygen. Antidysrhythmics and vasodilating drugs would be used only if the hypothermia caused symptomatic dysrhythmias and vasoconstriction. Sedatives and analgesics are not indicated for hypothermia.

12. b. On initial assessment in the PACU, the airway, breathing, and circulation (ABC) status is assessed using a standardized tool that usually includes consciousness, respiration, oxygen saturation, circulation, and activity. Increased or decreased respiratory rate, hypertension, and a SpO_2 below 92% indicate inadequate oxygenation that will be treated or managed in the PACU before discharging the patient to the next phase.

13. c, d, e, f. These problems are improved with ambulation. Other clinical problems could be potential complications: Risk for urinary retention, atelectasis, and pneumonia.

14. c. The stress response causes fluid retention during the first 1 to 3 days postoperatively, and fluid overload is possible during this time. Fluid retention results from secretion and release of antidiuretic hormone (ADH) and adrenocorticotropic hormone (ACTH) by the pituitary and activation of the renin-angiotensin-aldosterone system (RAAS). ACTH stimulates the adrenal cortex to secrete cortisol and aldosterone. The RAAS increases aldosterone release, which also increases fluid retention. Aldosterone causes renal potassium loss with possible hypokalemia and blood coagulation is enhanced by cortisol.

15. c. Slow progression to ambulation by slowly changing the patient's position will help prevent syncope. Monitoring vital signs after walking will not prevent or treat syncope. Monitor the patient's pulse and BP before, during, and after position changes. Elevate the patient's head, then slowly have the patient dangle, then stand by the bed to help determine if the patient is safe for walking. Eating will not have an effect on syncope. Deep breathing and coughing will not decrease syncope, although it will prevent respiratory complications.

16. c, e. The nasogastric tube and gastrointestinal tube drain gastric contents. The T-tube drains bile, the Penrose drains wound drainage, and the indwelling catheter drains urine from the bladder.

17. d. The Hemovac removes wound drainage, especially blood. Bile is drained by a T-tube, urine is drained by an indwelling urinary catheter, and gastric contents are drained by a nasogastric tube or a gastrointestinal tube.

18. a. 2; b. 5; c. 4; d. 1; e. 3. The nurse must be aware of drains, if used, and the type of surgery to help predict the expected drainage. Dressings over surgical sites are initially removed by the surgeon unless otherwise specified and should not be changed, although reinforcing the dressing is appropriate. Some drainage is expected for most surgical wounds, and the drainage should be evaluated and recorded to establish a baseline for continuing assessment. The surgeon should be notified of excessive drainage. Dressings will then be changed as ordered with assessment for infection being done as well.

19. d. During the first 24 to 48 postoperative hours, temperature elevations to 100.4°F (38°C) are a result of the inflammatory response to surgical stress. Dehydration and lung congestion or atelectasis in the first 2 days will cause a temperature elevation above 100.4°F (38°C). Wound infections usually do not become evident until 3 to 5 days postoperatively and manifest with temperatures above 100°F (37.8°C).

20. d. Before administering all analgesic medications, the nurse should first assess the nature and intensity of the patient's pain to determine if the pain is expected, prior doses of the medication have been effective, and any undesirable side effects are occurring. The administration of as needed analgesic medication is based on the nursing assessment. If possible, pain medication should be in effect during painful activities, but activities may be scheduled around medication administration.

21. c. All postoperative patients need discharge instructions regarding what to expect and what self-care can be assumed during recovery. Symptoms to report, instructions about medications, wound care, activities, diet, and follow-up care are individualized to the patient.

Case Study

1. **Indicated**: offer oral fluids, report gross hematuria to the HCP (this is unexpected and may cause clot formation blocking urinary elimination), use bladder scan if patient is unable to void (to determine urinary retention versus fluid deficit). **Contraindicated**: naloxone administration (use is not indicated and may negate any effects of opioids that are currently managing her pain), B&O suppository (can be used to treat bladder spasms but only for patients with indwelling urinary catheters as this will relax the bladder and cause urinary retention), contact ride-share to transport patient home (the patient must have a responsible adult accompany them home. This doesn't include ride-share drivers or public transportation drivers). **Non-essential**: SCD devices (are not necessary for the ambulatory patient who will be discharged home soon after surgery), observe dressing for drainage (cystoscopy patients don't have incisions or wounds that require dressings).

2. **Expected**: patient reports burning during urination (this is expected after cystoscopy), SpO_2 96% on room air (this is an acceptable finding), patient reports feeling sleepy (an expected finding after having sedation for the procedure), needs assistance during ambulation (protects patient's safety after having sedation); **Unexpected**: BP 95/45 mm Hg (could indicate hypotension resulting from fluid loss or active bleeding), HR 110 beats/min (tachycardia could indicate a fluid deficit or active bleeding), reports nausea with movement (indicates the patient isn't tolerating the activity possibly due to hypotension or fluid deficit, antiemetics should be administered); **Unrelated**: Temperature 37.9°C (this is unrelated to the patient's ability to ambulate and doesn't provide useful information for the situation), patient reports being thirsty (isn't an immediate concern or relevant information to care for the patient).

3. B., C., F., G., H., I. The patient should wait 24 hours to drive after anesthesia or sedation. There aren't any dressings after a cystoscopy. The patient doesn't have

to strain their urine, as this applies to patients having brachytherapy with implanted radioactive seeds or after a procedure to treat urinary (kidney) stones.

4. **Discharge home**: must be accompanied by an adult, patient is able to ambulate, is able to eat and drink without nausea or vomiting, understands postoperative self-care, IV is removed; **Discharge to clinical unit**: SBAR hand-off, patient is arousable but goes to sleep easily (patients don't need to be wide awake if staying in the hospital) **Both**: PO opioid administration 15 minutes before discharge (the nurse should wait at least 30 minutes after IV opioid administration before discharging the patient from PACU, but PO administration doesn't require a specific waiting period before discharge), pain is controlled or tolerable to the patient, vital signs are at baseline or stable for the patient

5. **Laryngospasm**: use bag-valve mask to apply positive pressure ventilation, administer oxygen; **Airway obstruction**: head-tilt-chin-lift or jaw thrust, stimulate the patient, insert artificial airway; **Atelectasis**: use incentive spirometry, ambulate patient, have patient cough and deep breath, administer oxygen. **Options not chosen**: furosemide treats pulmonary edema or fluid in the lungs causing respiratory distress; chest physiotherapy treats retained pulmonary secretions to help the patient mobilize and expectorate them.

CHAPTER 21

1. a. 2; b. 1; c. 2; d. 4; e. 1; f. 5; g. 2; h. 3 (See Table 68.2.)
2. d. During the primary survey of emergency care, assessment and immediate interventions are made for life-threatening problems affecting alertness and airway, breathing, circulation, disability, exposure and environmental control, facilitate adjuncts and family, and get resuscitation adjuncts. The triage system is used initially to determine the priority of care for patients and history of the illness or accident is part of the secondary survey. Any emergency department (ED) should be able to stabilize and initially treat a patient who requires specialized care before transferring to another facility if needed.
3. d. Asymmetric chest wall movement may indicate a flail chest, which requires bag-mask ventilation with 100% oxygen and may require intubation. A central pulse is checked, and pressure is applied to a wound when there is profuse bleeding. The cervical spine is stabilized if there is any suspicion of a head or neck injury.
4. a. Specific injuries are associated with specific types of accidents and events surrounding an incident and details of the incident. The trajectory of penetrating injuries is important in identifying and treating injuries. Alcohol use is assessed with blood testing, and although information may be used for regulatory agencies, the primary use of the information is for treatment of the patient.
5. b. During the "E" step (exposure and environmental control), the nurse will remove the patient's clothing and perform a thorough physical assessment. A full set of vital signs are obtained in the "F" step (facilitate adjuncts and family). The "C" step (circulation) includes assessing mental status and capillary refill for signs of shock. The "H" step of the secondary survey involves eliciting history and head-to-toe assessment.

6. b. A nasally placed tube is contraindicated if the patient has facial fractures or a possible basilar skull fracture because the tube could enter the brain. It would not be contraindicated in the other conditions.
7. c. The mnemonic SAMPLE stands for symptoms, allergies, medications, past health history, last meal, and events/environment leading to the illness or injury. These things will provide information to deal with the emergency situation. The other options will be assessed if pertinent, but not all of them relate to health history; many are physical assessments.
8. c. Tetanus and diphtheria toxoid with acellular pertussis vaccine (Tdap) provides active immunity for tetanus, diphtheria, and pertussis. It would be used after tetanus immunoglobulin (TIG) (for immediate passive immunity) in treatment of a tetanus-prone wound if patients have not had at least 3 doses of active tetanus toxoid or are unsure of their vaccination history. If the patient has fewer than 3 doses of tetanus toxoid and a non–tetanus-prone wound, only tetanus and diphtheria toxoid (Td) or Tdap would be given to initiate active immunity. In the actively immunized patient, Td or Tdap is given for tetanus-prone wounds if it has been more than 5 years since the last dose and is given for non–tetanus-prone wounds if it has been more than 10 years since the last dose.
9. b. Therapeutic hypothermia postcardiac arrest for 24 hours after the return of spontaneous circulation (postdefibrillation) improves mortality and neurologic outcomes. Patient "b" may benefit from this therapy. Patient "a" will need airway maintenance and evaluation of the cause of unconsciousness. Patient "c" should have airway, breathing, and circulation (ABCs) monitored and begin the cooling process. Watch for dysrhythmias and provide fluid and electrolyte replacement. Patient "d" will need mechanical ventilation and diuretics.
10. b. Organ procurement organizations are called to talk with families as they are trained to screen and counsel families, obtain informed consent, and harvest organs.
11. c. Heat cramps are related to physical exertion during hot weather without adequate fluid replacement. Heatstroke is from failure of hypothalamic thermoregulatory processes. Heat exhaustion is from prolonged exposure to heat over hours or days.
12. a, d, e. In heat exhaustion, volume and electrolyte depletion, increased rectal temperature, mild confusion, profuse diaphoresis, pupil dilation, and other symptoms occur. Heatstroke is characterized by an increased core temperature (above 104°F [40°C] without sweating), the need for oxygen administration and treatment with cooling methods, and a high risk of mortality and morbidity.
13. d. Rewarming of frostbitten tissue is extremely painful, and IV analgesia should be given during the process. Blisters form in hours to days following the injury and are not an immediate concern. The affected part is submerged in a 98.6°F to 104°F (37°C to 40°C) circulating water bath. Massage or scrubbing of the tissue should be avoided because of the potential for tissue damage.
14. c. Rigidity, bradycardia, and slowed respiratory rate are signs of moderate hypothermia. The ABCs are the initial priority. Active core rewarming is indicated for moderate to severe hypothermia. Axillary temperatures are inadequate

to monitor core temperature, so esophageal, rectal, or indwelling urinary catheter thermometers are used. The patient should be assessed for other injuries but should not be exposed to prevent further loss of heat.

15. b. Patients with profound hypothermia appear dead on presentation and have fixed, dilated pupils; difficult-to-detect vital signs; unconsciousness; and apnea. Shivering is seen in mild hypothermia. Moderate hypothermia is characterized by slowed respirations, BP obtainable only by Doppler, and rigidity.

16. d. With saltwater drowning, fluid is drawn from the vascular space into the alveoli, impairing alveolar ventilation and resulting in hypoxia. Surfactant destruction and noncardiogenic pulmonary edema occur with both saltwater and freshwater drowning. Water moves from the alveoli to the circulation with freshwater drowning.

17. b. Airway and oxygenation are the first priorities. A life-threatening consequence of drowning of any type is hypoxia from fluid-filled and poorly ventilated alveoli. Correction of acidosis occurs with effective ventilation and oxygenation. Lactated Ringer's solution or normal saline solution is started to manage fluid balance, and mannitol or furosemide may be used to treat free water and cerebral edema.

18. a. Wood ticks or dog ticks release a neurotoxin as long as the tick head is attached to the body. Tick removal is essential for effective treatment. Tick removal leads to return of muscle movement, usually within 48 to 72 hours. There is no antidote and hemodialysis is not known to remove the neurotoxin. Antibiotics are used to treat Lyme disease and Rocky Mountain spotted fever, which are infections spread by tick bites.

19. c. The priority care for a patient with an animal bite is to clean it with copious irrigation and debridement (if necessary). Antibiotics will be prescribed prophylactically because this patient is at greater risk for infection because of his age and because the bite occurred 8 hours ago. Caring for the patient should be done before reporting the bite to authorities, if required. Rabies prophylaxis would be needed only if the neighbor's dog had not been vaccinated. The neurotoxin virus that mammals carry is rabies and the dressing will not prevent this exposure.

20. c. Hemodialysis is reserved for patients who develop severe acidosis from ingestion of toxic substances (e.g., aspirin). Milk or water may be used for immediate dilution of acids, such as toilet bowl cleaners. Cathartics are given with activated charcoal for nonsevere/nonacute ingestion of aspirin. Whole bowel irrigation is controversial and can cause electrolyte imbalance.

21. a, b, d, e. Gastric lavage is used for patients who ingest bleach, aspirin, iron supplements, and tricyclic antidepressants (e.g., amitriptyline). Patients who ingest caustic agents, co-ingest sharp objects, or ingest nontoxic substances should not receive lavage.

22. d. Activated charcoal will absorb any of the medication left in the stomach. Cathartics are usually given with activated charcoal to increase elimination of the toxins absorbed by the charcoal. N-acetylcysteine will be administered for acetaminophen toxicity. GoLYTELY and gastric lavage would not be needed. Vomiting from Ipecac syrup should never be induced in a patient who is unconscious.

23. a. Botulism caused by *Clostridium botulinum* is a lethal neurotoxin that is treated by inducing vomiting, enemas, antitoxin, and mechanical ventilation. Smallpox is from a virus and causes skin lesions. Tularemia is a bacterium that primarily infects rabbits and causes influenza-like symptoms in humans. Mustard gas is a chemical with a garlic-like odor that irritates the eyes and causes skin burns and blisters.

24. d. There is no established treatment to cure the viruses that cause hemorrhagic fever. Plague, anthrax, and tularemia are effectively treated with antibiotics if there is a sufficient supply of the antibiotics and the organisms are not resistant to them.

25. d, f. There are currently vaccines available to protect against the biologic agents of terrorism of smallpox and some hemorrhagic fevers (e.g., yellow fever, Argentine hemorrhagic fever). The anthrax vaccine is only used for those exposed to anthrax because of their job, not as protection against terrorism. There are currently vaccines in development for plague, botulism, and tularemia.

26. b. Because hemorrhagic fever (e.g., Marburg virus, Ebola virus) causes hemorrhage of tissues and organs, care is primarily supportive. IM injections and anticoagulants are avoided. Care of the rodent or mosquito bite, if needed, is included in supportive treatment.

27. d. Disaster medical assistance teams are composed of members with health or medical skills and directly provide medical care in disaster situations. Triage is performed by first responders, such as police and designated emergency medical personnel. The hospital's emergency response plan is a specific plan that addresses how personnel and resources will be used at that facility in case of a disaster, and community emergency response teams provide training to communities in general to respond to disasters.

Case Study

1. **Indicated**: C-spine precautions (which includes a hard cervical collar because the patient fell off of the roof and could have suffered a spinal cord injury), establish large-bore IVs (to maximize fluid resuscitation), remove patient's clothing (to assess for visible injuries and treat hyperthermia), insert an indwelling urinary catheter (to monitor urine output which determines adequate fluid resuscitation), assess pupils (patient fell off of the roof and could have experienced a traumatic brain injury); **Contraindicated**: oxygen via 6 L/min nasal cannula (oxygen delivery should be administered using a nonrebreather mask at 12L/min or higher to treat severe hypoxemia), infuse normal saline 0.9% at 30 mL/hr (this is equivalent to 1 ounce per hour which is insufficient to treat the fluid deficit in this patient); **Non-essential**: clean and dress the abrasions and cuts (ABCs are the priority, this intervention is not a priority), auscultate bowel sounds (not a priority for this patient)

2. **Expected**: CT scan shows cerebral contusion (consistent with mechanism of injury and supports a TBI diagnosis), Na 120 mEq/L (occurs in heatstroke due to salt depletion which causes a change in LOC), K^+ 2.9 mEq/L (loss of potassium through sweat); **Unexpected**: Hct 22% (unless the patient is hemorrhaging which isn't mentioned, dehydration will cause a higher than normal hematocrit level because the blood becomes more viscous due to

severe fluid loss), creatinine 0.8 mg/dL (severe dehydration can cause acute kidney injury due to poor renal perfusion and rhabdomyolysis causing the creatinine to increase), PaO_2 85 mm Hg (tachypnea, shallow respirations, and ashen skin indicate that he is hypoxemic; plus, the patient suffered a traumatic fall which may have caused fractured ribs, a pulmonary contusion, or a pneumothorax all increasing the risk of hypoxemia)

3. A., C., E., F., H. The patient should be in an air conditioned room and fans should be used to cool patient not an AC unit blowing on him. Lavaging using cool fluids may be implemented but not lukewarm fluids. A Bair hugger machine is used to treat hypothermia.

4. **Fluid imbalance**: 1000 mL bolus of 0.9% normal saline (to treat dehydration), maintain urine output 1 mL/kg/hr (achieving this goal indicates adequate fluid resuscitation), maintain CVP ≥ 8 mm Hg (achieving this goal indicates adequate venous return which is an additional indicator of adequate fluid resuscitation); **Electrolyte imbalance**: administer KCL 10 mEq IVPB over 1 hour (to treat hypokalemia), continuous cardiac monitoring (dysrhythmias and ectopy can occur from electrolyte imbalances, specifically potassium), administer 3% saline as ordered (to treat hyponatremia); **Impaired mobility**: passive ROM every 4 hours (helps prevent contractures, circulates blood, and prevents VTE), place patient on kinetic bed (is a bed that moves 180° side-to-side to decrease the risks associated with immobility), apply sequential compression devices (to decrease risk of VTE from immobility); **Not used**: oxygen isn't applicable to improve any of these clinical problems.

5. A., B., E., F., G. If the patient experiences muscle cramps, it is recommended to wait 12 hours before resuming strenuous activities. Drinking alcoholic beverages after doing strenuous activity on a hot day can cause cellular dehydration exacerbating overall dehydration and cause acute kidney injury from rhabdomyolysis.

CHAPTER 22

1. a. lens; b. iris; c. cornea; d. anterior chamber; e. pupil; f. posterior chamber; g. ciliary body; h. vitreous humor; i. optic disc; j. optic nerve; k. retina; l. choroid; m. sclera

2. d. Vitreous humor fills the posterior cavity. The zonule connects the lens to the ciliary body. The cornea is a transparent external structure that is responsible for the majority of light refraction needed for clear vision. Aqueous humor fills the anterior and posterior chambers of the anterior cavity of the eye.

3. c. The sclera is the outer protective layer of the eyeball. Aqueous humor is produced from capillary blood in the ciliary body. The lens bends light rays so that they fall on the retina. Rods are the photoreceptor cells stimulated in dim lighting.

4. c. The conjunctiva is the transparent mucous membrane lining the eyclids. The junction of the eyelids is the medial and lateral canthi. The optic disc is the point where the optic nerve leaves the eyeball. The puncta drain the tears to the lacrimal canals.

5. c. Choroid nourishes the ciliary body, iris, and part of the retina. The pupil is the opening of the iris; the cones are photoreceptors sensitive to color in bright light; and the canal of Schlemm is the drainage path for aqueous humor.

6.
Eye Function	Cranial Nerve
Elevating eyelids	Open: CN III (oculomotor)
Closing eyelids	Close: CN VII (facial)
Elevating eyelids	CN II (optic)

7.
Assessment Finding	Cause
Floaters	Vitreous liquefaction and retinal holes or tears
Ectropion	Loss of orbital fat
Pinguecula	Chronic exposure to ultraviolet (UV) light or other environmental irritants
Arcus senilis	Cholesterol deposits in the peripheral cornea
Yellowish sclera	Deposition of lipids
Dry, irritated eyes	Decreased tear secretion or composition
Decreased pupil size	Increased rigidity of iris
Changes in color perception	Decrease in number of cones

8. a. The use of corticosteroids has been associated with the development of cataracts and glaucoma. Use of oral hypoglycemic agents alerts the nurse to the presence of diabetes and risk for diabetic retinopathy. β-Adrenergic blocking agents may cause additive effects in patients with glaucoma for whom these medications may be prescribed. Antihistamine and decongestant drugs may cause eye dryness.

9.
Functional Health Pattern	Risk Factor for or Response to Visual Problem
Health perception–health management	UV light exposure, age-related eye problems, improper contact lens care, family history of ocular problems, diseases affecting the eye, allergies causing eye problems
Nutritional-metabolic	Deficiencies of zinc or vitamins C and E
Elimination	Constipation and straining to defecate increases intraocular pressure
Activity-exercise	Work and leisure activities that increase eye strain or risk, lack of protective eyewear during sports, visual difficulties with activities
Sleep-rest	Lack of sleep
Cognitive-perceptual	Presence of eye pain, unable to read

Functional Health Pattern	Risk Factor for or Response to Visual Problem
Self-perception–self-concept	Decreased self-concept and self-image, loss of independence
Role-relationship	Loss of roles and responsibilities, occupational eye injuries
Sexuality-reproductive	Eye medications that may cause fetal abnormalities, change in sexual activity related to self-image, use of erectile dysfunction drugs in males
Coping–stress tolerance	Grief related to loss of vision, emotional stress, lack of support system
Value-belief	Values and beliefs that limit treatment decisions

10. With the right eye, the patient standing at 20 feet from a Snellen chart can read to the 40-foot line on the chart with 2 or fewer errors. With the left eye, the patient can read only to the 50-foot line on the chart. This patient can read at 20 feet what a person with normal vision can read at 40 and 50 feet.

11. d. *PERRLA* means pupils equal (in size), round, and react to light (pupil constricts when light shines into same eye and also constricts in the opposite eye) and accommodation (pupils constrict and converge with focus moved from a distant object to a near object). An oval pupil and dilation of pupil instead of constriction with light needs further assessment. Nystagmus on far lateral gaze is normal but is not part of the assessment of pupil function.

12.

Assessment Data	Assessment Technique
Peripheral vision field	Confrontation test
Extraocular muscle functions	Corneal light reflex and cardinal field of gaze
Near visual acuity	Jaeger chart
Visual acuity	Snellen chart
Intraocular pressure	Tono-Pen or other tonometry equipment

13. b. A normal yellowish hue to the normally white sclera is found in older adults. Infants and some older adults may exhibit a normal blue cast to the sclera because of thin sclera. Iris color does not affect the color of the sclera, and infections of the eye may cause dilation of small blood vessels in the normally clear bulbar conjunctiva, reddening the sclera and conjunctiva. Older adults with dark skin may have muddy-brown sclera.

14. b. Fluorescein dye is used topically to identify corneal irregularities; irregularities stain a bright green on application of the dye. A tonometer is used to measure intraocular pressure. Light from either a penlight or an ophthalmoscope often is not able to illuminate corneal injuries.

15. a, c. Abnormal assessment findings of the eyelids include ptosis, which is drooping of the upper lid, and blepharitis, which is redness, swelling, and crusting along the lid margins. Strabismus is seen with extraocular muscle assessment. Anisocoria is pupils that are unequal (see Table 20.5). The pinna is the outer part of the ear.

16. c. Exophthalmos, or protrusion of the eyeball, is seen with hyperthyroidism. Photophobia (light intolerance) is seen with inflammation or infection of the cornea or anterior uveal tract. Anisocoria is seen with central nervous system disorders, although some people normally have a slight difference in pupil size. Strabismus is seen with overaction or underaction of 1 or more extraocular muscles.

17. c. A break in the retina anywhere in the eye is abnormal and indicates a potential loss of vision. No blood vessels in the macula and depression of the center of the optic disc are normal findings. Pieces of liquefied vitreous are "floaters" and may be a normal finding, especially in older adults.

18. b. Although fluorescein dye can be used topically to identify corneal lesions, in angiography, the dye is injected IV and outlines the vasculature of the retina, locating areas of retinopathy. A keratometry is measurement of the corneal curvature, and intraocular pressure is measured indirectly with a tonometer.

19. a, d, e. Myopia is characterized by excessive light refraction, the image focused in front of the retina, and correction with a concave or divergent lens. Myopic people may have abnormally long eyeballs, not abnormally short ones, which occurs in hyperopia and is corrected with a convex lens. Unequal corneal curvature results in astigmatism.

20. d. Presbyopia is accommodation lost with aging. Absence of lens is aphakia. Myopia occurs with abnormally long eyeballs. Astigmatism is corrected with a cylinder lens.

21. a. A light shone at an angle over the cornea will illuminate a contact lens, and fluorescein should not have to be used. Cotton balls should not be placed on the cornea, and simply tensing the outer canthus will not dislodge the lens.

22. a, d, e. Surgical therapy includes laser-assisted in situ keratomileusis (LASIK), intraocular lens implants, and photorefractive keratectomy (PRK). Refractive errors are the most common visual problem and nonsurgical correction may include glasses and contact lenses.

23. d. A person who is legally blind has central visual acuity of 20/200 or less in the better eye with correction or a peripheral visual field of 20 degrees or less. There may be some usable vision that will benefit from vision enhancement techniques. A person with total blindness has no light perception and no usable vision, but that is not this person. As only a small percentage of blindness occurs suddenly from injuries, the grieving is probably already in process. Dependency on others from visual impairment is individual and cannot be assumed.

24. a. Address the patient, not others with the patient, in normal conversational tones. b. Face the patient and make eye contact. c. Introduce self when approaching the patient and let the patient know when you are leaving. d. Orient to sounds, activities, and physical surroundings. e. Use sighted-guide technique to ambulate and orient patient. (Other options: do not move objects positioned by the patient without the knowledge and consent of the patient, ask the patient what help is needed and how to provide it, facilitate approach magnification.)

25. c. Emergency management of foreign bodies in the eye includes stabilizing the foreign object by covering and shielding the eye, with no attempt to treat the injury, until

an ophthalmologist can evaluate the injury. Irrigations are performed as emergency management in chemical exposure. Pressure should never be applied because it could further injure the eye.

26. b. Acute bacterial conjunctivitis describes pinkeye. Pinkeye does not cause blindness. Epidemic keratoconjunctivitis is an ocular adenoviral disease. Chalazion is chronic inflammatory granuloma of sebaceous glands on the eyelid.

27. a. Keratitis is inflammation of the cornea. Blepharitis is inflammation of the eyelid. Hordeolum is an infection of the sebaceous glands in the lid margin. Conjunctivitis is infection or inflammation of the conjunctiva.

28. d. All infections of the conjunctiva or cornea are transmittable, and frequent, thorough hand washing is essential to prevent spread from 1 eye to the other or to other persons. Artificial tears are not normally used for eye infections. Photophobia is not experienced by all patients with eye infections. Warm or cool, not iced, compresses are indicated for some infections.

29. a, b, f. Ocular pain, photophobia, decreased visual acuity, and also headaches, reddened and swollen conjunctiva, and corneal edema occur with endophthalmitis. Eyelid edema, reddened sclera, and bleeding conjunctiva do not occur with endophthalmitis.

30. d. Vision enhancement techniques may be used until the patient feels the need for cataract surgery. Although cataracts do become worse with time, surgical extraction is considered an elective procedure. Surgical extraction is generally safe, but infections can occur. The patient will still need glasses for near vision and for any residual refractive error of the implanted lens. There are no proven measures to prevent cataract development or progression.

31. c. The lens opacity of cataracts causes a decrease in vision, abnormal color perception, and glare. Blurred vision, halos around lights, and eye pain are characteristic of glaucoma. Light flashes, floaters, and "cobwebs" or "hairnets" in the field of vision followed by a painless, sudden loss of vision are characteristic of detached retina.

32. a. Assessment of the visual acuity in the patient's nonoperative eye enables the nurse to determine how visually compromised the patient may be while the operative eye is patched and healing and to plan for assistance until vision improves. The patch on the operative eye is usually removed within 24 hours (if used), and although vision in the eye may be good, it is not unusual for visual acuity to be reduced immediately after surgery. Activities that are thought to increase intraocular pressure, such as bending, coughing, and lifting, are frequently restricted postoperatively.

33. a, d. Cryopexy (freezing the retinal break) and laser photocoagulation (creating an inflammatory reaction) are extraocular procedures used with scleral buckling to seal a retinal break. Vitrectomy is an intraocular procedure that removes vitreous to relieve tension on the retina. Pneumatic retinopexy is an intraocular procedure injecting gas to form a temporary bubble with photocoagulation or cryotherapy to close a retinal break. Penetrating keratoplasty is used for corneal scars or opacities and removes the cornea.

34. a. Postoperatively, the patient must position the head so that the bubble is in contact with the retinal break and may have to maintain this position for up to 16 hours a day for at least 5 days. The patient may go home within a few hours of surgery or may remain in the hospital for several days. No

matter what the type of repair, reattachment is successful in 90% of retinal detachments. If postoperative pain occurs, it is treated with analgesics.

35. b. The patient with dry age-related macular degeneration (AMD) can benefit from low-vision aids despite increasing loss of vision, and it is important to promote a positive outlook by not giving patients the impression that "nothing can be done" for them. Approach magnification can help, and vision-enhancing devices include desktop video magnification/closed circuit units, electronic hand-held magnifiers, text-to-speech scanners, e-readers and computer tablets with magnification, brighter screens, voice recognition, and verbal response. The American Foundation for the Blind can help as well. Limited treatment options include vitreal injections of selective inhibitors of endothelial growth factor slow vision loss in wet AMD. Photodynamic therapy is indicated for neovascularization in a small percentage of patients with wet AMD, but there is no treatment for the increasing deposit of extracellular debris (drusen) in the retinal pigment epithelium. Mineral and vitamin supplements may also be ordered.

36. c. Verteporfin, the dye used with photodynamic therapy to destroy abnormal blood vessels, is a photosensitizing drug that can be activated by exposure to sunlight or other high-intensity light. Patients must cover all of their skin to avoid chemical burns when exposed to sunlight until the drug has cleared the body. Blind spots occur with wet AMD. Head movements and position are not of concern following this procedure.

37. c. Because glaucoma develops slowly and without symptoms, it is important that intraocular pressure be evaluated every 2 to 4 years in persons between the ages of 40 and 64 years and every 1 to 2 years in those over 65-years-old. More frequent measurement of intraocular pressure should be done in a patient with a family history of glaucoma, black patients, and patients with diabetes or cardiovascular disease. The disease is chronic, but vision impairment is preventable in most cases with treatment.

38. a, d, f. Primary open-angle glaucoma (POAG) is associated with gradual loss of peripheral vision, increased production of aqueous humor, and resistance to aqueous outflow via trabecular meshwork. Treatment with iridotomy or iridectomy and cholinergic agents to facilitate aqueous humor outflow, as well as central vision loss with corneal edema, are associated with primary angle-closure glaucoma (PACG).

39. a, c, e, f. Acute PACG is caused by the lens blocking the papillary opening, which causes loss of central vision with corneal edema. Sudden severe eye pain and nausea and vomiting occur, and it is initially treated with hyperosmotic oral and IV fluids. Treatment with trabeculoplasty or trabeculectomy or β-adrenergic blockers are associated with POAG.

40.

Drug	Rationale for Use
Betaxolol	A β-adrenergic blocking agent that decreases aqueous humor production and intraocular pressure
Latanoprost	A prostaglandin agonist that increases the outflow of aqueous humor between the uvea and sclera and the usual exit through the trabecular meshwork

Drug	Rationale for Use
Pilocarpine	A miotic agent that stimulates ciliary muscle contraction, causing miosis and opening of trabecular meshwork, increasing aqueous outflow
Acetazolamide	A carbonic anhydrase inhibitor that decreases aqueous humor production

Case Study

1. **Expected**: loss of peripheral vision; IOP in POAG 22 mm Hg – 32 mm Hg; **Unexpected**: severe eye pain (POAG is painless and asymptomatic); blurred vision (occurs in AACG); light gray optic disc (found in chronic POAG); **Unrelated**: opacity of the lens (occurs in cataracts); eyelid ptosis (not relevant to glaucoma).

2. Abnormal ophthalmic findings include: IOP in right eye of 25 mm Hg and 28 mm Hg in left eye; small scattered retinal hemorrhages; loss of lateral 80-95 degrees peripheral vision in both eyes.

3. **Effective**: handwashing; waiting several minutes between eye drops; and using punctal occlusion to prevent systemic absorption since she is already taking another beta blocker for hypertension; **Ineffective**: the tip should remain clean and shouldn't touch the eyelid; there is no need to lay down to administer eye drops unless the patient prefers it; there is no need to keep the eyelids closed for any length of time after instilling eye drops.

4. A., C., D., F., H. Increased fatigue is unexpected. Betaxolol can cause bradycardia, not tachycardia. Respiratory distress is unexpected and the patient should seek medical care. Patients should keep all eye appointments to monitor her condition closely. Further loss of vision needs to be reported to the HCP as it could indicate her condition is getting worse or closed-angle glaucoma is occurring. Severe eye pain is unexpected in POAG and could indicate increased IOP

or closed-angle glaucoma which is a medical emergency. There is no need to sleep at a 30 degree angle. Dizziness or lightheadedness should be reported to the HCP as it may indicate the beta-blocker eye medication is being absorbed systemically causing hypotension or bradycardia. Glaucoma cannot be cured only treated; therefore, eye drops will be lifelong.

CHAPTER 23

1. d. Semicircular canals and the vestibule make up the organ of balance. The receptor organ for hearing is the cochlea. It contains the organ of Corti, whose tiny hair cells respond to stimulation according to pitch. The ossicular chain moves and transmits sound waves to the oval window.

2. c. The eustachian tube equalizes air pressure between the middle ear and throat. The other options have nothing to do with the eustachian tube. The vestibulocochlear nerve (CN VIII) transmits sound stimuli to the brain. The tympanic membrane sets the bones (ossicles) in motion. The semicircular canals are part of the organ of balance.

3. a, c, f. Atrophy of the eardrum, increased production and dryness of cerumen, and neuron degeneration are changes of aging that impair hearing. Increased hair growth occurs, but this does not cause hearing loss. The vestibular apparatus is less effective. There is a decrease in blood supply, which decreases cochlear efficiency.

4. d. Presbycusis is a sensorineural hearing loss that occurs with aging and is associated with decreased ability to hear high-pitched sounds. Tinnitus is present in some, but not all, cases of presbycusis. A sensation of fullness in the ears is related to a blocked eustachian tube, and difficulty understanding the meaning of words is associated with a central hearing loss occurring with problems arising from the cochlea to the cerebral cortex.

5.

Question	Significance
Do you have a history of childhood ear infections or ruptured eardrums?	Childhood middle ear infections with perforations and scarring of the eardrum lead to conductive hearing impairments in adulthood.
Do you use any OTC or prescription medications on a regular basis?	Many medications are ototoxic, causing damage to the auditory nerve. OTC agents, such as aspirin and nonsteroidal antiinflammatory drugs (NSAIDs) are potentially ototoxic, as are prescription diuretics, antibiotics, and chemotherapy drugs.
Have you ever been treated for a head injury?	A head injury can damage areas of the brain to which auditory and vestibular stimuli are transmitted, with a resultant loss of hearing or balance.
Is there a history of hearing loss in your parents?	Some congenital hearing disorders are hereditary, and the age of onset of presbycusis also follows a familial pattern.
Have you been exposed to excessive noise levels in your work or recreational activities?	It is well documented that exposure to loud noises causes damage to the auditory organs and hearing loss. Noise exposure earlier in life can also result in increased hearing loss with age.
Has the amount of social activities you are involved in changed?	Persons with hearing loss may withdraw from social relationships because of difficulty with communication. A hearing loss often leaves the patient feeling isolated and cut off from valued relationships.

6. a. Landmarks of the tympanic membrane include the umbo, handle of malleus, and a reflected cone of light. The tympanic retraction indicates negative pressure in the middle ear. The lack of landmarks and a bulging

eardrum describe acute otitis media. Straightening the ear canal by pulling the auricle downward and backward describes otoscope use for children; for adults, the auricle is pulled upward and backward to insert the otoscope.

7. a, d, f. Positive Rinne test, Weber lateralization to the good ear, and inner ear or nerve pathway pathology indicate sensorineural hearing loss, as does recruitment. Negative Rinne test, Weber lateralization to impaired ear, and external or middle ear pathology indicate conductive hearing loss.

8. b. Speaking in a normal tone of voice will be the best action. Hearing is most sensitive between 500 and 4000 Hz, and a 10-dB loss is not a loss at 8000 Hz. Lip-reading and a hearing aid will not be recommended. A 40- to 45-dB loss in the frequency between 4000 and 8000 Hz will cause difficulty in distinguishing high-pitched consonants.

9. b. The absence of nystagmus indicates that peripheral or central vestibular functions are impaired. An improvement in hearing would occur only if an obstruction of the ear canal was removed with irrigation, which would not be an indication for caloric testing. Severe pain upon irrigation would not be related to vestibular function. Irrigation of the external ear with cool water causes a disturbance in the endolymph that normally results in nystagmus directed opposite the side of instillation.

10.

Functional Health Pattern	Risk Factor for or Response to Hearing Problem
Health perception–health management	Gradual or sudden hearing loss, use of protective earwear for high-noise environments or with swimming
Nutritional-metabolic	Alcohol, sodium, and dietary supplements used. Changes in symptoms with food eaten, ear pain with chewing, grinding of the teeth
Elimination	Constipation and straining may increase intracranial and inner ear pressure
Activity-exercise	Changes in activity related to hearing or equilibrium problems
Sleep-rest	Tinnitus disturbs sleep, snoring may be caused by swelling in nasopharynx, which impairs eustachian tube function and causes the sensation of ear fullness or pain
Cognitive-perceptual	Pain and relief methods, inability to pay attention or hear and follow directions
Self-perception–self-concept	Effect on personal life, feelings about self, embarrassing social situations
Role-relationship	Strained family life, work, and social relationships. Dangerous situations with vertigo or dizziness
Sexuality-reproductive	Interference with establishing or maintaining a satisfactory sexual relationship
Coping–stress tolerance	Denial is common with hearing problems. Support system
Value-belief	Values and beliefs that limit treatment options

11. b. Patients receiving ototoxic drugs should be monitored for tinnitus, hearing loss, and vertigo to prevent further damage caused by the drugs. Ears should not be cleaned with anything but a washcloth, and finger and ear protection should be used in any environment with consistent noise levels above 85 dB. Exposure to the rubella virus during the first 8 weeks of pregnancy may cause fetal deafness, and the vaccine should never be given during pregnancy.

12. a. 5; b. 4; c. 3; d. 6; e. 1; f. 2. The highest risk is determined by the highest dB level per time.

13. Advanced age, use of 3 potentially ototoxic drugs (aspirin, quinidine, and furosemide)

14. d. Antibiotic eardrops for external otitis should be applied without touching the auricle to avoid contaminating the dropper and solution and the patient should hold the ear upward for several minutes to allow the drops to run down the canal. An ear wick may be placed in the external canal and remains in the ear for at least several days to deliver treatment. The use of irrigation or lubricating eardrops is performed for impacted cerumen. "Swimmer's ear" is best prevented by avoiding swimming in contaminated waters; prophylactic antibiotics are not used.

15. a, c, e. Antibiotics are used to treat bacteria identified with culture and sensitivity test. If antibiotic resistant, frequent evacuation of drainage and debris or surgery is needed. Effusion (collection of fluid in the middle ear) causes a full feeling and popping and may decrease hearing. Infection or sudden pressure changes disrupt the surgical repair during healing or cause facial nerve paralysis post-tympanoplasty. Both acute and chronic otitis media occur in the middle ear. A cholesteatoma, not acoustic neuroma, may form and enlarge to damage ossicles.

16. a. Otosclerosis is an autosomal dominant hereditary disease that causes fixation of the footplate of the stapes, leading to conductive hearing loss. Tuning fork testing in conductive hearing loss would result in a negative Rinne test and lateralization to the ear with greater hearing loss upon Weber testing. During a stapedectomy, the patient often reports an immediate improvement in hearing, but the hearing level decreases temporarily postoperatively.

17. b. Stimulation of the labyrinth intraoperatively may cause postoperative dizziness, increasing the risk for falls. Nystagmus on lateral gaze may result from perilymph disturbances but does not constitute a risk for injury. A tympanic graft is not performed in a stapedectomy nor is postoperative tinnitus common.

18. a, c, d. Vertigo, tinnitus, and sensorineural hearing loss are the triad of symptoms that occur with inner ear problems. Nausea may occur with vertigo but is not part of the triad of symptoms. Inflammation of the ear canal occurs with external otitis.

19. b. Nursing care should minimize vertigo by keeping the patient in a quiet, dark environment. Movement aggravates the whirling and roaring sensations, and the patient should be

moved only for essential care. Fluorescent lights or television flickering may also increase vertigo and should be avoided. Side rails should be raised to assist with safe movement when the patient is in bed, but padding is not indicated.

20. c. The benign acoustic neuroma can compress the trigeminal and facial nerves and arteries in the internal auditory canal and may expand into the cranium, but if it is removed when small, hearing and vestibular function can be preserved. During surgery for a tumor that has expanded into the cranium, preservation of hearing and the facial nerve is reduced.

21. b, c, e, f. The remaining answers are characteristics of sensorineural hearing loss.

22. a, c, e, f. The remaining answers are characteristics of conductive hearing loss.

23. c. Initial adjustment to a hearing aid should include voices and household sounds and experimenting with volume in a quiet environment. The next recommended exposure is small parties, the outdoors, and, finally, uncontrolled areas (e.g., shopping areas).

Case Study

1. **Expected**: sensorineural hearing loss, ear congestion, "drop attacks," nystagmus; **Unexpected**: symptoms began at 25 years of age (usually symptoms of this disease start between 40 and 60 years of age), conductive hearing loss (hearing loss in Ménière's disease is sensorineural); **Unrelated**: visual floaters and headaches (don't occur in Ménière's disease)

2. **Indicated**: restrict eating canned foods, chocolate (has caffeine), drinking alcoholic beverages (the patient should be advised to restrict these because they affect the amount of endolymph in the inner ear), audiology can help the patient learn vestibular exercises; **Contraindicated**: tea, coffee and colas should be avoided (all contain caffeine which affect the amount of endolymph in the inner ear), antibiotics are not indicated for this disease and by prescribing them it could cause antibiotic resistance); **Non-essential**: headaches (are not associated with this disease), riding as a passenger in a car (is not relevant to this disease).

3. 1=diphenhydramine; 2=vertigo; 3=before bed; 4=drowsiness; 5=drive; 6=dry mouth, fatigue, headaches

4. B., C., D., E. Sun exposure won't trigger or exacerbate symptoms of the disease. Patients should find a dark quiet room if experiencing vertigo. The patient should practice safety by avoiding heights, driving, and using machinery when experiencing vertigo or are prone to "drop attacks." Flickering lights from the TV can exacerbate symptoms. Patients should be able to work when not experiencing severe symptoms. Patients can watch movies in movie theaters as long as they are asymptomatic.

5. **Indicated**: maintain eye contact, use simple sentences, write if necessary; **Contraindicated**: exaggerate facial expressions (patients often read lips and rely on facial expressions), speak loudly in impaired ear (the nurse should use a normal voice to speak in the unimpaired ear); **Unrelated**: positioning upright or avoiding sudden position changes.

CHAPTER 24

1. a. hair shaft; b. stratum corneum; c. stratum germinativum; d. melanocyte; e. sebaceous gland; f. eccrine sweat gland; g. apocrine sweat gland; h. blood vessels; i. adipose tissue; j. nerves; k. hair follicle; l. arrector pili muscle; m. connective tissue; n. subcutaneous tissue; o. dermis; p. epidermis

2. c. In older adults, there are decreased surface lipids, apocrine and eccrine sweat gland and sebaceous gland activity, and fewer blood vessels that all cause dry skin. Some older people do not drink enough fluids, and this can also contribute to dry skin. Increased bruising from capillary fragility does not contribute to dry skin. Chronic ultraviolet (UV) light exposure leads to wrinkles.

3. d. A careful medication history is important because many medications cause dermatologic side effects and patients also use many OTC preparations to treat skin problems. Freckles are common in childhood and are not related to skin disease. Patterns of weight gain and loss are not significant, but the presence of obesity may cause skin problems in overlapping skin areas. Communicable childhood illnesses are not directly related to skin problems, although varicella viruses may affect the skin in adulthood.

4.

Functional Health Pattern	Risk Factor for or Patient Response to Skin Problem
Health perception–health management	Poor skin hygiene, excessive or unprotected sun exposure. Family history of alopecia, ichthyosis, psoriasis. History of skin cancer
Nutritional-metabolic	Decreased intake of vitamins A, D, E, or C. Malnutrition, food allergies, obesity
Elimination	Incontinence, fluid imbalances, pruritus
Activity-exercise	Exposure to carcinogens or chemical irritants, allergens
Sleep-rest	Itching that interferes with sleep
Cognitive-perceptual	Pain; decreased perception of heat, cold, and touch. Numbness
Self-perception–self-concept	Feelings of rejection, prejudice, loss of self-esteem, and decreased body image
Role-relationship	Altered relationships with others. Occupational exposure to irritants and allergens
Sexuality-reproductive	Changes in sexual intimacy because of appearance, pain, treatment effects
Coping–stress tolerance	Skin problems worsened by stress, coping strategies used
Value-belief	High social value placed on appearance and skin condition with tanning, use of cosmetics, religious beliefs

5. d. It is necessary for the patient to be completely undressed for an examination of the skin. Gowns should be provided, and exposure minimized as the skin is inspected generally first, followed by a lesion-specific examination. Skin temperature is best assessed with the back of the hand, and turgor is assessed by pinching the skin on the back of the hand.

6. a, d, f. Obesity affects skin with increased sweating that causes inflammation and dry skin, poor wound healing, and problems in skin folds. Photosensitivity occurs when certain chemicals absorb light from the sun and harm the skin. Benzophenones block both UVA and UVB rays. Vitamin A, not vitamin C, is critical in maintaining and repairing the structure of epithelial cells. Exposure to UV is important in the development of skin cancer. Chronic UV exposure from tanning beds causes the same damage as UV from the sun.

7. b. Discolored lesions that are caused by intradermal or subcutaneous bleeding do not blanch with pressure. Those caused by inflammation and dilated blood vessels will blanch and refill after palpation. Varicosities are engorged, dilated veins that may empty with pressure applied along the vein.

8. a. vesicles; b. discrete, localized to the chest and abdomen. c. color, size, height, shape, configuration, and odor

9. d. An excoriation is a focal loss of epidermis; it does not involve the dermis and, as such, does not scar with healing. Ulcers do penetrate into and through the dermis, and scarring does occur with these deeper lesions. Epidermal and dermal thinning is atrophy of the skin but does not involve a break in skin integrity. Both excoriations and ulcers have a break in skin integrity and may develop crusts or scabs over the lesions.

10. b. A shave biopsy is done for superficial lesions that can be scraped with a razor blade, removing the full thickness of the stratum corneum. An excisional biopsy is done when the entire removal of a lesion is desired. Punch biopsies are done with larger nodules to examine for pathology, as are incisional biopsies.

11. a. A culture can be performed to distinguish among fungal, bacterial, and viral infections. A Tzanck test is specific for herpesvirus infections, potassium hydroxide slides are specific for fungal infections, and immunofluorescent studies are specific for infections that cause abnormal antibody proteins.

12. b. Telangiectasia looks like small, superficial, dilated blood vessels. A small circumscribed, flat discoloration describes a macule. A benign tumor of blood or lymph vessels describes an angioma. Tiny purple spots resulting from tiny hemorrhages describes petechiae.

13. b. Fissures are linear cracks, such as athlete's foot. Scales are excess dead epidermal cells. A pustule is a circumscribed collection of leukocytes and free fluid. Comedo is associated with acne vulgaris.

14. b. Intertrigo is dermatitis in the folds of her skin. Thickening of the skin is lichenification. Loss of color in diffuse areas of skin is vitiligo. A firm, edematous area caused by fluid in the dermis is a wheal.

15. c. In dark-skinned persons, cyanosis is seen as ashen nail beds, conjunctiva, or mucous membranes. Vital signs, lung sounds, and cardiorespiratory history would be assessed after verifying cyanosis of mucous membranes. Palpating for rashes and assessing for jaundice and pallor would not be related to this patient's potential cyanosis.

16. a. These manifestations are all present with hyperthyroidism related to accelerated body processes. Alopecia, fatigue, and photosensitivity are seen with systemic lupus erythematosus. Tachycardia, redness of the soles of the feet, and edema are seen with vitamin B_1 (thiamine) deficiency. Human immunodeficiency (HIV) infection would more likely manifest as Kaposi sarcoma or eosinophilic folliculitis.

CHAPTER 25

1. b, c, d. Malignant melanomas are neoplastic growths of melanocytes, have the highest mortality rate of skin cancers, and are irregular color and asymmetric shape. Cutaneous T-cell lymphoma is related to chemical exposure. Squamous cell carcinoma (SCC) frequently occurs in previously damaged skin.

2. b. Basal cell carcinoma (BCC) is the most common skin cancer and has pearly borders. Actinic keratosis is an irregularly shaped, flat, slightly erythematous papule with indistinct borders and an overlying hard keratotic scale or horn. Malignant melanoma tumors are often dark brown or black. Malignant melanoma is the deadliest skin cancer and has an increased risk in people with dysplastic nevus syndrome. SCC is a malignant neoplasm of keratinizing epidermal cells.

3. a. BCC is nodular and ulcerative with pearly borders. Actinic keratosis is the most common premalignant skin lesion. Malignant melanoma is the deadliest skin cancer and has an increased risk in people with dysplastic nevus syndrome. SCC is a malignant neoplasm of keratinizing epidermal cells.

4. d. Dysplastic nevus syndrome involves atypical moles with irregular borders and various shades of color. Dysplastic nevus syndrome may be a precursor of malignant melanoma, although not directly related to sun exposure. There are frequently multiple nevi to monitor.

5. *A*symmetry: one half unlike the other half; *B*order: irregular and poorly circumscribed; *C*olor: change and varied within lesion; *D*iameter: larger than 6 mm; *E*volving: look and appearance is changing

6. d. Using the prescribed ointment to keep the wound moist and the bandage for protection will promote healing and less scarring. Radiation is not used after excision of BCC. Without treatment, BCC causes massive tissue destruction, but he has it treated. Laser surgery is not used for BCC, so this is not appropriate. The potential of keloid scarring may be included for this black patient.

7. b, c. In the early stages, surgical excision with a margin of normal skin is the initial treatment for malignant melanoma. Mohs surgery can also be used to treat malignant melanoma. A shave biopsy is used for diagnosis, not treatment. Radiation may be used for malignant melanoma after excision, depending on staging of the disease. Fluorouracil is used to treat actinic keratosis. Topical nitrogen mustard may be used for treatment of cutaneous T-cell lymphoma.

8. a. chronic disease; b. obesity; c. recent antibiotic therapy; d. recent corticosteroid therapy

9. d. A plantar wart is caused by human papillomavirus (HPV). A furuncle is a deep skin infection with staphylococci around the hair follicle. A carbuncle is multiple, interconnecting furuncles. Erysipelas is superficial cellulitis primarily involving the dermis.

10. b. Seborrheic keratoses are irregularly round or oval and are often verrucous (warty) papules or plaques. Candidiasis is a white, patchy yeast infection. Psoriasis is an excessive turnover of epithelial cells. Cellulitis is a deep inflammation of subcutaneous tissue.

11. a. In scabies, mites penetrate the skin and deposits eggs. An allergic reaction can result from the presence of eggs, feces, and mite parts. Streptococci or staphylococci cause impetigo with vesiculopustular lesions that develop a thick, honey-colored crust surrounded by erythema. Folliculitis is a small pustule at the hair follicle opening with minimal erythema caused by staphylococci. Pediculosis is lice.

12. c, e, f. Patients who are immunocompromised are at an increased risk for candidiasis (a fungal infection), herpes simplex 1 (caused by a virus), and Kaposi sarcoma (vascular lesions on the skin, mucous membranes, and viscera with wide range of presentation). The other options are not at increased risk with immunosuppression. Acne is caused by inflammation of sebaceous glands. Lentigo (also called *liver spots* or *age spots*) is caused by an increased number of normal melanocytes in the basal layer of epidermis. Herpes zoster, which is caused by an activation of the varicella-zoster virus, is a group of vesicles and pustules resembling chickenpox located in a linear distribution along a dermatome.

13. b. Urticaria (hives) is inflammation and edema in the upper dermis, most commonly caused by histamine released during an allergic reaction. The best treatment for all types of allergic dermatitis is avoidance of the allergen. Topical benzene hexachloride is used to treat pediculosis. Sunlight and warmth would increase the edema and inflammation. Antihistamines may be used for an acute outbreak but not to prevent the dermatitis.

14. a. Pediculosis (head lice and body lice) causes very small, red, noninflammatory lesions that progress to papular wheal-like lesions and cause severe itching. Lice live on the scalp and body and nits (tiny white eggs) are firmly attached to hair shafts. Sexually transmitted infections and ticks do not produce these manifestations. Burrows, especially in interdigital webs, are found with scabies.

15. c. A lotion is an emulsion of water, alcohol, and/or oil. Calamine has insoluble powder that has cooling and drying properties when the residual powder is left after water evaporation. It is useful when itching is present. Ointments and creams have an oil and water base that lubricate and ointments prevent drying. Creams protect skin and paste is a mixture of powder in an ointment base.

16. d. Psoralen is absorbed by the lens of the eye, and eyewear that blocks 100% of ultraviolet (UV) light must be used for 24 hours after taking the medication. Because UVA penetrates glass, the eyewear must also be worn indoors when near a bright window. Psoralen does not affect the accommodative ability of the eye.

17.

Medication	Nursing Instruction
Topical antibiotics	Clean skin. Thin film, dry dressings
Topical corticosteroids	Diagnosis of the lesion first. Thin layers. Massage in at prescribed frequency. Occlusive dressing

Medication	Nursing Instruction
Systemic antihistamines	Advise of side effects and potential risks associated with driving or operating heavy machinery
Topical fluorouracil	Avoid sunlight. Causes photosensitivity. Warn patient that it will cause painful, eroded dermatitis before healing
Topical immunomodulators	Heat may be felt at application site. Red, swelling, blistering, excoriation, itching, peeling, and burning may occur.

18. a. 4; b. 1, 2, 3, 5; c. 1, 3; d. 2, 3, 6; e. 2, 3, 6

19. a. Compresses used to treat pruritic lesions should be cool to cause vasoconstriction and have an antiinflammatory effect. Water is most commonly used, and it does not need to be sterile. Acetic acid solutions are bactericidal and are used to treat skin infections. Potassium permanganate compresses are questionable.

20. b. Tepid or warm solutions should be used when the purpose is debridement, and saline is a common debridement solution. Warm baths of oatmeal and sodium bicarbonate are used for itching of large areas of the body. Magnesium sulfate is used in baths or compresses for inflammation.

21.

Intervention	Rationale
Cool environment	Vasoconstriction
Topical menthol, camphor, or phenol	Decreased inflammation and blood flow, numbing of itch receptor
Soaks and baths	Vasoconstriction and stopping itch sensation

22. b. Defining characteristics for reduced self-concept problems include verbalization of self-disgust and reluctance to look at lesions, as evidenced in this patient. Social isolation is indicated only if there is evidence of decreased social activities and of anxiety by verbalization of anxiety or frustration. Although impaired health maintenance may be a problem, it is not indicated in this situation.

23. a. Lichenification is thickening of the skin caused by chronic scratching or rubbing and can be prevented by controlling itching. It is not an infection, nor is it contagious, as the other options indicate.

24. a. Improvement of self-image is the most common reason for undergoing cosmetic surgery; appearance is an important part of confidence and self-assurance. Acne scars, pigmentation problems, and wrinkling can be treated with cosmetic surgery but the surgery does not prevent the skin changes associated with aging.

25. d. Laser surgery reduces fine wrinkles and removes facial lesions. A facelift is used for preauricular lesions and redundant soft tissue reduction. Liposuction is used for obesity with subcutaneous fat accumulation.

26. a. Skin flaps as grafts include moving skin and subcutaneous tissue to another part of the body and are used to cover wounds with poor vascular beds, add

padding, and cover wounds over cartilage and bone. Free grafts transfer the epidermis and part or all of the dermis or include establishment of circulation as well. Soft tissue extension involves placement of an expander under the skin, which stretches the skin over time to provide extra skin to cover the desired area.

27. b. The appearance of candidiasis on the skin shows diffuse papular erythematous rash with pinpoint satellites around the affected area. Height and weight would indicate that the patient is obese, but it would be better to ask if the areas affected are moist. Chemotherapy could contribute to candidiasis, but it doesn't matter if the chemotherapy treatments are finished. If she is experiencing side effects from medications, it is likely to be systemic and not confined to the groin and under her breasts.

28. a, d, e, f. Corticosteroid excess can cause acne and decreased subcutaneous fat over the extremities. Diabetes can cause erythematous plaques of the shins, and both corticosteroids and diabetes can impair or delay wound healing. Increased sweating is seen with hyperthyroidism and coarse, brittle hair is seen with hypothyroidism.

Case Study

1. **1**=cellulitis; **2**=Streptococci and *Staphylococcus aureus;* **3**=subcutaneous; **4**=gangrene and septicemia

2. **Indicated:** measure the size and depth of the cut (for documentation), use sterile saline to flush the wound, use an arm sling to elevate the extremity (also reminds the patient to rest and immobilize it); **Contraindicated:** cleanse the wound with alcohol (alcohol will be very painful and could be cytotoxic; it is best for the patient to use soap and water at home and sterile irrigant in the acute care setting), apply a clean dressing to the wound (the dressing should be sterile, a.k.a. aseptic, to reduce introducing additional bacteria), arrange for casting of the arm (this is unnecessary and could be harmful because casts create a dark moist environment which promotes bacterial growth); **Non-essential:** pack the cut with xeroform gauze (this is unnecessary, if the wound is deep enough and warrants packing normal saline soaked gauze would be used)

3. A., D., E., G., H., I. Antibiotics should be taken until completely gone to adequately treat infection and prevent antibiotic resistance. Ice packs are not recommended because ice will vasoconstrict and limit blood flow and other mediators fighting the infection. Fluorouracil is a topical cytotoxic agent with selective toxicity for sun-damaged cells, used to treat precancerous lesions.

4. **Sepsis**: tachycardia (compensatory response to improve tissue perfusion), hypotension (due to vasodilation), leukocytosis (increased WBCs), confusion (due to decreased perfusion to the brain as well as metabolic acidosis that often occurs due to infection); **Gangrene**: absent radial pulse (occurs if perfusion to the extremity is completely compromised), fingers are cold and numb (indicates decreased or no perfusion), arm is pale (indicates decreased perfusion); **Not used**: anemia and hemorrhage (are unrelated to both of these complications unless sepsis causes DIC)

CHAPTER 26

1. b. An electrical injury causes tissue damage from intense heat generated by the electrical current passing through tissue, including muscle contractions that can fracture long bones and vertebrae. Myoglobin is released into the circulation when massive muscle damage occurs. The electric shock can even cause cardiac standstill or dysrhythmias as well as delayed dysrhythmias during the first 24 hours after injury.

2. d, e. With chemical burns, removing the chemical from the skin is important. Lavaging the skin with water or saline solution for 20 minutes to 2 hours postexposure may be needed. Alkali tends to adhere to skin and causes prolonged damage with protein hydrolysis and liquefaction. Metabolic asphyxiation is from the inhalation of carbon monoxide or hydrogen cyanide. Metabolic acidosis is most common in electrical burns, as is the "iceberg effect" of tissue injury below the skin.

3. a. Dry, waxy white, leathery, or hard skin is characteristic of full-thickness burns in the emergent phase, and it may turn brown and dry in the acute phase. Deep partial-thickness burns in the emergent phase are red and shiny and have blisters. Edema may not be as extensive in full-thickness burns because of thrombosed vessels.

4. a. $3\frac{1}{2}+1+6\frac{1}{2}+2+1\frac{1}{2}+3\frac{1}{2}=18\%$ TBSA (total body surface area)

   b. $4\frac{1}{2}+9+4\frac{1}{2}+4\frac{1}{2}=22\frac{1}{2}\%$ TBSA

   c. No, because edema and inflammation obscure the demarcation of zones of injury.

5. a. 2; b. 4; c. 3; d. 1. The first intervention in emergency management of a burn injury is to remove the burn source and stop the burning process. Airway maintenance would be second, then establishing IV access, followed by assessing for other injuries.

6. b. The emergent phase usually lasts up to 72 hours after the time the burn occurred and focuses on fluid resuscitation. The acute phase is after the emergent phase and may last weeks to months after the burn occurred but begins when the extracellular fluid is mobilized and diuresis occurs. There is no postacute phase. The rehabilitative phase begins weeks to months after the injury, when the wounds have healed and the patient participates in self-care.

7. a. With increased capillary permeability, water, sodium, and plasma proteins leave the plasma and move into the interstitial spaces, decreasing serum sodium and albumin. Serum potassium is elevated because injured cells and hemolyzed red blood cells (RBCs) release potassium from cells. An elevated hematocrit is caused by water loss into the interstitium, creating a hemoconcentration.

8. a. Although all of the selections add to the hypovolemia that occurs in the emergent burn phase, the initial and most pronounced effect is caused by fluid shifts out of the blood vessels as a result of increased capillary permeability.

9. c. Burn injury causes widespread impairment of the immune system, with impaired white blood cell (WBC) functioning, bone marrow depression, and a decrease in circulating immunoglobulins, which allows microorganisms to grow.

10. b. Shivering often occurs in a patient with a burn as a result of chilling that is caused by heat loss, anxiety, or pain. Fever is a sign of infection in later burn phases. Severe pain is not common in full-thickness burns, nor is unconsciousness unless other factors are present.

11. d. In circumferential burns, circulation to the extremities can be severely impaired, and pulses should be monitored closely for signs of obstruction by edema. Swelling of the arms would be expected, but it becomes dangerous when it occludes blood vessels. Pain and eschar are also expected.

12. c. Patients with major injuries involving burns to the face and neck require intubation within 1 to 2 hours after burn injury to prevent the need for emergency tracheostomy, which is done if symptoms of upper respiratory obstruction occur. Carbon monoxide poisoning is treated with 100% oxygen and eschar constriction of the chest is treated with an escharotomy.

13. To calculate fluid replacement, the patient's weight in pounds must be converted to kilograms: 132 lb = 60 kg.
    a. lactated Ringer's solution; 4 mL × 60 × 40 = 9600 mL
    b. 4800 mL between 10:15 PM and 5:30 AM; 2400 mL between 5:30 AM and 1:30 PM; 2400 mL between 1:30 PM and 9:30 PM
    c. 720–1200 mL (0.3 to 0.5 mL/kg/% TBSA or 0.3 or 0.5 mL × 60 × 40)
    d. urine output (0.5 to 1 mL/kg/hr = 30 to 50 mL/hr) and vital signs (systolic BP 90, HR < 120 bpm, RR 16 to 20).

14. b. When the patient's wounds are exposed with the open method, the staff must wear caps, masks, gowns, and gloves. Sterile water is not necessary in the debridement tank. If dressings are used with the open method, they are removed and wounds are washed with clean gloves. Topical antiinfective agents should be applied with sterile gloves to prevent infection.

15. a. Morphine is the drug of choice for pain control, and during the emergent phase it should be administered IV because gastrointestinal (GI) function is impaired and IM injections will not be absorbed adequately. Amnesia from midazolam is not needed for pain control.

16. b. The patient with large burns often develops paralytic ileus within a few hours, and a nasogastric tube is inserted and connected to low, intermittent suction. After GI function returns, feeding tubes may be used for nutritional supplementation, and H₂ histamine blockers may be used to prevent Curling's ulcers. Free water is not given to drink because of the potential for water intoxication.

17. c. Patients with ear burns are not allowed to use pillows because of the danger of the burned ear sticking to the pillowcase, and patients with neck burns are not allowed to use pillows because contractures of the neck can occur.

18. b, c, e. There is a hypermetabolic state proportional to the size of the burn, which increases the core temperature. Massive catabolism can occur and leads to malnutrition and delayed healing without adequate calorie and protein supplementation. The electrolyte imbalance has more effect on the fluid resuscitation than the nutritional needs.

19. c. At the end of the emergent phase, fluid mobilization moves potassium back into the cells and sodium returns to the vascular space, causing hypokalemia and hypernatremia. As diuresis in the acute phase continues, sodium will be lost in the urine and potassium will continue to be low unless it is replaced. Free oral water intake and prolonged hydrotherapy can cause a decrease in both sodium and potassium. Excessive fluid replacement with 5% dextrose in water without potassium supplementation can cause hyponatremia with hypokalemia.

20. b. The limited range of motion (ROM) in this situation is related to the patient's inability or reluctance to exercise the joints because of pain and the appropriate intervention is to help control the pain so that exercises can be performed. The patient is probably never without some pain. Teaching about prevention of contractures with exercise and enlisting the help of the physical therapist are important, but neither of these interventions addresses the cause.

21. a. Early signs of sepsis include an elevated temperature and increased pulse and respiratory rate accompanied by decreased BP and, later, decreased urine output and perhaps paralytic ileus. A burn wound may become locally infected without causing sepsis.

22.

Body System	Complication
Neurologic	Confusion or delirium
Gastrointestinal	Curling's (stress) ulcer
Endocrine	Hyperglycemia

23. a. cultured epithelial autograft; b. eschar (or necrotic tissue); autograft; c. aspirating the fluid with a tuberculin syringe, performed by individuals trained in this skill

24. a. Midazolam is useful when patients' anticipation of the pain experience increases their pain because it causes a short-term memory loss and, if given before a dressing change, the patient will not recall the event. A dosage range of morphine is useful, as is patient-controlled analgesia, but seldom will these doses effectively relieve the discomfort of dressing changes. Buprenorphine is an opioid agonist/antagonist and cannot be used with other opioids.

25. a. After wound healing, pressure garments help keep scars flat and prevent elevation and enlargement above the original burn injury area. Avoidance of sunlight is necessary for at least 3 months to prevent hyperpigmentation and sunburn injury to healed burn areas. Water-based lotions and splinting are used to prevent contractures.

26. c. There is a tremendous psychologic impact with a burn injury. Open communication with caregivers, close friends, and the burn team about fears regarding loss of life as she once knew it, loss of function, temporary or permanent deformity and disfigurement, return to routine life, financial burdens, rehabilitation, and her future are all essential. Simply convincing her to have the wound cared for ignores her psychologic, emotional, and perhaps spiritual needs.

27. a. 3; b. 2; c. 1; d. 4. Face and neck burns are frequently associated with airway inhalation. Therefore this patient requires airway assessment (priority = airway, breathing and circulation [ABCs]). Severe pain would be the next priority (high physiologic need). The patient returning from the postanesthesia care unit (PACU) will need to be seen soon to assess vital signs, level of consciousness, IV fluids, and wounds. However, at the current time the transport personnel should be with her. The 18-year-old is not at risk related to ABCs, and it will probably take a few minutes to talk with him about why he does not want to go for the dressing change.

Case Study

1. **1**=27% (9% for each arm to include anterior and posterior x2 + 9% for the chest); **2**=25% (6% for each arm to include anterior and posterior x2 + 13% for chest); **3**=3750-4050 (depending on which TBSA chart is used); **4**=1950

(½ during the 1st 8 hours); **5**=975 (¼ during 2nd and 3rd 8 hours); **6**=75; **7**=100 (Urine output goals are higher for electrical burn patients [75-100 mL/hr]).

2. **Indicated**: cardiac monitoring and 12-lead ECG (patient had an electrical burn which can cause dysrhythmias as indicated by an irregular rhythm); urine for urinalysis (to detect myoglobinuria due to skeletal muscle damage from electrical burn); administer lactated Ringer's bolus (isotonic fluid used for fluid resuscitation); insert urinary catheter (urine output will be evaluated to determine the adequacy of fluid resuscitation); **Contraindicated**: oropharyngeal airway (OPA) (patient is awake, if an OPA is inserted it is likely to stimulate the gag reflex and cause vomiting increasing the risk for aspiration pneumonia); **Non-essential**: collect blood for coagulation studies (unnecessary as electrical burns can cause coagulation but do not tend to cause bleeding tendencies ; perform active ROM (unnecessary in the emergent phase of care).

3. **Acute kidney injury (AKI)**: myoglobinuria (occurs due to damage to skeletal muscle which can clog kidneys leading to an intrarenal cause of AKI); urine output 25 mL/hr (urine output < 30 mL/hr or < 0.5 mL/kg/hr is considered oliguria which may indicate AKI); creatinine 2.8 mg/dL (increased creatinine levels are indicative of renal injury). **Compartment syndrome**: absent right radial pulse; pale and cool right hand (consider the 6 Ps: pain, paresthesia, pallor, pulseless, poikilothermia, paralysis). **Myocardial injury**: elevated troponin levels (a cardiac enzyme that is released when myocardial cells are damaged); ST segment elevation (a change in the ECG that indicates myocardial injury); frequent PVCs (ventricular ectopy that could indicate myocardial injury).

4. **Effective**: MAP 66 mm Hg (a goal of fluid resuscitation); 1+ radial pulses (indicate peripheral perfusion); HR 82 beats/min (has decreased from 110 beats/min indicating adequate fluid resuscitation); **Ineffective**: urine output 40 mL/hr (not sufficient as the goal for an electrical burn patient is 75-100 mL/hr); irregular heart rhythm (indicates a dysrhythmia that hasn't resolved); temperature 38.3°C (may indicate infection which burn patients are prone to developing); **Unrelated**: headache of 4 out of 10 (irrelevant to the burn); 5/5 dorsiplantar flexion (irrelevant as the patient's injuries involved her arms and torso).

5. A., B., E., F., H., I. Burn patients are not routinely prescribed anticoagulants when discharged home, unless they are considered at high risk for VTE. Anticoagulant therapy is usually only used in the acute care setting because of the increased risk of developing VTE due to bedrest. A burn patient's diet should consist of normal to high protein to promote healing. Reporting any pain to the HCP is unnecessary, unless it is severe pain that may indicate infection or compartment syndrome; otherwise, pain from the injuries is expected.

CHAPTER 27

1. a. 9; b. 6; c. 7; d. 8; e. 5; f. 1; g. 12; h. 3; i. 2; j. 13; k. 4; l. 10; m. 11

2. b, e. This patient is older and short of breath. To obtain the most information, auscultate the posterior to avoid breast tissue and start at the base because of her respiratory difficulty and the chance that she will tire easily. Important sounds may be missed if the other strategies are used first.

3. b. Surfactant is a lipoprotein that lowers the surface tension in the alveoli. It reduces the pressure needed to inflate the alveoli and decreases the tendency of the alveoli to collapse. The other options do not maintain inflation of the alveoli. The carina is the point of bifurcation of the trachea into the right and left bronchi. Empyema is a collection of pus in the thoracic cavity. The thoracic cage is formed by the ribs and protects the thoracic organs.

4. c. Alveolar sacs are terminal structures of the respiratory tract, where gas exchange takes place. The visceral pleura lines the lungs and forms a closed, double-walled sac with the parietal pleura. Turbinates warm and moisturize inhaled air. The 150 mL of air is dead space in the trachea and bronchi.

5. b. The epiglottis is a small flap closing over the larynx during swallowing. The trachea connects the larynx and the bronchi. The turbinates in the nose warm and moisturize inhaled air. The parietal pleura is a membrane that lines the chest cavity.

6. a. Normal findings in arterial blood gases (ABGs) in the older adult include a small decrease in PaO_2 and arterial oxygen saturation (SaO_2) but normal pH and $PaCO_2$. No interventions are necessary for these findings. PaO_2 levels between 80-100 mm Hg are expected in patients 60 years of age or younger.

7. d. Normal venous blood gas values reflect the normal uptake of oxygen from arterial blood and the release of carbon dioxide from cells into the blood, resulting in a much lower PaO_2 and an increased $PaCO_2$. The pH is decreased in mixed venous blood gases because of the higher partial pressure of carbon dioxide in venous blood ($PvCO_2$). Normal mixed venous blood gases also have a much lower partial pressure of oxygen in venous blood (PvO_2) and venous oxygen saturation (SvO_2) than ABGs. Mixed venous blood gases are used when patients are hemodynamically unstable to evaluate the amount of oxygen delivered to the tissue and the amount of oxygen consumed by the tissues.

8. c. Pulse oximetry is inaccurate if the probe is loose, if there is low perfusion, or when skin color is dark. Before other measures are taken, the nurse should check the probe site. If the probe is intact at the site and perfusion is adequate, an ABG analysis may be ordered by the HCP to verify accuracy, and oxygen may be necessary depending on the patient's condition and the assessment of their respiratory and cardiac status.

9. c. Poor peripheral perfusion that occurs with hypovolemia or other conditions that cause peripheral vasoconstriction will cause inaccurate pulse oximetry, and ABGs may have to be used to monitor oxygenation status and ventilation status in these patients. Pulse oximetry would not be affected by fever or anesthesia and is a method of monitoring arterial oxygen saturation in patients who are receiving oxygen therapy.

10. d. The respiratory rate, pulse rate, and BP will all increase to compensate for a decreased oxygenation as compared to the patient's own normal results. The position of the oximeter should also be assessed. The oxygenation status with a stress test would not assist the nurse in caring for the patient now. Hyperkalemia is not occurring and will not directly affect oxygenation initially. The arterial oxygen saturation by pulse oximetry (SpO_2), compared with normal values, will not be helpful in this older patient

or in a patient with respiratory disease as the patient's expected normal will not be the same as standard normal values.

11. d. A SpO_2 of 88% and a PaO_2 of 55 mm Hg indicate inadequate oxygenation and are the criteria for continuous oxygen therapy (see Table 27.10). These values may be adequate for patients with chronic hypoxemia if no cardiac problems occur but will affect the patients' activity tolerance.

12. c. A combination of excess CO_2 and H_2O results in carbonic acid, which lowers the pH of cerebrospinal fluid and stimulates an increase in the respiratory rate. Peripheral chemoreceptors in the carotid and aortic bodies also respond to increases in $PaCO_2$ to stimulate the respiratory center. Excess CO_2 does not increase the amount of hydrogen ions available in the body but does combine with the hydrogen of water to form an acid.

13. c. Ciliary action impaired by smoking and increased mucus production may be caused by the irritants in tobacco smoke, leading to impairment of the mucociliary clearance system. Smoking does not directly affect filtration of air, the cough reflex, or reflex bronchoconstriction, but it does impair the respiratory defense mechanism provided by alveolar macrophages.

14. a, b. Decreased functional cilia and decreased force of cough from declining muscle strength cause decreased secretion clearance. The other options contribute to other age-related changes. Decreased compliance contributes to barrel chest appearance. Early small airway closure contributes to decreased PaO_2. Decreased immunoglobulin A (IgA) decreases the resistance to infection.

15.

Functional Health Pattern	Risk Factor for or Response to Respiratory Problem
Health perception–health management	Tobacco use history, gradual change in health status, family history of lung disease, sputum production, no immunizations for influenza or pneumococcal pneumonia received, travel to developing countries
Nutritional-metabolic	Decreased fluid intake, anorexia and rapid weight loss, obesity
Elimination	Constipation, incontinence
Activity-exercise	Decreased exercise or activity tolerance, dyspnea on rest or exertion, sedentary habits
Sleep-rest	Sleep apnea. Awakening with dyspnea, wheezing, or cough. Night sweats
Cognitive-perceptual	Decreased cognitive function with restlessness, irritability. Chest pain or pain with breathing
Self-perception–self-concept	Inability to maintain lifestyle, altered self-esteem
Role-relationship	Loss of roles at work or home, exposure to respiratory toxins at work
Sexuality-reproductive	Sexual activity altered by respiratory symptoms
Coping–stress tolerance	Dyspnea-anxiety-dyspnea cycle, poor coping with stress of chronic respiratory problems
Value-belief	Noncompliance with treatment plan, conflict with values

16. c. Dullness and hyperresonance are found in the lungs using percussion, not the other assessment techniques.

17. c, d, e. Palpation identifies tracheal deviation, limited chest expansion, and increased tactile fremitus. Stridor is identified with auscultation. Finger clubbing and accessory muscle use are identified with inspection.

18. c. To assess the extent and symmetry of chest movement, the nurse places the hands over the lower anterior chest wall along the costal margin and moves them inward until the thumbs meet at the midline and then asks the patient to breathe deeply and observes the movement of the thumbs away from each other. The palms are placed against the chest wall to assess tactile fremitus. To determine the tracheal position, the nurse places the index fingers on either side of the trachea just above the suprasternal notch and gently presses backward.

19. b. An increased anteroposterior (AP) diameter is characteristic of a barrel chest, in which the AP diameter is about equal to the side-to-side diameter. Normally the AP diameter should be ⅓ to ½ the side-to-side diameter. A prominent protrusion of the sternum is the pectus carinatum and diminished movement of both sides of the chest indicates decreased chest excursion. Lack of lung expansion caused by kyphosis of the spine results in shallow breathing with decreased chest expansion.

20. d. Pleural friction rub occurs with pneumonia and is a grating or creaking sound. Stridor is a continuous musical or crowing sound and unrelated to pneumonia. Bronchophony occurs with pneumonia but is a spoken or whispered word that is more distinct than normal on auscultation. Course crackles sound like blowing through a straw under water and occur in pneumonia when there is severe congestion. See Table 27.8 for more thorough descriptions of these sounds and their possible etiologies and significance.

21. a. 7; b. 6; c. 5; d. 8; e. 1; f. 2; g. 4; h. 3

22. d. A 10-mm red indurated injection site could be a positive result for a nurse as an employee in a high-risk setting. Because antibody production in response to infection with the tuberculosis (TB) bacillus may not be sufficient to produce a reaction to TB skin testing immediately after infection, 2-step testing is recommended for individuals likely to be tested often, such as health care professionals. An initial negative skin test should be repeated in 1 to 3 weeks and if the second test is negative, the individual can be considered uninfected. All other answers indicate a negative response to skin testing.

23. c. Samples for ABGs must be iced to keep the gases dissolved in the blood (unless the specimen will be analyzed in < 1 minute) and taken directly to the laboratory. The syringe used to obtain the specimen is rinsed with heparin before the specimen is taken and pressure is applied to the arterial puncture site for at least 5 minutes after obtaining the specimen. Changes in oxygen therapy or interventions

should be avoided for 15 minutes before the specimen is drawn because these changes might alter blood gas values.

24. a. A pulmonary angiogram involves the injection of an iodine-based radiopaque dye, and iodine or shellfish allergies should be assessed before injection. A bronchoscopy requires NPO status for 6 to 12 hours before the test, and invasive tests (e.g., bronchoscopy, mediastinoscopy, biopsies) require informed consent that the HCP should obtain from the patient. Nuclear scans use radioactive materials for diagnosis, but the amounts are very small and no radiation precautions are indicated for the patient.

25. a. 6; b. 1; c. 7; d. 2; e. 5; f. 4; g. 3. The nurse will gather the supplies as soon as the order to do a thoracentesis is given. Hopefully the family will have some time to discuss this before they are instructed to leave the room, unless it is an emergency. The patient is positioned and instructed not to talk or cough to avoid damage to the lung. Observing for hypoxia is done to keep the HCP informed. Breath sounds in all lobes are verified to be sure that there was no damage to the lung. This is done before sending the sample to the laboratory if there is no one else who can send the sample to the laboratory.

26. a. The greatest chance for a pneumothorax occurs with a thoracentesis because of the possibility of lung tissue injury during this procedure. Ventilation-perfusion scans and positron emission tomography (PET) scans involve injections, but no manipulation of the respiratory tract is involved. Pulmonary function tests are noninvasive.

27. d. A pulmonary angiogram outlines the pulmonary vasculature and is useful to diagnose obstructions or pathologic conditions of the pulmonary vessels, such as a pulmonary embolus. The tissue changes of TB and cancer of the lung may be diagnosed by chest x-ray or CT scan, MRI, or positron emission tomography (PET) scans. Airway obstruction is most often diagnosed with pulmonary function testing.

28. a. 3; b. 7; c. 2; d. 4; e. 5; f. 6; g. 1; h. 8 (see Tables 27.17 and 27.18).

CHAPTER 28

1. a. Suction control chamber or dry suction regulator; b. water-seal chamber; c. air leak monitor; d, collection chamber; e. suction monitor bellows

2.

Chamber	Function
Water-seal	This chamber contains 2 cm of water, which acts as a 1-way valve. Incoming air enters from the collection chamber and bubbles up through the water. The water prevents backflow of the air into the patient from the system
Suction control	This chamber applies suction to the chest drainage system. The water suction type system contains a column of water with the top end vented to the atmosphere to control the amount of suction, with bubbles to indicate it is working. The amount of suction applied is controlled by the amount of water in the chamber (usually -20 cm H_2O), not by the wall suction applied to it. The dry suction device contains no water and uses a regulator to dial the desired negative pressure.
Collection	This chamber receives fluid and air from the pleural or mediastinal space. Nurses keep track of the amount of drainage and can mark the container for easy measuring.
Suction monitor bellows	The dry model has the suction monitor bellows, which expands to show that the suction is operating, as this model does not make the bubbling noise made by the models that control the suction with water.

3. a. The water-seal chamber should bubble intermittently as air leaves the lung with exhalation in a spontaneously breathing patient. Continuous bubbling indicates a leak. The water in the suction control chamber will bubble continuously and the fluid in the water-seal chamber fluctuates (tidaling) with the patient's breathing. Water in the suction control chamber, and perhaps in the water-seal chamber, evaporates and may have to be replaced periodically.

4. c. If chest tubes are to be milked or stripped, this procedure should be done only by the professional nurse. This procedure is no longer recommended, as it may dangerously increase pleural pressure, but there is no indication to milk the tubes when there is no bloody drainage, as in a pneumothorax. The AP can loop the chest tubing on the bed to promote drainage and secure the drainage container in an upright position. An AP can remind patients to cough and deep breathe at least every 2 hours to aid in lung reexpansion.

5. b. Decortication is the stripping of a thick fibrous membrane. A lobectomy is the removal of 1 lung lobe. A thoracotomy is the incision into the thorax. A wedge resection is used to remove a small localized lesion.

6. d. During video-assisted thoracic surgery (VATS), a video scope is inserted into the thorax to assess, diagnose, and treat intrathoracic injuries. A pneumonectomy is the removal of an entire lung. A wedge resection is the removal of a lung segment with localized lesions. Lung volume reduction surgery is the removal of lung tissue by excising multiple wedges.

7. d. A thoracotomy incision is large and involves cutting into muscle, cartilage, and possibly the sternum, resulting in significant postoperative pain, interfering with deep-breathing and coughing. The patient should be provided analgesics before attempting these activities. Water intake is important to liquefy secretions but is not indicated in this case, nor should a patient with chest trauma or surgery be placed in Trendelenburg position, because it increases intrathoracic pressure. Auscultating before and after coughing evaluates effectiveness of airway clearance but does not facilitate it.

8. c. With a tracheostomy (versus an endotracheal [ET] tube), patient comfort is increased because there is no tube in the mouth. Because the tube is more secure, mobility is improved. The ET tube is more easily inserted

in an emergency situation. It is preferable to perform a tracheostomy in the operating room because it requires careful dissection, but it can be performed with local anesthetic in the intensive care unit (ICU) or in an emergency. With a cuff, tracheal pressure necrosis is as much a risk with a tracheostomy tube as with an ET tube, and infection is also as likely to occur because the defenses of the upper airway are bypassed.

9. e, f. The fenestrated tracheostomy tube has openings on the outer cannula to allow air to pass over the vocal cords to allow speaking. If the steps of using the fenestrated tracheostomy tube are not completed in the correct order, severe respiratory distress may result. The cuff of the tracheostomy tube with a foam-filled cuff passively fills with air and does require pressure monitoring, although cuff integrity must be assessed daily. The speaking tracheostomy tube has 2 tubes attached. One tube allows air to pass over the vocal cords to enable the person to speak with the cuff inflated.

10. b. An inner cannula is a second tubing that fits inside the outer tracheostomy tube. Disposable inner cannulas are frequently used, but nondisposable ones can be removed and cleaned of mucus that has accumulated on the inside of the tube. Many tracheostomy tubes do not have inner cannulas because when humidification is adequate, accumulation of mucus should not occur. Cuff deflation is no longer recommended. When signs of airway obstruction occur, suction is needed.

11. d, e. Changing the tracheostomy ties soon after placement of the tracheostomy will be irritating to the trachea and could contribute to dislodgement of the tracheostomy tube. Suctioning should be done when increased secretions are evident in the tube to prevent the patient from severe coughing, which could cause tube dislodgement. Tracheostomy care is done every 8 hours. Keeping the patient in a semi-Fowler's position will not prevent dislodgement. Keeping an extra tube at the bedside will speed reinsertion if the tracheostomy tube is dislodged, but it will not prevent dislodgement. The physician will not change the tracheostomy tube until the insertion site is healed, approximately 3 to 5 days after original insertion.

12. a, b, c. LPNs may determine the need for suctioning, suction the tracheostomy, and determine whether the patient has improved after the suctioning when caring for stable patients. They also may perform tracheostomy care using sterile technique. The patient's swallowing ability is assessed by a speech therapist, videofluoroscopy, or fiberoptic endoscopic evaluations. The RN will teach the patient about home tracheostomy care.

13. b. Cuff pressure should be monitored at least every 8 hours to ensure that an air leak around the cuff does not occur and that the pressure is not too high to allow adequate tracheal capillary perfusion. Respiratory therapists in some institutions will record the cuff pressure, but the nurse must be able to assess cuff pressure and identify if there is a problem maintaining cuff pressure. Tracheostomy tubes are changed monthly when needed for long-term use. Mouth care should be performed a minimum of every 8 hours and more often as needed to remove dried secretions. Arterial blood gases (ABGs) are not routinely assessed with tracheostomy tube placement unless symptoms of respiratory distress continue.

14. a. If a tracheostomy tube is dislodged, the nurse should immediately attempt to replace the tube by using hemostats to spread the opening. The obturator is inserted in the replacement tube, water-soluble lubricant is applied to the tip, and the tube is inserted in the stoma at a 45-degree angle to the neck. The obturator is immediately removed to provide an airway. If the tube cannot be reinserted, the HCP should be notified and the patient should be assessed for the level of respiratory distress, positioned in semi-Fowler's position, and ventilated with a manual resuscitation bag (MRB) only if necessary, until assistance arrives.

15. c. A nasal endotracheal (ET) tube is longer and smaller in diameter than an oral ET tube, creating more airway resistance and increasing the work of breathing. Suctioning and secretion removal are also more difficult with nasal ET tubes and they are more subject to kinking than are oral tubes. Oral tubes may require a bite block to stop the patient from biting the tube and may cause more laryngeal damage because of their larger size.

16. a. The patient is positioned with the head extended and the neck flexed in the "sniffing position," but the head must not hang over the edge of the bed. The patient may be asked to extrude the tongue during nasal intubation, if possible. Speaking is not possible during intubation or while the oral ET tube is in place because the tube separates the vocal cords.

17. a. 5, b. 4, c. 1, d. 3, e. 2. The first action of the nurse is to use an end tidal CO_2 detector. If no CO_2 is detected, the tube is in the esophagus. The second action by the nurse following ET intubation is to auscultate the chest to confirm bilateral breath sounds and observe to confirm bilateral chest expansion. If this evidence is present, the tube is secured and connected to an O_2 source. Then the placement is confirmed immediately with x-ray, and the tube is marked where it exits the mouth. The patient should be suctioned as needed.

18. c. The minimal occluding volume (MOV) involves adding air to the ET tube cuff until no leak is heard at peak inspiratory pressure but ensures that minimal pressure is applied to the tracheal wall to prevent tracheal necrosis from high cuff pressure. The MOV should be between 20 and 25 cm H_2O of pressure to prevent tracheal injury. The cuff does not secure the tube in place but rather prevents escape of ventilating gases through the upper airway.

19. 100 to 120 mm Hg

20. c. Suctioning an ET tube is performed when adventitious sounds over the trachea or bronchi confirm the presence of secretions that can be removed by suctioning. Visible secretions in the ET tube, respiratory distress, suspected aspiration, increase in peak airway pressures, and changes in oxygen status are other indications. Peripheral wheezes or crackles are not an indication for suctioning. Suctioning as a means of inducing a cough is not recommended because of the complications associated with suctioning.

21. c. Nursing care for a patient with an ET tube includes: (1) hyperoxygenation before and after suctioning, (2) keeping suctioning equipment and a self-inflating bag-valve-mask (BVM) at the bedside, and (3) using either 1-time use sterile suction catheters for open suction technique or a suction catheter that is enclosed in a plastic sleeve connected directly to the patient ventilator circuit, which is changed per facility protocol for the closed suction technique. Tracheostomy trays and used suction catheters are not left at the bedside.

22. d. If new dysrhythmias occur during suctioning, the suctioning should be stopped and the patient should be hyperoxygenated via BVM with 100% oxygen until the dysrhythmia subsides. Patients with bradycardia should not be suctioned excessively. Ventilation of the patient with slow, small-volume breaths using the BVM is performed when severe coughing results from suctioning.

23. a, d. To prevent dislodgement of the oral ET tube during care, 2 nurses work together; one holds the tube while it is unsecured and the other performs care. After completion of care, confirm the presence of bilateral breath sounds to ensure that the position of the tube was not changed and reconfirm cuff pressure. Suction pressure <120 mm Hg will prevent tracheal mucosal damage. Humidified inspired gas helps thin secretions. Secretions are moved to larger airways with turning, postural drainage, and percussion. None of these other actions will prevent or detect tube dislodgement.

24. b, c, e. Because the patient with an ET tube cannot protect the airway from aspiration and cannot swallow, the cuff should always be inflated and the head of the bed (HOB) elevated while the patient is receiving tube feedings or mouth care is being done. The HOB elevated 30 to 45 degrees reduces risk of aspiration. The mouth and oropharynx should be suctioned with Yankauer or tonsil suction to remove accumulated secretions that cannot be swallowed. Clearing the ventilatory tubing of condensed water is important to prevent ventilator-associated pneumonia (VAP).

25. a, b. Sedation may be appropriate. As well, having someone the patient knows at the bedside talking to him and reassuring him may decrease his anxiety and calm him. Restraints have not been shown to be an absolute deterrent to self-extubation, and the patient will need ongoing and frequent assessment of need. Reminding the patient of the need for the tube may help, but it may not be enough to prevent him from pulling out the tube if he becomes extremely anxious. Moving the patient near the nurses' station will not be enough to prevent self-extubation because it can be done so quickly.

26. b, e. Cystic fibrosis and acute respiratory distress syndrome (ARDS) are the most likely of these diagnoses to need mechanical ventilation related to severe hypoxia or respiratory muscle fatigue. Other indications for mechanical ventilation are apnea or impending inability to breathe and acute respiratory failure.

27. a, d. Positive pressure ventilators require an artificial airway and are most frequently used with acutely ill patients. Although they are frequently used in the home, the other options describe negative pressure ventilators.

28. a, c, e. Positive pressure ventilation has a predetermined peak inspiratory pressure, which increases the risk for hyperventilation and hypoventilation because the volume delivered varies based on the selected pressure and the patient's lung compliance. The other options describe volume ventilation.

29. d. Synchronized intermittent mandatory ventilation (SIMV) is described. Assist-control ventilation (ACV) has a preset tidal volume delivered at a set frequency and more frequently when the patient attempts to inhale. Pressure support ventilation (PSV) applies positive pressure only during inspiration with a rapid flow of gas with spontaneous respirations. Pressure-controlled inverse ratio ventilation (PC-IRV) delivers prolonged inspiration and shortened expiration to promote alveolar expansion and prevent collapse.

30. a. Positive pressure ventilation, especially with positive end-expiratory pressure (PEEP), increases intrathoracic pressure with compression of thoracic vessels, resulting in decreased venous return to the heart, decreased left ventricular end-diastolic volume (preload), decreased CO, and lowered BP. None of the other factors is related to increased intrathoracic pressure.

31. d. Decreased CO associated with positive pressure ventilation and PEEP results in decreased renal perfusion, release of renin, and increased aldosterone secretion, which causes sodium and water retention. Antidiuretic hormone (ADH) may be released because of stress, but ADH is responsible only for water retention. Increased intrathoracic pressure will decrease, not increase, the release of atrial natriuretic factor, causing sodium retention. There is decreased, not increased, insensible water loss via the airway during mechanical ventilation.

32. a. LPN; b. RN; c. LPN; d. AP; e. RN; f. LPN; g. RN; h. AP; i. RN; j. AP

33. c. Neuromuscular blocking agents produce a paralysis that facilitates ventilation, but they do not sedate the patient. It is important for the nurse to remember that the patient can hear, see, feel, and think and should be addressed and given explanations accordingly. Communication with the patient is possible, especially from the nurse, but visitors for an anxious and agitated patient should provide a calming, restful effect on the patient.

34. c. The patient is experiencing effects of inadequate nutrition: anemia, delayed ventilator weaning with decreased respiratory strength, decreased resistance to infection, and prolonged recovery. Hypoxemia is related to anemia. Enteral feeding would provide needed nutrition. Decreased activity may be related to muscle weakness from lack of nutrition.

35. b. A leaking cuff can lower tidal volume or respiratory rates. A SIMV rate that is too low, the presence of lung secretions, or obstruction can decrease tidal volume. Dysrhythmias can occur with either hyperventilation or hypoventilation. A decreased partial pressure of carbon dioxide in arterial blood ($PaCO_2$) and increased pH indicate a respiratory alkalosis from hyperventilation.

36. b. A variety of ventilator weaning methods is used, but all should provide weaning trials with adequate rest between trials to prevent respiratory muscle fatigue. Weaning is usually carried out during the day, with the patient ventilated at night until there is sufficient spontaneous ventilation without excess fatigue. If the patient becomes hypoxemic, ventilator support is indicated.

37. a. Care of a ventilator-dependent patient in the home requires that the caregiver know how to manage the ventilator and take care of the patient on it. Before final decisions and arrangements are made, the nurse should ensure that caregivers understand the potential sacrifices they may have to make and the impact that home mechanical ventilation will have over time. Placement in long-term care facilities is not usually necessary unless the caregiver can no longer manage the care or the patient's condition deteriorates.

Case Study

1. **Expected**: increase in SpO_2, decrease in BP (hypotension), increase in PaO_2, increase in SVR (compensatory response to decrease in BP); **Unexpected**: increase in cardiac output

(PEEP causes a decrease in CO), decrease in ICP (causes an increase), decrease in FRC (PEEP increases FRC)

2. **Indicated**: monitor $EtCO_2$ (end-tidal CO_2 should be monitored in patients on mechanical ventilation to assess for airway patency and adequacy of ventilation), document RASS score while on sedation (most patients on mechanical ventilation require sedation which should be monitored using some type of sedation score to ensure adequate sedation without causing oversedation), explain procedures while patient is sedated or on neuromuscular blockades (patients can still hear despite sedation and paralytics, therefore all procedures should be explained before performing them); **Contraindicated**: assess the need for ETT suction every 4 hours (the need should be assessed every hour), insert an oropharyngeal airway to prevent biting on ETT tube (a bite block should be used versus an OPA which is designed to keep the upper airway patent by moving the tongue; this is not necessary in intubated patients and may stimulate the gag reflex risking aspiration), use 4-point restraints while intubated (this type of restraint is used for patients with behavioral issues that may cause harm to themselves or others; it is not necessary for intubated patients especially if a patient is on sedation; 2-point restraints are common); **Non-essential**: auscultate bowel sounds (even though this is part of a routine physical assessment, it isn't specific to those on mechanical ventilation), monitor for new heart murmurs (isn't specific to a patient on mechanical ventilation)

3. B., C., D., G., H. Patients on AC cannot determine their own V_T as it is preset by the ventilator. The patient will receive the set RR and cannot go below this preset rate. Patients can initiate a spontaneous breath over the set RR but the ventilator will determine the V_T. There is a potential for hyperventilation on this mode which may require sedation or changes to the settings. It is the most common mode used in mechanical ventilation. Peak inspiratory pressures are used to determine V_T in pressure control ventilation. AC is preferred in patients without acute lung injury (ALI) or ARDS. It uses volume control ventilation versus other modes which use pressure control ventilation. Patients who have a drive to breathe, as evidenced by spontaneous breathing, would be more comfortable on different modes like SIMV.

4. **Indicated**: extubate as soon as medically possible (VAP can occur in 48 hours after intubation), obtain sputum cultures (can identify microorganisms which can be treated with specific antibiotics), keep HOB 30-45° (decreases the risk of GI aspiration, especially if on tube feedings), drain ventilator condensation away from the patient (condensate contains a high concentration of pathogenic bacteria); **Contraindicated**: oral care once daily (chlorhexidine can be used for oral care, but oral care should occur more frequently, often every 2-4 hours); keep the patient on bedrest (this promotes VAP, early mobilization is recommended if the patient is stable), change the ventilator circuit tubing every 48 hours (it is contraindicated to routinely change the circuitry as it exposes the system to microorganisms); **Non-essential**: put patient on contact isolation (this is unnecessary unless there is an indication like *C-difficile*), monitor urine output hourly (this is not relevant to reducing the risk of VAP)

5. Data that do not support extubation: Bibasilar rhonchi (the patient must be able to manage and clear secretions after extubation, information about secretions may cause concern about extubation), HR 103 (this patient's HR was 80 beats/min, tachycardia may indicate anxiety and agitation during the weaning trial), RR 32 breaths/min (tachypnea may indicate an increased work of breathing), PEEP 10 mm Hg (higher PEEP setting than is recommended to wean from the ventilator), pH 7.30 (acidosis, recommendation is $\geq$ 7.35), HCO_3^- 20 mEq/L (metabolic acidosis likely from sepsis which may cause Kussmaul breathing if the patient is extubated), NIP -15 mm Hg (more negative than -25 is recommended; this value indicates weak intercostal muscle strength), moist skin (could indicate diaphoresis as a result of increased work of breathing or anxiety/agitation)

CHAPTER 29

1. a. Direct pressure on the entire soft lower portion of the nose against the nasal septum for 5 to 15 minutes is indicated for epistaxis. In addition, have the patient sit upright and leaning forward to prevent swallowing or aspirating blood.

2. d. All of the assessments are appropriate, but the most important is the patient's oxygen status. After the posterior nasopharynx is packed, some patients, especially older adults, experience a decrease in PaO_2 and an increase in $PaCO_2$ because of impaired respiration, and the nurse should monitor the patient's respiratory rate and rhythm and SpO_2.

3. b. The most important factor in managing allergic rhinitis is identification and avoidance of triggers of the allergic reactions. Immunotherapy may be indicated if specific allergens are identified and cannot be avoided. Drug therapy is an alternative to avoidance of the allergens, but long-term use of decongestants can cause rebound nasal congestion.

4. d. Dyspnea and severe sinus pain as well as tender swollen glands, severe ear pain, or significantly worsening symptoms or changes in sputum characteristics in a patient who has a viral upper respiratory infection (URI) indicate lower respiratory involvement and a possible secondary bacterial infection. Bacterial infections are indications for antibiotic therapy, but unless symptoms of complications are present, injudicious administration of antibiotics may produce resistant organisms. Cough, sore throat, low-grade elevated temperature, myalgia, and purulent nasal drainage at the end of a cold are common symptoms of viral rhinitis and influenza.

5. a. The injected inactivated influenza vaccine is recommended for individuals 6 months of age and older and those at increased risk for influenza-related complications, such as people with chronic medical conditions or those who are immunocompromised, residents of long-term care facilities, health care workers, and providers of care to at-risk persons. The live attenuated influenza vaccine is given intranasally and is recommended for all healthy people between the ages of 2 and 49 years but not for those at increased risk of complications or HCPs. The immunity will not protect for several years, as new strains of influenza may develop each year. Antiviral agents will help reduce the duration and severity of influenza in those at high risk, but immunization is the best control.

6. c. Although inadequately treated β-hemolytic streptococcal infections may lead to rheumatic heart disease or glomerulonephritis, antibiotic treatment is not recommended until strep infections are definitely diagnosed with culture or antigen tests. The manifestations of viral, fungal, and bacterial infections are similar, and appearance is not diagnostic except when the white, irregular patches on the oropharynx suggest that candidiasis is present.

7. a, b, c. With partial airway obstruction, choking, stridor, use of accessory muscles, suprasternal and intercostals retraction, flaring nostrils, wheezing, restlessness, tachycardia, cyanosis, and change in level of consciousness may occur. Partial airway obstruction may progress to complete obstruction without prompt assessment and treatment.

8. b. The primary risk factors associated with head and neck cancers are heavy tobacco and alcohol use. Oral cancer may cause a change in the fit of dentures, but denture use is not a risk factor for oral cancer. Chronic infections are not known to be risk factors, although cancers in patients younger than age 50 years have been associated with human papillomavirus (HPV) infection.

9. a. If laryngeal tumors are small, radiation is the treatment of choice because it can be curative and can preserve voice quality. Surgical procedures are used if radiation treatment is not successful or if larger or advanced lesions are present.

10. a. With removal of the larynx, the patient will not be able to communicate verbally, and it is important to arrange with the patient a method of communication before surgery so that postoperative communication can take place. Dry mouth and stomatitis result from radiation therapy. Vigorous coughing is not encouraged immediately postoperatively, and information related to community resources is usually introduced during the postoperative period.

11. a. Following a radical neck dissection, drainage tubes are often used to prevent fluid accumulation in the wound as well as possible pressure on the trachea. A nasal endotracheal tube would not be useful. The patient has placement of a nasogastric tube to suction immediately after surgery, which will later be used to administer tube feedings until swallowing can be accomplished. A tracheostomy tube is in place, but mechanical ventilation is usually not indicated.

12. b. Suctioning of the tracheostomy with the use of a mirror is a self-care activity taught to the patient before discharge. Voice rehabilitation is usually managed by a speech therapist or speech pathologist, but the nurse should discuss the various types of voice rehabilitation and the advantages and disadvantages of each option. The laryngectomy stoma should be covered with a shield during showering and covered with light scarves or fabric when aspiration of foreign materials is likely.

13. b. Transesophageal puncture provides the most normal voice reproduction but requires a surgical fistula made between the esophagus and the trachea and a valve prosthesis. Esophageal speech involves air trapped in the esophagus and expelled past the pharyngoesophageal segment, but it is difficult, takes a lot of time, and voice quality is reduced. The electrolarynx, whether placed in the mouth or held to the neck, allows speech that has a metallic or robotic sound.

Case Study

1. **Infection**: ambulate the patient at least 3x/day (promotes circulation for healing and oxygenation of the lungs preventing atelectasis which can lead to lung infections like pneumonia), using incentive spirometer and deep breathing and coughing (prevents atelectasis from turning into pneumonia), performing sterile dressing changes (reduces the chance of microorganisms being introduced into the wound); **Venous thromboembolism**: ambulating the patient 3x/day and apply sequential compression devices to BLE while in bed (promotes circulation and decreases venous pooling of blood which leads to clot formation); **Atelectasis**: ambulate the patient at least 3x/day, use the incentive spirometer, deep breath and cough (all promotes oxygenation of the lungs preventing atelectasis); **Not used**: neutropenic precautions (are unnecessary unless there is evidence that the patient is immunocompromised which increases their susceptibility to contracting infections), applying ice (reduces swelling and may reduce pain, but isn't an applicable intervention for these potential complications)

2. **1**=3rd, **2**=basilar skull fracture; **3**=cerebrospinal fluid; **4**=glucose; **5**=airway obstruction, epistaxis (nosebleed), septal hematoma; (note: crepitus is a manifestation not a complication) **6**=septoplasty and rhinoplasty, respectively.

3. The nurse will implement the use of **incentive spirometry** due to signs of **atelectasis** which is a result of **rib fractures** sustained in the motor vehicle accident 5 days ago. **Rationale**: The nurse should always consider *ABCs* when prioritizing care. Respiratory evidence includes: sharp pain with deep breathing, RR 26 breaths/min, SpO$_2$ 91%, and diminished bibasilar breath sounds. A headache reported as a 5 is moderate and expected with facial trauma. Rib fractures will cause pain, but this pain should be treated (not necessarily with opioids) to optimize the patient to perform deep breathing and incentive spirometry. BP may be slightly elevated due to pain. Temperature may indicate infection, but there is no other evidence supporting this conclusion. It is normal to have serous fluid weep from an incision several days after surgery, as long as it isn't purulent. Decreased circulation, as evidenced by a dorsalis pedis pulse of +1, being cool and pale when compared to the left lower extremity, is expected after trauma to this leg. There are no other signs of poor circulation or compartment syndrome which would require more aggressive interventions.

4. **Indicated**: apply nasal sling with gauze under the nose (a dressing to capture drainage following a rhinoplasty), apply ice to periorbital areas (will reduce swelling and may help with pain; ice should not be applied to the bridge of the nose because it may be too heavy for a weak reconstructed nasal bone); **Contraindicated**: HOB less than 30 degrees (the HOB should be greater than 30 degrees to protect the airway and reduce swelling), apply heat packs to nose (heat will vasodilate and increase the risk of bleeding), insert a nasopharyngeal airway (nothing should be inserted in the nares after nasal surgery and reconstruction); **Non-essential**: avoid stimulating the patient (the patient may need to be stimulated after surgery to breathe and wake-up from anesthesia, but this may not be necessary if the patient is accomplishing these on his own), pinch nostrils for scant sanguineous drainage (scant to small amounts of

bleeding are expected after nasal reconstruction surgery; if the bleeding is profuse then pinching the nostrils for 5-15 minutes may be necessary to stop active bleeding)

5. A., C., D., F., H., J. Nasal rinses will help clean the nostrils from dried blood and moisten the turbinates. If the patient has nosebleeds, they should sit upright and lean forward, not lie down and hyperextend their neck. Visual changes are unexpected and should be reported to the HCP. Phenylephrine nasal spray may be used to treat minor continuous nosebleeds, major bleeding should be reported to the HCP. Patients can use frozen vegetables, like peas or corn, or crushed ice to reduce swelling and bruising but the weight of these should not be placed directly on the bridge of the nose as it could cause a displaced fracture. Patients should sleep with their head elevated approximately 30 degrees to reduce swelling and protect their airway from the nasal bleeding that will drain into the upper airway. Steamy hot showers can loosen the nasal splints that are often applied externally as well as increase the risk of bleeding. Blowing their nose can cause bleeding as it dislodges clots that have tamponaded the bleeding. Aspirin, and often times NSAIDs, are not recommended as they can increase the risk of bleeding. Don't do any heavy lifting, usually more than 10 lbs, because this will increase blood pressure and predispose the patient to an increased risk of bleeding.

CHAPTER 30

1. a, c, e. Microorganisms that cause pneumonia reach the lungs by aspiration from the nasopharynx or oropharynx, inhalation of microbes in the air, and hematogenous spread from infections elsewhere in the body. The other causes of infection do not contribute to pneumonia.

2. c. Pneumonia that has its onset in the community is usually caused by different microorganisms than pneumonia that develops related to hospitalization and treatment can be empiric—based on observations and experience without knowing the exact causative organism. Frequently, a causative organism cannot be identified from cultures, and treatment is based on experience.

3. b. People at risk for opportunistic pneumonia include those with altered immune responses. *Pneumocystis jiroveci* rarely causes pneumonia in healthy individuals but is the most common cause of pneumonia in persons with human immunodeficiency (HIV) disease. Cytomegalovirus (CMV) occurs in people with an impaired immune response. Necrotizing pneumonia is caused by *Staphylococcus, Klebsiella,* and *Streptococcus.* Hospital-acquired pneumonia (HAP) is frequently caused by *Pseudomonas aeruginosa, Escherichia coli, Klebsiella,* and *Acinetobacter.* Community-acquired pneumonia (CAP) is most commonly caused by *Streptococcus pneumonia.*

4. a, c, e, f. CAP and HAP are both associated with *Klebsiella, Staphylococcus aureus, Pseudomonas aeruginosa,* and *Streptococcus pneumoniae. Acinetobacter* is only associated with HAP. *Mycoplasma pneumoniae* is only associated with CAP.

5. a. 4; b. 3; c. 1; d. 2. With most pneumonia-causing organisms the inflammatory response results in increased blood flow and neutrophils to engulf the offending organisms. The alveoli are filled with extra fluid from increased blood flow and capillary permeability from surrounding vessels, which leads to hypoxia. Mucus production is increased and can further obstruct airflow. With bacterial pneumonia consolidation occurs when the alveoli fill with fluid and debris. Macrophages lyse and process the debris so that normal gas exchange returns.

6. a. Confusion possibly related to hypoxia may be the only finding in older adults. Although CAP is most commonly caused by *S. aureus* and is associated with an acute onset with fever, chills, productive cough with purulent or bloody sputum, and pleuritic chest pain, the older patient may not have classic symptoms. A recent loss of consciousness or altered consciousness is common in those pneumonias associated with aspiration, such as anaerobic bacterial pneumonias. Other causes of pneumonia have a more gradual onset with dry, hacking cough; headache; and sore throat.

7. d. Prompt treatment of pneumonia with appropriate antibiotics is important in treating bacterial and mycoplasma pneumonia, and antibiotics are often administered on the basis of the history, physical examination, and a chest x-ray indicating a typical pattern characteristic of a particular organism without further testing. It is more significant if it is CAP or HAP than the severity of pneumonia symptoms. Blood and sputum cultures take 24 to 72 hours for results, and microorganisms often cannot be identified with either Gram stain or cultures.

8. d. A sputum specimen for Gram stain and culture should be obtained before starting antibiotic therapy and while waiting for the antibiotic to be delivered from the pharmacy in a hospitalized patient with suspected pneumonia. Then antibiotics should be started without delay. If the sputum specimen cannot be obtained rapidly, the chest x-ray will be done to assess the typical pattern characteristic of the infecting organism. Blood cell tests will not be altered significantly by delaying the tests until after the first dose of antibiotics.

9.

Clinical Situation	Nursing Intervention
Patient with altered consciousness	Position to side, protect airway
Patient with a feeding tube	Check placement of the tube before feeding and residual feeding; keep head of bed up after feedings or continuously with continuous feedings
Patient with local anesthetic to throat	Check gag reflex before feeding or offering fluids
Patient with difficulty swallowing	Cut food in small bites, encourage thorough chewing, and provide soft foods that are easier to swallow than liquids

10. a. Oxygen saturation obtained by pulse oximetry should be >94%. An arterial oxygen saturation by pulse oximetry (SpO_2) lower than 95% indicates hypoxemia and impaired gas exchange. Crackles, fever, and purulent sputum are all manifestations of pneumonia but do not necessarily relate to impaired gas exchange.

11. b. Clear lung sounds indicate that the airways are clear. SpO_2 of 95% to 100% indicates appropriate gas exchange. Tolerating walking in the hallway indicates appropriate

gas exchange and activity tolerance, not improved airway clearance. Deep breaths are necessary to move mucus from distal airways, but this is not an outcome for this clinical problem.

12. a. He should receive his first dose of PCV13, followed at least 1 year later by a dose of PPSV23. Influenza vaccine should be taken each year. Antibiotic therapy is not appropriate for all upper respiratory infections unless secondary bacterial infections develop.

13. b. Drug-resistant strains of tuberculosis (TB) have developed because TB patients' compliance with drug therapy has been poor, and there has been general decreased vigilance in monitoring and follow-up of TB treatment. TB can be diagnosed effectively with sputum cultures. Antitubercular drugs are almost exclusively used for TB infections. The incidence of TB is at epidemic proportions in patients with HIV, but this does not account for multidrug-resistant strains of TB.

14. b. A patient with class 3 TB has clinically active disease, and airborne infection isolation is required for active disease until the patient is noninfectious, indicated by negative sputum smears. Cardiac monitoring and observation will be done with the patient in isolation. The nurse will administer the antitubercular drugs after the patient is in isolation. There should be no need for suction or extra linens after the TB patient is receiving drug therapy.

15. b. TB usually develops insidiously with fatigue, malaise, anorexia, low-grade fevers, and night sweats, a dry cough, and unexplained weight loss. Pleuritic pain, flu-like symptoms, and a productive cough may occur with an acute sudden presentation; but dyspnea and hemoptysis are late symptoms.

16. a, c, d, f. For the first 2 months, a 4-drug regimen consists of isoniazid, pyrazinamide, rifampin (Rifadin), and ethambutol (Myambutol). Rifabutin (Mycobutin) and levofloxacin may be used if the patient develops toxicity to the primary drugs. Rifabutin may be used as first-line treatment for patients receiving medications that interact with rifampin (e.g., antiretrovirals, estradiol, warfarin).

17. a. Notification of the public health department is required. If drug compliance is questionable, follow-up of patients can be made by directly observed therapy by a public health nurse. A patient who cannot remember to take the medication usually will not remember to come to the clinic daily or will find it too inconvenient. Additional teaching or support from others is not usually effective for this type of patient.

18. b. Although all of the precautions identified in this question are appropriate in decreasing the risk of occupational lung diseases, using masks and effective ventilation systems to reduce exposure is the most efficient and affects the greatest number of employees. The safety inspections are required.

19. a, b, e. Smoking by women is taking a great toll, as reflected by the increasing incidence and deaths from lung cancer in women, who develop lung cancer at a younger age than men. Nonsmoking women are at greater risk of developing lung cancer than nonsmoking men. Men still have a worse prognosis than women from lung cancer. White women have a higher rate of lung cancer than other ethnic groups.

20. d. Adults ages 55 to 77 years with a history of smoking (30-pack year smoking history or currently smoke) or who quit smoking but <15 years ago should have annual screening for lung cancer. Screening is done using low-dose CT. The use of x-ray has also been shown to detect lung cancer at earlier stages when it is suspected. Sputum cytology may be used, but malignant cells are seldom present in sputum. A patient who has a smoking history always has an increased risk for lung cancer compared with an individual who has never smoked, but the risk decreases to that of a nonsmoker after 15 years of nonsmoking.

21. a. Although chest x-rays, lung tomograms, CT scans, MRI, and positron emission tomography (PET) can identify tumors and masses, a definitive diagnosis of a lung cancer requires identification of malignant cells in a biopsy or cytologic study of bronchial washings.

22. a. 3; b. 6; c. 8; d. 7; e. 1; f. 9; g. 5; h. 2; i. 4; j. 10

23. b. Before making any judgments about the patient's statement, it is important to explore what meaning they find in the pain. It may be that the patient feels the pain is deserved punishment for smoking, but further information must be obtained from the patient. Immediate referral to a counselor negates the nurse's responsibility in helping the patient, and there is no indication that the patient is not dealing effectively with their feelings.

24. d. Spontaneous pneumothorax is seen from the rupture of small blebs on the surface of the lung in patients with lung disease or smoking, as well as in tall, thin males with a family history of or a previous spontaneous pneumothorax. Tension pneumothorax occurs with mechanical ventilation and with blocked chest tubes. Iatrogenic pneumothorax occurs because of the laceration or puncture of the lung during medical procedures. Traumatic pneumothorax can occur with penetrating or blunt chest trauma.

25. b. A tension pneumothorax causes many of the same manifestations as other types of pneumothoraxes, but severe respiratory distress from collapse of the entire lung with movement of the mediastinal structures and trachea to the unaffected side is present in a tension pneumothorax. Percussion dullness on the injured site indicates the presence of blood or fluid, and decreased movement and diminished breath sounds are characteristic of a pneumothorax. Muffled and distant heart sounds indicate a cardiac tamponade.

26. d. Flail chest may occur when 2 or more ribs are fractured, causing an unstable segment. The chest wall cannot provide the support for ventilation, and the injured segment will move paradoxically to the stable portion of the chest (in on expiration; out on inspiration). Hypotension occurs with a number of conditions that impair cardiac function, and chest pain occurs with a single fractured rib and will be important with flail chest. Absent breath sounds occur following pneumothorax or hemothorax.

27. a. 8; b. 7; c. 2; d. 3; e. 6; f. 1; g. 9; h. 4; i. 5

28. a. All of the activities are correct, but the first thing to do is to raise the head of the bed to facilitate breathing in the patient who is dyspneic. The HCP would not be called until the nurse has assessment data relating to vital signs, pulse oximetry, and any other patient complaints.

29. c. A spiral (helical) CT scan is the most frequently used test to diagnose pulmonary emboli (PE) because it allows illumination of all anatomic structures and produces a

3-dimensional picture. If a patient cannot have contrast media, a ventilation-perfusion scan is done. Although pulmonary angiography is most sensitive, it is invasive, expensive, and carries more risk for complications. D-dimer is neither specific nor sensitive for small PE, especially in this patient with deep vein thrombosis. Chest x-rays do not detect PE until necrosis or abscesses occur.

30. a. Chronic obstructive pulmonary disease (COPD) causes pulmonary capillary and alveolar damage increasing pressure, as does scleroderma. Sarcoidosis is a granulomatous disease, pulmonary fibrosis stiffens the pulmonary vasculature, and PE obstructs pulmonary blood flow, but alone, these would not cause secondary pulmonary arterial hypertension.

31. b. High pressure in the pulmonary arteries increases the workload of the right ventricle and eventually causes right ventricular hypertrophy, known as *cor pulmonale*, and eventual heart failure. Eventually, decreased left ventricular output may occur because of decreased return to the left atrium, but it is not the primary effect of pulmonary hypertension. Alveolar interstitial edema is pulmonary edema associated with left ventricular failure. Pulmonary hypertension does not cause systemic hypertension.

32. d. If possible, the primary management of cor pulmonale is treatment of the underlying pulmonary problem that caused the heart problem. Low-flow oxygen therapy will help prevent hypoxemia and hypercapnia, which cause pulmonary vasoconstriction. The treatments used will be individualized for the patient.

33. c. Acute rejection may occur as early as 5 to 10 days after surgery and is manifested by low-grade fever, fatigue, and oxygen desaturation with exertion. Complete remission of symptoms can be accomplished with high doses of IV corticosteroids followed by high doses of oral prednisone. Cytomegalovirus and other infections can be fatal but usually occur weeks after surgery and manifest with symptoms of pneumonia. Obliterative bronchiolitis is a late complication of lung transplantation, reflecting chronic rejection.

Case Study

1. **Expected**: jugular vein distention, hepatomegaly, weight gain (all are right-sided heart failure manifestations); **Unrelated**: syncope, crackles in the lungs, renal insufficiency, confusion (all are left-sided heart failure manifestations)

2. 1=diltiazem; 2=phosphodiesterase enzyme inhibitor; 3=2.5 mcg inhaled every 4 hours; 4=dilates systemic and pulmonary artery (PA) vasculature; 5=blocks constriction of pulmonary artery; 6=furosemide; 7=40 mg PO once daily; 8=vitamin K antagonist

3. **Indicated:** "You will not be a candidate if having cancer within the past 2 years." (Patients having cancer recently will be predisposed to recurrence when put on immunosuppressants), "You will need to take immunosuppressants for the rest of your life." (To avoid organ rejection), "Lung transplant recipients are prioritized based on a lung allocation score." (Patients who are more acutely ill will be higher on the recipient list than those being well-managed on medications), "You will need adequate financial resources to afford post-transplant care and drugs." (Insurance may cover care,

but if the patient loses their insurance coverage they may not have alternative resources to cover these expenses); **Contraindicated**: "You may travel while waiting for an organ." (Patients need to stay close to home or within the region where the transplant will occur as time from harvest to transplantation is of the essence), "There is a low risk of postoperative complications." (There is a high risk of complications including acute rejection, especially during the first year.); **Non-essential**: "You will be considered permanently disabled and will not be able to be employed." (This is unnecessary to include when doing preoperative teaching as no one knows if this will be true or if the patient can regain gainful employment)

4. 1=thoracotomy; 2=pulmonary veins, bronchus, and pulmonary artery; 3=sternum; 4=heart-lung; 5=lobar; 6=relatives

5. A., D., E., F., H. Acute rejection usually occurs within 5-10 days after transplant but is common within the 1st year. A bronchoscopy will be performed to obtain lung biopsies for acute rejection. Dyspnea and other clinical manifestations should be reported to the HCP to rule-out rejection. Home spirometry to measure lung function and enrolling in rehabilitation to improve physical endurance are recommended and encouraged. Patients who are on immunosuppressants should avoid crowded events and wear a mask as they are more susceptible to contagions. There aren't any restrictions post-transplant to fly on airplanes. Deep breathing, chest physiotherapy, and coughing are important postoperatively to maintain airway clearance.

CHAPTER 31

1. d. Respiratory infections are one of the most common precipitating factors of an acute asthma attack. Sensitivity to food and drugs may also precipitate attacks, and exercise-induced asthma occurs after exercise, especially in cold, dry air. Psychologic factors may interact with the asthmatic response to worsen the disease, but it is not a psychosomatic disease.

2. b. Decreased or absent breath sounds may indicate a significant decrease in air movement resulting from exhaustion and an inability to generate enough muscle force to ventilate and is an ominous sign. The other symptoms are expected in an asthma attack but are not life threatening.

3. c. Early in an asthma attack, an increased respiratory rate and hyperventilation create a respiratory alkalosis with increased pH and decreased $PaCO_2$, accompanied by hypoxemia. As the attack progresses, pH shifts to normal, then decreases, with arterial blood gases (ABGs) that reflect respiratory acidosis with hypoxemia. During the attack, high-flow oxygen should be provided. Breathing in a paper bag, although used to treat some types of hyperventilation, would increase the hypoxemia.

4.

Agent	Role for or Relationship to Asthma
Salicylic acid	Associated with the asthma triad: (1) people with nasal polyps, (2) asthma, and (3) sensitivity to salicylic acid and nonsteroidal antiinflammatory drugs (NSAIDs)

Agent	Role for or Relationship to Asthma
Nonselective β-adrenergic blockers	Contraindicated for patients with asthma because they inhibit bronchodilation
Beer and wine	Contain sulfiting agents as preservatives and are common triggers of asthma

5. b. Peak expiratory flow rates (PEFRs) are normally up to 600 L/min and in a severe asthma attack may be as low as 100 to 150 L/min. An arterial oxygen saturation (SaO_2) of 85% and a forced expiratory volume in 1 second (FEV_1) of 85% of predicted are typical of mild to well controlled asthma. A flattened diaphragm may be present in the patient with long-standing asthma but does not reflect current bronchoconstriction.

6. d. The albuterol nebulizer will rapidly cause bronchodilation and be easier to use in an emergency than an inhaler. It will be used every 20 minutes to 4 hours as needed. The tiotropium inhaler is only approved for chronic obstructive pulmonary disease (COPD). Oral or inhaled corticosteroids will be used to decrease the inflammation and provide better symptom control after the emergency is over.

7. c, f, g, i. These are the corticosteroids described. Zileuton (Zyflo CR) and montelukast (Singulair) are leukotriene modifiers that interfere with the synthesis or block the action of the leukotriene inflammatory mediators that cause bronchoconstriction. Omalizumab (Xolair) is a monoclonal antibody to immunoglobulin (Ig)E, which prevents IgE from attaching to mast cells and prevents the release of chemical mediators. Salmeterol (Serevent) is a long-acting β2-adrenergic agonist bronchodilator. Theophylline is a methylxanthine used when other long-term bronchodilators are not available or affordable.

8. d. Storing the dry powder inhaler (DPI) in the bathroom will expose it to moisture, which could cause clumping of the medication and an altered dose. The other statements show patient understanding.

9. a, f. With asthma, salmeterol (Serevent) should not be taken without inhaled corticosteroids. Gastroesophageal reflux disease (GERD) medications help asthma, but asthma medications may make GERD symptoms worse by relaxing the lower esophageal sphincter. The rest of the statements show patient understanding.

10. b. The patient in an acute asthma attack is very anxious and fearful. It is best to stay with the patient and interact in a calm, unhurried manner. Helping the patient breathe with pursed lips will facilitate expiration of trapped air and help the patient gain control of breathing. Pursed-lip breathing is also used with COPD for this same reason. The other options will not decrease the panic of an acute asthma attack.

11. c. A yellow zone reading with the peak flow meter indicates that the patient's asthma is getting worse and quick-relief medications should be used. The meter is routinely used each morning before taking medications after the personal best peak flow number has been determined. It does not always have to be on hand. The meter measures the ability to empty the lungs and involves blowing through the meter.

12. b. Nonprescription drugs should not be used by patients with asthma because of dangers associated with rebound bronchospasm, interactions with prescribed drugs, and undesirable side effects. All the other responses are appropriate for the patient with asthma.

13. d. Increased risk of infection, hyperplasia of mucous glands, cancer, chronic cough, chronic bronchitis, and COPD are the long-term effects of smoking. Bronchospasm and hoarseness are acute effects of smoking.

14. a. A; b. C; c. C; d. C; e. C; f. C; g. B; h. B; i. C; j. A

15. b. Constriction of the pulmonary vessels, leading to pulmonary hypertension, is caused by alveolar hypoxia and the acidosis that results from hypercapnia. Polycythemia is a contributing factor in cor pulmonale because it increases the viscosity of blood and the pressure needed to circulate the blood but does not cause vasoconstriction. Long-term low-flow oxygen therapy dilates pulmonary vessels and is used to treat cor pulmonale. High oxygen administration is not related to cor pulmonale.

16. d. Smoking cessation is one of the most important factors in preventing further damage to the lungs in COPD, but prevention of infections that further increase lung damage is also important. The patient is very susceptible to infections, and these infections make the disease worse, creating a vicious cycle. Bronchodilators, inhaled corticosteroids, and lung volume–reduction surgery help control symptoms, but these are symptomatic measures.

17. a. A Venturi mask is helpful to administer low, constant O_2 concentrations to patients with COPD and can be set to administer a varied percentage of O_2. The amount of O_2 inhaled via the nasal cannula depends on room air and the patient's breathing pattern. The simple face mask must have a tight seal and may generate heat under the mask. The non-rebreather mask is more useful for short-term therapy with patients needing high O_2 concentrations.

18. b. The partial rebreather mask has O_2 flow into the reservoir bag and mask during inhalation. The O_2-conserving cannula is used for long-term therapy at home versus during hospitalization. The Venturi mask can deliver the highest concentrations of O_2. The nasal cannula is the most comfortable and mobile delivery device.

19. c. Oxygen concentrators or extractors continuously supply O_2 concentrated from the air. Portable liquid O_2 units will hold about 6 to 8 hours of O_2, but because of the expense, they are only used for portable and emergency use. Portable O_2-conserving units slow the use of oxygen. Compressed O_2 comes in various tank sizes. It requires weekly deliveries of 4 to 5 large tanks to meet a 7- to 10-day supply.

20. c. Pursed lip breathing prolongs exhalation and prevents bronchiolar collapse and air trapping. Huff coughing is a technique used to increase coughing patterns to remove secretions. Thoracic breathing is not as effective as diaphragmatic breathing and is the method most naturally used by patients with COPD. Diaphragmatic breathing emphasizes the use of the diaphragm to increase maximum inhalation, but it may increase the work of breathing and dyspnea.

21. c. Many postural drainage positions require placement in Trendelenburg position, but patients with head injury, heart disease, hemoptysis, chest trauma, and others should not be placed in these positions. Postural drainage should be done 1 hour before and 3 hours after meals if possible. Coughing, percussion, and vibration are all done after the patient has been positioned.

22. b. Eating is an effort for patients with COPD, and often these patients do not eat because of fatigue, dyspnea, altered taste, and decreased appetite. Foods that require much chewing cause more exhaustion and should be avoided. A low-carbohydrate diet is indicated if the patient has hypercapnia because carbohydrates are metabolized into carbon dioxide. Cold foods seem to give less of a sense of fullness than hot foods, and fluids should be avoided at meals to prevent a full stomach.

23. a. Assistance with positioning and activities of daily living (ADLs) is within the training of AP. Teaching, assessing, and planning are all part of the RN's practice.

24. d. Indacaterol (Arcapta Neohaler) is a β_2-adrenergic agonist administered via DPI that is used only for COPD. Roflumilast (Daliresp) is an oral medication used for COPD. Salmeterol (Serevent) is a DPI, but it is also used in asthma with inhaled corticosteroids. Ipratropium (Atrovent HFA) is used for COPD, but it is delivered via metered-dose inhaler or nebulizer.

25. d. The tripod position with an elevated backrest and supported upper extremities to fix the shoulder girdle maximizes respiratory excursion and an effective breathing pattern. Staying with the patient and encouraging pursed lip breathing also helps. Rescue short-acting, not routine bronchodilators, will be ordered but can also increase nervousness and anxiety. Postural drainage is not tolerated by a patient in acute respiratory distress, and oxygen is titrated to an effective rate based on ABGs because of the possibility of carbon dioxide narcosis.

26. d. Specific guidelines for sexual activity help preserve energy and prevent dyspnea, and maintenance of sexual activity is important to the healthy psychologic well-being of the patient. Open communication between partners is needed so that the modifications can be made with consideration of both partners.

27. c. Shortness of breath usually increases during exercise, but the activity is not being overdone if breathing returns to baseline within 5 minutes after stopping. Bronchodilators can be administered 10 minutes before exercise but should not be administered for at least 5 minutes after activity to allow recovery. Patients are encouraged to walk 15 to 20 minutes per day with gradual increases, but actual patterns will depend on patient tolerance. Dyspnea most often limits exercise and is a better sign of exercise tolerance than is heart rate in the patient with COPD.

28. b. These results show worsening respiratory function and failure with the pH at 7.34, the lower PaO_2, and the higher $PaCO_2$. The pH results of 7.35 and 7.42 show potential normal results for the patient described. The pH of 7.46 shows alkalosis, respiratory with the low $PaCO_2$, but the HCO_3^- results are needed to be sure.

29. b, d, e. Decreasing depression, fear of exercise, and hospitalizations along with improving exercise capacity are benefits of pulmonary rehabilitation (PR). Decreased FEV_1 and increased oxygen need are not beneficial.

30. c. Cystic fibrosis (CF) is an autosomal recessive, multisystem disease involving gene mutations that make secretions of the lungs, pancreas, intestines low in sodium chloride and thus water, so they are abnormally thick and sticky. This leads to a chronic, diffuse, obstructive pulmonary disorder in almost all patients. Exocrine pancreatic insufficiency occurs in about 85% to 90% of patients with CF. Fibrosis occurs in the subepithelium of the lungs and pancreas, which plugs the exocrine ducts. Bronchiectasis occurs when bronchial walls are changed.

31. d. The major goals of therapy in CF are to relieve airway obstruction and control infection. Airway clearance techniques (ACT) are the mainstay of treatment. Aerobic exercise is effective in clearing the airways, requiring increased nutrition and fluid, plus salt loss replacement. Antibiotics are used for early signs of infection, and long courses are necessary, but they are not used prophylactically. Bronchodilators have shown no long-term benefit. Although CF has become a leading indication for heart-lung transplant, this treatment option may not be available for many patients.

32. b. The presence of a chronic disease that is present at birth, delayed sexual development, difficulty in marrying and having children, and the many treatments needed by those with CF affects all relationships and development of these patients. Although a lung transplant may be needed, not all CF patients need one. Not all children will inherit CF (e.g., 25% chance for offspring with both parents having the defective gene). Many men with CF are sterile. Women may have difficulty becoming pregnant. Educational and vocational goals may be met in those who maintain treatment programs and health.

33. d. In adults, most forms of bronchiectasis are associated with bacterial infections that damage the bronchial walls. In children, CF is the prominent cause of bronchiectasis. The incidence of bronchiectasis has decreased with the use of measles and pertussis vaccines and better treatment of lower respiratory tract infections.

34. d. Mucus production is increased in bronchiectasis and collects in the dilated, pouched bronchi. A major goal of treatment is to promote drainage and removal of the mucus, primarily through ACT, including deep breathing, coughing, and especially postural drainage. Pleuritic chest pain and prevention of coughing will occur with the removal of mucus. The disease is not contagious.

35. d. α_1-Antitrypsin (AAT) deficiency is an autosomal recessive disorder that is a genetic risk factor for COPD with symptoms (often by age 40 years) in people with no tobacco use and family history of COPD or liver disease. AAT occurs in about 3% of people diagnosed with COPD. Although CF occurs in 1 in 3000 white births, legislation requires babies to be screened at birth, so it would have been previously diagnosed. Asthma is a multifactorial genetic disorder.

Case Study

1. **Related**: peak expiratory flow rate (measures the maximum rate of airflow after a forceful exhalation and determines lung function), jugular vein distention (would be present if there are signs of right-sided heart failure), serum IgE levels (to determine if the asthma attack is related to an allergy mediated response), history of heartburn (could be a trigger); **Unrelated**: blood cultures (are irrelevant unless there are indications of infection), recent UTI (recent URIs are significant, not UTIs) history of migraines (are irrelevant)

2. **Indicated**: administer oxygen via non-rebreather (patient is in respiratory distress as indicated by agitation, restlessness, RR 34 breaths/min, HR 126 beats/min,

SpO_2 88% with PaO_2 66 mm Hg requiring the delivery of high concentrations of oxygen), administer albuterol/ipratropium nebulizer (both medications will bronchodilate opening up the airways to promote oxygenation and exhalation of CO_2), administer hydrocortisone (a corticosteroid which will reduce inflammation of the airway); **Contraindicated**: administer labetalol to treat tachycardia (tachycardia is a compensatory response and should not be treated until the underlying cause is treated, labetalol is a nonselective beta-blocker which is contraindicated in patients with history of asthma as it could trigger or exacerbate asthma attacks), administer lorazepam to treat anxiety (patient is anxious because she is struggling to breathe; her underlying issue should be addressed which may resolve the agitation and restlessness); **Non-essential**: have the patient breathe into a paper bag (treats hyperventilation related to excessive exhalation of CO_2, but isn't used to treat hyperventilation related to an asthma attack), obtain a spiral CT scan (this test is performed to identify a pulmonary embolism)

3. **Mild to Moderate**: sitting upright, audible wheezing, $PaCO_2$ 36 mm Hg, dyspnea (all are evidence of an asthma attack that can be treated on an outpatient basis); **Severe**: use of accessory muscles, HR 126 beats/min, 1- to 3-word sentences, breath sounds absent in bilateral bases, SpO_2 88% (all are evidence of an attack that requires hospitalization and access to emergency care)

4. **1**=ipratropium; **2**=montelukast; **3**=Advair; **4**= β2-Adrenergic Agonist; **5**=corticosteroid; **6**=bronchodilator; **7**=anti-IgE; **8**=tachycardia is a side effect; **9**= rinse mouth after use to prevent fungal infections; **10**= don't use in an acute asthma attack

5. A., C., D., F., G. It is recommended that patients with asthma measure their daily peak expiratory flow rate (PEFR) to obtain a baseline and determine if there is a change that requires interventions. Rescue inhalers, like albuterol, need to be carried at all times regardless of their PEFR in case they experience an asthma attack that requires a bronchodilator. It is recommended that people with medical conditions, like asthma, wear a MedicAlert bracelet to alert first responders about their medical condition if they are unable to communicate. Patients should use the Asthma Control Test online to determine what "good control" is for them. Patients need to adhere to all medications prescribed to treat asthma. Corticosteroids play an integral role in preventing patients from experiencing severe asthma attacks and should not be abruptly stopped or weaned without the advice of their HCP. Patients with a history of asthma should undergo allergy testing to identify possible triggers of an asthma attack. Support groups online and in the community are great resources for patients and families to learn more about their disease. If symptoms of asthma wake patients up at night, they should consult with their HCP as this indicates that their asthma is not well controlled.

CHAPTER 32

1. d. *Acute respiratory failure* (ARF) occurs when oxygenation, ventilation, or both are inadequate. It results when the transfer of oxygen or carbon dioxide function in the respiratory system is impaired. The major factor in respiratory failure is inadequate gas exchange. Absence of ventilation is respiratory arrest and partial airway obstruction may not necessarily cause respiratory failure. Acute hypoxemia may be caused by factors other than a lung problem.

2. b, c, e, f. The main problem in hypoxemic respiratory failure is inadequate oxygen transfer. There is a risk of inadequate oxygen saturation of hemoglobin. It is often caused by ventilation-perfusion (V/Q) mismatch and shunt. It exists when the partial pressure of oxygen in arterial blood (PaO_2) is 60 mm Hg or less, even though oxygen is given at 60% or more. Ventilatory failure is hypercapnic respiratory failure. Hypercapnic respiratory failure results from an imbalance between ventilatory supply and ventilatory demand and the body is unable to compensate for the acidemia of increased partial pressure of carbon dioxide in arterial blood ($PaCO_2$).

3. c. Intrapulmonary shunt occurs when blood flows through the capillaries in the lungs without taking part in gas exchange (e.g., acute respiratory distress syndrome [ARDS], pneumonia). Obstruction impairs the flow of blood to the ventilated areas of the lung in a V/Q mismatch ratio >1 (e.g., pulmonary embolus). Blood passes through an anatomic channel in the heart and bypasses the lungs with anatomic shunt (e.g., ventricular septal defect). Gas exchange across the alveolar capillary interface is compromised by thickened or damaged alveolar membranes in diffusion limitation (e.g., pulmonary fibrosis, ARDS).

4. c. There will be more ventilation than perfusion (V/Q ratio >1) with a pulmonary embolus. Pain and atelectasis will cause a V/Q ratio <1. A ventricular septal defect causes an anatomic shunt as the blood bypasses the lungs.

5. b. Diffusion limitation in pulmonary fibrosis is caused by thickened alveolar-capillary interface, which slows gas transport. Anatomic shunt is often congenital. Blood passes through an anatomic channel in the heart and bypasses the lungs. An intrapulmonary shunt occurs when blood flows through the pulmonary capillaries, but gas exchange does not occur as with ARDS. In V/Q mismatch the amount of air (ventilation) is not matched to the amount of blood flow (perfusion).

6. b. Hypercapnic respiratory failure is associated with alveolar hypoventilation with increases in alveolar and arterial CO_2 and often is caused by problems outside the lungs. A patient with slow, shallow respirations is not exchanging enough gas volume to eliminate CO_2. Deep, rapid respirations reflect hyperventilation and often accompany lung problems that cause hypoxemic respiratory failure. Large airway resistance and pulmonary edema cause obstruction of oxygenation and result in a V/Q mismatch or shunt typical of hypoxemic respiratory failure.

7. d. In a patient with normal lung function, respiratory failure is defined as a $PaO_2 \leq 60$ mm Hg or a $PaCO_2 > 45$ mm Hg, or both. However, because the patient with chronic pulmonary disease normally maintains low PaO_2 and high $PaCO_2$, acute respiratory failure in these patients can be defined as an acute decrease in PaO_2 or an increase in $PaCO_2$ from the patient's baseline parameters, accompanied by an acidic pH. The pH of 7.28 reflects an acidemia and a loss of compensation in the patient with chronic lung disease.

8. c, d, e, f. Morning headache, respiratory acidosis, the use of tripod position, and rapid, shallow respirations would

be expected. Cyanosis occurs late in hypoxemia, and metabolic acidosis occurs if hypoxemia is severe and the cells use anaerobic metabolism but have run out of sodium bicarbonate to buffer the removal of CO_2.

9. a. Because the brain is very sensitive to a decrease in oxygen delivery, restlessness, confusion, agitation, and combative behavior are early signs of hypoxemia, for which the nurse should be alert. Mild hypertension is also an early sign, accompanied by tachycardia. Central cyanosis is an unreliable, late sign of hypoxemia. Dysrhythmias also occur later.

10. a, e, f. Changes from aging that increase the older adult's risk for respiratory failure include alveolar dilation, decreased respiratory muscle strength, and diminished elastic recoil in the airways. Although delirium can complicate ventilator management, it does not increase the older patient's risk for respiratory failure. The older adult's BP and heart rate (HR) increase, but this does not affect the risk for respiratory failure. The ventilatory capacity is decreased and the larger air spaces decrease the surface area for gas exchange, which also increase the risk.

11. d. The increase in respiratory rate needed to blow off accumulated CO_2 predisposes to respiratory muscle fatigue. The slowing of a rapid rate in a patient in acute distress shows tiring and the possibility of respiratory arrest unless ventilatory assistance is provided. Orthopnea, accessory muscle use, and decreased inspiratory-expiratory (I/E) ratio are common findings in respiratory distress but do not necessarily signal respiratory fatigue or arrest. Abdominal muscle use is normal.

12. a. Patients with a shunt are usually more hypoxemic than patients with a V/Q mismatch because the alveoli are filled with fluid, which prevents gas exchange. Hypoxemia from an intrapulmonary shunt is usually not responsive to high O_2 concentrations. The patient will usually need positive pressure ventilation. Hypoxemia associated with a V/Q mismatch usually responds favorably to O_2 at 1 to 3 L/min by nasal cannula. Removing secretions with coughing and suctioning is generally not effective in reversing an acute hypoxemia resulting from a shunt.

13. a. When there is impaired function of 1 lung, the patient should be positioned with the unaffected lung in the dependent position to promote perfusion to the functioning tissue. If the diseased lung is positioned dependently, more V/Q mismatch occurs. The head of the bed may be elevated or a reclining chair may be used, with the patient positioned on the unaffected side, to maximize thoracic expansion if the patient has increased work of breathing.

14. b. Augmented coughing is done by applying pressure on the abdominal muscles at the beginning of expiration. This type of coughing helps increase abdominal pressure and expiratory flow to assist the cough to remove secretions in the patient who is exhausted. An oral airway is used only if there is a possibility that the tongue will obstruct the airway. Huff coughing prevents the glottis from closing during the cough and works well for patients with chronic obstructive pulmonary disease (COPD) to clear central airways. Slow pursed lip breathing allows more time for expiration and prevents small bronchioles from collapsing.

15. c. For the patient with a history of heart failure, current acute respiratory failure, and thick secretions, the best

intervention is to liquefy the secretions with either aerosol mask or using normal saline given by a nebulizer. Excess IV fluid may cause cardiovascular distress. The patient likely would not tolerate postural drainage with her history. Suctioning thick secretions without thinning them is difficult and increases the patient's difficulty in maintaining oxygenation. With copious secretions, suction can be done after thinning the secretions.

16. a. It is most important to assess the patient for the cause of the restlessness and agitation (e.g., pain, hypoxemia, electrolyte imbalances) and treat the underlying cause before sedating the patient. Although sedation, analgesia, and neuromuscular blockade are often used to control agitation and pain, these treatments may contribute to prolonged ventilator support and hospital days.

17. d. Hemodynamic monitoring with a pulmonary artery catheter is instituted in severe respiratory failure to determine the amount of blood flow to tissues and the response of the lungs and heart to hypoxemia. Continuous BP monitoring may be used, but BP reflects cardiac activity, which can be determined by the pulmonary artery catheter findings. Arterial blood gases (ABGs) are important to evaluate oxygenation and ventilation status and detect potential V/Q mismatches.

18. a, c, d. Morphine and nitroglycerin will decrease pulmonary congestion caused by heart failure; IV diuretics (e.g., furosemide) are also used. Ceftriaxone and azithromycin (Zithromax) are used to treat pulmonary infections. Inhaled albuterol or metaproterenol sulfate will relieve bronchospasms. Methylprednisolone (Solu-Medrol), an IV corticosteroid, will reduce airway inflammation. Morphine is also used to decrease anxiety, agitation, and pain.

19. d. Noninvasive positive pressure ventilation (NIPPV) involves the application of a face mask and delivery of a volume of air under inspiratory pressure. Because the device is worn externally, the patient must be able to cooperate in its use and frequent access to the airway for suctioning or inhaled medications must not be necessary. It is not indicated when high levels of oxygen are needed, or respirations are absent.

20. a. A sedation holiday is needed to assess the patient's condition and readiness to extubate. A hypermetabolic state occurs with critical illness. Enteral or parenteral nutrition is started within 24 to 48 hours. With these medications, the patient will be assessed for cardiopulmonary depression. Venous thromboembolism prophylaxis will be used, but there is no reason to keep the legs still. Repositioning the patient every 2 hours may help decrease discomfort and agitation.

21. a. Although ARDS may occur in the patient who has any severe illness and may be both a cause and a result of systemic inflammatory response syndrome (SIRS), the most common precipitating injuries of ARDS are sepsis, gastric aspiration, and severe massive trauma.

22. a, c, d. The injury or exudative phase is the early phase of ARDS when atelectasis and interstitial and alveolar edema occur. Hyaline membranes composed of necrotic cells, protein, and fibrin line the alveoli. Together, these decrease gas exchange capability and lung compliance. Shortness of breath occurs but it is not a physiologic change. The increased inflammation and proliferation of

fibroblasts occurs in the reparative or proliferative phase of ARDS, which occurs 1 to 2 weeks after the initial lung injury.

23. c. In the fibrotic phase of ARDS, diffuse scarring and fibrosis of the lungs occur, resulting in decreased surface area for gas exchange and continued hypoxemia caused by diffusion limitation. Although edema is resolved, lung compliance is decreased because of interstitial fibrosis. Long-term mechanical ventilation is needed. The patient has a poor prognosis for survival.

24. a. Refractory hypoxemia, hypoxemia that does not respond to increasing concentrations of oxygenation by any route, is a hallmark of ARDS and is always present. Bronchial breath sounds may be associated with the progression of ARDS. $PaCO_2$ levels may be normal until the patient is no longer able to compensate in response to the hypoxemia. Pulmonary artery wedge pressure (PAWP) that is normally increased in cardiogenic pulmonary edema is normal in the pulmonary edema of ARDS.

25. b. Early signs of ARDS are insidious and difficult to detect, but the nurse should be alert for any early signs of hypoxemia, such as dyspnea, tachypnea, cough, and restlessness in patients at risk for ARDS. Later, tachycardia, diaphoresis, mental status changes, cyanosis, and pallor may be present. Abnormal findings on physical examination or diagnostic studies, such as worsened lung sounds and respiratory distress, respiratory alkalosis, or decreasing PaO_2, are usually indications that ARDS has progressed beyond the initial stages.

26. b. Ventilator-associated pneumonia (VAP) is one of the most common complications of ARDS. Early detection requires frequent monitoring of sputum smears and cultures and assessment of the quality, quantity, and consistency of sputum. Prevention of VAP is done with strict infection control measures and ventilator bundle protocol. Blood in gastric aspirate may show a stress ulcer and subcutaneous emphysema of the face, neck, and chest occurs with barotrauma during mechanical ventilation. Oral infections may result from prophylactic antibiotics and impaired host defenses but are not common.

27. a. Because ARDS is precipitated by a physiologic insult, a critical factor in its prevention and early management is treatment of the underlying condition. Prophylactic antibiotics, treatment with diuretics and fluid restriction, and mechanical ventilation are used as ARDS progresses.

28. a. Positive end-expiratory pressure (PEEP) used with mechanical ventilation applies positive pressure to the airway and lungs at the end of exhalation, keeping the lung partially expanded and preventing collapse of the alveoli and helping open collapsed alveoli. Permissive hypercapnia is allowed when the patient with ARDS is ventilated with smaller tidal volumes to prevent barotrauma. Extracorporeal membrane oxygenation and extracorporeal CO_2 removal involve passing blood across a gas-exchanging membrane outside the body and then returning oxygenated blood to the body.

29. b. There is often a dramatic decrease in BP with decreased preload (CVP) and cardiac output (CO). PEEP increases intrathoracic and intrapulmonary pressures and reduces blood return to both the right and left sides of the heart. Increased PaO_2 is an expected effect of PEEP.

30. d. When a patient with ARDS is supine, alveoli in the posterior areas of the lung are dependent and fluid-filled and the heart and mediastinal contents place more pressure on the lungs, predisposing to atelectasis. If the patient is turned prone, air-filled nonatelectatic alveoli in the anterior part of the lung receive more blood and perfusion may be better matched to ventilation, causing less V/Q mismatch. Lateral rotation therapy is used to stimulate postural drainage and help mobilize pulmonary secretions.

31. P/F ratio is calculated by dividing the PaO_2 by the fractional inspired oxygen concentration (FIO_2)
    a. P/F ratio = 117; (PaO_2 of 70 divided by 0.60)
    b. P/F ratio = 200; (PaO_2 of 80 divided by 0.40)
    c. P/F ratio = 271; (PaO_2 of 95 divided by 0.35)
    d. All show signs of hypoxemia, but the patient with the most severe hypoxemia and likely to be diagnosed with ARDS is the one with a P/F ratio of 117.

32. b. Permissive hypercapnia is contraindicated in patients with increased intracranial pressure as increased CO_2 levels will cause an increase in cerebral flow worsening the patient's intracranial pressure.

33. d. Low tidal volume ventilation is calculated using 4 to 8 mL/kg. The patient weighs 79.5 kg (175 lbs divided by 2.2). Using 4 mL/kg the tidal volume would equal 318 mL; 5 mL/kg equals 398 mL; 6 mL/kg equals 477 mL; 7 mL/kg equals 557 mL and 8 mL/kg equals 636 mL.

Case Study

1. **1**=shortness of breath, pursed-lip breathing, and tripod positioning; **2**= hypercapnic **3**=pneumonia; **4**=combined acidosis; **5**=impaired respiratory function
   Rationale: The patient has hypercapnic respiratory failure as evidenced by a $PaCO_2$ of 55, dyspnea on exertion, shortness of breath, pursed lip breathing and tripod positioning. The tripod position helps decrease the work of breathing (WOB) because propping the arms up increases the anterior-posterior diameter of the chest and changes pressures in the thorax. Pursed lip breathing causes an increase in arterial oxygen saturation (SaO_2) because it slows respiration, allows more time for expiration, and prevents the small bronchioles from collapsing. The main contributing factor to P.C.'s onset of acute respiratory failure is the pneumonia, with inflammation, edema, and hypersecretion of exudates in the bronchioles and obstructed airways causing a V/Q mismatch. Other factors include the presence of chronic lung disease, her age, and immunosuppression with corticosteroids. Since the pH, $PaCO_2$ and HCO_3^- are all acidic, the ABG results should be documented as a combined acidosis, which includes metabolic and respiratory components. The PaO_2 indicates mild hypoxemia. Impaired respiratory function is the priority clinical problem based on the assessment data. Fatigue, activity intolerance, and anxiety are applicable, but result from the acute respiratory failure. Infection is an applicable clinical problem, but isn't a priority when someone is in acute respiratory distress. The patient doesn't have ARDS.

2. **Effective:** SpO_2 92% (The oxygen saturation improved from 84% to 92%.); ambulates in hallway (If the patient can ambulate in the hallway, her ability to breathe is improving.); $EtCO_2$ 48 mm Hg (This value shows a

decrease in $PaCO_2$ as the $PaCO_2$ upon admission was 55 mm Hg.) **Ineffective**: Temp. 38.5°C (The temperature increased from 38.1°C to 38.5°C); reports pain during inspiration (This may be an expected finding in patients with pneumonia, but it indicates infection is still present.) **Unrelated**: bilateral +1 edema in ankles (This is unrelated to acute respiratory failure and is more applicable for cardiac assessment.); no JVD (This is unrelated to acute respiratory failure and is more applicable for cardiac assessment.); voiding 100 mL/hr (This isn't relevant to respiratory failure.)

3. **Indicated**: keep the HOB greater than 30 degrees (This intervention will improve respiratory effort.); perform FSBG checks every 4 hours (The patient is on corticosteroids which can cause hyperglycemia even in non-diabetic patients.); educate the patient about the incentive spirometer (The patient should be encouraged to deep breathe, cough, and use the I.S. to mobilize secretions and promote oxygenation.); **Contraindicated**: place the patient on a fluid restriction (2-3 L/day are recommended to help liquefy secretions and treat pneumonia.); use a non-rebreather mask to deliver oxygen (This patient has a history of severe COPD. Therefore, high FiO_2 levels should be avoided unless absolutely necessary, as too much oxygen can negate this patient's drive to breathe.) **Non-essential**: place the patient on Droplet Precautions (It isn't necessary to place this patient on droplet precautions as her condition doesn't require it.); weigh the patient daily (This isn't necessary as it doesn't offer much relevant information to treat this patient.)

4. **1** = tachycardia and hypertension; **2** = benzodiazepines; **3** = fluoroquinolone

5. A, C, E, H. Optimizing hydration (2 to 3 L/day if cardiac and renal status can tolerate it) and nutrition are important to decrease her risk by making secretions easier to expel. Corticosteroids should be tapered and never abruptly stopped. Antibiotics should be taken as directed until gone to avoid recurring infection and antibiotic resistant infections. Albuterol should be used as needed when P.C. is short of breath or when she feels that her airways are narrowed as evidenced by wheezing or difficulty breathing. Any signs of infection should be immediately reported to her HCP because she takes corticosteroids which cause immunosuppression and increases her risk of infection. She should continue to use her home oxygen, using the appropriate amount and delivery device to prevent blunting of her respiratory drive. P.C. should increase her activity as tolerated and shouldn't limit ambulation just to the bathroom. Annual influenza vaccines are recommended to prevent developing pneumonia and associated complications.

CHAPTER 33

1. a, b, c, f. These characteristics are evident with neutrophils. Platelets arise from megakaryocytes and are stored in the spleen. Eosinophils are increased in individuals with allergies and make up 2% to 4% of white blood cells (WBCs).

2. c. Increased reticulocytes, or immature red blood cells (RBCs), indicate an increased rate of erythropoiesis or stimulation of erythrocyte (RBC) production by the bone marrow. Basophils are stimulated by granulocyte colony-stimulating factor in response to an antigen or by tissue injury. Monocytes and lymphocytes respond to tissue injury, including infection.

3. a, c, d. Basophils, eosinophils, and neutrophils are the granulocytic leukocytes. Lymphocytes are the agranular leukocytes that form the basis of the cellular and humoral immune responses. Monocytes are agranulocytes that are potent phagocytic cells. Thrombocytes are not granulocytes or agranulocytes, and they initiate the clotting process.

4. a. Lymphedema is the obstruction of lymph flow that results in accumulation of lymph fluid for the patient in the right arm following a right-sided breast mastectomy. The other options are not hematologic problems that would cause extreme swelling.

5. a, b, c, e. Although all of the listed nutrients are helpful, iron, folic acid, vitamin C, and cobalamin (vitamin B_{12}) are essential for erythropoiesis.

6. a. 2; b. 3; c. 4; d. 5; e. 6; f. 1

7. d. Proteins C and S are examples of anticoagulants that are involved in clot retraction and dissolution. Fibrinolysis also keeps blood in its fluid form by thrombin-activating conversion of plasminogen to plasmin. Plasmin attacks fibrin or fibrinogen and splits it into smaller elements known as *fibrin split products* (FSPs) or *fibrin degradation products* (FDPs).

8. a, b, e. The abdominal organs that are primarily involved in hematologic function are the liver, spleen, and lymph nodes. The liver filters the blood, produces procoagulants, and stores iron. The spleen's functions are hematopoietic (RBCs produced during fetal development); filtration (removes old and defective erythrocytes, iron for reuse, and bacteria); immunologic (supplies lymphocytes, monocytes, and stored immunoglobulins); and storage (RBCs and platelets). The lymph nodes filter pathogens and foreign particles from lymphatic circulation.

9. b. During fibrinolysis by plasmin, the fibrin clot is split into smaller molecules known as *FSPs* or *FDPs*. Increased FSPs impair platelet aggregation, reduce prothrombin, prevent fibrin stabilization, and lead to bleeding.

10. c. As a person ages the partial thromboplastin time (PTT) is normally decreased, so an abnormally high PTT of 60 seconds is an indication that bleeding could readily occur. Platelets are unaffected by aging and 150,000/μL is a normal count. Serum iron levels are decreased and the erythrocyte sedimentation rate (ESR) is significantly increased with aging, as are reflected in these values.

11. a, b, d. The myeloblast is a committed hematopoietic cell found in the bone marrow from which granulocytes develop. A disorder in which myeloblasts are overproduced would result in increased basophils, eosinophils, and neutrophils.

12. a. The parietal cells of the stomach secrete intrinsic factor, a substance necessary for the absorption of cobalamin (vitamin B_{12}), and if all or part of the stomach is removed, the lack of intrinsic factor can lead to impaired RBC production and pernicious anemia. Recurring infections indicate decreased WBCs and immune response, and corticosteroid therapy may cause a neutrophilia and lymphopenia. Oral contraceptive use is strongly associated with changes in blood coagulation.

13.

Functional Health Pattern	Risk Factor for or Response to Hematologic Problem
Health perception–health management	Ethnic background, family history of hematologic disorders. Use of alcohol, illicit drugs, and cigarettes
Nutritional-metabolic	Weight. History of anorexia, nausea, vomiting, or oral discomfort. Deficiencies of iron, vitamin B_{12}, and folic acid. Gastrointestinal (GI) bleeding, petechiae or bruising of the skin, fever, lymph node swelling
Elimination	Frankly bloody or dark, tarry stools, dark or bloody urine
Activity-exercise	Fatigue, weakness, change in ability to perform normal exercise or activities of daily living
Sleep-rest	Fatigue unrelieved by sleep
Cognitive-perceptual	Pain, especially in joints or bones. Paresthesias, numbness, or tingling. Changes in hearing, vision, taste, or mental status
Self-perception–self-concept	Altered self-perception because of lymph node enlargement or skin changes
Role-relationship	Home or work exposure to radiation or chemicals. Military history; change in role or responsibility
Sexuality-reproductive	Menstrual history and characteristics of bleeding. Intrapartum or postpartum bleeding problems. Impotence
Coping–stress tolerance	Lack of support to meet daily needs. Methods of coping with stress
Value-belief	Values conflict with treatment, especially blood product or bone marrow transplants

14. a. Superficial lymph nodes are evaluated by light palpation, but they are not normally palpable. It may be normal to find small (< 1.0 cm), mobile, firm, nontender nodes. Deep lymph nodes are detected radiographically.

15. b. Petechiae are small, flat, red, or reddish-brown pinpoint microhemorrhages that occur on the skin when platelet levels are low. When petechiae are numerous, they group, causing reddish bruises known as *purpura*. Sternal tenderness is associated with leukemias. Jaundice occurs when anemias are of a hemolytic origin, resulting in accumulation of bile pigments from RBCs. Enlarged, tender lymph nodes are associated with infection or cancer.

16. b. A smooth, shiny, reddened tongue is an indication of iron-deficiency anemia or pernicious anemia that would be reflected by a decreased hemoglobin level. The decreased neutrophils would be indicative of neutropenia. The increased WBC count could be indicative of an infection and the increased RBC count of polycythemia.

17. c. Any platelet count < 150,000/μL is considered thrombocytopenia and could place the patient at risk for bleeding, necessitating special consideration in nursing care. Chemotherapy may cause bone marrow suppression and a depletion of all blood cells. The other factors are all within normal range.

18.

Laboratory Finding	Possible Etiology
Serum iron 40 mcg/dL (7 μmol/L)	Iron-deficiency anemia
ESR 30 mm/hr	Inflammatory conditions of any kind
Increased band neutrophils	Infection
Activated partial thromboplastin time 60 sec	Heparin therapy
Indirect bilirubin 2.0 mg/dL (34 μmol/L)	Hemolysis of RBCs
Bence Jones protein in urine	Multiple myeloma

19. b. A patient with type O Rh⁺ blood has no A or B antigens on the RBC but does have anti-A and anti-B antibodies in the blood and has an Rh antigen. Type AB Rh⁻ blood has both A and B antigens on the RBC but no Rh antigen and no anti-A or anti-B antibodies. If the type AB Rh⁻ blood is given to the patient with type O Rh⁺ blood, the antibodies in the patient's blood will react with the antigens in the donor blood, causing hemolysis of the donor cells. There will be no Rh reaction because the donor blood has no Rh antigen.

20. a. A contrast CT scan involves the use of an iodine-based dye that could cause a reaction if the patient is sensitive to iodine. Metal implants or internal appliances and claustrophobia should be determined before MRI. Prior blood transfusions are not a factor in this diagnostic test.

21. c. The aspiration of bone marrow content is done with local anesthesia at the site of the puncture, but the aspiration causes a suction pain that is quite painful but very brief. There is generally only residual soreness following the test.

22. d. Lymph node biopsy is usually done to determine whether malignant cells are present in lymph nodes and can be used to diagnose lymphomas as well as metastatic spread from any malignant tumor in the body. Leukemias may infiltrate lymph nodes, but biopsy of the nodes is more commonly used to detect any type of neoplastic cells.

23. c. Pancytopenia is decreased RBCs, WBCs, and platelets. Hemolysis is RBC destruction. Leukopenia is WBC < 5000/μL. Thrombocytosis is increased platelets, and thrombocytopenia is decreased platelets.

24. b, c. Bone marrow and lymph node biopsies are preferred methods to obtain the sample for gene analysis. If a large number of abnormal cells are circulating in the blood, peripheral blood may be used. The other options will not provide the desired information.

CHAPTER 34

1.

Type or Cause of Anemia	Etiology	Morphology
Malaria	3	4
Thalassemia	1	6
Acute trauma	2	4
Aplastic anemia	1	4
Pernicious anemia	1	5
Sickle cell anemia	3	4
Anemia of gastritis	2	4
Anemia of leukemia	1	4
Iron-deficiency anemia	1	6
Anemia of renal injury	1	4
Glucose-6-phosphate dehydrogenase (G6PD)	3	4
Anemia associated with prosthetic heart valve	3	4

2. b. The patient's hemoglobin (Hgb) level indicates a moderate anemia, and at this severity, additional findings usually include dyspnea and fatigue. Pallor, smooth tongue, and sensitivity to cold usually manifest in severe anemia when the Hgb level is below 6 g/dL (60 g/L).

3. c. Keeping the top bedside rails up and the call bell within reach will facilitate safety and safe mobility for this patient. In the older adult, confusion, ataxia, fatigue, and weakness are common manifestations of anemia and place the patient at risk for injury. Nursing interventions should include safety precautions to prevent falls and injury when these symptoms are present. The nurse, not the patient's family, is responsible for the patient, and although a quiet room may promote rest, it is not as important as protection of the patient.

4. d. Dyspnea at rest indicates that the patient is making an effort to provide adequate amounts of oxygen to the tissues. If oxygen needs are not met, angina, myocardial infarction, heart failure, and pulmonary and systemic congestion can occur. The other manifestations are present in severe anemia, but they do not reflect hypoxemia, a priority problem.

5. b. Aplastic anemia has a decrease of all blood cell types and hypocellular bone marrow. Thalassemia is characterized by inadequate production of normal Hgb and decreased erythrocyte production. Megaloblastic anemias (cobalamin deficiency and folic acid deficiency anemias) are caused by impaired DNA synthesis, which results in the presence of large red blood cells (RBCs). Anemia of chronic disease occurs with chronic inflammation, autoimmune and infectious disorders, heart failure, malignancies, or bleeding episodes. It manifests with underproduction of RBCs and shortened RBC survival.

6. c, d, f. Iron-deficiency anemia is the most common type of anemia and occurs with chronic blood loss or malabsorption in the duodenum so it may occur with duodenal removal. The other options are associated with cobalamin deficiency.

7. d. Folic acid deficiency megaloblastic anemia is related to dietary deficiency as seen in anorexia and with the use of oral contraceptives and antiseizure medications. The other anemias are unrelated to this patient's history.

8.

Finding	Explanation
Reticulocyte counts are increased in chronic blood loss but decreased in cobalamin (vitamin B_{12}) deficiency.	The hypoxia resulting from loss of RBCs in chronic blood loss stimulates the kidney to release erythropoietin, stimulating production of RBCs and reticulocytes. However, in pernicious anemia, normal reticulocytes are not produced because of the lack of cobalamin.
Bilirubin levels are increased in sickle cell anemia but are normal in acute blood loss.	Sickle cell anemia is a hemolytic anemia involving an accelerated RBC breakdown, leading to increased serum bilirubin levels, whereas acute blood loss results in loss of the RBC and the bile pigments from the body.
Mean corpuscular volume (MCV) is increased in folic acid deficiency but decreased in iron-deficiency anemia.	The MCV is a determination of the relative size of an RBC and macrocytic anemias, such as folic acid deficiency and cobalamin deficiency, are characterized by the production of large, immature RBCs that would reflect an increased MCV. In iron-deficiency anemia, the MCV is low because of the lack of Hgb in the cells.

9. a. Constipation is a common side effect of oral iron supplementation, and increased fluids and fiber should be consumed to prevent this effect. Because iron is best absorbed in an acid environment and can be bound in the gastrointestinal (GI) tract by food, it should be taken before meals, unless gastric side effects of the supplements necessitate its ingestion with food. Taking iron with ascorbic acid or orange juice enhances absorption of the iron, but enteric-coated iron often is ineffective because of unpredictable release of the iron in areas of the GI tract where it can be absorbed. Black stools are an expected result of oral iron preparations.

10. b. Pernicious anemia is a type of cobalamin (vitamin B_{12}) deficiency that results when parietal cells in the stomach fail to secrete enough intrinsic factor to absorb ingested cobalamin. Folic acid deficiency may contribute to folic acid deficiency anemia, not pernicious anemia. Extrinsic factor may be a factor in some cobalamin deficiencies but not in pernicious anemia. Lack of cobalamin intake can cause cobalamin deficiency but not pernicious anemia. Increasing cobalamin intake cannot improve pernicious anemia without intrinsic factor to aid its absorption.

11. c. Neurologic manifestations of weakness, paresthesia of the feet and hands, and impaired thought processes are characteristic of cobalamin deficiency and pernicious anemia. Hepatomegaly and jaundice often occur with hemolytic anemia. The patient with cobalamin deficiency often has achlorhydria or decreased stomach acidity and would not experience effects of gastric hyperacidity.

12. a. Without cobalamin replacement, individuals with pernicious anemia will die in 1 to 3 years, but the disease can be controlled with cobalamin supplements for life. Hematologic manifestations can be completely reversed with therapy, but long-standing neuromuscular complications may not be reversed. Because pernicious anemia results from an inability to absorb cobalamin, dietary intake of the vitamin is not a treatment option, nor is a bone marrow transplant.

13. d. Because red meats are the primary dietary sources of cobalamin, a strict vegetarian is most at risk for cobalamin deficiency anemia. Meats are also an important source of iron and folic acid, but whole grains, legumes, and green leafy vegetables also supply these nutrients. Thalassemia is not related to dietary deficiencies.

14. a, c, e. Aplastic anemia may cause an inflamed, painful tongue. Oxygen is not delivered without RBCs. The thrombocytopenia may contribute to blood-filled bullae in the mouth and gingival bleeding. The leukopenia may lead to stomatitis and oral ulcers and infections. MCV will be normal or slightly increased. Ferritin and coagulation factors are not affected in aplastic anemia.

15. b. Hemorrhage from thrombocytopenia and infection from neutropenia are the greatest risks for the patient with aplastic anemia. The patient will experience fatigue from anemia, but bleeding and infection are the major causes of death in aplastic anemia.

16. a, d, e. With rapid blood loss, hypovolemic shock may occur. Clinical manifestations, such as postural hypotension and increased heart rate, will be more reliable than laboratory values as they reflect the body's attempt to meet oxygen requirements. As the percentage of blood loss increases, clinical manifestations worsen.

17. b. Because RBCs become abnormal related to hypoxia or infection in sickle cell anemia, the spleen accelerates RBC breakdown as the sickling increases. Antibody reactions with RBCs may be seen in other types of hemolytic anemias but are not present in sickle cell anemia.

18. b. During a sickle cell crisis, the sickling cells clog small capillaries, and the resulting hemostasis promotes a self-perpetuating cycle of local hypoxia, deoxygenation of more erythrocytes, and more sickling. Administration of oxygen may reverse sickling at first, but eventually the sickling becomes irreversible because of cell membrane damage from recurrent sickling.

19. d. Because pain is the most common symptom with a sickle cell crisis and may last for 4 to 6 days, pain control is an essential part of treatment. Rest is indicated to reduce metabolic needs. Although thrombosis does occur in capillaries, antiembolism stockings that primarily affect venous circulation are not indicated; anticoagulants are more effective. Fluids and electrolytes are administered to reduce blood viscosity and maintain renal function.

20. d. The patient with sickle cell disease is particularly prone to upper respiratory infection, and infection can precipitate a sickle cell crisis. Patients should seek medical attention quickly to counteract upper respiratory infections because pneumonia is the most common infection in patients with sickle cell disease. Fluids should be increased to decrease blood viscosity, which may precipitate a crisis. Moderate activity is permitted. Dehydration in hot weather may precipitate a sickling episode, but humid weather alone will not do so.

21. a, c, d. Platelet deficiencies lead to internal and external hemorrhage. Immune thrombocytopenic purpura (ITP) is characterized by increased platelet destruction by the spleen. Thrombotic thrombocytopenic purpura (TTP) is characterized by decreased platelets and RBCs with enhanced agglutination of the platelets. ITP is the most common acquired thrombocytopenia. Petechiae, not ecchymosis, is a common manifestation of thrombocytopenia.

22. b. The symptoms describe hemochromatosis, which is treated with iron chelating agents to remove accumulated iron via the kidneys. Thalassemia involves inadequate production of normal hemoglobin, is asymptomatic or has growth and development deficits, and is treated with blood transfusion and chelating agents (e.g., deferasirox). Myelodysplastic syndrome has disordered and ineffective hematopoiesis and is treated supportively with hematologic monitoring, antibiotic therapy, transfusions, iron chelators, or intensive chemotherapy and/or hematopoietic stem cell transplantation (HSCT). Delayed transfusion reactions exhibit delayed hemolytic reactions, infections, and iron overload and have no acute treatment unless severe enough to warrant further transfusions.

23. b. Active or passive leg exercises and ambulation should be implemented to prevent thrombus formation. Thrombus and embolization are the major complications of polycythemia vera because of hypervolemia and hyperviscosity. Isolation is not needed and falls are not expected. Hydration therapy is important to decrease blood viscosity. However, because the patient already has hypervolemia, a careful balance of intake and output must be maintained and fluids are not increased injudiciously.

24. b. Corticosteroids are used in initial treatment of ITP because they suppress the phagocytic response of splenic macrophages, decreasing platelet destruction. They also depress autoimmune antibody formation and reduce capillary leakage. All of the other therapies may be used but only in patients who are unresponsive to corticosteroid therapy and severely reduced platelet counts.

25. c. The major complication of thrombocytopenia is hemorrhage, and it may occur in any area of the body. Cerebral hemorrhage may be fatal, and evaluation of mental status for central nervous system (CNS) alterations to identify CNS bleeding is very important. Fever is not a common finding in thrombocytopenia. Protection from injury to prevent bleeding is an important nursing intervention, but strict bed rest is not indicated. Oral care is performed very gently with minimum friction and soft swabs.

26. Any 5 of these are appropriate: Heparin administration must be discontinued and expect a direct or indirect thrombin inhibitor to be ordered. Monitor for signs and symptoms of bleeding (check IV sites, wounds, any secretions). Monitor ordered coagulation studies. Avoid injections. Use an electric razor. Protect the patient from trauma. Administer ordered blood products. Instruct the patient and caregiver to avoid aspirin and other anticoagulants. Instruct the patient to avoid high-contact activities (many sports).

27. d. A prolonged PTT occurs when there is a deficiency of clotting factors, such as factor VIII associated with hemophilia A. Factor IX is deficient in hemophilia B and prolonged bleeding time, and decreased platelet counts are associated with platelet deficiencies.

28. c. Although whole blood and fresh frozen plasma contain the clotting factors that are deficient in hemophilia, specific coagulation factors have been developed that are purer and safer in preventing infection transmission. Thromboplastin is factor III and is not deficient in patients with hemophilia.

29. b. During an acute bleeding episode in a joint, it is important to rest the involved joint totally and slow bleeding with application of ice. Drugs that decrease platelet aggregation, such as aspirin or nonsteroidal antiinflammatory drugs (NSAIDs), should not be used for pain. As soon as bleeding stops, mobilization of the affected area is encouraged with range-of-motion (ROM) exercises and physical therapy.

30. d. This description is characteristic of von Willebrand disease with prolonged bleeding time occurring because of defective platelets, which does not occur with either type of hemophilia. Although inherited thrombocytopenia is believed to be autosomal dominant, the number of platelets is decreased.

31. a. 4; b. 7; c. 3; d. 5; e. 2; f. 6; g. 1

32. a. Yes, as the WBC count is below 4000/μL. b. The absolute neutrophil count (ANC) is 2300 × 40% = 920/μL. c. Yes, as the ANC is <1000/μL. d. Yes, the patient is at moderate risk of infection with opportunistic pathogens and nonpathogenic organisms from normal body flora because normal phagocytic mechanisms are impaired.

33. a. An elevated temperature is of most significance in recognizing the presence of an infection in the neutropenic patient because there is little leukocytic response to injury with low WBC count. Minor reports of pain or other symptoms should also be reported. Monitoring WBC count will not identify infection. Cultures are indicated if the temperature is elevated but are not used to monitor for infection.

34. d. Despite its seeming simplicity, hand washing before, during, and after care of the patient with neutropenia is the major method to prevent transmission of harmful pathogens to the patient. IV antibiotics are administered when febrile episodes occur. Some oral antibiotics may be used prophylactically in some neutropenic patients. High-efficiency particulate air (HEPA) filtration will be used for the neutropenic patient at home to reduce the number of aerosolized pathogens.

35. a. Myelodysplastic syndromes, like leukemias, are a group of disorders in which hematopoietic stem cells of the bone marrow undergo clonal change and may cause eventual bone marrow failure. However, the primary difference from leukemias is that myelodysplastic cells have some degree of maturation, and the disease progression is slower than in acute leukemias.

36. d. Acute myelogenous leukemia (AML) is seen in 80% of adults with acute leukemia and is characterized by hyperplasia of the bone marrow with uncontrolled proliferation of myeloblasts, the precursors of granulocytes. Hairy cell leukemia is a rare cancer with hairy-looking abnormal lymphocytes. Biphenotypic leukemia is a rare form of both types of acute leukemia. Acute lymphocytic leukemia (ALL), the other acute leukemia, is most common in children and is characterized by small, immature lymphocytes, primarily of B-cell origin, proliferated in the bone marrow.

37. a, c, f. Chronic lymphocytic leukemia (CLL) is the most common leukemia in adults in Western countries. It is a neoplasm of activated B lymphocytes that are mature appearing but functionally inactive. As it progresses, pressure on nerves from enlarged lymph nodes causes pain and paralysis. Mediastinal node enlargement leads to pulmonary symptoms. The other characteristics are related to chronic myelogenous leukemia (CML).

38. c. Almost all leukemias cause some degree of hepatosplenomegaly because of infiltration of these organs as well as the bone marrow, lymph nodes, bones, and CNS by excessive WBCs in the blood.

39. c. Whether the donor bone marrow is from a human leukocyte antigen (HLA)-matched donor or taken from the patient during a remission for later use, HSCT always involves the use of chemotherapy and/or total-body radiation to eliminate leukemic cells and the patient's bone marrow stem cells totally before IV infusion of the donor cells. A severe pancytopenic period follows the transplant, during which the patient must be in protective isolation and during which RBC and platelet transfusions may be given.

40. a. Non-Hodgkin lymphoma (NHL); b. Hodgkin lymphoma (HL); c. B; d. NHL; e. HL; f. NHL; g. B; h. HL; i. B

41. b. The patient is monitored for infection because leukopenia and thrombocytopenia may develop from the disease or usually as a consequence of treatment. Staging of Hodgkin's disease is important to determine treatment. Multiple myeloma is characterized by proliferation of malignant activated B cells that destroy the bones. The intervention of increasing fluid to manage hypercalcemia is used with multiple myeloma.

42. c. Splenectomy may be indicated for treatment for ITP, and when the spleen is removed, platelet counts increase significantly in most patients. In any of the disorders in which the spleen removes excessive blood cells, splenectomy will most often increase peripheral RBC, WBC, and platelet counts.

43. c, e, f. Because he has hypercalcemia, adequate hydration and ambulation, not bed rest, are implemented to dilute calcium and prevent protein precipitates from causing renal tubular obstruction and help bones resorb some calcium with weight bearing. Assessing for infection must be done because the excess plasma cells are monoclonal and ineffective against infection. Privacy would be provided for all patients. Although this patient may need dialysis in the late states of multiple myeloma, it is not needed at this time. Analgesia for rib pain will be provided as prescribed by the HCP.

44. a. Chills and fever are symptoms of an acute hemolytic or febrile transfusion reaction, and if these develop, the nurse should stop the transfusion, infuse saline through the IV line, notify the HCP and blood bank immediately, recheck the ID tags, and monitor vital signs and urine output. The addition of a leukocyte reduction filter may prevent a febrile reaction but is not helpful once the reaction has occurred. Mild and transient allergic reactions indicated by itching and hives may permit restarting the transfusion after treatment with antihistamines.

45. b. Because platelets adhere to the plastic bags, the bag should be gently agitated throughout the transfusion. Platelets do not have A, B, or Rh antibodies, and ABO compatibility is not a consideration. Baseline vital signs should be taken before the transfusion is started, and the nurse should stay with the patient during the first

15 minutes. Platelets are stored at room temperature for 1 to 5 days.

46. c. Febrile nonhemolytic reaction is the most common transfusion reaction. Allergic reactions occur with sensitivity to foreign plasma proteins and can be treated prophylactically with antihistamines. Acute hemolytic reactions are related to the infusion of ABO-incompatible blood or components with 10 mL or more of RBCs. Massive blood transfusion reactions occur when patients receive more RBCs or blood than the total blood volume.

47. a, c, d. ABO incompatibility, destruction of donor RBCs, and acute kidney injury may occur in an acute hemolytic transfusion reaction. Hypothermia, hypocalcemia, and hyperkalemia are most likely to occur in massive blood transfusion reactions. Epinephrine may be used for severe allergic transfusion reactions, and the infusion may be restarted after treatment with antihistamines in mild cases.

48. a. 1; b. 3; c. 4; d. 2; e. 6; f. 7; g. 10; h. 9; i. 8; j. 5.

Case Study

1. The following laboratory results are **Expected** in DIC: decreased fibrinogen levels (formation of clots consumes and depletes fibrinogen); increased (not decreased) FSPs (produced from fibrinolysis); PTT is prolonged (indicating an increased risk of bleeding); factor VIII is decreased (depleted when forming clots); the INR is increased or prolonged (indicating an increased risk of bleeding); antithrombin III levels are decreased; thrombocytopenia occurs; decreased (not increased) hematocrit level (if the patient with DIC is actively bleeding). Calcium and potassium levels are not related in diagnosing DIC.

2. Nursing actions that are **Indicated** (necessary to treat a patient with DIC) are: transfusing platelets to treat thrombocytopenia; administering oxygen using 6 L/min simple face mask to improve oxygenation to tissues; administering 2 units of FFP to replace antithrombin III and clotting factors; monitoring for signs of active bleeding or oozing around invasive catheters which occurs in DIC; massaging the fundus to promote uterine contractions (addresses a boggy fundus which is a predisposition to active bleeding); **Contraindicated** (could be harmful) actions: warfarin (is an anticoagulant and would increase the risk of bleeding); suppository medications (due to an increased risk of rectal injury causing rectal bleeding); administering D_5W (physiologically acts as a hypotonic solution; boluses of isotonic crystalloids to treat hypotension are warranted using 0.9% normal saline or lactated Ringer's); **Non-essential** actions: administering ondansetron (is an antiemetic); cooling blanket (would be indicated to treat hyperthermia, but isn't applicable for this patient)

3. **1**=decreased LOC, ecchymosis, and oliguria; **2**=Heparin; **3**=Cryoprecipitate; **4**=antithrombin; **5**=impaired tissue perfusion

4. A, C, E, G, H. IM routes are not recommended unless absolutely necessary due to increased risk of bleeding. Excedrin contains aspirin which is contraindicated in DIC due to the increased risk of bleeding. Sanitary pads are acceptable, but tampons are contraindicated.

5. **Indicated**: when transfusing multiple blood products, it is recommended to have at least 2 IV sites that are 18G-20G (or larger) catheters (this will provide emergency access if the patient have a blood transfusion reaction), the nurse should stay with the patient for the first 15 minutes of the blood transfusion (to monitor for any adverse reactions), FFP can be infused over 15-30 minutes, if the patient has any adverse reactions, the blood transfusion should be stopped and reported to the blood bank and the health care provider; **Contraindicated**: one blood product should be administered at a time in case there is an adverse reaction, only 0.9% normal saline should be used to prime the Y-type blood tubing as well as flushing the blood into the patient as other solutions will cause RBC hemolysis, blood products need to be checked by 2 licensed health care providers and assistive personnel are not licensed; **Non-essential**: cryoprecipitate is compatible with all ABO types, an IO route is only necessary in an emergency situation when IV access cannot be obtained, passive leg raise aids in assessing fluid responsiveness in sepsis patients

CHAPTER 35

1. a. Pulmonic (semilunar) valve; b. tricuspid valve; c. interventricular septum; d. papillary muscle; e. chordae tendineae; f. mitral valve; g. aortic (semilunar) valve

2. a. Aorta; b. superior vena cava; c. right atrium; d. right coronary artery; e. right marginal artery; f. posterior descending artery; g. right ventricle; h. left ventricle; i. left marginal artery; j. left anterior descending artery; k. circumflex artery; l. left atrium; m. left coronary artery; n. pulmonary trunk; o. aorta; p. superior vena cava; q. right atrium; r. small cardiac vein; s. middle cardiac vein; t. right ventricle; u. left ventricle; v. great cardiac vein; w. coronary sinus; x. posterior vein; y. left atrium; z. pulmonary trunk

3. c, d, f. The left circumflex and left anterior descending arteries branch from the left coronary artery. The left coronary artery and right coronary artery arise from the aorta to supply the atria, ventricles, and interventricular septum.

4. a. 4; b. 7; c. 3; d. 5; e. 8; f. 1; g. 2; h. 6

5. a. P; b. Q; c. R; d. S; e. T; f. U; g. PR interval; h. QRS interval; i. QT interval

6. a. 2; b. 4; c. 2; d. 4; e. 5; f. 3; g. 3; h. 1 (see Table 39.2).

7.

Situation	Stroke Volume Factor	Cardiac Output
Valsalva maneuver	Preload, ↓	↓
Venous dilation	Preload, ↓	↓
Hypertension	Afterload, ↑	↓
Administration of epinephrine	Contractility, ↑	↑
Obstruction of pulmonary artery	Preload, ↓ (left ventricle)	
	↑ (right ventricle)	↓
Hemorrhage	Preload, ↓	↓

8. b, d, f. The sympathetic nervous system increases the heart rate, the speed of impulse conduction through the atrioventricular (AV) node, and the force of atrial and ventricular contractions via the β-adrenergic receptors.

9.

Cardiovascular Problem	Physiologic Change
Widened pulse pressure	Loss of vascular elasticity and distensibility, increased sensitivity to antidiuretic hormone
Decreased cardiac reserve	Increased collagen and decreased elastin
Increased dysrhythmias	Decrease in sinoatrial (SA) node cells, conduction cells in the internodal tracts, the bundle of His, and bundle branches
Decreased response to sympathetic stimulation	Decreased number and function of β-adrenergic receptors
Aortic or mitral valve murmurs	Valvular lipid accumulation, collagen degeneration and fibrosis

10. d. Recreational or abused drugs, especially stimulants, such as cocaine and methamphetamine, are a growing cause of dysrhythmias and problems associated with tachycardia. IV injection of abused drugs is a risk factor for inflammatory and infectious conditions of the heart. Although calcium is involved in the contraction of muscles, calcium supplementation is not a significant factor in heart disease, nor is metastatic cancer. Streptococcal, but not viral, pharyngitis is a risk factor for rheumatic heart disease.

11.

Functional Health Pattern	Risk Factor for or Response to Cardiovascular Problem
Health perception–health management	Family history of coronary artery disease (CAD), cardiomyopathy, familial cardiovascular disease, or hypertension. Patient's history of hyperlipidemia, hypertension, tobacco use, obesity, or sedentary or stressful lifestyle. History of diabetes, alcohol use or use of recreational drugs. Experience of drug, allergic, or anaphylactic reaction
Nutritional-metabolic	Underweight or obesity, high intake of sodium and saturated fat
Elimination	Dependent edema, incontinence or constipation, use of diuretics with increased urinary output
Activity-exercise	Lack of aerobic exercise, decreased activity tolerance, symptoms during exercise
Sleep-rest	Attacks of shortness of breath interrupting sleep, use of several pillows to sleep, sleep apnea
Cognitive-perceptual	Vertigo, syncope, language, memory problems, or other cognitive changes
Self-perception–self-concept	Loss of self-esteem resulting from fatigue and decreased activity tolerance
Role-relationship	Stress or conflict in roles
Sexuality-reproductive	Change in sexual activity caused by shortness of breath or fatigue, impotence, and medications taken for erectile dysfunction. Oral contraceptives, hormone therapy for menopause, or medications for breast cancer
Coping–stress tolerance	Depression, high stress, or anxiety. Support system. Denial, anger, or hostility as coping mechanisms
Value-belief	Diagnosis or treatment conflict with value system

12. d. A palpable vibration of a blood vessel is called a *thrill* and usually indicates a narrowed or bulging vessel wall. A weak, thready pulse has little pressure and is difficult to palpate. A bruit is an abnormal buzzing or humming sound that may be auscultated over diseased blood vessels, and a bounding pulse is an extra full, hard pulse that may occur with atherosclerosis or hypervolemia.

13. a. Angle of Louis; b. Aortic area; c. Mitral area (apex) and point of maximal impulse (PMI); d. Tricuspid area; e. Erb's point; f. Pulmonic area

14. a. S_1; b. S_2; c. S_1; d. S_2; e. S_2; f. S_1

15. b, d, f. The heart murmurs are produced by turbulent blood flow across diseased heart valves, S_3 is heard with mitral valve regurgitation, and S_4 is heard with aortic stenosis. Arterial bruits are from turbulent peripheral blood flow. Pulsus alternans, seen in heart failure, is a variation in the strength of each pulse when palpated. Pericardial friction rub is the sound heard with pericarditis.

16. c. The bell of the stethoscope will enable better hearing of the low-pitched extra heart sounds. Having the patient lean forward best enables hearing the aortic and pulmonic areas; having the patient on the left side will enhance the mitral area sounds; both of these positions bring the heart closer to the chest wall. Having the patient supine or prone will not improve the auscultation.

17. b. Central cyanosis is evident with a blue tinge in the lips, conjunctiva, or tongue. Finger clubbing results from endocarditis, congenital defects, or prolonged O_2 deficiency. Peripheral cyanosis is evident with blue-tinged extremities or in the nose and ears. Decreased capillary refill may be seen in reduced capillary perfusion or anemia.

18. a. In an exercise nuclear imaging scan, a radioisotope is injected at the maximum heart rate on a bicycle or treadmill and used to evaluate blood flow in different parts of the heart. Insertion of electrodes into the heart chambers via the venous system to record intracardiac electrical activity is an electrophysiology study. Simply monitoring electrocardiogram (ECG) activity during exercise is an exercise stress test, and an echocardiogram uses transducers to bounce sound waves off of the heart.

19. d. All actions will be done but to perform a transesophageal echocardiogram (TEE). The throat must be numbed. Until sensation returns, as evidenced by the gag reflex, the patient is at risk of aspiration, so this action has the highest priority (priority related to airway—airway, breathing and circulation [ABCs]).

20. b. Holter monitoring involves placing electrodes on the chest attached to a recorder that will record ECG rhythm for 24 to 48 hours while the patient engages in normal activities of daily living (ADLs). The recording is later analyzed for dysrhythmias. Serial ECGs are frequent but not continuous ECGs. The 6-minute walk test measures the distance walked in 6 minutes to determine response to treatments and functional capacity for ADLs. An event monitor or loop recorder is used to record infrequent rhythm disturbances when the patient activates the recording with symptom occurrence.

21. c. An absence of pulses distal to the catheter insertion site indicates that clotting is occluding blood flow to the extremity and is an emergency that requires immediate medical attention. Some swelling and pain at the site are expected, but the site is also monitored for bleeding, and a pressure dressing or compression device may be applied. Hives may occur as a result of iodine sensitivity and will require treatment but the priority is the lack of pulses.

22. d. A risk assessment for CAD is determined by comparing the total cholesterol to high-density lipoprotein (HDL), and a ratio can be calculated by dividing the total cholesterol level by the HDL level. The ratio provides more information than either value alone, and an increased ratio indicates an increased risk. The female patient has a ratio of 3.57, which is average risk, compared with the male patient's ratio of 6.25, which is increased risk.

23. a, c. Copeptin is detected immediately with acute coronary syndrome (ACS) and increased levels of cardiac troponin T (cTnT) are detected within hours. Increased CK-MM is most commonly associated with skeletal muscle injury. Increased b-type natriuretic peptide (BNP) is a marker for heart failure. Increased C-reactive protein (CRP) occurs with acute inflammation as in atherosclerosis. Increased lipoprotein-associated phospholipase A_2 (Lp-PLA$_2$) indicates increased risk for CAD.

24. b. Decreased heart rate (HR) causes decreased cardiac output (CO). The other options contribute to an increased CO.

25. d. Impedance cardiography (ICG) is noninvasive and transmits continuous or intermittent electric current through the chest that travels through the path of least resistance: the blood. Thoracic fluid status or impedance-based hemodynamic parameters (CO, stroke volume [SV], and systemic vascular resistance [SVR]) are calculated from the average impedance of fluid in the thorax. ICG measures the change in impedance in the ascending aorta and left ventricle over time. Generalized edema or third spacing interferes with accurate signals because of the excess volume.

26. c. Increased fluid administration increases preload, which will increase CO. Diuretics will decrease preload. Dopamine does not affect preload but increases CO with increased cardiac contractility. Calcium channel blockers do not affect preload but decrease contractility.

27. c. CO is dependent on HR and SV. SV is determined by preload, afterload, and contractility. If CO is decreased and HR is unchanged, SV is the variable factor. If the preload (determined by pulmonary artery wedge pressure [PAWP]) and the afterload (determined by SVR) are unchanged, the factor that is changed is the contractility of the myocardium.

28. a. Referencing hemodynamic monitoring equipment means positioning the monitoring equipment so that the zero reference point is at the vertical level of the left atrium of the heart. The stopcock nearest the transducer is placed at the phlebostatic axis, the external landmark of the left atrium. The phlebostatic axis is the intersection of 2 planes: a horizontal line midaxillary, halfway between the outermost anterior and posterior surfaces, transecting a vertical line through the fourth intercostal space at the sternum.

29. c. The pressure obtained when the balloon of the pulmonary artery catheter is inflated reflects the preload of the left ventricle. The pulmonary artery flow–directed catheter's balloon floats from the right atrium into the pulmonary artery. In the absence of mitral valve impairment, the left ventricular end-diastolic pressure or left ventricular preload is reflected by the PAWP. The low pressure alarm in the arterial catheter placed for arterial blood gas (ABG) sampling detects disconnection of the line, which is a medical emergency.

30. d. During insertion of a pulmonary artery catheter, it is necessary to monitor the electrocardiogram (ECG) continuously because of the risk for dysrhythmias, particularly when the catheter reaches the right ventricle. The RN also notes the patient's electrolyte, acid-base, oxygenation, and coagulation status. During the catheter insertion, the patient is placed supine with the head of the bed flat. It is the HCP's responsibility to obtain informed consent regarding the catheter insertion. An Allen test to confirm adequate ulnar artery perfusion is performed before insertion of an arterial catheter in the radial artery for arterial pressure monitoring.

31. c. Arterial pressure–based CO (APCO) monitoring is used because of decreased risk with this less invasive technology than pulmonary artery pressure (PAP) monitoring. PAP monitoring is contraindicated for patients with coagulopathy and mechanical tricuspid or pulmonic valves.

32. a. Mean arterial pressure (MAP): 75 mm Hg = (90 mm Hg + 136 mm Hg)/3
   Pulmonary artery mean pressure (PAMP): 26 mm Hg = (38 mm Hg + 40 mm Hg)/3
   SV: 25.8 mL/beat = (3.2 L/min × 1000 mL)/124 bpm
   SVR: 1525 dynes/sec/cm^{-5} = (75 mm Hg − 14 mm Hg × 80/3.2 L/min)

   b. All of the changes in the hemodynamic parameters are characteristic findings in the patient with heart failure: increased pulmonary congestion reflected by increased PAP; increased pressure in the left atrium and ventricle (PAWP); increased SVR; and decreased SV, CO, and systemic BP. Increased central venous pressure (CVP) may result from the effects of left ventricular heart failure or biventricular heart failure.

33. b. The normal central venous oxygen saturation/mixed venous oxygen saturation (ScvO$_2$/SvO$_2$) of 60% to 80% becomes decreased with decreased arterial oxygenation, low CO, low hemoglobin, or increased oxygen consumption. With normal CO, arterial oxygenation, and hemoglobin, the factor that is responsible for decreased ScvO$_2$/SvO$_2$ is increased oxygen consumption, which can result from increased metabolic rate, pain, movement, fever, or shivering.

34. d. When a PAP tracing indicates a wedged waveform while the balloon is deflated, this indicates that the catheter has

advanced and has become spontaneously wedged. If the catheter is not repositioned immediately, a pulmonary infarction or a rupture of a pulmonary artery may occur. If the catheter is becoming occluded, the pressure tracing becomes blunted. Pulmonary edema and increased pulmonary congestion increase the pulmonary artery waveform. Balloon leaks found when injected air does not flow back into the syringe do not alter waveforms.

CHAPTER 36

1.

	Increasing Cardiac Output	Increasing Systemic Vascular Resistance	Mechanisms Causing Increases
β_1-Adrenergic stimulation	X	X	Increased rate and contractility of the heart increases cardiac output (CO). Peripheral artery vasoconstriction. Stimulation of renin production that activates the renin-angiotensin-aldosterone system (RAAS).
α_1-Adrenergic stimulation	X	X	Peripheral arteriole vasoconstriction and increased contractility of the heart
α_2-Adrenergic stimulation		X	Constriction of selected vascular beds
Endothelin release		X	Vasoconstriction
Angiotensin II		X	Arteriole vasoconstriction
Aldosterone release	X		Increased vascular volume
Antidiuretic hormone (ADH) release	X		Increased vascular volume

2. The vasoconstriction caused by the α_1-adrenergic agent raises the BP, stimulating the baroreceptors. The baroreceptors send impulses to the sympathetic vasomotor center in the brainstem, which inhibits the sympathetic nervous system, resulting in a decreased heart rate (HR), decreased force of contraction, and vasodilation.

3. The drug will lower BP because of decreased stroke volume and decreased HR, both of which decrease CO.

4. a, c, d, e. Hypertension progresses with increasing age. It is more prevalent in men before early middle age and above the age of 64 years in women. Blacks have a higher incidence of hypertension than do whites. Children and siblings of patients with hypertension should be screened and taught about healthy lifestyles.

5. c. Secondary hypertension has an underlying cause that will be treated, in contrast to primary or essential hypertension, which has no single known cause. Isolated systolic hypertension occurs when the systolic BP (SBP) is consistently equal to or over 130 mm Hg and the diastolic BP (DBP) is consistently equal to or over at 80 mm Hg.

6. a. Hypertension is often asymptomatic, especially if it is mild or moderate, and has been called the *silent killer*. The absence of symptoms often leads to noncompliance with medical treatment and a lack of concern about the disease in patients. With severe hypertension, symptoms may include fatigue, palpitations, angina, dyspnea, and dizziness.

7. b. Elevated BP causes endothelial damage, which causes the inner lining of arterioles to become thickened and stiffened and affects coronary circulation, cerebral circulation, peripheral vessels, and renal and retinal blood vessels. The narrowed vessels lead to ischemia and ultimately to damage of these organs.

8. b. The increased systemic vascular resistance (SVR) of hypertension directly increases the workload of the heart, and heart failure occurs when the heart can no longer pump effectively against the increased resistance. The heart may be indirectly damaged by atherosclerotic changes in the blood vessels, as are the brain, retina, and kidney.

9.

Laboratory Test Result	Significance
Blood urea nitrogen (BUN): 48 mg/dL (17.1 mmol/L) Creatinine: 4.3 mg/dL (380 mmol/L)	Elevated BUN and creatinine may indicate destruction of glomeruli and tubules of the kidney resulting from hypertension.
Serum K^+: 3.1 mEq/L (3.1 mmol/L)	Serum potassium levels are decreased when hypertension is associated with hyperaldosteronism.
Serum uric acid: 9.2 mg/dL (547 mmol/L)	An increased uric acid level may be caused by diuretics used to treat hypertension.
Fasting blood glucose: 183 mg/dL (10.2 mmol/L)	Fasting glucose levels are elevated when hypertension is associated with glucose intolerance and insulin resistance.
Low-density lipoproteins (LDL): 154 mg/dL (4.0 mmol/L)	An elevated LDL level indicates an increased risk for atherosclerotic changes in the patient with hypertension.

10. a. Dietary modifications to increase fruits, vegetables, fat-free milk, whole grains, fish, poultry, beans, seeds, and nuts; and restrict sodium, cholesterol, and saturated fat; maintain intake of potassium, calcium, vitamin D, and omega-3 fatty acids; and promote weight reduction if overweight b. Daily moderate-intensity physical activity for

at least 30 minutes on most days of the week c. Cessation of tobacco use (if a user) d. Moderation or cessation of alcohol intake

Usually medications, monitoring BP at home, and psychosocial risk factors must also be addressed.

11. c. Cardioselective β-adrenergic blockers decrease CO, reduce sympathetic vasoconstrictor tone, and decrease renin secretion by kidneys. Calcium channel blockers reduce BP by causing blocked movement of calcium into cells, which causes vasodilation of arterioles. Spironolactone blocks the effect of aldosterone. Central adrenergic antagonists, such as clonidine (Catapres) inhibit sympathetic outflow from the central nervous system (CNS).

12. d. Valsartan (Diovan) is an angiotensin II receptor blocker (ARB). ARBs prevent the action of angiotensin II, produce vasodilation, and increase salt and water excretion. Angiotensin-converting enzyme (ACE) inhibitors prevent the conversion of angiotensin I to angiotensin II. Direct vasodilators act directly on smooth muscle of arterioles to cause vasodilation. Thiazide diuretics decrease extracellular fluid volume by increasing Na^+ and Cl^- excretion with water.

13. d. Hydrochlorothiazide is a thiazide diuretic that causes sodium and potassium loss through the kidneys. High-potassium foods should be included in the diet, or potassium supplements may be used to prevent hypokalemia. Enalapril and spironolactone may cause hyperkalemia by inhibiting the action of aldosterone, and potassium supplements should not be used by patients taking these drugs. As a combined α/β-blocker, labetalol does not affect potassium levels.

14. b. Chlorothiazide is a thiazide diuretic that causes orthostatic hypotension. Prazosin is an α-adrenergic blocker that causes dilation of arterioles and veins and causes orthostatic hypotension. The patient may feel dizzy, weak, and faint when assuming an upright position after sitting or lying down and should be taught to change positions slowly, avoid standing for long periods, do leg exercises to increase venous return, and lie or sit down when dizziness occurs. Direct-acting vasodilators often cause fluid retention; dry mouth may occur with diuretic use, and centrally acting α- and β-blockers may cause bradycardia.

15. c. Sexual dysfunction, which can occur with many of the antihypertensive drugs, including thiazide and potassium-sparing diuretics and β-adrenergic blockers, can be a major reason that a male patient does not adhere to his treatment regimen. It is helpful for the nurse to raise the subject because sexual problems may be easier for the patient to discuss and handle once it has been explained that the drug may be the source of the problem.

16. a, c, e, f. The age-related changes that contribute to hypertension include decreased renal function, increased peripheral vascular resistance, increased collagen and stiffness of the myocardium, and decreased elasticity in large arteries from arteriosclerosis. The baroreceptor reflexes are blunted. The adrenergic receptor sensitivity and renin response are both decreased with aging.

17. a. Centrally acting α-adrenergic blockers may cause severe rebound hypertension if the drugs are abruptly discontinued, and patients should be taught about this effect because many are not consistently compliant with drug therapy. Diuretics should be taken early in the day

to prevent nocturia. The profound orthostatic hypotension that occurs with first-dose peripheral acting α-adrenergic blockers can be prevented by taking the initial dose at bedtime. Aspirin use may decrease the effectiveness of ACE inhibitors.

18. d. Correct technique in measuring BP includes taking and averaging 2 or more readings at least 1 minute apart. Initially BP measurements should be taken in both arms to detect any differences. If there is a difference, the arm with the higher reading should be used for all subsequent BP readings. The patient may be supine or sitting. The important points are that the arm being used is at the heart level and the cuff needs to fit snugly.

19. b. The AP may check postural changes in BP as directed. The LPN may administer antihypertensive medications to stable patients. The RN must monitor the patient receiving IV sodium nitroprusside, as the patient is in a hypertensive crisis. The RN must also do the teaching related to home BP monitoring.

20. c. Hypertensive emergency, a type of hypertensive crisis, is a situation in which a patient's BP is severely elevated with evidence of acute target organ disease (e.g., cerebrovascular, cardiovascular, renal, or retinal). The neurologic manifestations are often similar to the presentation of a stroke but do not show the focal or lateralizing symptoms of stroke. Hypertensive crises are defined by the degree of organ damage and how rapidly the BP rises, not by specific BP measurements. A hypertensive urgency is a less severe crisis, in which a patient's BP becomes severely elevated over hours or days but there is no evidence of target organ damage.

21. d. Hypertensive crises are treated with IV administration of antihypertensive drugs, including the vasodilators sodium nitroprusside, fenoldopam, and nicardipine; adrenergic blockers, such as labetalol, esmolol, and phentolamine; the ACE inhibitor enalaprilat; the calcium channel blocker clevidipine; nitroglycerin for myocardial ischemia; hydralazine with other medications; and oral captopril. Sodium nitroprusside is the most effective parenteral drug for hypertensive emergencies.

22. a. Initially, the treatment goal in hypertensive emergencies is to reduce the mean arterial pressure (MAP) by no more than 20% to 25% in the first hour, with further gradual reduction over the next 24 hours. In this case, the MAP is $222 + 2(148)/3 = 172$, so decreasing it by 25% equals 129. Lowering the BP too far or too fast may cause a stroke, myocardial infarction (MI), or renal failure. Only when the patient has an aortic dissection, angina, or signs of an ischemic stroke does the SBP have to be lowered to 100 to 120 mm Hg or less as quickly as possible.

23. d. Hypertensive urgencies are often treated with oral drugs on an outpatient basis, but it is important for the patient to be seen by a HCP within 24 hours to evaluate the effectiveness of the treatment. Hourly urine measurements, titration of IV drugs, and Electrocardiogram (ECG) monitoring are indicated for hypertensive emergencies.

Case Study

1. B., C., E., F., H. The arm should be rested at heart level. The arm with the highest BP should be used to measure BPs. The patient only needs to rest for 5 minutes before measuring BP.

2. **Triamterene**= potassium-sparing diuretic; **lisinopril**=ACE inhibitor; **metoprolol**= cardioselective β-blocker; **hydralazine**=direct vasodilator; **nicardipine**=dihydropyridine; **diltiazem**; non-dihydropyridine; **losartan**= angiotensin II receptor blocker; **carvedilol**= mixed α- and β-blocker

3. **Indicated**: referral to a dietician (to help choose appropriate foods); using Mrs. Dash substitute to replace salt; monitoring BP at home and keeping a record; **Contraindicated**: exercising for 20 minutes per week (the recommendation is 150 minutes of moderate exercise or 75 minutes of vigorous exercise per week); advising 2 glasses of red wine per day (the recommendation is 1 alcoholic drink per day for women); stop taking antihypertensive medications when BP is less than 120/80 mm Hg (BP medications should not be abruptly stopped, plus the medication is likely the reason the BP is less than 120/80); **Non-essential**: refer to an occupational therapist (there isn't any indication that K.J. needs this referral)

4. **Effective**: reading labels; working with a physical therapist; one alcoholic beverage per day; grief counseling are all recommended for this patient; **Ineffective**: training for a half marathon (this is too vigorous for this patient; she should gradually increase her exercise); weighing herself daily (is too frequent and could cause frustration when trying to lose weight; there is no need to report weight gain); 3 grams of salt per day (2300 mg of salt per day is recommended for adults but 1500 mg or less will reduce BP even more); **Unrelated**: eating more fiber or taking a fiber supplement (will not affect BP)

5. **Fenoldopam**=use cautiously in patients with glaucoma; **hydralazine**=contraindicated in patients with CAD; **nifedipine**=don't use sublingual in hypertensive emergencies; **methyldopa**=may cause daytime drowsiness; **verapamil**=don't use in 2nd degree or 3rd degree heart blocks; **captopril**=may increase serum creatinine levels; **propranolol**=contraindicated in patients with asthma history; **sodium nitroprusside**=monitor thiocyanate levels

CHAPTER 37

1. c. The fibrous plaque stage has progressive changes that can be seen by age 30 years. Collagen covers the fatty streak and forms a fibrous plaque in the artery. The thrombus adheres to the arterial wall in the complicated lesion stage. Rapid onset of coronary artery disease (CAD) with hypercholesterolemia may be related to familial hypercholesterolemia, not a stage of CAD development. The fatty streak stage is the earliest stage of atherosclerosis and can be seen by age 20 years.

2. b. The etiology of CAD includes atherosclerosis as the major cause. The pathophysiology of atherosclerosis development and resulting atheromas is related to endothelial injury and inflammation, which can be the result of tobacco use, hyperlipidemia, hypertension, toxins, diabetes, high homocysteine levels, and infection causing a local inflammatory response in the inner lining of the vessel walls. Partial or total occlusion occurs in the complicated lesion stage. Extra collateral circulation occurs in the presence of chronic ischemia. Therefore it is more likely to occur in an older patient.

3. b. This white woman has 1 unmodifiable risk factor (age) and 2 major modifiable risk factors (hypertension and physical inactivity). Her gender risk is as high as a man's because she is 75 years of age. The white man has 1 unmodifiable risk factor (gender), 1 major modifiable risk factor (smoking), and 1 contributing modifiable risk factor (stressful lifestyle). The Asian woman has only 1 major modifiable risk factor (hyperlipidemia), and Asians in the United States have fewer myocardial infarctions (MIs) than do whites. The Hispanic man has an unmodifiable risk factor related to age and 1 major modifiable risk factor (obesity). Hispanics have slightly lower rates of CAD than non-Hispanic whites or blacks.

4. d. CAD is the number-one killer of American women, and women have a much higher mortality rate within 1 year following MI than do men. Smoking carries specific problems for women because smoking has been linked to a decrease in natural estrogen levels and to early menopause, and it has been identified as the most powerful contributor to CAD in women under the age of 50 years. Fewer women than men present with classic manifestations, and women delay seeking care longer than men. Estrogen replacement does not always reduce the risk for CAD, even though natural estrogen lowers low-density lipoprotein (LDL) and raises high-density lipoprotein (HDL) cholesterol.

5. b, c, e. LDLs contain more cholesterol than the other lipoproteins, have an attraction for arterial walls, and correlate most closely with increased incidence of atherosclerosis and CAD. HDLs increase with exercise and carry lipids away from arteries to the liver for metabolism. A high HDL level is associated with a lower risk of CAD.

6. b. High fasting triglyceride levels are associated with cardiovascular disease and diabetes. Apolipoproteins are found in varying amounts on the HDLs and activate enzyme or receptor sites that promote removal of fat from plasma, which is protective. The apolipoprotein A and apolipoprotein B ratio must be done to predict CAD. High total serum cholesterol must be calculated with HDL for a ratio over time to determine an increased risk of CAD. High HDLs are associated with a lower risk of CAD.

7. d. All the results are abnormal. The patient in option "c" is close to being at risk; if this patient is a woman, the HDL is too low and the other results are at or near the cut off for being normal. The other patients' results are at acceptable levels.

8. b. Increased exercise without an increase in caloric intake will result in weight loss, reducing the risk associated with obesity. Exercise increases lipid metabolism and increases HDL, thus reducing CAD risk. Exercise may indirectly reduce the risk of CAD by controlling hypertension, promoting glucose metabolism in diabetes, and reducing stress. While high blood levels of homocysteine are linked to an increased risk for CAD, reducing homocysteine levels has not been shown to reduce the risk of heart disease.

9. a, c, e. Therapeutic Lifestyle Changes diet recommendations emphasize reduction in saturated fat and cholesterol intake. Whole milk products, red meats, and eggs as well as butter, stick margarine, lard, and solid shortening should be reduced or eliminated from diets. If triglyceride levels are high, alcohol and simple sugars should be reduced.

10. b. The Therapeutic Lifestyle Changes diet includes recommendations for all people, not just those with risk factors, to decrease the risk for CAD.

11. c. Without the total serum cholesterol and HDL results, diet therapy and smoking cessation are indicated for this patient without CAD who has prehypertension and an LDL level ≥ 130 mg/dL. When the patient's LDL level is 75 to 189 mg/dL with a 10-year risk for cardiovascular disease (CVD) of 7.5% or above, drug therapy would be added to diet therapy. Because tobacco use is related to increased BP and LDL level, the benefit of smoking cessation is almost immediate. Exercise is indicated to reduce risk factors throughout treatment.

12. c, d, e. Unstable angina, ST-segment-elevation myocardial infarction (STEMI), and non–ST-segment-elevation myocardial infarction (NSTEMI) are conditions that are manifestations of acute coronary syndrome (ACS). The other options are not manifestations of ACS.

13. b, d, e, f. Increased oxygen demand is caused by increasing the workload of the heart, including left ventricular hypertrophy with hypertension, sympathetic nervous stimulation, and anything precipitating angina. Hypovolemia, anemia, and narrowed coronary arteries contribute to decreased oxygen supply.

14. c. When the coronary arteries are occluded, contractility ceases after several minutes, depriving the myocardial cells of glucose and oxygen for aerobic metabolism. Anaerobic metabolism begins, and lactic acid accumulates, irritating myocardial nerve fibers that then transmit a pain message to the cardiac nerves and upper thoracic posterior roots. The other factors may occur during vessel occlusion but are not the source of pain.

15. c, d. Prinzmetal angina and microvascular angina may occur in the absence of CAD but with arterial spasm in Prinzmetal angina or abnormalities of the coronary microcirculation. Silent ischemia is prevalent in persons with diabetes and contributes to asymptomatic myocardial ischemia. Nocturnal angina occurs only at night. Chronic stable angina refers to chest pain that occurs with the same pattern of onset, duration, and intensity intermittently over a long period of time.

16. b, d. Unstable angina is new-onset angina occurring at rest or with minimal exertion and increases in frequency, duration, or severity. Chronic stable angina is usually precipitated by exertion. Angina decubitus occurs when the person is recumbent. Prinzmetal's angina is often caused by a coronary artery spasm.

17. d. An increased heart rate (HR) decreases the time the heart spends in diastole, which is the time of greatest coronary blood flow. Unlike other arteries, coronary arteries are perfused when the myocardium relaxes and blood backflows from the aorta into the sinuses of Valsalva, which have openings to the right and left coronary arteries. Thus the heart has a decreased oxygen supply at a time when there is an increased oxygen demand. Tachycardia may also lead to ventricular dysrhythmia. The other options are incorrect.

18. a, b, c. Nitrates decrease preload and afterload to decrease the coronary workload and dilate coronary arteries to increase coronary blood supply. The other options are not attributed to nitrates.

19. a. Captopril would be added. It is an angiotensin-converting enzyme (ACE) inhibitor that vasodilates and decreases endothelial dysfunction and may prevent ventricular remodeling. Clopidogrel (Plavix) is an antiplatelet agent used as an alternative for a patient unable to use aspirin. Diltiazem (Cardizem), a calcium channel blocker, may be used to decrease vasospasm but is not known to prevent ventricular remodeling. Metoprolol (Lopressor) is a β-adrenergic blocker that inhibits sympathetic nervous stimulation of the heart.

20. a. A common complication of nitrates is dizziness caused by orthostatic hypotension, so the patient should sit or lie down and place the tablet under the tongue. The tablet should be allowed to dissolve under the tongue. To prevent the tablet from being swallowed, water should not be taken with it. The recommended dose for the patient for whom nitroglycerin (NTG) has been prescribed is 1 tablet taken sublingually (SL) or 1 metered spray for symptoms of angina. If symptoms are unchanged or worse after 5 minutes, the patient should contact the emergency medical system (EMS) before taking more NTG. If symptoms are significantly improved by 1 dose of NTG, teach the patient or caregiver to repeat NTG every 5 minutes for a maximum of 3 doses and contact EMS if symptoms have not resolved completely. Headache is a common complication of nitrates but usually resolves with continued use of nitrates. It may be controlled with mild analgesics.

21. a. Orthostatic hypotension may cause dizziness and falls in older adults taking antianginal agents that decrease preload. Patients should be cautioned to change positions slowly. Daily exercise programs are indicated for older adults and may increase performance, endurance, and ability to tolerate stress. A change in lifestyle behaviors may increase the quality of life and reduce the risks of CAD, even in the older adult. Aspirin is often used in these patients and is not contraindicated.

22. c. Unstable angina is associated with the rupture of a once-stable atherosclerotic plaque, exposing the intima to blood and stimulating platelet aggregation and local vasoconstriction with thrombus formation. Patients with unstable angina need immediate hospitalization and monitoring because the lesion is at increased risk of complete thrombosis of the lumen with progression to MI. Any type of angina may be associated with severe pain, electrocardiogram (ECG) changes, and dysrhythmias. Prinzmetal's angina is characterized by coronary artery spasm.

23. a. One of the primary differences between the pain of angina and the pain of an MI is that angina pain is usually relieved by rest or NTG, which reduces the oxygen demand of the heart, while MI pain is not. Both angina and MI pain can cause a pressure or squeezing sensation; may or may not radiate to the neck, back, arms, fingers, and jaw; and may be precipitated by exertion.

24. b. An exercise stress test will reveal ECG changes that indicate impaired coronary circulation when the oxygen demand of the heart is increased. A single ECG is not conclusive for CAD, and negative findings do not rule out CAD. Coronary angiography can detect narrowing of coronary arteries but is an invasive procedure. Echocardiograms of various types may identify abnormalities of myocardial wall motion under stress but are indirect measures of CAD.

25. d. The subjective report of the pain from an MI is usually severe. It usually is unrelieved by NTG, rest, or position

change and usually lasts more than the 15 or 20 minutes typical of angina pain. All the other symptoms may occur with angina as well as with an MI.

26. c. At 10 to 14 days after MI, the new scar tissue is weak and is vulnerable to increased stress because of the unstable state of healing at this point, as well as the increasing physical activity of the patient. At 2 to 4 days, removal of necrotic tissue is taking place by phagocytic cells. By 4 to 10 days, the necrotic tissue has been cleared and a collagen matrix for scar tissue has been deposited. Healing with scar-tissue replacement of the necrotic area is usually complete in 6 weeks.

27. c. The most common complication of MI is dysrhythmias. Continuous cardiac monitoring allows identification and treatment of dysrhythmias that may cause further deterioration of the cardiovascular status or death. Measurement of hourly urine output and vital signs is indicated to detect symptoms of the complication of cardiogenic shock. Crackles, dyspnea, and tachycardia may indicate the onset of heart failure (HF).

28. b. Left-sided HF, which can escalate to cardiogenic shock, initially occurs and manifests as mild dyspnea, restlessness, agitation, pulmonary congestion with crackles, and/or S_3 or S_4 heart sounds. Right-sided HF includes jugular vein distention, hepatic congestion, or lower extremity edema. Pericarditis is a common complication identified with chest pain that is aggravated by inspiration, coughing, and moving the upper body. Ventricular aneurysm is manifested with HF, dysrhythmias, and angina. Papillary muscle dysfunction is suspected with a new systolic apical murmur.

29. c. Cardiac-specific troponin T and troponin I have a greater sensitivity and specificity for myocardial injury than creatine kinase MB (CK-MB), are released 4 to 6 hours after the onset of MI, peak in 10 to 24 hours, and return to baseline over 10 to 14 days. CK-MB levels begin to rise 6 hours after an acute MI, peak in about 18 hours, and return to normal within 24 to 36 hours. ECG changes are often not apparent immediately after infarct and may be normal when the patient seeks medical attention. An enlarged heart, determined by x-ray, indicates cardiac stress but is not diagnostic of acute MI.

30. c. A differentiation is made between MIs that have ST-segment elevations on ECG and those that do not because chest pain accompanied by ST-segment elevations is associated with prolonged and complete coronary thrombosis and is treated with reperfusion therapy. The other options are incorrect.

31. c. Transmyocardial laser revascularization (TMR) is a treatment used for patients with inoperable CAD. It uses a high-energy laser to create channels in the heart to allow blood to flow to the ischemic area and can be done using a left anterior thoracotomy incision or with coronary artery bypass graft (CABG) surgery. A stent is the structure used to hold vessels open and requires anticoagulation following the procedure. Surgical construction of new vessels is done with CABG surgery.

32. d. Emergent percutaneous coronary intervention (PCI) is the first treatment for patients with a confirmed MI within 90 minutes of arriving at the facility with an interventional cardiac catheterization laboratory. TMR, stent placement, and CABG are usually done to facilitate circulation in nonemergency situations.

33. b. The AP can check vital signs and report results to the RN. The other actions include assessment, teaching, and monitoring of IV fluids, which are all responsibilities of the RN.

34. c. The most common method of coronary artery bypass involves leaving the internal mammary artery attached to its origin from the subclavian artery but dissecting it from the chest wall and anastomosing it distal to an obstruction in a coronary artery. Other grafts options include using the saphenous vein, and/or radial artery.

35. c. An NSTEMI is an ACS that indicates a transient thrombosis or incomplete coronary artery occlusion. Treatment involves intensive drug therapy with antiplatelets, glycoprotein IIb/IIIa inhibitors, antithrombotics, and heparin to prevent clot extension. In addition, IV NTG is used. Reperfusion therapy using thrombolytics, CABG, or PCI is used for treatment of STEMI.

36. c. Decreasing level of consciousness (LOC) may reflect hypoxemia resulting from internal bleeding, which is always a risk with thrombolytic therapy. Oozing of blood is expected, as are reperfusion dysrhythmias. BP is low but not considered abnormal because the pulse is within normal range. Idioventricular dysrhythmias are common with reperfusion.

37. a. If chest pain is unchanged, it is a sign that reperfusion was not successful. Indications that the occluded coronary artery is patent and blood flow to the myocardium is reestablished following thrombolytic therapy include return of ST-segment to baseline on the ECG; relief of chest pain; marked, rapid rise of the CK-MB within 3 hours of therapy; and the presence of reperfusion dysrhythmias. Bleeding is a complication of thrombolytic therapy but does not indicate lack of success or successful reperfusion.

38. a. Morphine sulfate decreases anxiety and cardiac workload as a vasodilator and reduces preload and myocardial O_2 consumption, which relieves chest pain. Calcium channel blockers, amiodarone, and angiotensin-converting enzyme (ACE) inhibitors will not relieve chest pain related to an MI.

39. b. Docusate sodium (Colace) is a stool softener, which prevents straining and provoking dysrhythmias. It does not do any of the other options. Antidysrhythmics are used to control ventricular dysrhythmias; morphine sulfate is used to decrease anxiety and cardiac workload; and glycoprotein IIb/IIIa inhibitors and antiplatelets prevent the binding of fibrinogen to platelets.

40. b. It is recommended that patients with hypertension and after an MI be on β-adrenergic blockers indefinitely to decrease oxygen demand. They inhibit sympathetic nervous stimulation of the heart; reduce heart rate, contractility, and BP; and decrease afterload. Although calcium channel blockers decrease heart rate, contractility, and BP, they are not used unless the patient cannot tolerate β-adrenergic blockers. ACE inhibitors and angiotensin II receptor blockers (ARBs) are used for vasodilation.

41. a. This patient is indicating positive coping with a realization that recovery takes time and that lifestyle changes can be made as needed. The patient who is "just going to get on with life" is likely in denial about the seriousness of the condition and the changes that must be made. Nervous questioning about the expected duration and

effect of the condition indicates the presence of anxiety, as does the statement about the HCP's role in treatment.

42. a. 6; b. 3; c. 2; d. 1; e. 5; f. 4. A patient having chest pain needs to have the pain assessed and relieved as quickly as possible. Applying oxygen may help relieve the pain. Following an assessment of the vital signs, it is important to know if the pain is accompanied by ECG changes. Then perform a detailed assessment of the pain using PQRST and medicate as ordered. Perform a focused assessment of the heart and lungs before reporting the findings to the provider.

43. d. Anger about the MI may be directed at family, staff, or the medical regimen. Stating that the chest pain is no big deal is denial. Relaying an inability to care for self relates to dependency. Questioning what will happen if there is another attack is expressing anxiety and fear. Depression may be expressed related to changes in lifestyle. Realistic acceptance is seen with actively engaging in changing modifiable risk factors.

44. a. Golfing is a moderate-energy activity that expends about 5 metabolic equivalent units (METs). It is within the 3 to 6 METs activity level desired for a patient by the time of discharge from the hospital following an MI. Walking at 5 mph and mowing the lawn using a push mower are high-energy activities. Cycling at 13 mph is an extremely high–energy activity.

45. a. Any activity or exercise that causes dyspnea and chest pain should be stopped in the patient with CAD. The training target for a healthy 58-year-old is 80% of maximum HR, or 130 bpm. HR, rather than respiratory rate, determines the parameters for exercise.

46. b. Resumption of sexual activity is often difficult for patients to approach. It is reported that most cardiac patients do not resume sexual activity after MI. The nurse can give the patient permission to discuss concerns about sexual activity by introducing it as a physical activity when other physical activities are discussed. HCPs may have preferences about the timing of resumption of sexual activity. The nurse should discuss this with the HCP and the patient but addressing the patient's concerns is a nursing responsibility. Patients should be taught that impotence after MI is common but that it usually disappears after several attempts.

47. b. It is common for a patient who has chest pain on exertion to have some angina during sexual stimulation or intercourse. Teach the patient to use NTG prophylactically. Positions during intercourse are a matter of individual choice, and foreplay is desirable because it allows a gradual increase in HR. Sildenafil (Viagra) should be used cautiously in men with CAD and should not be used with nitrates.

48. a. Many patients who have a sudden cardiac death (SCD) experience because of CAD do not have an acute MI but have dysrhythmias that cause death. This is probably because of electrical instability of the myocardium. To identify and treat those specific dysrhythmias, continuous monitoring is important. The other assessments can be done but are not the most important after an episode of SCD.

Case Study

1. **Indicated:** apply supplemental oxygen (improves oxygen delivery to myocardial tissue); perform a pain assessment (will provide important information about intensity, location, radiation, and characteristics of patient's pain); obtain a 12-lead ECG (will identify cardiac rhythm as well as ST segment status which indicates myocardial ischemia, injury, or infarction); obtain a chest x-ray (will identify fluid in the lungs related to heart failure and other possible causes of chest pain, such as pericarditis); **Contraindicated**: administer NTG SL (This patient doesn't have baseline vital signs, including BP. Since NTG causes hypotension, it is essential to obtain the BP prior to administration.); administer a non-cardioselective beta blocker (This patient has a history of asthma which can be exacerbated by the administration of a non-cardioselective beta blocker. If a beta blocker is prescribed, it should be the cardioselective type.) **Non-essential:** perform a head-to-toe assessment (It isn't necessary to perform a head-to-toe assessment. The nurse should perform a focused assessment pertaining to the cardiovascular system.)

2. **Metoprolol**: Purpose: increases ventricular filling time by decreasing heart rate; Common Side/Adverse Effect: bradycardia (use cautiously if the HR is < 60 bpm). **Atorvastatin**: Purpose: prevent atherosclerosis; Common Side/Adverse Effect: muscle pain, tenderness, weakness. **Morphine sulfate**: Purpose: not only does it treat pain, it also decreases myocardial oxygen consumption; Common Side/Adverse Effect: decreases respiratory effort. **Captopril**: Purpose: prevent ventricular remodeling; Common Side/Adverse Effect: is an ACE inhibitor which targets the angiotensin converting enzyme produced in the lungs which may cause a persistent cough. **Aspirin**: Purpose: prevents platelet aggregation; Common Side. Adverse Effect: can increase the risk of bleeding, especially GI bleeding which can manifest as black tarry stools.

3. **Stable angina**: chest pain with activity that is relieved with rest; **Unstable angina**: chest pain at rest, ST segment elevation, elevated cardiac biomarkers; **Myocardial infarction**: chest pain at rest, ST segment elevation, elevated cardiac biomarkers, ventricular remodeling

4. B, C, E, G. Bibasilar crackles could indicate left ventricular heart failure due to myocardial infarction. Nausea could indicate hypotension or be an atypical sign of angina or MI. Elevated troponin levels (normal is < 0.04 ng/mL) indicate damage to myocardial tissue as a result of myocardial injury and infarction. Tachycardia isn't a definitive sign of an MI but could be a result of angina, heart failure, or anxiety and fear stemming from ACS. The nurse should follow-up about tachycardia because it increases myocardial oxygen consumption as well as decreases ventricular filling time which negatively impacts cardiac output. The patient may have a fever up to 100.4°F (38°C) as a result of a systemic inflammatory response, but the fever won't be treated unless it is > 38°C. Oxygen saturation of 96% on 2 L/min nasal cannula is acceptable. The patient's productive cough and low back pain aren't related to her cardiac condition, but the mid and upper back are common sites of radiating pain.

5. **Potential conditions**: unstable angina and acute coronary syndrome; **Actions to take**: apply oxygen 2 L/min; administer aspirin 325 mg chewed; perform 12-lead ECG; administer 0.4 mg NTG SL; **Parameters to monitor**: ECG rhythm; urinary output; cardiac enzymes; vital signs; pain assessment; breath sounds. **Rationale**: Heart failure isn't associated with intense pain that radiates. The evidence doesn't support the following conditions: acute renal

injury, asthma attack, panic attack, anaphylaxis, sepsis, hypertensive crisis, or pulmonary embolism. Therefore, the following actions are not warranted: albuterol, blood cultures, diphenhydramine, lorazepam, normal saline bolus, or hydralazine. The following parameters to monitor are not applicable or relevant to the clinical data provided nor the patient's condition: temperature, FSBS, peripheral pulses, and ABGs.

CHAPTER 38

1. a, b. Heart failure with preserved ejection fraction (HFpEF) (diastolic failure) is characterized by abnormal resistance to ventricular filling. Hypertension, coronary artery disease (CAD), advanced age, and diabetes are all risk factors for heart failure (HF). Ejection fraction (EF) is decreased in systolic HF. Decreased cardiac output (CO) and increased workload and oxygen requirements of the myocardium precipitate HF because of left ventricle dysfunction.

2.

Compensatory Mechanism	↑ Cardiac Output	Detrimental Effect
Cardiac dilation	Increased force of contraction by stretching of cardiac muscle	Overstrains the muscle fibers; mitral valve incompetence
Ventricular myocyte hypertrophy	Increased ventricular mass and increased contractile force of muscle	Increased myocardial oxygen need, then poor contractility
Neurohormonal response		
• Renin-angiotensin-aldosterone system (RAAS)	Increased fluid and sodium retention and vasoconstriction to maintain BP	Increased preload and afterload
• Antidiuretic hormone (ADH)	Increased water retention	Increased blood volume when already overloaded
• Sympathetic nervous system (SNS) stimulation	Increased BP, heart rate (HR) and contractility; increased preload	Increased myocardial oxygen need; overwhelming preload; increased afterload

3. c. Both natriuretic peptides and nitric oxide contribute to vasodilation, decreased BP, and decreased afterload. The natriuretic peptides also increase excretion of sodium by increasing glomerular filtration rate and diuresis (renal effects) as well as interfere with ADH release and inhibit aldosterone and renin secretion (hormonal effects).

4. d. FACES is used to teach patients to identify early HF symptoms. F = Fatigue; A = Activity limitations; C = Chest congestion/cough; E = Edema; S = Shortness of breath. The other options are not correct.

5. b. In left-sided HF, blood backs up into the pulmonary veins and capillaries. This increased hydrostatic pressure in the vessels causes fluid to move out of the vessels and into the pulmonary interstitial space. When increased lymphatic flow cannot remove enough fluid from the interstitial space, fluid moves into the alveoli, resulting in pulmonary edema and impaired alveolar oxygen and carbon dioxide exchange. Initially the right side of the heart is not involved.

6. a. Early clinical manifestations of acute left-sided HF are those of interstitial edema, with bubbling crackles and tachycardia, as well as tachypnea. Later frothy, blood-tinged sputum; severe dyspnea; and orthopnea develop with alveolar edema. Severe tachycardia and cool, clammy skin are present as a result of stimulation of the SNS from hypoxemia. Systemic edema reflected by jugular vein distention, peripheral edema, and hepatosplenomegaly are characteristic of right-sided HF.

7. d. Paroxysmal nocturnal dyspnea (PND) is awakening from sleep with a feeling of suffocation and a need to sit up to be able to breathe. Patients learn that sleeping with the upper body elevated on several pillows helps prevent PND. Behavior changes are seen in late stages of HF. Nocturia occurs with HF as fluid moves back into the vascular system during recumbency, increasing renal blood flow. Dependent edema does not indicate PND.

8. a. Arterial oxygen saturation by pulse oximetry (SpO$_2$) of 84% on 2 L/min via nasal cannula indicates impaired oxygen saturation. The patient is having trouble with gas exchange. Airway and breathing are the priority (follow airway, breathing and circulation [ABCs]). b. The nurse should place the patient in high Fowler's position, assess the patient immediately, recheck SpO$_2$, auscultate breath sounds, assess level of consciousness (LOC), check the oxygen connection and rate setting (2 L/min), and talk with the patient about her or his breathing.

9. b. Thrombus formation occurs in the heart when the chambers do not contract normally and empty completely. Both atrial fibrillation and very low left ventricular output (LVEF < 20%) lead to thrombus formation, which is treated with anticoagulants to prevent the release of emboli into the circulation as well as antidysrhythmics or cardioversion to control atrial fibrillation.

10. c. b-type natriuretic peptide (BNP) is released from the ventricles in response to increased blood volume in the heart and is a good marker for HF. If BNP is elevated, shortness of breath is caused by HF; if BNP is normal, dyspnea is caused by pulmonary disease. BNP opposes the actions of the RAAS, resulting in vasodilation and reduction in blood volume. Exercise stress testing and cardiac catheterization are more important tests to diagnose CAD, and although the blood urea nitrogen (BUN) may be elevated in HF, it is a reflection of decreased renal perfusion. (See Table 31.6.)

11. d. Isosorbide dinitrate and hydralazine (Bidil) is recommended for use in black patients with HFrEF to treat hypertension and angina. Captopril is used for hypertension by all patients. Nitroglycerin is used with hydralazine for patients who cannot tolerate RAAS inhibitors (angiotensin-converting enzyme [ACE] inhibitors or angiotensin II receptor blocker [ARBs]) for HF management. Spironolactone (Aldactone) is used for hypertension.

12. d. Diuretics are the first line for treating patients with volume overload. They decrease sodium reabsorption at various sites within the kidneys, enhancing sodium and water loss. Decreasing intravascular volume with diuretics reduces volume returning to the LV (preload). This allows for more efficient LV pumping, decreased pulmonary vascular pressures, and improved alveolar gas exchange. IV Nesiritide is a recombinant form of BNP used for short-term treatment of acute decompensated heart failure (ADHF) after a failed response to IV diuretics. Digoxin requires a loading dose and time to work, so it is not recommended for emergency treatment of ADHF. Morphine sulfate relieves dyspnea but has more adverse effects.

13. a. Dopamine is a β-adrenergic agonist that is a positive inotrope given IV, not orally, and used for acute HF. Losartan (Cozaar) is an angiotensin II receptor blocker used for patients who do not tolerate ACE inhibitors. Carvedilol (Coreg) is the β-adrenergic blocker that blocks the sympathetic nervous system's negative effects on the failing heart. Hydrochlorothiazide is the diuretic.

14. b, d. Furosemide is a diuretic that eliminates potassium and spironolactone is a potassium-sparing diuretic that retains potassium. The other treatments and medications are used for patients with HF, but they do not directly affect serum potassium levels.

15. b. Hypokalemia is one of the most common causes of digitalis toxicity because low serum potassium levels enhance ectopic pacemaker activity. When a patient is receiving potassium-excreting diuretics, such as hydrochlorothiazide or furosemide, it is essential to monitor the patient's serum potassium levels to prevent digitalis toxicity. Monitoring the HR assesses for complications related to digoxin but does not prevent toxicity.

16. a. Spironolactone is a potassium-sparing diuretic, and when it is the only diuretic used in the treatment of HF, moderate to low levels of potassium intake should be maintained to prevent development of hyperkalemia. Sodium intake is usually reduced to at least 2400 mg/day in patients with HF, but salt substitutes cannot be freely used because many contain high concentrations of potassium. Calcium intake is not increased.

17. d. Although all of these drugs may cause hypotension, nitroprusside is a potent dilator of both arteries and veins and may cause such marked hypotension that an inotropic agent (e.g., dobutamine) administration may be necessary to maintain the BP during its administration. Furosemide may cause hypotension because of diuretic-induced depletion of intravascular fluid volume. Milrinone has a positive inotropic effect in addition to peripheral vasodilation. Nitroglycerin is a vasodilator and can decrease BP but not as severely as nitroprusside. It primarily dilates veins and increases myocardial oxygen supply.

18. c. Not adding salt to foods will not eliminate enough sodium for the 2400-mg sodium diet. All foods that are high in sodium should be eliminated in a 2400-mg sodium diet, in addition to the elimination of salt during cooking. Examples include obviously salted foods as well as unexpected sodium sources that are identified by reading the label of prepared foods and medicines.

19.

Cardiovascular Condition Leading to HF	Preventive Measures
Hypertension	Use drugs, diet, and exercise to control
Valvular defects	Surgical replacement if contributing to HF and symptoms; prophylactic antibiotics
CAD	Coronary revascularization procedures; fibrinolytic therapy for occlusions
Dysrhythmias	Antidysrhythmic agents, pacemakers, or defibrillators to control; also, adequate treatment of pulmonary hypertension, hyperthyroidism, or myocarditis

20. c. Successful treatment of HF is indicated by an absence of symptoms of pulmonary edema and hypoxemia, such as clear lung sounds and a normal HR. Weight loss and diuresis, warm skin, less fatigue, and improved level of consciousness (LOC) may occur without resolution of pulmonary symptoms. Chest pain is not a common finding in HF unless coronary artery perfusion is impaired.

21. d. Further teaching is needed if the patient believes a weight gain of 2 to 3 pounds in 2 days is an indication for dieting. In a patient with HF, this type of weight gain reflects fluid retention and is a sign of HF that should be reported to the HCP. The other options show patient understanding of the HF management teaching (see Table 34.10).

22. d. The 52-year-old woman does not have any contraindications for cardiac transplantation, even though she lacks the indication of adequate financial resources. The 24-year-old man does not have a current cardiac diagnosis. The postoperative transplant regimen is complex and rigorous, and patients who have not been compliant with other treatments or who may not have the means to understand the care would not be good candidates. A history of drug or alcohol abuse is usually a contraindication to heart transplant.

23. a. In the first year after transplant, with the need for long-term immunosuppressant therapy to prevent rejection, the patient with a transplant is at high risk for infection, a leading cause of death in transplant patients. Acute rejection episodes may also cause death in patients with transplants, but many can be treated successfully with augmented immunosuppressive therapy. Malignancies occur in patients with organ transplants after taking immunosuppressants for a number of years.

24. d. The counterpulsation of the intraaortic balloon pump (IABP) increases diastolic arterial pressure, forcing blood back into the coronary arteries and main branches of the aortic arch, increasing coronary artery perfusion pressure and blood flow to the myocardium. The IABP also causes a drop in aortic pressure just before systole, decreasing afterload and myocardial oxygen consumption. These effects make the IABP valuable in treating unstable angina, acute myocardial infarction with cardiogenic shock, and a variety of surgical heart situations. Its use is contraindicated in incompetent aortic valves, dissecting

aortic and thoracic aneurysms, and generalized peripheral vascular disease.

25. d. During intraaortic counterpulsation, the balloon of the IABP is inflated during diastole and deflated during systole. This causes decreased HR, decreased peak systolic pressure, and decreased afterload. (See Table 65.6.)

26. c. Because the IABP is inserted into the femoral artery and advanced to the descending thoracic aorta, compromised distal extremity circulation is common and requires that the cannulated extremity be extended at all times. Repositioning the patient to prevent pneumonia is limited to side-lying or supine positions with the head of the bed elevated <45 degrees. Assessment for bleeding is important because the IABP may cause platelet destruction (not arterial trauma) and occlusive dressings are used to prevent site infection.

27. d. Weaning from the IABP involves reducing the pumping to every second or third heartbeat until the IABP catheter is removed. The pumping and infusion flow are continued to reduce the risk for thrombus formation around the catheter until it is removed.

28. b, c. Ventricular assist devices (VADs) are temporary devices that can partially or totally support circulation until the heart recovers and can be weaned from cardiopulmonary bypass, until a donor heart can be obtained, or for New York Heart Association Class IV heart disease patients who have failed medical therapy. An implantable artificial heart can now sustain the body's circulatory system for patients who are ineligible for a transplant.

Case Study

1. **Right-sided HF**: JVD, weight gain, peripheral edema, hepatomegaly; **Left-sided HF**: dyspnea, PMI displacement, hypotension, hypoxemia, blood-tinged frothy sputum (evidence of pulmonary edema); **Both**: tachycardia; **Unrelated**: pharyngitis, sleep apnea

2. **Indicated**: 12-lead ECG (patient has dysrhythmia), echocardiogram (can measure EF and assess valvular function and contractility), administer oxygen (to improve SpO_2), administer furosemide 20 mg IV (treats pulmonary edema); **Contraindicated**: place the patient in the supine position with legs raised (patient has difficulty breathing and hypoxemia which this position will exacerbate, in addition this position will increase preload to a heart that is experiencing failure and overload), place sequential compression devices on BLE (increases venous return and preload), administer 0.4 mg nitroglycerin SL (patient is hypotensive which NTG will worsen); **Non-essential**: ice chips, indwelling urinary catheter (is medically unnecessary and increases risk of infection)

3. **1**=bumetanide; **2**=50 mg PO once daily; **3**=ACE inhibitor; **4**=decreases preload; **5**=dabigatran; **6**=5 mg PO once daily (with a diuretic); **7**=cardiac glycoside; **8**=positive inotrope

4. **Effective**: EF 55% (normal is 55-65%), urine output 100 mL/hr (indicates adequate renal perfusion from adequate cardiac output), PAWP 8 mm Hg (represents normal LVEDP, normal is 6-12 mm Hg), SVR 1000 dynes/sec/cm^5 (normal is 800-1200 dynes/sec/cm^5, represents normal afterload); **Ineffective**: CVP 12 mm Hg (normal is 2-8 mm Hg, this CVP could indicate right-sided heart failure), MAP 55 mm Hg (normal is at least 65 mm Hg,

this MAP indicates decreased cardiac output), creatinine 2.5 (indicates acute kidney injury from decreased cardiac output and perfusion to the kidneys); **Unrelated**: temperature 99.0°F (37.2°C) (isn't relevant to heart failure), normal skin turgor (represents adequate fluid volume and hydration unrelated to heart failure)

5. A., C., D., F., H. The patient should be taught about adhering to the DASH diet which includes a sodium restriction. This patient should limit their sodium intake to 1500 mg/day. Activity should not be restricted and should be increased as tolerated. Vaping (or e-cigarettes) has nicotine and is not considered a good alternative to smoking tobacco products.

CHAPTER 39

1. c. The V_1 leads are placed toward each limb and centrally at the fourth intercostal space to the right of the sternal border. Depolarization of the ventricular cells produces the QRS interval on the electrocardiogram (ECG). The T wave is produced by repolarization of the ventricular cells. Abnormal cardiac impulses from the atria, ventricles, or atrioventricular (AV) junction create ectopic beats. Artifacts are seen with leads or electrodes that are not secure, with muscle activity or electrical interference. The rate produced by the AV node pacing in a junctional escape rhythm is 40 to 60 bpm. If the His-Purkinje system is blocked, the heart rate is 20 to 40 bpm.

2. d, f. The expected PR interval is 0.12 to 0.20 seconds and is measured from the beginning of the P wave to the beginning of the QRS complex. The T wave is 0.16 seconds, the QRS interval is < 0.12 seconds, the P wave is 0.06 to 0.12 seconds, and the QT interval is the time of depolarization and repolarization of the ventricles.

3. 4 (beats per 3 seconds) + 4 = 8 beats per 6 seconds × 10 = 80 bpm

4. 1500 ÷ 20 = 75 bpm

5. d. Automaticity describes the ability to discharge an electrical impulse spontaneously. Excitability is a property of myocardial tissue that enables it to be depolarized by an impulse. Contractility is the ability of the chambers to respond mechanically to an impulse. Conductivity is the ability to transmit an impulse along a membrane.

6. b. Refractory phase is the period in which heart tissue cannot be stimulated. Ectopic foci produce abnormal electrical impulses. Reentrant excitation causing premature beats may occur when areas of the heart do not repolarize simultaneously with depressed conduction. Depolarization of cardiac cells occurs when sodium migrates rapidly into the cell.

7. d. The normal PR interval is 0.12 to 0.20 seconds and reflects the time taken for the impulse to spread through the atria, AV node and bundle of His, the bundle branches, and Purkinje fibers. A PR interval of 6 small boxes is 0.24 second and indicates that the conduction of the impulse from the atria to the Purkinje fibers is delayed.

8. d. Electrophysiologic study (EPS) involves electrical stimulation to various areas of the atrium and ventricle to determine the inducibility of dysrhythmias and often induces ventricular tachycardia or ventricular fibrillation. The patient may have "near-death" experiences and requires emotional support if this occurs. Dye and anticoagulants are used for coronary angiograms.

9. d. In type II second-degree AV block, a P wave is nonconducted without progressive PR interval lengthening. It is usually from a block in a bundle branch, occurs in a ratio of 2 P waves–to–1 QRS complex, 3:1, and so on. Asystole is absence of ventricular activity. Atrial fibrillation has a chaotic P wave. First-degree AV block is a prolonged AV conduction time, so the PR interval is prolonged.

10. d. Pulseless electrical activity (PEA) occurs when there is electrical activity on the ECG but no mechanical activity on assessment and therefore no pulse. PEA is the most common dysrhythmia seen after defibrillation and may be caused by hypovolemia, hypoxia, metabolic acidosis, altered potassium level, hypoglycemia, hypothermia, toxins, cardiac tamponade, thrombosis, tension pneumothorax, and trauma. Dissociated atria and ventricles is a third-degree AV block.

11. c. The premature atrial contraction (PAC) has a distorted P wave that may feel like a skipped beat to the patient. Atrial flutter is an atrial tachydysrhythmia with recurring, regular, saw-toothed flutter waves from the same focus in the right or possibly left atrium. Sinus bradycardia has a regular heart rate <100 bpm. Paroxysmal supraventricular tachycardia (PSVT) starts in an ectopic focus above the bundle of His and may be triggered by PAC. If seen, the P wave may have an abnormal shape and has a spontaneous start and termination with a rate of 150 to 220 bpm.

12. b. Third-degree or complete heart block is recognized with the atrial and ventricular dissociation and treated with a pacemaker. Sinus bradycardia does not have atrial and ventricular dissociation. Atrial fibrillation does not have normal P waves, as they are stimulated by ectopic foci. In type I second-degree AV heart block, the PR interval gradually lengthens and a QRS complex is dropped. Then the cycle begins again.

13. b. When premature ventricular contraction (PVC) falls on the T wave of the preceding beat, R-on-T phenomenon occurs. Because the ventricle is repolarizing and there is increased excitability of cardiac cells, there is an increased risk of ventricular tachycardia or ventricular fibrillation. The other options do not increase this risk.

14. d. Although many factors can cause a sinus tachycardia, in the patient who has had an acute myocardial infarction (MI), tachycardia increases myocardial oxygen need in a heart that already has impaired circulation and may lead to increasing angina and further ischemia and necrosis.

15. a. A distorted P wave with normal conduction of the impulse through the ventricles is characteristic of a PAC. In a normal heart, this dysrhythmia is frequently associated with emotional stress or the use of caffeine, tobacco, or alcohol. Sedatives rarely slow the heart rate (HR). Aerobic conditioning and holding of breath during exertion (Valsalva maneuver) often cause bradycardia, but the P wave is not distorted.

16. a. A rhythm pattern that is normal except for a prolonged PR interval is characteristic of a first-degree heart block. First-degree heart blocks are not treated but are observed for progression to higher degrees of heart block. Atropine is administered for bradycardia. Synchronized cardioversion is used for atrial fibrillation with a rapid ventricular response or PSVT. Pacemakers are used for higher-degree heart blocks.

17. b. Symptoms of decreased cardiac output (CO) related to dysrhythmias include a sudden drop in BP and symptoms of hypoxemia, such as decreased mentation, chest pain, and dyspnea. Peripheral pulses are weak and the HR may be increased or decreased, depending on the type of dysrhythmia present.

18. c. Multifocal PVCs in a patient with an MI indicate significant ventricular irritability that may lead to ventricular tachycardia or ventricular fibrillation. Preparing to administer antidysrhythmics, such as β-adrenergic blockers, procainamide, amiodarone, or lidocaine, is the priority to control the dysrhythmias. Valsalva maneuver may be used to treat PSVT. The nurse must always be ready to perform cardiopulmonary resuscitation (CPR), but drugs may prevent this need.

19. a. PVC is an ectopic beat that causes a wide, distorted QRS complex ≥ 0.12 second because the impulse is not conducted normally through the ventricles. Because it is premature, it precedes the P wave and the P wave may be hidden in the QRS complex, or the ventricular impulse may be conducted retrograde and the P wave may be seen following the PVC, but the rhythm is not regular. Continuous wide QRS complexes with a ventricular rate between 150 and 250 bpm are seen in ventricular tachycardia, whereas saw-toothed P waves are characteristic of atrial flutter.

20. c. The intent of defibrillation is to apply an electrical current to the heart that will depolarize the cells of the myocardium so that subsequent repolarization of the cells will allow the SA node to resume the role of pacemaker. An artificial pacemaker provides an electrical impulse that stimulates normal myocardial contractions. Synchronized cardioversion involves delivery of a shock that is programmed to occur during the QRS complex of the ECG, but this cannot be done during ventricular fibrillation because there is no normal ventricular contraction or QRS complex.

21. a. In preparation for defibrillation the nurse should apply conductive materials (e.g., saline pads, electrode gel, defibrillator gel pads) to the patient's chest to decrease electrical impedance and prevent burns. For defibrillation, the initial shock is 120 to 200 joules with biphasic defibrillators, 360 joules with monophasic, and the synchronizer switch used for cardioversion must be turned off. Be sure all staff are clear of the patient and bed before defibrillating. Sedatives may be used before cardioversion if the patient is conscious, but the patient in ventricular fibrillation is unconscious.

22. b. If the implanted cardioverter-defibrillator delivers a shock, the patient has experienced a lethal dysrhythmia and needs to notify the cardiologist. The patient will want to lie down to allow recovery from the dysrhythmia. In the event that the patient loses consciousness or there is repetitive firing, a call should be placed to the emergency response system (ERS) by anyone who finds the patient.

23. b. The patient should avoid standing near antitheft devices in doorways of department stores and libraries but walking through them at normal pace is fine. High-output electrical generators or large magnets, such as those used in MRI, can reprogram pacemakers and should be avoided unless the pacemaker is MRI safe. Microwave ovens pose no problems to pacemaker function, but the affected arm should not be raised above the shoulder until approved by cardiologist. The pacing current of an implanted pacemaker

is not felt by the patient, but an external transcutaneous pacemaker may cause uncomfortable chest muscle contractions.

24. a. Until the defibrillator is available, the patient needs CPR. Defibrillation is needed as soon as possible, so someone should bring the crash cart to the room. Amiodarone is an antidysrhythmic that is part of the advanced cardiac life support (ACLS) protocol for ventricular fibrillation. Defibrillation would be with 360 joules for monophasic defibrillators and 120 to 200 joules for biphasic defibrillators.

25. c. Catheter ablation therapy uses radiofrequency energy to ablate or "burn" accessory pathways or ectopic sites in the atria, AV node, or ventricles that cause tachydysrhythmias. It is not used for sinus arrest, heart blocks, or premature ventricular beats.

26. c. ST segment elevation indicates injury or infarction of an area of the heart. A widened QRS occurs with second-degree AV block, type II and antidysrhythmic drugs. Occasional PVCs may be normal or may be the result of electrolyte imbalance or hypoxia. They require continued observation. A PR interval of 0.18 second is within normal range.

27. d. One of the most common causes of syncope is cardioneurogenic syncope, or "vasovagal" syncope. In this type of syncope, there is accentuated adrenergic activity in the upright position, with intense activation of cardiopulmonary receptors resulting in marked bradycardia and hypotension, cerebral hypoperfusion, and syncope. Normally testing with the head-up tilt-test causes activation of the renin-angiotensin-aldosterone system and compensation to increase CO and maintain BP when blood pools in the extremities.

28. d. ST segment elevation is seen in myocardial injury. An absent or buried P wave can occur with PVCs, ventricular tachycardia, or ventricular fibrillation. A wide pathologic QT interval affects repolarization and is caused by drugs and electrolyte imbalances. Tall, peaked T waves may be seen with electrolyte imbalance.

29. a. Third-degree block, characterized by atrial and ventricular dissociation with regular atrial rate b. Atrial flutter, saw-toothed flutter waves from same ectopic foci c. PVC, unifocal bigeminal, early occurrence of wide, distorted QRS complex every other beat d. Sinus bradycardia with ST depression, rate <60 bpm e. Second-degree block, type I, progressively lengthening PR interval until a QRS complex is blocked; left bundle branch block f. PAC, irregular rate and rhythm and different P wave shape g. Second-degree block, type II, regular atrial rate and PR interval, ventricular rate irregular with blocked QRS complexes h. Sinus tachycardia, rate >100 bpm but <180 bpm i. First-degree block, PR interval >0.20; QRS is >0.12 which indicates a bundle branch block j. Ventricular fibrillation, irregular chaotic waveforms of varying shapes and amplitude k. PVC, trigeminal, unifocal, early occurrence of wide, distorted QRS complex every third beat l. Atrial fibrillation, accelerated atrial rate with chaotic fibrillatory waves and irregular ventricular rate; controlled ventricular response as HR is <101 bpm m. Normal sinus rhythm with a run of PSVT; atrial and ventricular rate increases to 375 bpm briefly before normal conduction resumes; PSVT run could be caused by an atrial

dysrhythmia, such as atrial fibrillation or atrial flutter n. Normal sinus rhythm, starts at sinoatrial (SA) node with rate of 60 to 100 bpm and follows normal conduction pathway o. Monomorphic ventricular tachycardia, rate of 150 to 250 bpm with wide distorted QRS complex

Case Study

1. **Anticipated**: oxygen via simple mask (patient is short of breath and has RR 32 breaths/min); facilitate an echocardiogram (to assess blood flow through the cardiac chambers and estimate ejection fraction); position HOB at 45 degrees (to address respiratory difficulty); **Contraindicated**: atropine (is used to treat symptomatic bradycardia and causes an increase in HR which is contraindicated in a patient who has atrial fibrillation with a HR of 150); **Non-essential**: ambulate the patient to the bathroom (this activity isn't relevant to managing this patient's condition; plus, if the patient is orthostatic, ambulation would be unsafe); cardiac enzymes (there is no evidence supporting a coronary artery obstruction or MI).

2. **Pulmonary edema**: chest x-ray (would identify fluid in the lungs); furosemide (is a loop diuretic that is used to treat pulmonary edema); **Angina**: 12-lead ECG (a diagnostic tool to identify ST elevation and other causes of angina); nitroglycerin (treats angina); **Embolus**: warfarin (an anticoagulant to prevent blood clot formation); neurologic assessment (identifies signs and symptoms of stroke if embolus travels to the brain). Incentive spirometer isn't relevant as it won't help pulmonary edema.

3. A., B., E., G., H. IV access will be necessary to administer sedation and any emergency medications if necessary. Multifunction pads will be necessary to deliver the electricity for cardioversion. Paddles can be used, but using multifunction pads is the safest and most beneficial delivery method. Synchronization is necessary for cardioversion so the energy is delivered on the R wave and not on the T wave. Synchronization is contraindicated when defibrillating. The energy selection for synchronized cardioversion should start at 50 joules and increase to 100 joules if necessary. The electricity may cause minor skin burns and irritation. The nurse should assess for signs and apply lotions or other ointments if necessary to treat the burn. Sedation is administered via the IV route as PO sedation will take too long to take effect and will not wear off as quickly. Before delivery of any energy from the defibrillator, the person discharging the energy should announce "all clear, everyone clear" and look to make sure no one is touching the patient or any part of the bed. Patients may become incontinent during the procedure, so having them void prior to the procedure may prevent them from urinating on themselves. CPR is only necessary if the patient experiences pulselessness during the procedure.

4. **Effective**: HR 98 beats/min (is lower than the HR upon admission which was 150 beats/min); breath sounds are clear (indicates pulmonary edema has resolved and may indicate the heart is pumping blood effectively instead of blood regurgitating into the lungs); patient can stand without dizziness (indicates that cardiac output is sufficient to meet the patient's activity); **Ineffective**: rhythm is irregular and the patient reports palpitations (may indicate the patient is still in atrial fibrillation); **Unrelated**: patient is oriented x3 (this doesn't pertain to the patient's cardiac

condition); urine output is 100 mL/hr (this doesn't indicate that the patient's condition has changed or improved).

5. **1**=digoxin; **2**=125 mcg once daily; **3**=heart rate control; **4**=0.25 mg/kg IV once; **5**=enoxaparin; **6**=ACE inhibitor; **7**=anticoagulant.

CHAPTER 40

1. a, b, c, d, e. Recent dental, urologic, surgical, or gynecologic procedures and history of IV drug abuse, heart disease, cardiac catheterization or surgery, renal dialysis, and infections all increase the risk of infective endocarditis.

2. a. Three positive blood cultures drawn over a 1-hour period from 3 different sites are the primary diagnostic tool for infective endocarditis. Although a complete blood count (CBC) will reveal a mild leukocytosis, this is a nonspecific finding. Cardiac catheterization is used when surgical intervention is being considered. Transesophageal echocardiograms can identify vegetations on valves but are used when blood cultures are negative.

3. a. Petechiae from fragmentation and microembolization of vegetative lesions are seen as small hemorrhages in the conjunctiva, lips, and buccal mucosa and over the ankles, feet, and antecubital and popliteal areas. Roth's spots are hemorrhagic retinal lesions seen with funduscopic examination. Osler's nodes are lesions on the fingertips or toes. The cause of Roth's spots and Osler's nodes is not clear. Splinter hemorrhages are black longitudinal streaks that occur on nail beds. They may be caused by vessel damage from vasculitis or microemboli.

4. d. Janeway's lesions are flat, painless, small red spots found on the fingertips, palms of hands, the soles of feet, and toes. Hemorrhagic retinal lesions are Roth's spots. Black streaks on the nails are splinter hemorrhages. Painful lesions on the fingertips and toes are Osler's nodes.

5. b. Early valve replacement followed by prolonged antibiotic and anticoagulant therapy is recommended for these patients. Drug therapy for patients who develop endocarditis of prosthetic valves is often unsuccessful in eliminating the infection and preventing embolization.

6. c. The dyspnea, crackles, and restlessness that the patient is manifesting are manifestations of heart failure and decreased cardiac output (CO) that occurs in up to 80% of patients with aortic valve endocarditis because of aortic valve incompetence. Pulmonary emboli occur in right-sided endocarditis. Vegetative embolization from the aortic valve occurs throughout the arterial system and may affect any body organ.

7. d. The patient with outpatient antibiotic therapy needs vigilant home nursing care. It is most important to determine the adequacy of the home environment for successful management of the patient. The patient is at risk for life-threatening complications, such as embolization and pulmonary edema, and must be able to access a hospital if needed. Bed rest will not be necessary for the patient without heart damage. Avoiding infections and planning diversional activities are indicated for the patient but are not the most important factors while he is on outpatient antibiotic therapy.

8. d. Prophylactic antibiotic therapy should be started before invasive dental, medical, or surgical procedures to prevent recurrence of endocarditis. Symptoms of infection should be treated promptly, but antibiotics are not used for exposure to infection. Continuous antibiotic therapy is indicated only in patients with implanted devices or ongoing invasive procedure.

9. d. The stethoscope diaphragm at the lower left sternal border with the patient leaning forward is the best method to use to hear the high-pitched, grating sound of a pericardial friction rub. The sound does not radiate widely and occurs with the heartbeat. To differentiate a pericardial friction rub from a pleural friction rub, have the patient hold their breath. The rub will still be heard if it is cardiac in nature.

10. b. The patient is experiencing cardiac tamponade that consists of excess fluid in the pericardial sac, which compresses the heart and the adjoining structures, preventing normal filling and cardiac output. A scarred and thickened pericardium, adherent pericardial membranes, and fibrin accumulation occur in chronic constrictive pericarditis.

11. b, e. Pulsus paradoxus is measured with a manually operated sphygmomanometer. The cuff is deflated slowly until the first Korotkoff sound during expiration is heard and the number is noted. The slow deflation of the cuff is continued until sounds are heard throughout the respiratory cycle and that number is subtracted from the first number. When the difference is > 10 mm Hg, cardiac tamponade may be present. The difference is normally < 10 mm Hg.

12. b. Pneumothorax may occur as a needle is inserted into the pericardial space to remove fluid for analysis and relieve cardiac pressure with pericardiocentesis. Other complications could include dysrhythmias, further cardiac tamponade, pneumomediastinum myocardial laceration, and coronary artery laceration. Pneumonia, myocardial infarction (MI), and cerebrovascular accident (CVA) would not be expected.

13. d. Relief from pericardial pain is often obtained by sitting up and leaning forward. Pain is increased by lying flat. Antiinflammatory medications may also be used to help control pain, but opioids are not usually indicated. The pain has a sharp, pleuritic quality that changes with respiration, and patients take shallow breaths.

14. b. Viruses are the most common cause of myocarditis in the United States, and early manifestations of myocarditis are often those of systemic viral infections. Myocarditis may also be associated with autoimmune disorders as well as with other microorganisms, drugs, or toxins. The patient with myocarditis is predisposed to drug-related dysrhythmias and toxicity with digoxin, so it is used very cautiously, if at all, in treatment of the condition, but digoxin does not lead to myocarditis. A streptococcal infection is more likely to lead to rheumatic fever.

15. d. Adequate treatment of group A streptococcal pharyngitis can prevent initial attacks of rheumatic fever and the development of rheumatic heart disease. Because

streptococcal infection accounts for only about 20% of acute pharyngitis, cultures should be done to identify the organism and direct antibiotic therapy. Viral infections should not be treated with antibiotics. Prophylactic therapy is indicated in those who have valvular heart disease or have had rheumatic heart disease.

16. a. Two major criteria; 1 major and 2 minor criteria plus laboratory evidence of a preceding group A streptococcal infection indicate rheumatic fever. Major criteria for the diagnosis of rheumatic fever include evidence of carditis, polyarthritis, erythema marginatum, Sydenham's chorea (often very late), and subcutaneous nodules. Minor criteria include ↑ erythrocyte sedimentation rate (ESR) and/or ↑ C-reactive protein (CRP), fever, arthralgia.

17.

Drug	Rationale for Use
Antibiotics	To eliminate any residual group A β-hemolytic streptococci; prevent spread of infection; prevent recurrent infection
Aspirin	Antiinflammatory effect to control fever and arthritic and joint manifestations
Corticosteroids	Antiinflammatory effect to control fever and inflammation of severe carditis
Nonsteroidal antiinflammatory drugs (NSAIDs)	Antiinflammatory effect to control fever and joint manifestations

18. b. When carditis is present in the patient with rheumatic fever, ambulation is postponed until any symptoms of heart failure are controlled with treatment, and activity cannot be resumed until acute inflammation has subsided. In the patient without cardiac involvement, ambulation may be permitted as soon as acute symptoms have subsided, and normal activity can be resumed when antiinflammatory therapy is discontinued.

19. d. Valvular regurgitation causes a backward flow of blood and volume overload in the preceding chamber. Without treatment, eventually hypertrophy of that chamber occurs. Stenosis causes a pressure gradient difference and decreased blood flow and hypertrophy of the preceding chamber. A pericardial friction rub is not related to valvular regurgitation but would be heard at the lower left sternal border of the chest.

20. c. Monitoring vital signs before and after ambulation is the collection of data. Instructions should be provided to the LPN about what changes in these vital signs should be reported to the RN. The other actions listed are RN responsibilities.

21. c. Mitral valve prolapse is the buckling of the valve leaflets into the left atrium during ventricular systole. The rapid onset that prevents left chamber dilation and the rapid development of pulmonary edema and cardiogenic shock occur with acute mitral regurgitation. Pulmonary hypertension may contribute to tricuspid valve disease.

22. d. Acute aortic regurgitation causes a sudden cardiovascular collapse. With mitral valve stenosis, dyspnea is a prominent symptom, and embolization may result from chronic

atrial fibrillation. With tricuspid and pulmonic valve diseases, stenosis occurs more often than regurgitation. Tricuspid valve stenosis results in right atrial enlargement and elevated systemic venous pressures. Pulmonic valve stenosis results in right ventricular hypertension and hypertrophy.

23. b. Aortic valve stenosis is identified with the triad of angina, syncope, and dyspnea on exertion, as well as the systolic murmur and prominent S$_4$ heart sound. Mitral valve stenosis manifests as exertional dyspnea, hemoptysis, fatigue, atrial fibrillation, and a diastolic murmur. Acute mitral valve regurgitation has a new systolic murmur with pulmonary edema and cardiogenic shock rapidly developing. Chronic mitral valve regurgitation is identified with weakness, fatigue, exertional dyspnea, palpitations, an S$_3$ gallop, and holosystolic murmur.

24. b. Patients with mechanical valves have an increased risk for thromboembolism and require long-term anticoagulation to prevent systemic or pulmonary embolization. Nitrates are contraindicated for the patient with aortic stenosis because an adequate preload is necessary to open the stiffened aortic valve. Antidysrhythmics are used only if dysrhythmias occur and β-adrenergic blocking drugs may be used to control the heart rate if needed.

25. b. Dysrhythmias often cause palpitations, lightheadedness, and dizziness and the patient should be carefully attended to prevent falls. Hypervolemia and paroxysmal nocturnal dyspnea (PND) would be apparent in the patient with heart failure. Exercises will not prevent dysrhythmias.

26. c. This procedure has been used for repair of mitral, tricuspid, and pulmonic stenosis and less often for aortic stenosis. It is usually used for older patients and for those patients who are poor surgical risks because it is relatively easy and has good results and few complications.

27. c. Repair of mitral or tricuspid valves has a lower operative mortality rate than does replacement and is usually the surgical procedure of choice for these valvular diseases. Open repair is more precise than closed repair and requires cardiopulmonary bypass during surgery. All types of valve surgery are palliative, not curative, and patients require lifelong health care. Anticoagulation therapy is used for all valve surgery for at least some time postoperatively.

28. c. Mechanical prosthetic valves require long-term anticoagulation, and this is a factor in deciding about the type of valve to use for replacement. Patients who cannot take anticoagulant therapy, such as patients at risk for hemorrhage, women of childbearing age, patients who may not be compliant with anticoagulation therapy, and patients over age 65 years may be candidates for the less durable biologic valves.

29. d. The greatest risk to a patient who has an artificial valve is the development of endocarditis with invasive medical or dental procedures, not bleeding. Before any of these procedures, antibiotic prophylaxis is necessary to prevent infection. Planning of an exercise program and monitoring anticoagulant therapy will be done.

30. b. A secondary cause of restrictive cardiomyopathy (CMP) is radiation treatment to the thorax with stiffness of the ventricular wall occurring. Dilated CMP may have a genetic link, follow infectious myocarditis, or be related to an autoimmune process or excess alcohol ingestion. Takotsubo CMP is an acute stress-related syndrome that mimics acute coronary syndrome. It is most common in postmenopausal women. Hypertrophic CMP has a genetic link in about one-half of all cases and is often seen in young athletic individuals.

31. d, e, f. Dilated CMP, the most common type of CMP, reveals cardiomegaly with thin ventricular walls on echocardiogram, as there is no ventricular hypertrophy, and may follow an infective myocarditis. In addition, stasis of blood in the ventricles may contribute to systemic embolization. Restrictive CMP is the least common type and is characterized by ventricular stiffness. Hypertrophic CMP is characterized by massive ventricular hypertrophy and rapid, forceful contraction of the left ventricle, impaired relaxation (diastole), and obstructed aortic valve outflow.

32. c. Nursing interventions for the patient with hypertrophic CMP are to improve ventricular filling by reducing ventricular contractility and relieving left ventricular outflow obstruction to relieve symptoms and prevent complications. Strenuous activity and dehydration will increase systemic vascular resistance and should be avoided. Atrioventricular pacing will allow the septum to move away from the left ventricular wall and reduce the degree of outflow obstruction. Vasodilators may decrease venous return and further increase obstruction of blood flow from the heart. The surgery that could be done involves cutting into the thickened septal wall and removing some of the ventricular muscle.

33. a, c, d, e, f. These topics can apply to any patient with CMP. Going to the gym could only be included within the exercise guidelines from the HCP and balanced with rest.

Case Study

1. The following diagnostic results are abnormal and should be followed up by the nurse and reported to the health care provider: C-reactive protein (indicates inflammation), echocardiogram (vegetation is abnormal), 12-lead ECG results (heart block is abnormal), WBC (leukocytosis indicates infection), neutrophils (indicates infection), hemoglobin (indicates anemia), creatinine (indicates renal insufficiency or injury). Troponins are abnormal but are not likely elevated enough to indicate an MI. They should be rechecked in 3-6 hours.

2. Appropriate interventions for **hyperthermia** include administering acetaminophen since it is an antipyretic and administering a fluid bolus since fever can cause insensible fluid loss, vasodilation, and dehydration. Appropriate interventions for **impaired mobility** include an every 2-hour turning scheduled while on bedrest to prevent pressure injuries, apply sequential compression devices to promote lower extremity circulation and prevent VTE, and advocating for physical therapy to perform ROM exercises and assist with mobility when the patient is able to participate. Appropriate interventions for **infection** include administering antibiotics and monitoring for signs of infection by taking the patient's temperature. A

dietary consult and monitoring FSBG before meals aren't interventions that are relevant to any of these clinical problems.

3. **1**=*Staphylococcus aureus;* **2**=vegetations (fragmenting and embolizing); **3**=murmurs (if aortic valve is involved) and fever (the most common patient presentation); **4**=55% (50% to 60% require valvular surgery); **5**=renal failure, CVA, limb infarctions (left-sided vegetations) and pulmonary emboli (right-sided vegetations).

4. **Effective** assessment findings include: temperature of 37.9°C as this is lower than his previous temperature of 39.4°C; urine output greater than 1 mL/kg/hour indicates adequate perfusion to the kidneys; respiratory rate of 18 breath/min are normal for an adult and also less than 26 breaths/min during the previous assessment. **Ineffective** assessment findings include: crackles in bilateral bases which indicates fluid in the lungs possibly caused by impaired cardiac function; bilateral lower extremities that are cool and pale with greater than 3 seconds capillary refill indicate decreased tissue perfusion possibly caused by impaired cardiac function. **Unrelated** findings include negative urine ketones, which would be evaluated in patients with diabetes, and positive Trousseau sign, which indicates serum calcium abnormalities.

5. B, C, E, H. The patient shouldn't be on complete bedrest unless they have a fever or complications of infective endocarditis (e.g., heart damage). Signs and symptoms of cardiac dysfunction, such as difficulty breathing, or infection, such as fever, chills, arthralgias, etc., should be reported to the HCP in addition to any signs and symptoms of cold, flu, or upper respiratory infection. Nitroglycerin tablets would not be prescribed to this patient, unless he experienced heart damage, like an MI. Any invasive procedures, such as dental procedures, may require prophylactic antibiotics; therefore, the dentist should be informed. Steps to prevent infection, like hand washing and mask wearing, would be recommended. Fluids wouldn't routinely be restricted unless the patient was in congestive heart failure.

CHAPTER 41

1. d. Regardless of the location, atherosclerosis is responsible for peripheral arterial disease (PAD) and is related to other cardiovascular disease and its risk factors, such as coronary artery disease (CAD) and carotid artery disease. Venous thrombosis, venous stasis ulcers, and pulmonary embolism are diseases of the veins and are not related to atherosclerosis.

2. $102 \div 132 = 0.77$; mild (see Table 41.3)

3. c. Pentoxifylline allows blood cells to pass through small vessels, but there are no blood tests related to it. Warfarin (Coumadin), which needs international normalized ration (INR) blood tests, is not recommended for prevention of cardiovascular disease (CVD) events in patients with PAD. All the other statements are correct in relation to treatment of PAD.

4. b, c, e. Protecting feet and legs from injury is important. Walking exercise increases oxygen extraction in the legs and improves skeletal muscle metabolism. The patient with PAD should walk at least 30 minutes a day, at least 3 times per week. Exercise should be stopped when pain

occurs and resumed when the pain subsides. The lower extremities should be assessed at regular intervals for changes. Cold compresses and nicotine in all forms causes vasoconstriction and should be avoided.

5. b. PAD occurs as a result of atherosclerosis and the risk factors are the same as for other diseases associated with atherosclerosis, such as CAD, cerebrovascular disease, and aneurysms. Major risk factors are tobacco use, hyperlipidemia, elevated C-reactive protein, diabetes, obesity, and uncontrolled hypertension. The risk for amputation is high in patients with severe occlusive disease, but this is not the best approach to encourage patients to make lifestyle modifications.

6. c. Loss of palpable pulses, numbness and tingling of the extremity, extremity pallor, cyanosis, or cold are indications of occlusion of the bypass graft and need immediate medical attention. Pain, redness, and serous drainage at the incision site are expected postoperatively. Ankle brachial index measurements are not recommended because of increased risk for graft thrombosis, but this would decrease with occlusion.

7. a. Pain; b. pallor; c. pulselessness; d. paresthesia; e. paralysis; f. poikilothermia. The HCP requires immediate notification to begin immediate intervention to prevent tissue necrosis and gangrene.

8. b, d, f. Arterial leg ulcers and/or gangrene of the leg caused by PAD and chronic ischemic rest pain lasting more than 2 weeks characterize critical limb ischemia. Optimal therapy is revascularization via bypass surgery.

9. a, b, c, d, f. Raynaud's phenomenon is predominant in young females and may be associated with autoimmune disorders (e.g., rheumatoid arthritis, scleroderma, systemic lupus erythematosus). Incidents occur with cold, emotional upsets, and caffeine or tobacco use because of vasoconstrictive effects. Small cutaneous arteries are involved and cause color changes of the fingertips or toes. When conservative management is ineffective, it may be treated with nifedipine (Procardia).

10. d. The fusiform aneurysm is circumferential and relatively uniform in shape. The false aneurysm or pseudoaneurysm is not an aneurysm but a disruption of all the arterial wall layers with bleeding that is contained by surrounding anatomic structures. Saccular aneurysms are the pouchlike bulge of an artery.

11. c. Although most abdominal aortic aneurysms (AAAs) are asymptomatic, on physical examination a pulsatile mass in the periumbilical area slightly to the left of the midline may be detected and bruits may be audible with a stethoscope placed over the aneurysm. Hoarseness and dysphagia may occur with aneurysms of the ascending aorta and the aortic arch. Severe back pain with flank ecchymosis is usually present on rupture of an AAA and neurovascular loss in the lower extremities may occur from pressure of a thoracic aneurysm.

12. d. A CT scan is the most accurate test to determine the length and diameter of the aneurysm and whether a thrombus is present. The other tests may also be used, but the CT scan yields the most descriptive results.

13. b. Increased systolic BP (SBP) continually puts pressure on the diseased area of the artery, promoting its expansion. Small aneurysms can be treated by decreasing BP, modifying atherosclerosis risk factors, and monitoring

the size of the aneurysm. Anticoagulants are used during surgical treatment of aneurysms, but physical activity is not known to increase their size. Calcium intake is not related to calcification in arteries.

14. b. Because atherosclerosis is a systemic disease, the patient with an AAA is likely to have cardiac, pulmonary, cerebral, or lower extremity vascular problems that should be noted and monitored throughout the perioperative period. Postoperatively, the BP is balanced: high enough to keep adequate flow through the artery to prevent thrombosis but low enough to prevent bleeding at the surgical site.

15. a. With the aortic cross-clamping proximal and distal to the aneurysm, the open aneurysm repair (OAR) above the renal artery may cause kidney injury from lack of blood flow during the surgery. The saccular aneurysm may involve excising only the weakened area of the artery and suturing the artery closed, but this will not decrease renal blood flow. Renal blood flow will not be directly obstructed using the bifurcated graft or the minimally invasive endovascular aneurysm repair.

16. a. Usually aortic surgery patients will have a bowel preparation, skin cleansing with an antimicrobial agent on the day before surgery, nothing by mouth after midnight on the day of the surgery, and IV antibiotics immediately before the incision is made. Patients with a history of CVD will receive a β-adrenergic blocker preoperatively to reduce morbidity and mortality. Each surgeon's protocol may be different.

17. c. The BP and peripheral pulses are evaluated every hour in the acute postoperative period to ensure that BP is adequate to maintain graft patency and that extremities are being perfused. BP is kept within normal range. If BP is too low, thrombosis of the graft may occur; if it is too high, it may cause leaking or rupture at the suture line. Hypothermia is induced during surgery, but the patient is rewarmed as soon as surgery is over. Fluid replacement to maintain urine output at 100 mL/hr would increase the BP too much and only 30 mL/hr of urine is needed to show adequate renal perfusion.

18. c. During repair of an ascending aortic aneurysm, the blood supply to the carotid arteries may be interrupted, leading to neurologic complications manifested by a decreased level of consciousness (LOC) and altered pupil responses to light as well as changes in facial symmetry, speech, upper extremity movement, and hand grasp quality. The thorax is opened for ascending aortic surgery, and shallow breathing, poor cough, and decreasing chest drainage are expected. Lower limb pulses may normally be decreased or absent for a short time following surgery.

19. d. Decreased or absent pulses in conjunction with cool, painful extremities below the level of repair indicate graft thrombosis. Dysrhythmias or chest pain indicates myocardial ischemia. Absent bowel sounds, abdominal distention, diarrhea, or bloody stools indicate bowel infarction. Increased temperature and white blood cells (WBCs), surgical site inflammation, or drainage indicates graft infection.

20. b. The decreasing urine output is evidence that either the patient needs volume replacement or there is reduced renal blood flow. The HCP will want to be notified as soon as possible of this change in condition and will request results of daily blood urea nitrogen (BUN) and serum creatinine levels. The other options are incorrect.

21. d. Patients are taught to palpate peripheral pulses to identify changes in their quality or strength, but the rate is not a significant factor in peripheral perfusion. The color and temperature of the extremities are important for patients to observe. The remaining statements are true.

22. c. A Type B aortic dissection involves the distal descending aorta and is usually characterized by a sudden, severe, tearing pain in the back. As it progresses down the aorta, the kidneys, abdominal organs, and lower extremities may begin to show evidence of ischemia. Type A aortic dissections of the ascending aorta and aortic arch may affect the heart and circulation to the head, with the development of cerebral ischemia, murmurs, ventricular failure, and pulmonary edema.

23. a. Immediate surgery is indicated when complications (such as occlusion of the carotid arteries) occur. Otherwise, initial treatment for aortic dissection involves a period of lowering the BP and myocardial contractility to diminish the pulsatile forces in the aorta. Anticoagulants would prolong and intensify the bleeding. Blood is given only if the dissection ruptures.

24. a. Relief of pain is a sign that the dissection has stabilized, and it may be treated conservatively for an extended time with drugs that lower the BP and decrease myocardial contractility. Surgery is usually indicated for Type A aortic dissection or if complications occur.

25. b, d, e, f. PAD is manifested as thick, brittle nails; decreased peripheral pulses; pallor when the legs are elevated; ulcers over bony prominences on the toes and feet; and paresthesia. The other options are characteristic of venous disease and paresthesia could occur with venous thromboembolism (VTE).

26. b. If left untreated, a superficial vein thrombosis (SVT) may extend to deeper veins and VTE may occur. VTE may embolize to the lungs and have tenderness to pressure and edema. SVTs usually occur in superficial leg veins and have tenderness, itchiness, redness, warmth, pain, inflammation, and induration along the course of the superficial vein.

27. a, b, d, e, f. This patient is a smoker and on hormone therapy, both of which increase blood hypercoagulability. She will have an IV, and her fractured hip can cause VTE by damaging the venous endothelium. She is an older patient who has had an orthopedic surgery and may have experienced prolonged immobility postinjury and through her "lengthy hip replacement surgery," which contributes to venous stasis. These are representative of Virchow's triad in this patient. The other options are also related to Virchow's triad but not present in this patient via the transfer report.

28. a. With manifestations of a VTE, the Duplex ultrasound is most widely used to diagnose VTE by identifying where a thrombus is found and its extent. D-dimer may also be drawn to determine if a VTE exists.

29. c. The RN could delegate to the AP the task to remind the patient to flex and extend the legs and feet every 2 hours while in bed. Measuring for elastic compression stockings may be delegated to the LPN. The RN must assess and teach the patient.

30. d. With acute VTE, prevention of emboli formation, decreased edema and pain can be achieved initially by bed rest and limiting movement of the involved extremity. Ambulation will be the next priority. Dangling the legs promotes venous stasis and further clot formation. Elevating the affected limb will promote venous return, but it does not prevent embolization.

31. d. Low-molecular-weight heparin (LMWH) (enoxaparin [Lovenox]) is only given subcutaneously and does not need routine coagulation testing. Unfractionated heparin is the only other indirect thrombin inhibitor option. It can be given subcutaneously or IV and therapeutic effects must be monitored with coagulation testing.

32. a, e. Warfarin (Coumadin) is a vitamin K antagonist, so vitamin K is the antidote. It is monitored with the INR. It is only given orally. Protamine sulfate is the antidote for unfractionated heparin (UH) and LMWH. UH can be given subcutaneously or IV. It is monitored with activated partial thromboplastin time (aPTT). Hirudin derivatives are given IV or subcutaneously, do not have an antidote, and are monitored with aPTT. Argatroban, a synthetic thrombin inhibitor, is given only IV and is monitored with aPTT. Factor Xa inhibitor, fondaparinux (Arixtra), is given subcutaneously and does not need routine coagulation testing. Rivaroxaban (Xarelto), another factor Xa inhibitor, is given orally.

33. b. Anticoagulant therapy with heparin or warfarin (Coumadin) does not dissolve clots but prevents propagation of the clot, development of new thrombi, and embolization. Clot lysis occurs naturally through the body's intrinsic fibrinolytic system or by the administration of thrombolytic agents.

34. d. Exercise programs for patients recovering from VTE should emphasize swimming, which is particularly beneficial because of the gentle, even pressure of the water. Coumadin will not blacken stools. If this occurs, it could be a sign of gastrointestinal bleeding. Dark green and leafy vegetables have high amounts of vitamin K and should not be increased during Coumadin therapy, but they do not need to be restricted. The legs must not be massaged because of the risk for dislodging any clots that may be present.

35. a. During walking, the muscles of the legs continuously knead the veins, promoting movement of venous blood toward the heart. Walking is the best measure to prevent venous stasis and will be increased gradually. Elevating the legs will decrease edema. The other methods will help venous return, but they do not provide the benefit that ambulation does.

36. a. 2; b. 7; c. 9; d. 1; e. 6; f. 4; g. 5; h. 3; i. 8

37. c. Although leg elevation, moist dressings, and systemic antibiotics are useful in treatment of venous stasis ulcers, the most important factor is compression, which minimizes venous stasis, venous hypertension, and edema and prevents recurrence. Compression may be applied with various methods including stockings, elastic bandages or wraps, or a Velcro wrap, among others.

Case Study

1. **Anticipated**: abdominal CT scan; CBC; abdominal x-ray; cholesterol studies; BUN and creatinine levels; **Non-essential**: echocardiogram; coagulation studies; blood glucose; 12-lead ECG; liver function tests. **Rationale**: This patient has an abdominal aortic aneurysm that was being monitored annually. Diagnostics that would provide valuable information are those of the abdomen which

include an abdominal CT scan and abdominal x-ray to identify the size and severity of the aneurysm. A CBC, which includes hemoglobin and hematocrit levels, would provide information about hemorrhage (or leaking from the aneurysm). Cholesterol levels are important since cholesterol contributes to the development of aortic aneurysms. BUN and creatinine levels identify renal disease associated with impaired perfusion caused by abdominal aortic aneurysms. An echocardiogram would be indicated if the aneurysm was thoracic because it would evaluate the function of the aortic valve. Coagulation studies would be indicated if the patient was taking certain anticoagulants, which may predispose the patient to hemorrhage. Blood glucose levels would be applicable if the patient had a history of diabetes. Liver function tests do not pertain to this patient's situation. An ECG could rule out an MI since thoracic aneurysms can mimic angina.

2. **Anticipated**: The nurse keeps the patient NPO (This is expected prior to surgery.); The HCP orders 1000 mL of 0.9% NSS (The patient is bleeding, as evidenced by the hypotensive BP, which warrants fluid resuscitation.); Insert an indwelling urinary catheter (Since an AAA can cause impaired renal perfusion, the urine output should be closely monitored.); The nurse gets the surgical consent signed by the patient (Once the patient agrees to the surgery, the nurse should get the consent form signed.); The nurse documents a baseline creatinine level (Since an AAA can cause impaired renal perfusion, renal function should be closely monitored.); The HCP orders to type and crossmatch 4 units of PRBCs (The patient is showing symptoms of hemorrhage and, with surgery, may require blood transfusions.)
Contraindicated: The nurse provides informed consent (This is not within the scope of the nurse as it is the responsibility of the surgeon.); The nurse ambulates the patient to the bathroom prior to transfer to the OR suite (The patient is hypotensive and should not be ambulating to the bathroom due to safety concerns, like falls.); The nurse requests an order for an enema (This is a vascular emergency, not one that involves the bowels. Therefore, an enema is unnecessary and may increase the risk of AAA rupture.) **Non-essential**: The nurse obtains an order to insert a nasogastric tube (An NG tube is expected postoperatively, but not preoperatively.); The nurse performs an abdominal assessment (This is unnecessary at this time as it doesn't provide any additional or beneficial information.)

3. Capillary refill > 3 sec in BLE; bilateral dorsalis pedis pulses are not palpable but present by Doppler; reports numbness and tingling in BLE; BLE are cool and pale; urine output is 25 mL/hr and is tea-colored; BP 100/58 mm Hg. **Rationale:** The nurse should report the decreased pedal pulses and the change in sensation, color, and temperature of the lower extremities as these are all signs of impaired tissue perfusion resulting from the AAA repair or complications from surgery. Decreased urine output also indicates impaired renal perfusion. This BP could be hypotensive for this patient and should be reported to the HCP as a higher blood pressure may be required to perfuse the kidneys and the lower extremities.

4. **1**=enoxaparin; **2**=CBC; **3**=subcutaneous; **4**=protamine sulfate (Refer to Table 41.11)

5. B, D, F, H. The nurse should teach the patient about risk factors contributing to aortic aneurysms and ways to decrease these risk factors which include smoking cessation, treating hypertension (which includes promoting the DASH diet), exercising several times per week, and eating foods low in fat and cholesterol. Alcohol can be consumed in moderation. If the patient is a diabetic, then close monitoring of blood glucose several times per day would be recommended as well as maintaining an A_1C below 7%.

CHAPTER 42

1. d. Although all the factors may be present, the end result is decreased supply of oxygen and nutrients to body cells from decreased tissue perfusion.

2. b. Obstructive shock occurs when a physical obstruction impedes the filling or outflow of blood, resulting in reduced cardiac output (CO). Distributive shock is evident with massive vasodilation and impaired cellular metabolism (neurogenic shock) or increased capillary permeability (anaphylactic shock). Cardiogenic shock occurs when the systolic or diastolic dysfunction of the heart's pumping action results in reduced CO. Hypovolemic shock is the absolute or relative loss of blood or fluid.

3. a, b, e, f. Hypovolemic shock occurs when there is a loss of intravascular fluid volume from fluid loss (e.g., hemorrhage or severe vomiting and diarrhea), fluid shift (e.g., burns or ascites), or internal bleeding (e.g., with a ruptured spleen). Vaccines and insect bites would precipitate the anaphylactic type of distributive shock.

4. a. Older adults with chronic diseases and malnourished or debilitated patients are at risk of developing septic shock, especially when they have an infection (e.g., pneumonia, urinary tract infection) or indwelling lines or catheters. Fever, hypothermia, tachycardia, tachypnea, altered mental status, significant edema, or hyperglycemia without diabetes are criteria for diagnosis of sepsis.

5. b. Hemodynamic monitoring in cardiogenic shock will reveal increased pulmonary artery wedge pressure (PAWP) and decreased CO. The characteristic signs of neurogenic shock are bradycardia and hypotension. Hypovolemic shock is characterized by increased systemic vascular resistance (SVR), decreased CO, and decreased PAWP. Septic shock manifests with decreased SVR and increased CO.

6. a, d, e. After sympathetic nervous system (SNS) activation of vasoconstriction, blood flow to nonvital organs, such as skin, kidneys, and the gastrointestinal (GI) tract is diverted or shunted to the most essential organs of the heart and brain. The patient will feel cool and clammy, the renin-angiotensin-aldosterone system will be activated, and the patient may develop a paralytic ileus.

7. d. Angiotensin II vasoconstricts both arteries and veins, which increases BP. It stimulates aldosterone release from the adrenal cortex, which results in sodium and water reabsorption and potassium excretion by the kidneys. The increased sodium raises serum osmolality and stimulates the pituitary gland to release antidiuretic hormone (ADH), which increases water reabsorption, which further increases blood volume, leading to an increase in BP and CO.

8. a, c, f. In the compensatory stage of shock the patient's skin will be pale and cool (α-adrenergic stimulation).

There may also be a change in level of consciousness, but the person will be responsive, the BP will be lower than baseline, bowel sounds will be hypoactive (α-adrenergic stimulation), and tachypnea and tachycardia (β-adrenergic stimulation) will occur. Unresponsiveness and moist crackles in the lungs occur in the progressive stage of shock.

9. b. Thrombocytopenia can occur. When sepsis is the cause of shock, endotoxin stimulates a cascade of inflammatory responses that start with the release of tumor necrosis factor (TNF) and interleukin-1 (IL-1), which stimulate other inflammatory mediators. The release of platelet-activating factor causes formation of microthrombi and vessel obstruction. There is vasodilation, increased capillary permeability, neutrophil and platelet aggregation, and adhesion to the endothelium. The process does not occur in other types of shock until late stages of shock.

10. d. Decreased myocardial perfusion leads to dysrhythmias and myocardial ischemia, further decreasing CO and oxygen delivery to cells. The kidney's renin-angiotensin-aldosterone system activation causes arteriolar constriction that decreases perfusion. In the lung, vasoconstriction of arterioles decreases blood flow and a ventilation-perfusion mismatch occurs. Areas of the lung that are oxygenated are not perfused because of the decreased blood flow, resulting in hypoxemia and decreased oxygen for cells. Increased capillary permeability and vasoconstriction cause increased hydrostatic pressure that contributes to the fluid shifting to interstitial spaces, but this is not a change in the heart.

11. b. During both the compensatory and progressive stages of shock, the SNS is activated in an attempt to maintain CO and SVR. In the refractory stage of shock, the SNS can no longer compensate to maintain homeostasis and a loss of vasomotor tone leading to profound hypotension affects perfusion to all vital organs, causing increasing cellular hypoxia, metabolic acidosis, and cellular death. Respiratory alkalosis occurs in early shock. Unresponsiveness and absent peripheral pulses can occur for many reasons and in earlier shock.

12. d. In every type of shock, there is a deficiency of oxygen to the cells, and high-flow oxygen therapy is indicated. Fluids would be started next, blood cultures would be done before any antibiotic therapy, and laboratory specimens could also be drawn.

13. b. In early compensatory shock, activation of the renin-angiotensin-aldosterone system stimulates the release of aldosterone, which causes sodium reabsorption and potassium excretion by the kidney, elevating serum sodium levels and decreasing serum potassium levels. Metabolic

acidosis does not occur until the progressive stage of shock. At this stage, compensatory mechanisms become ineffective and anaerobic cellular metabolism causes lactic acid production. Blood glucose levels are elevated during the compensatory stage of shock in response to catecholamine stimulation of the liver, which releases its glycogen stores in the form of glucose.

14. d. In late refractory shock, progressive cellular destruction causes changes in laboratory findings that indicate organ damage. Increasing ammonia levels indicate impaired liver function. Metabolic acidosis is usually severe as cells continue anaerobic metabolism and the respiratory alkalosis that may occur in the compensatory stage has failed to compensate for the acidosis. Potassium levels increase and blood glucose decreases.

15. a. Lactated Ringer's solution may increase lactate levels, which a damaged liver cannot convert to bicarbonate. This may worsen metabolic lactic acidosis that occurs in progressive shock, necessitating careful attention to the patient's acid-base balance. Sodium and potassium levels as well as hemoglobin (Hgb) and hematocrit (Hct) levels should be monitored in all patients receiving fluid replacement therapy.

16. b. The endpoint of fluid resuscitation in septic and hypovolemic shock is a central venous pressure (CVP) of 15 mm Hg or a PAWP of 10 to 12 mm Hg. This CO is too low and this heart rate is too high to indicate adequate fluid replacement.

17. a. A decreased mixed venous oxygen saturation (SvO_2) indicates that the patient has used the venous oxygen reserve and is at greater risk for anaerobic metabolism. The SvO_2 decreases when more oxygen is used by the cells, as in activity or hypermetabolism. All of the other values indicate an improvement in the patient's condition.

18. d. As a vasopressor, norepinephrine may cause severe vasoconstriction. This would further decrease tissue perfusion, especially if fluid replacement is inadequate. Vasopressors generally cause hypertension, reflex bradycardia, and decreased urine output because of decreased renal blood flow. They do not directly affect acid-base balance.

19. c. Vasoactive drugs are those that can either dilate or constrict blood vessels and are used in various stages of shock treatment. When using either vasodilators or vasoconstrictors, it is important to maintain a mean arterial pressure (MAP) >65 mm Hg to maintain adequate perfusion. The goal for urine output is ≥ 0.5 mL/kg/hr. The other goals would be appropriate only with either vasodilators or vasoconstrictors, not with all vasoactive drugs.

20.

Type of Shock	Medical Therapies
Cardiogenic	Restore coronary artery blood flow with thrombolytic therapy, angioplasty, emergency revascularization; increase CO with inotropic agents; reduce workload by dilating coronary arteries, decreasing preload and afterload; use circulatory assist devices, such as an intraaortic balloon pump; treat dysrhythmias
Hypovolemic	Fluid and/or blood replacement, control of bleeding with pressure, surgery
Septic	Fluid resuscitation, antimicrobial agents, inotropic agents with vasopressors
Anaphylactic	Epinephrine, inhaled bronchodilators, colloidal fluid replacement, diphenhydramine, corticosteroids

21.

Drug	Action
Diuretics (e.g., furosemide [Lasix])	Decrease the workload of the heart by decreasing fluid volume and reducing preload.
Dopamine	Increases myocardial contractility, automaticity, atrioventricular conduction, heart rate, CO, BP, and MAP
Nitroglycerin	Primarily dilates veins, reducing preload.
Nitroprusside	Acts as a potent vasodilator of veins and arteries and may increase or decrease CO, depending on the extent of preload and afterload reduction.
β-adrenergic blockers	Reduce heart rate and contractility when there is not a low ejection fraction

Others: angiotensin-converting enzyme (ACE) inhibitors

22. c. Prevention of shock necessitates identification of persons who are at risk and a thorough baseline nursing assessment with frequent ongoing assessments to monitor and detect changes in patients at risk. Frequent monitoring of all patients' vital signs is not necessary. Aseptic technique for all invasive procedures should always be implemented but will not prevent all types of shock. Health promotion activities that reduce the risk for precipitating conditions, such as coronary artery disease or anaphylaxis, may help prevent shock in only some cases.

23. a, b, c, e, f. Skin (color, temperature, moisture), urine output, level of consciousness, vital signs (including pulse oximetry), and peripheral pulses with capillary refill should be monitored to evaluate tissue perfusion.

24. c. If the metabolic acidosis is compensated, the pH will be within the normal range. If the patient is hyperventilating to blow off carbon dioxide to reduce the acid load of the blood, partial pressure of carbon dioxide in arterial blood ($PaCO_2$) will be decreased.

25. c, d, e, f. Antihistamines, oxygen supplementation, and colloid volume expansion are used to treat anaphylactic shock. Crystalloids may also be used. Epinephrine, a vasopressor, is often used. Only septic shock is treated with antibiotics. Vasodilators and inotropes are only used for cardiogenic shock. Volume expansion fluids vary with each type of shock.

26. d. Although some patients in shock may be treated with antianxiety and sedative drugs to control anxiety and apprehension, the nurse should always acknowledge the patient's feelings, explain procedures before they are carried out, and inform the patient of the plan of care and its rationale. Visits by family may have a therapeutic effect for some patients but may increase stress in others. Offering to call a member of the clergy is appropriate, but they should be called only if the patient requests or agrees to a visit.

27. d. A common initial mediator that causes endothelial damage leading to systemic inflammatory response syndrome (SIRS) and/or multiple organ dysfunction syndrome (MODS) is endotoxin. MODS results from SIRS. Not all patients with septic shock develop MODS, although they do have SIRS. The respiratory system is often the first to show evidence of SIRS and MODS.

28. d. The ischemic or necrotic tissue mechanism triggers SIRS with myocardial infarction, pancreatitis, and vascular disease. The abscess formation mechanism occurs with intraabdominal and extremity abscesses. The microbial invasion trigger is related to bacteria, viruses, fungi, or parasites. Global perfusion deficits are seen postcardiac resuscitation and in shock states.

29. a, b, e. Mechanical tissue trauma triggering of SIRS occurs with burns, crush injuries, and surgical procedures.

30. a. Early enteral feedings in the patient in shock increase the blood supply to the GI tract and help prevent translocation of GI bacteria and endotoxins into the blood, preventing initial or additional infection. Surgical removal of necrotic tissue, especially from burns, eliminates a source of infection in critically ill patients, as does the use of strict aseptic technique in all patient procedures. Known infections are treated with specific agents and broad-spectrum agents are used only until organisms are identified.

31. b. In general, the first body system affected by mediator-induced injury in MODS is the respiratory system. Adventitious sounds and areas with absent breath sounds will be present. Other organ damage occurs but lungs are usually first.

32. b. The presence of MODS is confirmed when there is defined clinical evidence of failure of 2 or more organs. Elevated serum bilirubin indicates liver dysfunction, a serum creatinine of 3.8 mg/dL indicates kidney injury, and a platelet count of 15,000/μL indicates hematologic failure. Other criteria include urine output <0.5 mL/kg/hr, blood urea nitrogen (BUN) ≥ 100 mg/dL, upper or lower GI bleeding, Glasgow Coma Scale (GCS) score ≤ 6, and Hct ≤ 20%. A respiratory rate of 45 breaths/min, $PaCO_2$ of 60 mm Hg, and chest x-ray with bilateral diffuse patchy infiltrates indicate respiratory failure but no other organ damage.

Case Study

1. **1**=nitrate (angina) and thiazide diuretic (HCTZ); **2**=100 mg once daily; **3**=isosorbide (nitrate that treats angina) and lisinopril (ACE inhibitor); **4**=hypertension

2. **Impaired tissue perfusion**=decreased LOC (occurs due to hypoxia to the brain); tachycardia (occurs because of activation of the sympathetic nervous system with β-adrenergic stimulation); tachypnea (occurs due to a compensatory response for hypoxemia and hypoxia); oliguria (occurs because of decreased perfusion to the kidneys); **Metabolic acidosis**=tachypnea (occurs because of a compensatory response to exhale excess CO_2); decreased SVR (occurs because metabolic acidosis contributes to vasodilation); **Vasodilation**=warm, dry, and flushed skin; decreased SVR; increased cardiac output (CO) (occurs in hyperdynamic phase of septic shock); oliguria (impaired tissue perfusion occurs due to blood

pooling in blood vessels); **Gram-negative infection**=fever; leukocytosis

3. **Anticipated**: monitor vital signs every hour (vital signs may be monitored more frequently when titrating vasoactive drugs); provide oral care every 4 hours and PRN (to prevent ventilator-associated pneumonia); administer antibiotics as prescribed (treats the underlying cause of sepsis); frequent FSBG monitoring (the patient is a diabetic and is hyperglycemic from the infection); administer norepinephrine to keep MAP $\geq$ 65 mm Hg (this drug is recommended in septic shock); **Contraindicated**: administer KCL 40 mEq IVPB over 1 hour (the patient's potassium level is 4.5 mEq/L which is within normal range); administer nitroglycerin IV infusion (this drug will cause vasodilation and exacerbate hypotension); transfuse 1 unit PRBCs over 2 hours (the patient's hemoglobin and hematocrit levels do not warrant a blood transfusion); **Non-essential**: advocate for physical therapy (the patient is too ill and unstable to participate in PT); complete a dietary assessment (this isn't a priority); obtain an order for an echocardiogram (there isn't an indication for this diagnostic test).

4. A, E, G, I, J. Neurologic assessments should be performed more frequently, every 1-2 hours. The $PaCO_2$ is 28 which indicates the patient is exhaling too much CO_2 due to tachypnea. The respiratory rate should be decreased to correct this lab value. Phenylephrine will vasoconstrict and increase BP, but it isn't a recommended drug in septic shock. Sodium nitroprusside is a vasodilator and will decrease the SVR which is contraindicated in septic shock. The patient is tachycardic due to compensatory mechanisms of shock, which should not be treated with a beta-blocker as this will interfere with compensation.

5. 1=central venous pressure and mean arterial pressure; 2= proton pump inhibitors; 3= enoxaparin (prevent VTE) and dobutamine (to increase O_2 delivery and increase SvO_2) 4= angiotensin II

CHAPTER 43

1. a. Parotid gland; b. submandibular saliva gland; c. pharynx; d. trachea; e. esophagus; f. diaphragm; g. liver; h. gallbladder; i. transverse colon; j. ascending colon; k. small intestine; l. cecum; m. vermiform appendix; n. anal canal; o. rectum; p. sigmoid colon; q. descending colon; r. stomach; s. spleen; t. larynx; u. sublingual gland; v. tongue

2. a. Right lobe of liver; b. right hepatic duct; c. cystic duct; d. common bile duct; e. gallbladder; f. pancreas (head); g. ampulla of Vater; h. duodenum; i. main pancreatic duct; j. pancreas (tail); k. stomach; l. left lobe of liver

3. c. The parasympathetic nervous system stimulates activity of the gastrointestinal (GI) tract, increasing motility and secretions and relaxing sphincters to promote movement of contents. A drug that blocks this activity decreases secretions and peristalsis, slows gastric emptying, and contracts sphincters. The enteric nervous system of the GI tract is modulated by sympathetic and parasympathetic influence.

4. d. Cholecystokinin is secreted by the duodenal mucosa when fats and amino acids enter the duodenum and stimulate the gallbladder to release bile to emulsify the fats

for digestion. The bile is produced by the liver but stored in the gallbladder. Secretin stimulates pancreatic bicarbonate secretion. Gastrin increases gastric motility and acid secretion.

5. c. The stomach secretes intrinsic factor, necessary for cobalamin (vitamin B_{12}) absorption in the intestine. When part or all the stomach is removed, cobalamin must be supplemented for life. The other options will not be a problem.

6. d. When food enters the stomach and duodenum, the gastrocolic and duodenocolic reflexes are started and are more active after the first daily meal. Additional laxatives or laxative abuse contribute to constipation in older adults. Decreasing food intake is not recommended, as many older adults have a decreased appetite. Fiber and fluids should be increased.

7. b, c. Pepsinogen is changed to pepsin by acidity of the stomach, where it begins to break down proteins. Gastrin stimulates gastric acid secretion and motility and maintains lower esophageal sphincter tone. The stomach also secretes lipase for fat digestion. Bile is secreted by the liver and stored in the gallbladder for emulsifying fats. Maltase is secreted in the small intestine and converts maltose to glucose. Secretin is secreted by the duodenal mucosa and inhibits gastric motility and acid secretion. Amylase is secreted in the small intestine and by the pancreas for carbohydrate digestion.

8. a. Bacteria in the colon: (1) synthesize vitamin K, which is needed to produce prothrombin by the liver; and (2) deaminate undigested or nonabsorbed proteins, producing ammonia, which is converted to urea by the liver. A reduction in normal flora bacteria by antibiotic therapy can lead to decreased vitamin K, resulting in decreased prothrombin and coagulation problems. Bowel bacteria do not influence protein absorption or the secretion of mucus.

9. c. The ampulla of Vater is the site where the pancreatic duct and common bile duct enter the duodenum and the opening and closing of the ampulla is controlled by the sphincter of Oddi. Because bile from the common bile duct is needed for emulsification of fat to promote digestion and pancreatic enzymes from the pancreas are needed for digestion of all nutrients, a blockage at this point would affect the digestion of all nutrients. Gastric contents pass into the duodenum through the pylorus or pyloric valve.

10. The bilirubin from hemoglobin (Hgb) is insoluble (unconjugated) and attached to albumin in the blood, removed by the liver, combined with glucuronic acid to become soluble (conjugated), and excreted in bile into the intestine. Bowel bacteria convert some of the bilirubin to urobilinogen. Urobilinogen is absorbed into the blood and a small amount of urobilinogen is excreted by the kidneys in urine, with the rest being removed by the liver and reexcreted in the bile.

11. d. There is decreased tone of the lower esophageal sphincter with aging and regurgitation of gastric contents back into the esophagus occurs, causing heartburn and belching. There is a decrease in hydrochloric acid secretion with aging. Jaundice and intolerance to fatty foods are symptoms of liver or gallbladder disease and are not normal age-related findings.

12.

Functional Health Pattern	Risk Factor for or Response to GI Problem
Health perception–health management	Excessive alcohol intake, smoking, exposure to hepatotoxins, recent foreign travel, family history of colorectal cancer, inflammatory bowel disease or breast cancer
Nutritional-metabolic	Anorexia and weight loss, excessive weight gain, inadequate diet, food intolerances
Elimination	Change in bowel patterns, laxative or enema use, decreased fluid or fiber intake, external drainage systems
Activity-exercise	Immobility, weakness, fatigue, inability to obtain and prepare food, inability to feed self
Sleep-rest	Interruption of sleep with GI symptoms
Cognitive-perceptual	Changes in taste or smell, use of pain medications, sensory problems that interfere with food preparation or intake
Self-perception–self-concept	Self-esteem and body image problems related to weight, symptoms affecting appearance
Role-relationship	Loss of employment because of chronic illness, altered relationships with others
Sexuality-reproductive	Anorexia, obesity, alcohol intake, decreased acceptance by sexual partner
Coping–stress tolerance	GI problems or symptoms induced by stress, depression
Value-belief	Religious dietary restrictions, vegetarianism

13. c. A thin, white coating of the dorsum (top) of the tongue is normal. A red, slick appearance is characteristic of cobalamin deficiency, and scattered red, smooth areas on the tongue are known as *geographic tongue*. The uvula should remain in the midline while the patient is saying "Ahh."

14. b. The pulsation of the aorta in the epigastric area is a normal finding. Bruits indicate that blood flow is abnormal, the liver is percussed in the right midclavicular line, and a normal spleen cannot be palpated.

15. b. The body of the pancreas is in the left upper quadrant, the liver is in the right upper quadrant, the appendix is in the right lower quadrant, and the gallbladder is in the right upper quadrant.

16. a. Borborygmi are loud gurgles (stomach growling) that indicate hyperperistalsis. Normal bowel sounds are relatively high-pitched and are heard best with the diaphragm of the stethoscope. High-pitched, tinkling bowel sounds occur when the intestines are under tension, as in bowel obstructions. If you do not hear bowel sounds, note the amount of time you listened in each quadrant without hearing bowel sounds.

17. a. The abdomen should be assessed in the following sequence: inspection, auscultation, percussion, palpation. The patient should empty their bladder before assessment begins.

18.

Procedure	(1) NPO	(2) Bowel	(3) Consent	(4) Allergy
Upper GI series	X			
Barium enema	X	X		
Percutaneous transhepatic cholangiogram	X		X	X
Gallbladder ultrasound	X			
Hepatobiliary scintigraphy	X		X	
Esophagogastroduodenoscopy (EGD)	X		X	
Colonoscopy	X	X	X	
Endoscopic retrograde cholangiopancreatography (ERCP)	X		X	X

19. c. The aspartate aminotransferase (AST) level is elevated in liver disease but it is important to note that it is also elevated in damage to the heart and lungs and is not a specific test for liver function. Measurement of most of the transaminases involves nonspecific tests unless isoenzyme fractions are determined. Hepatic encephalopathy is related to elevated ammonia levels.

20. c, d, f. Because the liver is a vascular organ, vital signs are monitored to assess for internal bleeding. Prevention of bleeding is the reason for positioning on the right side for at least 2 hours and for splinting the puncture site. Again, because of the vasculature of the liver, coagulation status is checked before the biopsy is done.

White stools occur with upper gastrointestinal (UGI) or barium swallow tests. The bowel must be cleared before a lower GI or barium enema, a virtual colonoscopy, or a colonoscopy. Rectal bleeding may occur with a sigmoidoscopy or colonoscopy.

21. a. Left upper quadrant (LUQ) pain, nausea, and vomiting could occur from perforation. The return of gag reflex is essential to prevent aspiration after an ERCP. A perforation may occur with an EGD, ERCP, or peritoneoscopy. The gag reflex is also assessed with an EGD. These are not relevant assessments for the colonoscopy, barium swallow, or defecography.

CHAPTER 44

1. a.

2.

Nutrient	Percentage of Total Calories From Nutrient
Protein	120 g × 4 cal/g = 480 cal 480/3000 = 16% of 3000 cal
Fat	160 g × 9 cal/g = 1440 cal 1440/3000 = 48% of 3000 cal
Carbohydrates	270 g × 4 cal/g = 1080 cal 1080/3000 = 36% of 3000 cal

   b. Not enough carbohydrates (should be 45%–65%) and too much fat (should be 20%–35%).

   c. An average adult requires an estimated 20 to 35 calories per kilogram of body weight per day. In this patient, recommended calories would be between 1600 (80 kg × 20) and 2800 (80 kg × 35) calories per day.

   d. Without knowing the activity level of the patient, the intake should be 2400 calories for a sedentary man and 3000 calories for an active man. Increase breads, cereals, rice, and pasta as sources of complex carbohydrate; increase fruits to 2 to 2.5 cups and vegetables to 3.5 cups per day. Decrease the meat and egg group to 7 oz per day in 3 servings each day to lower protein and fat. Use 3 cups of low-fat milk to lower fat intake. Use all fats, oils, and sweets sparingly.

3. b. Patients who have surgery on the gastrointestinal (GI) tract may be at risk for vitamin deficiencies because of inability to absorb or metabolize them. The strict vegan diet most often lacks cobalamin (vitamin B_{12}) and iron. Vitamin deficiencies in adults also have neurologic manifestations. Although the high intake of fat is a major nutritional problem in the United States, vitamin deficiencies are rare in developed countries except in people with eating disorders or chronic alcohol abuse.

4. d. In the United States, where protein intake is high and of good quality, chronic disease–related or secondary protein-calorie malnutrition most commonly results from problems of the GI system. In developing countries, adequate food sources may not exist, the inhabitants may not be well educated about nutritional needs, and economic conditions can prevent purchase of balanced diets.

5.

Time Frame	Metabolism of Nutrients
First 18 hours	Carbohydrates stored in the liver and muscles in the form of glycogen are used and may be depleted quickly.
18 hours to 5 to 9 days	Protein, primarily the amino acids alanine and glutamine, is converted to glucose for energy and a negative nitrogen balance occurs.
In 5 to 9 days for up to 6 weeks	Body fat is mobilized and used as the primary source of energy, conserving protein.
Over 6 weeks	Fat stores are usually depleted in 4 to 6 weeks and body or visceral proteins, including those in internal organs and plasma, are used because they are the only source of energy available.

6. c. The sodium-potassium pump uses 20% to 50% of all calories ingested. When energy sources are decreased, the pump fails to function, sodium and water are left in the cell, and potassium remains in extracellular fluids. Hyperkalemia, as well as hyponatremia, can occur.

7. a. With surgery a patient will recover more rapidly with a balanced nutritional status before the surgery and increased protein is needed for healing after the surgery. Following a vegan diet does not put the patient at risk of low protein intake. A fever will increase protein-calorie needs. Following religious and cultural beliefs would not be expected to affect an increased need for protein.

8. a, b, c, e, f. In malnutrition, metabolic processes are slowed, leading to increased sensitivity to cold, decreased heart rate (HR) and cardiac output (CO), and decreased neurologic function. Because the immune system is weakened, susceptibility to respiratory infections is increased. Because of slowed GI motility and absorption, the abdomen becomes distended and protruding and bowel sounds are decreased. Skin is rough, dry, and scaly and bone structures protrude because of muscle loss. Neurologic effects of malnutrition include decreased reflexes, lack of attention, irritability, syncope, and peripheral neuropathy.

9. d. Malnutrition that results from a decreased intake of food is most common in individuals with severe anorexia where there is a decreased desire to eat. Infections create a hypermetabolic state that increases nutritional demand, malabsorption causes less availability of nutrients that are ingested, and draining decubitus ulcers (although treated) are examples of disorders that cause both loss of protein and hypermetabolic states.

10. c. Serum transferrin is a protein that is synthesized by the liver and used for iron transport and decreases when there is protein deficiency. An increase in the protein would indicate a more positive nitrogen balance with amino acids available for synthesis. Decreased lymphocytes and serum prealbumin are indicators of protein depletion and increased serum potassium shows continuing failure of the sodium-potassium pump.

11. d. Anthropometric measurements, including mid-upper arm circumference and triceps skinfold measurements, are good indicators of lean body mass and skeletal protein reserves and are valuable in evaluating persons who may have been or are being treated for acute protein malnutrition. The other measurements do not specifically address muscle mass.

12. a. The breakfast with the eggs provides 24 g of complete protein, compared with 14 g for the protein-fortified cream of wheat and milkshake breakfast. Whole milk instead of skim milk helps meet the calorie requirements. The toast has 10 g of protein and the pancakes have about 6 g. Bacon is considered a fat rather than a meat serving.

13. b. Although calorie intake should be decreased in the older adult because of decreased activity, lean muscle mass and basal metabolic rate, the need for specific nutrients, such as proteins and vitamins, does not change.

14. a. Socioeconomic conditions frequently have the greatest effect on the nutritional status of the healthy older adult. Limited income and social isolation can result in the "tea

and toast" meals of the older adult. The other options do not interfere with nutritional status.

15. a. Standard nasogastric (NG) tubes are only used for enteral nutrition (EN) for short-term feeding problems because prolonged therapy can result in irritation and erosion of the mucosa of the upper GI tract. Gastric reflux and the potential for aspiration can occur with both NG and gastrostomy feeding tubes. Both tubes deprive the patient of the sensations associated with eating and can become displaced.

16.

Desired Outcome	Nursing Intervention
Prevention of aspiration	X-ray confirmation of tube location before feeding. Recheck the tube's insertion length at regular intervals. Position the patient with the head of the bed elevated 30 to 45 degrees during feedings. Following intermittent feedings, keep the head of the bed elevated for 30 to 60 minutes. Measuring gastric residuals is per institutional policy as there is a lot of disagreement about whether gastric residuals should be checked. Monitor for sensation of fullness, nausea, and vomiting. Promotility medications may be prescribed.
Prevention of diarrhea	Start feedings with small amounts and/or decrease rate of infusion. Refrigerate and date opened solutions to prevent bacterial growth but warm them to room temperature before administration; discard outdated formula; use closed systems; use sterile water to flush for immunocompromised patients; check for medications that may cause diarrhea; and provide free water with feedings to compensate for high-concentration EN. Use high-fiber formula.
Maintenance of tube patency	Flush the tube with 30 mL water before and after feedings and medication administration. Only administer medications that can be crushed and be sure that they are dissolved in water before administration. In continuous feedings, flush the tube with water every 4 hours; flush after residual measurements, if performed.
Maintenance of tube placement	Confirm placement initially with chest x-ray; mark exit point of tube following x-ray confirmation and routinely assess for changes in the external length of the tube. If lengthened, assess color and pH of aspirate (< 5 desired).

Desired Outcome	Nursing Intervention
Administration of medication	Stop feeding. Check tube placement. Flush with 15 mL of water, dilute medications, and use clean oral syringe to administer medications; flush again taking into account the patient's fluid status; separately dilute and administer each medication; use liquid forms of medications, if available; use immediate release form, if liquid not available. Check to see if medications are to be given with meals or on an empty stomach and hold feeding if necessary.

17. a. LPN; b. AP; c. RN; d. LPN; e. AP; f. AP; g. RN; h. AP
18. a. peripheral parenteral nutrition (PPN); b. central parenteral nutrition (CPN); c. CPN; d. PPN; e. CPN; f. PPN; g. CPN
19. c. In malabsorption syndromes, foods that are ingested into the intestinal tract cannot be digested or absorbed and tube feedings infused into the intestinal tract would not be absorbed. All of the other conditions can be treated with enteral or parenteral nutrition, depending on the patient's needs.

20.

Complication	Preventive Measure
Infection	Refrigerate solutions until 30 minutes before use; aseptically change dressing to catheter site per institutional protocol and assess for signs of infection; label date and time started; change filter and tubing every 24 hours if lipids are being administered or every 72 hours if amino acids and dextrose are being administered, and label tubing with date and time attached; do not infuse solution in 1 bottle more than 24 hours; do not add anything to the solution.
Hyperglycemia	Start infusions slowly, gradually increasing rate for 24 to 48 hours; check capillary blood glucose levels every 4 to 6 hours; provide sliding-scale insulin as prescribed; do not speed up infusion rates or remove infusion from infusion controllers and pumps; visually check the amount infused every 30 to 60 minutes.
Air embolism	Place patient supine before changing the dressing with sterile technique; clamp the infusion line before changing the injection cap with sterile technique; if the line cannot be clamped, instruct the patient to perform the Valsalva maneuver when the catheter is open to air; do not inject air when flushing the catheter lumen(s).

21. a. Remaining solution should be discarded. Bacterial growth occurs at room temperature in nutritional solutions. Therefore solutions must not be infused for longer than 24 hours. Speeding up the solution may cause hyperglycemia and should not be done. The HCP does not need to be notified as the rate is determined to meet the patient's nutritional needs.

22. a. AB; b. A; c. B; d. B; e. AB; f. A; g. A; h. B

23. d. The potential life-threatening cardiac complications related to the hypokalemia are the most important immediate considerations in the patient's care. The other clinical problems are important for the patient's care but do not pose the immediate risk that the hypokalemia does.

Case Study

1. **Expected**: calculating the BMI (part of anthropometric measurements when assessing nutrition); obtaining a prealbumin level (a negative acute phase protein that is decreased in inflammatory states due to decreased liver synthesis); collecting a food intake history (evaluates the foods the patient is consuming to assess nutritional value); peripheral edema (when patient loses plasma oncotic pressure, albumin and fluid leak into the interstitial spaces causing edema); pale skin (due to anemia as evidenced by the decreased Hgb/Hct levels). **Unexpected**: pink mucous membranes (they are expected to be pale); hyperactive bowel sounds (expected to be hypoactive); **Unrelated**: bone density scan (this assesses for osteoporosis but there is no evidence for this patient); obtaining coagulation studies (is unnecessary and doesn't pertain to this patient)

2. **1**=nutritionally compromised (fatigue is also applicable, but this patient's nutritional status is likely a contributing factor to being fatigued); **2**=936 (*Women*: 10 × weight (kg) + 6.25 × height (cm) − 5 × age (yr) − 161); **3**=1123 (take the energy expenditure formula and multiply by 1.200 for sedentary activity); **4**=dietary

3. **Chicken**: B6, B12; **tofu**: B6; **carrots**: vitamin A; **milk**: B12, calcium, vitamin A (with fortified milk); **spinach**: magnesium, vitamins A & E; **legumes**: magnesium, zinc; **salmon**: B6, B12, calcium; **meat**: B6, B12, zinc, vitamin A; **grains**: zinc, vitamin E

4. A., C., D., E., F., H.; Meals should be high in calories from protein and carbohydrates; instructions should be provided in Spanish as the patient doesn't read English well; water should be consumed after a meal so it doesn't interfere with fullness.

5. **Indicated**: use a 0.22 micron filter; fat emulsion can be mixed with PN or infused separately or concurrently with PN; 2 RNs should verify the PN and its infusion rate; blood glucose should be monitored while on PN due to the high concentrations of glucose in PN; **Contraindicated**: The nurse should never refrigerate the PN. (TPN should be kept refrigerated up to 30 minutes prior to infusion, but can be at room temperature during the 24 hours it will infuse); The nurse should change the IV tubing every 72 hours.(IV tubing should be changed every 24 hours when a new bag is started); if the PN infusion runs out before a new bag can be started, dextrose 5% should be started for peripheral IVs. (dextrose 10% or greater should be used if central PN is being administered); The nurse should add insulin to the PN if the patient is hyperglycemic.(nothing should be added to the PN once the pharmacy has prepared

the solution); **Non-essential**: The nurse should monitor potassium levels during PN administration. (glucose should be monitored but monitoring potassium isn't essential during PN administration); keep patient NPO (it isn't necessary to keep the patient NPO just because they are receiving PN)

CHAPTER 45

1. a. $202 × 703 = 142,006 ÷ 4225 (65 × 65) = 33.6$ kg/m^2; classified as obesity b. $32 ÷ 36 = 0.89$; an increased risk for health complications

2. b. Twin studies and studies with adopted children have shown that body shape and weight gain are influenced by genetics, but more research is needed. Older obese people do have exacerbated aging problems related to declines in physical function, not genetics. Blacks and Hispanics have a higher incidence of obesity than whites. Women have a higher incidence of obesity and more difficulty losing weight than men because women have a higher percentage of metabolically less active fat.

3. b. The 56-year-old woman has a body mass index (BMI) of 38 kg/m^2 (obese, Class II) with a waist-to-hip ratio of 1.1 with android obesity is more at risk (very high) than the other patients. The 30-year-old woman has the least risk with a BMI of 27.3 kg/m^2 (overweight) and gynoid shape. The 42-year-old man has a BMI of 24.2 kg/m^2 (normal weight) with 1 risk factor in the waist-to-hip ratio of 1.0 and the 68-year-old man has a BMI of 27.9 kg/m^2 (overweight) with a waist-to-hip ratio of 0.9.

4. b. A patient who is obese (BMI of 32.2 kg/m^2) but has a waist-to-hip ratio of <0.8, indicating gynoid obesity, has an increased risk for osteoporosis. The other conditions are risks associated with android obesity (see Table 40.6).

5. a. Motivation is essential. Focus on the reasons for wanting to lose weight. The rest of the options will assist in planning the weight loss if the patient is motivated.

6. a, b, c, d, e, f. Normally ghrelin and neuropeptide Y stimulate appetite. Leptin suppresses appetite and hunger. Insulin decreases appetite. Peptide YY and cholecystokinin inhibit appetite by slowing gastric emptying and sending satiety signals to the hypothalamus.

7. a, c. To restrict dietary intake so that it is below energy requirements, the moderately obese woman should limit or avoid alcohol intake because it increases caloric intake and has low nutritional value. Portion sizes have increased over the years and are larger than they should be. Teach the patient to determine portion sizes by weight or learn equivalencies, such as a serving of fruit is the size of a baseball. A progressive exercise program will increase energy requirements and a diet with an initial 800- to 1200-calorie limit would decrease calorie intake. Overeaters Anonymous would not restrict dietary intake below energy requirements, although it may offer support for the patient. Parking farther away will increase walking and use calories but not restrict intake.

8. c. Progressively increasing physical activity helps decrease weight, cholesterol, BP, and glucose levels for the obese person. Although psychosocial components (i.e., using food for comfort or reward and inability to buy high–nutritional quality food) may have an influence on weight gain, these factors along with lack of physical exercise,

overestimation of portion size, and genetics contribute to weight gain. Weekly weighing is recommended as a more reliable indicator of weight loss because daily weighing shows frequent fluctuation from retained water (including urine) and elimination of feces. Men are able to lose weight more quickly than women because women have a higher percentage of metabolically less active fat.

9. b. Plateau periods during which no weight is lost are normal occurrences during weight reduction and may last for several days to several weeks but weight loss will resume if the prescribed weight reduction plan is continued. Weight loss may stop if former eating habits are resumed but this is not the most common cause of plateaus.

10. d. A chicken breast the size of a deck of cards is about 3 oz, a recommended portion size of meat. Other normal portions include a 3-inch bagel, 1/2 cup of chopped vegetables, and a piece of cheese the size of 6 dice.

11. b. Medications are used only as adjuncts to diet and exercise programs in the treatment of obesity. Drugs do not cure obesity; without changes in food intake and physical activity, weight gain will occur when the medications are discontinued. The medications used work in a variety of ways to control appetite but over-the-counter (OTC) drugs are probably the least effective and most abused of these drugs.

12. a. Qsymia is a combination of phentermine and topiramate. It must not be used in patients with glaucoma or hyperthyroidism.

13. d. People who have undergone behavior therapy are more successful in maintaining weight losses over time because most programs deemphasize the diet, focus on how and when the person eats, and provide support from others. Weighing daily is not recommended, and plateaus may not allow for consistent weight loss. A goal for weight loss must be set, and 1 to 2 pounds a week is realistic. A more rapid loss often causes skin and underlying tissue to lose elasticity and become flabby folds of tissue. Exercising more often depresses appetite and exercise need not be limited.

14. c. The Roux-en-Y gastric bypass is a common combination of restrictive (limiting the size of the stomach) and malabsorptive (less food is absorbed) surgery. Lipectomy is used to remove unsightly flabby folds of adipose tissue. Adjustable gastric banding is the most common restrictive procedure. Sleeve gastrectomy is a restrictive procedure that preserves stomach function.

15. b, e. The adjustable gastric banding procedure is reversible and allows a change in gastric stoma size by inflation or deflation of the band around the fundus of the stomach. The sleeve gastrectomy removes about 75% of the stomach and eliminates the hormones produced in the stomach that stimulate hunger. The biliopancreatic diversion is a malabsorptive surgery that prevents absorption of nutrients, including fat-soluble vitamins. The Roux-en-Y gastric bypass reduces the stomach size with a gastric pouch anastomosed to the small intestine, so it is both restrictive and malabsorptive.

16. c. Special considerations are needed for the care of the patient with extreme obesity because most hospital units are not prepared with beds, chairs, BP cuffs, and other equipment that will have to be used with the very obese patient. Consideration of all aspects of care should be made before implementing care for the patient, including extra time and assistance for positioning, physical assessment, and transferring the patient.

17. c, d, f. Obese patients are at higher risk for cancer, sleep apnea and sleep deprivation, type 2 diabetes, gastroesophageal reflux disease (GERD), nonalcoholic steatohepatitis, osteoarthritis, and cardiovascular problems. The other options are not related to obesity.

18. b. Patients with histories of untreated depression or psychosis are not good candidates for surgery. All other historical information includes medical complications of extreme obesity that would help qualify the patient for the surgery.

19. d. Turning, coughing, and deep breathing are essential to prevent postoperative complications. Protecting the incision from strain is important since wound dehiscence is a problem for obese patients. If a nasogastric (NG) tube that is present following gastric surgery for extreme obesity becomes blocked or needs repositioning, the HCP should be notified. Ambulation is usually started on the evening of surgery, and additional help will be needed to support the patient. Respiratory function is promoted by keeping the head of the bed elevated at an angle of 35 to 40 degrees.

20. a. Fluids and foods high in carbohydrates tend to promote diarrhea and symptoms of dumping syndrome in patients with gastric bypass surgery. The diet generally should be high in protein and low in carbohydrates, fat, and roughage and consist of 6 small feedings a day because of the small stomach size. Liquid diets are likely to be used longer for the patient with a gastroplasty.

21. b. Three of the following 5 measures are needed for a woman to be diagnosed with metabolic syndrome: waist circumference $\geq$ 35 in, triglycerides > 150 mg/dL, high-density lipoproteins < 50 mg/dL, BP $\geq$ 130 mm Hg systolic or $\geq$ 85 mm Hg diastolic, fasting blood glucose $\geq$ 100 mg/dL. Although the other options have some abnormal measures, none has all 3 measures in the diagnostic ranges. The criteria for metabolic syndrome for both women and men are listed in Table 40.12.

22. a, c, d, e. Patients with metabolic syndrome need to lower their risk factors by smoking cessation, increasing physical activity, establishing healthy diet habits, and reducing and maintaining weight. Some patients with metabolic syndrome are diabetic and would need to monitor glucose levels frequently. When monitoring weight reduction, it is recommended to check weight weekly, not daily.

23. c. Insulin resistance is the main underlying risk factor for metabolic syndrome. Aging is associated with metabolic syndrome. High cholesterol, hypertension, and increased clotting risk are characteristics of metabolic syndrome.

Case Study

1. **Indicates** (metabolic syndrome): Triglycerides 312 mg/dL, HDL 30 mg/dL, fasting blood glucose 146 mg/dL, waist circumference 56 in, BP 172/96 mm Hg; **Unrelated**: weight 296 lbs., height 68 in, HR 88 beats/min, total cholesterol 250 mg/dL. (Refer to Table 45.11 Diagnostic Criteria for Metabolic Syndrome)

2. **Indicates** (a complication): uses a CPAP machine (indicates sleep apnea which is common in obese patients), prescribed metformin (a medication to treat type II diabetes), chest pain when climbing stairs (indicates coronary artery

disease), blood in stools (a sign of colorectal cancer); **Unrelated**: urinating 550 mL/day (normal amount of urine per day), loss of hearing in left ear (unrelated), abdominal pain after eating bread (may indicate gluten intolerance)

3. **1**=gastric banding; **2**=90 mL; **3**=gastric sleeve; **4**=75%; **5**=Roux-en-Y; **6**=dumping syndrome; **7**=gastric pacemaker

4. **Indicated:** keep HOB $\geq$ 45 degrees, splint the incision when coughing (to avoid dehiscence and promote comfort), administer IV fluids until PO of 500 mL (keeps the patient hydrated until PO fluids are tolerated); **Contraindicated**: drinking through a straw (to reduce swallowing air), allow patient to drink up to 90 mL initially (the recommendation is to start with 15 mL of fluid every 10-15 minutes gradually increasing to 90 mL every 30 minutes), keep patient on bedrest until postop day #2 (increasing activity is important and starts on postop day #0); **Non-essential**: measure abdominal girth (is performed for patients who have ascites fluid or is at risk for compartment syndrome which are not applicable to this patient), palpate peripheral pulses (will be included in a physical assessment but isn't essential or specific to bariatric surgery)

5. A., C., E., F., G., H. Wound edges that are separating indicate a possible dehiscence and should be evaluated by the HCP. Heavy lifting should be avoided and is usually less than 10-20 lbs. to avoid dehiscence during healing of the incision. Cobalamin supplementation will be lifelong because of bypassing the stomach and small intestine where cobalamin is extracted and absorbed. Stools may appear black because of iron supplements which are required because of bypassing the duodenum where iron is absorbed. Iron that isn't absorbed by the body is excreted in the stool causing the stool color to be black. Patients are on a full-liquid diet for the first 10-14 days before advancing to a soft diet. Patients are told to eat small frequent meals and stop when they feel full, which occurs sooner than it did prior to the surgery. When taking narcotics for pain management, driving is unsafe and would be considered under the influence (or driving while intoxicated). Diets should be high in protein and low in carbohydrates to avoid dumping syndrome and diarrhea. A Roux-en-Y is not reversible.

CHAPTER 46

1. d. The parasympathetic nervous system causes increased salivation and gastric mobility as well as relaxation of the lower esophageal sphincter. The acid-base imbalance that occurs with vomiting is metabolic alkalosis from the loss of hydrochloric acid (HCl). The vomiting center in the chemoreceptor trigger zone (CTZ) can be caused by chemical stimuli of drugs, toxins, and labyrinthine stimulation. Vomiting requires the coordination of closing the glottis, deep inspiration with contraction of the diaphragm in the inspiratory position, closure of the pylorus, relaxation of the stomach and lower esophageal sphincter, and contraction of abdominal muscles.

2. c. The loss of gastric HCl causes metabolic alkalosis and an increase in pH; loss of potassium, sodium, and chloride; and loss of fluid, which increases the hematocrit.

3. b. The patient with severe or persistent vomiting requires IV replacement of fluids and electrolytes until able to tolerate oral intake to prevent serious dehydration and electrolyte imbalances. Oral fluids are not given until vomiting has been relieved and parenteral antiemetics are often not used until a cause of the vomiting can be established. Nasogastric (NG) intubation may be needed in some cases, but fluid and electrolyte replacement are the first priority.

4. a. Water is the fluid of choice for rehydration by mouth. Very hot or cold liquids are not usually well tolerated. Although broth and Gatorade have been used for the patient with severe vomiting, these substances are high in sodium and should be administered with caution.

5. d. Ondansetron (Zofran) is one of several serotonin antagonists that act both centrally and peripherally to reduce vomiting: centrally on the vomiting center in the brainstem and peripherally by promoting gastric emptying. Dronabinol (Marinol) is an orally active cannabinoid that causes sedation and has a potential for abuse and it is used when other therapies are ineffective. Antihistamines used as antiemetics also cause sedation.

6. b. Implementing safety precautions (placement close to the nurses' station, call bell in reach, hourly visual checks) is the priority. The patient would not be kept in a flat position because of the potential for aspiration of vomitus. Keeping the patient NPO would be done for all patients but is not the priority with this older patient. Because the older patient is more likely to have cardiac or renal insufficiency, the patient's fluid and electrolyte status are monitored more closely (laboratory, intake and output). Monitor vital signs along with breath sounds. Assess mucous membranes, skin turgor, and color to assess for dehydration. Assess level of consciousness closely. Check dosing of antiemetics. Assess for weakness and fatigue.

7. a. When gingivitis is untreated, abscesses form, and teeth are loosened with periodontitis. Herpes simplex is a viral infection related to the upper respiratory system and has shallow, painful vesicular ulcerations of lips and mouth. Aphthous stomatitis has infectious ulcers of the mouth and lips with a defined erythematous base occurring because of systemic disease.

8. b. Stomatitis is inflammation of the mouth related to systemic diseases and cancer chemotherapy medications. There is excessive salivation, halitosis, and a sore mouth. Parotitis is a *Staphylococcus* infection that may occur with prolonged NPO status and results in decreased saliva and ear pain. Oral candidiasis is seen with prolonged antibiotic or corticosteroid therapy; it has white membranous lesions on the mucosa of the mouth and larynx. Vincent's infection is a bacterial infection predisposed to by fatigue, stress, and poor oral hygiene. There are painful, bleeding gums and increased metallic-tasting saliva.

9. c. A positive history of use of tobacco and alcohol is the most significant etiologic factor in oral cancer. Excessive exposure to ultraviolet radiation from the sun is a factor in the development of cancer of the lip. Herpes simplex infections have not been associated with oral cancer. Difficulty swallowing and ear pain are symptoms of advanced oral cancer, not risk factors.

10. b. Because surgical treatment of oral cancers involves extensive excision, a tracheostomy is usually performed with the radical dissections. The first goal of care is that the patient will have a patent airway. The other goals are appropriate but of lesser priority.

11. b. Measures to assess and treat withdrawal from alcohol should be implemented with patients who have

heavy use of alcohol because alcohol withdrawal can be life threatening. Tobacco withdrawal may also be uncomfortable for the patient. Nutritional needs may have to be addressed with tube feedings postoperatively, and pain medications may have to be increased because of cross-tolerance. Counseling about lifestyle changes is not a priority in the early postoperative course.

12. a, c, e, f. Alcohol, chocolate, fatty foods, and cola sodas (caffeine) as well as peppermint and spearmint will decrease lower esophageal sphincter (LES) pressure. Root beer and herbal tea do not have caffeine. Citrus fruits will not affect LES pressure.

13. c. The use of blocks to elevate the head of the bed facilitates gastric emptying by gravity and is strongly recommended to prevent nighttime reflux. Liquids should be taken between meals to prevent gastric distention with meals. Small meals should be eaten frequently, but patients should not eat at bedtime or lie down for 2 to 3 hours after eating. Activities that involve increasing intraabdominal pressure, such as bending over, lifting, or wearing tight clothing, should be avoided.

14. d. Eating a high-calorie, high-protein diet, perhaps in liquid form, is the highest priority preoperatively. Because of dysphagia, the patient often has poor nutritional status because of the inability to ingest adequate amounts of food before surgery. An esophageal stent may be placed to improve the nutritional status. Turning and deep breathing will be done. The patient will need to know about postoperative care, but these are not the preoperative priorities. Meticulous oral care is done but with swabs or gauze pads to prevent the injury and pain brushing may incur.

15. b. Following esophageal surgery, the patient should be positioned in semi-Fowler's or Fowler's position to prevent reflux and aspiration of gastric sections. NG drainage is expected to be bloody for 8 to 12 hours postoperatively. Abdominal distention is not a major concern following esophageal surgery, and even though the thorax may be opened during the surgery, clear breath sounds should be expected in all areas of the lungs.

16. b. Barrett's esophagus is an esophageal metaplasia primarily related to gastroesophageal reflux disease (GERD). Achalasia is a rare chronic disorder with delayed emptying of the lower esophagus and is associated with squamous cell cancer. Esophageal strictures are narrowing of the esophagus from scarring by many causes. Esophageal diverticula are saclike outpouchings of 1 or more layers of the esophagus. They often occur above the esophageal sphincter.

17. d. Eosinophilic esophagitis is swelling of the esophagus caused by infiltration of eosinophils in response to food triggers or environmental allergens. Esophageal cancer is usually caused by adenocarcinoma. The rest are squamous cell tumors. Esophageal varices are dilated veins in the esophagus caused by portal hypertension. Esophagitis is inflammation of the esophagus commonly seen with GERD.

18. a. Acute gastritis is most likely to occur with an isolated drinking binge. Chronic gastritis is usually caused by *Helicobacter pylori* or viral and fungal infections. Autoimmune gastritis is an inherited condition.

19. a. A nonirritating diet with 6 small meals a day is recommended to help control the symptoms of gastritis.

Antacids are often used for control of symptoms but have the best neutralizing effect if taken after meals. Alcohol and caffeine should be eliminated entirely because they may precipitate gastritis. Nonsteroidal antiinflammatory drugs (NSAIDs) are often as irritating to the stomach as aspirin and should not be used in the patient with gastritis.

20. a, c, f. Duodenal ulcers have increased HCl gastric secretion, which causes the burning and cramping in the midepigastric area; the pain is relieved with food. The other options occur with both duodenal and gastric ulcers.

21. a. The 55-year-old female smoker experiencing nausea and vomiting is more likely to have a gastric ulcer. The other patients are not in the highest-risk age range or do not have enough risk factors. Although lower socioeconomic status, smoking, and drug use increase the risk of gastric ulcers, these patients are more likely to have duodenal ulcers but further assessment is needed.

22. c. Corticosteroids decrease the rate of mucous cell renewal. *H. pylori* produces the enzyme urease. Alcohol ingestion increases the secretion of HCl. Aspirin and NSAIDs inhibit the synthesis of mucus and prostaglandins.

23. a. The ultimate damage to the tissues of the stomach and duodenum, precipitating ulceration, is acid back diffusion into the mucosa. The gastric mucosal barrier is protective of the mucosa but without the acid environment and damage, ulceration does not occur. Ammonia formation by *H. pylori* and release of histamine impair the barrier but are not directly responsible for tissue injury.

24. c. There is no specific diet used for the treatment of peptic ulcers, and patients are encouraged to eat as normally as possible, eliminating foods that cause discomfort or pain. Eating 6 meals a day prevents the stomach from being totally empty and is recommended. Caffeine and alcohol should be eliminated from the diet because they are known to cause gastric irritation. Milk and milk products do not have to be avoided but they can add fat content to the diet.

25. d. NG intubation is used with acute exacerbation of peptic ulcer disease (PUD) to remove the stimulation for HCl and pepsin secretion by keeping the stomach empty. Stopping the spillage of GI contents into the peritoneal cavity is used for peritonitis. Removing excess fluids and undigested food from the stomach is the rationale for using NG intubation for gastric outlet obstruction.

26. b, c, f. Antacids provide a quick, short-lived relief of heartburn by neutralizing HCl in the stomach that prevents the conversion of pepsinogen to pepsin. Antacids may be given hourly, orally or through an NG tube, after an acute phase of GI bleeding to neutralize HCl in the stomach. Amoxicillin/clarithromycin/omeprazole are used in patients with verified *H. pylori*. Sucralfate (Carafate) covers the ulcer to protect it from acid erosion. The side effects are manageable.

27. a, c, d. Famotidine (Pepcid) reduces HCl secretion by blocking histamine and omeprazole (Prilosec) decreases gastric acid secretion by blocking adenosine triphosphatase (ATPase) enzyme. Misoprostol (Cytotec) has antisecretory effects. Sucralfate (Carafate) coats the ulcer to protect it from acid erosion. Bethanechol (Urecholine) for GERD increases LES pressure and facilitates gastric emptying.

28. c. Increased vagal stimulation from emotional stress causes hypersecretion of HCl, and stress reduction is an important part of the patient's management of peptic ulcers, especially

duodenal ulcers. If side effects to medications develop, the patient should notify the HCP before altering the drug regimen. Although effective treatment will promote pain relief in several days, the treatment regimen should be continued until there is evidence that the ulcer has healed completely. Interchanging brands and preparations of antacids and histamine (H_2)-receptor blockers without checking with HCPs may cause harmful side effects, and patients should take only prescribed medications.

29. c. Perforation of an ulcer causes sudden, severe abdominal pain that becomes generalized and may be referred to the back, accompanied by a rigid, boardlike abdomen, shallow respirations, and a weak rapid heart rate. Vomiting of blood indicates hemorrhage of an ulcer. Gastric outlet obstruction is characterized by projectile vomiting of undigested food, hyperactive stomach sounds, and upper abdominal swelling.

30. a. If symptoms of gastric outlet obstruction, such as nausea, vomiting, and stomach distention, occur while the patient is on NPO status or has an NG tube, the patency of the NG tube should first be assessed. A recumbent position should not be used in a patient with a gastric outlet obstruction because it increases abdominal pressure on the stomach. Vital signs and circulatory status assessment are important if hemorrhage or perforation is suspected. Deep breathing and relaxation may help some patients with nausea, but not when stomach contents are obstructed from flowing into the small intestine.

31. d. Abdominal pain that causes the knees to be drawn up and shallow, grunting respirations in a patient with peptic ulcer disease are characteristic of perforation and the nurse should assess the patient's vital signs and abdomen before notifying the HCP. Irrigation of the NG tube should not be done because the added fluid may be spilled into the peritoneal cavity and the patient should be placed in a position of comfort, usually on the side with the head slightly elevated.

32. a. 3; b. 4; c. 2; d. 1

33. d. Because there is no sphincter control of food taken into the stomach following a Billroth II procedure, concentrated food and fluid move rapidly into the small intestine, creating a hypertonic environment that pulls fluid from the bowel wall into the lumen of the intestine, reducing plasma volume and distending the bowel. Postprandial hypoglycemia occurs when the concentrated carbohydrate bolus in the small intestine results in hyperglycemia and the release of excessive amounts of insulin into the circulation, resulting in symptoms of hypoglycemia. Irritation of the stomach by bile salts causes epigastric distress after meals, not dumping syndrome.

34. a. Dietary control of dumping syndrome includes small, frequent meals with low carbohydrate content and elimination of fluids with meals. The patient should also lie down for 30 to 60 minutes after meals. These measures help delay stomach emptying, preventing the rapid movement of a high-carbohydrate food bolus into the small intestine.

35. d. If the patient's NG tube becomes obstructed following a gastrectomy with an intestinal anastomosis, gastric secretions may put a strain on the sutured anastomosis and cause serious complications. Be sure that the suction is working and because of the danger of perforating the gastric mucosa or disrupting the suture line, the nurse

should notify the surgeon. Periodic gentle irrigation with normal saline solution may be ordered or the surgeon may choose to reposition or replace the NG tube.

36. b. A total gastrectomy removes the parietal cells responsible for secreting intrinsic factor necessary for absorption of cobalamin. Lifelong IM administration of cobalamin is necessary to prevent the development of pernicious anemia. Wound healing is usually impaired in the patient with a total gastrectomy performed for gastric cancer because of impaired nutritional status before surgery. Following a total gastrectomy, the patient needs diet modifications because of dumping syndrome and postprandial hypoglycemia. Peptic ulcers are not a common finding after total gastrectomy.

37. a. Melena is black, tarry stools from slow bleeding from an upper gastrointestinal (GI) source when blood passes through the GI tract and is digested. Occult blood is the presence of guaiac-positive stools or gastric aspirate. Coffee-ground emesis is blood that has been in the stomach for some time and has reacted with gastric secretions. Profuse bright-red hematemesis is arterial blood that has not been in contact with gastric secretions, as in esophageal or oral bleeding.

38. b. Although all the interventions may be indicated when a patient has upper GI bleeding, the first nursing priority with bright-red (arterial) blood is to perform a focused assessment of the patient's condition, with emphasis on BP, pulse, and peripheral perfusion to determine the presence of hypovolemic shock.

39. d. IV esomeprazole (Nexium) is a proton pump inhibitor (PPI) that is used to decrease acid secretion and prevent interference with clotting as a bolus before endoscopy and then a continuous infusion. Nizatidine is a histamine (H_2)-receptor blocker that decreases acid secretion but is not as effective as PPIs. Epinephrine injection during endoscopy is effective for acute hemostasis. Vasopressin has a vasoconstriction action useful in controlling upper GI bleeding but does not facilitate clotting.

40. b. All OTC drugs should be avoided because their contents may include drugs that are contraindicated because of the irritating effects on the gastric mucosa. Patients are taught to test suspicious vomitus or stools for occult blood, but all stools do not have to be tested. Antacids cannot be taken with all medications because they prevent the absorption of many drugs. Patients with a history of ulcers who must take low-dose aspirin are prescribed misoprostol to protect the gastric mucosa.

41. d. The patient's blood urea nitrogen (BUN) is usually elevated with a significant hemorrhage because blood proteins are subjected to bacterial breakdown in the GI tract. With control of bleeding, the BUN will return to normal. During the early stage of bleeding, the hematocrit (Hct) is not always a reliable indicator of the amount of blood lost or the amount of blood replaced and may be falsely high or low. A urinary output of ≤ 20 mL/hr indicates impaired renal perfusion and hypovolemia and a urine specific gravity of 1.030 indicates concentrated urine typical of hypovolemia.

42. b. Food poisoning caused by *Escherichia coli* O147:H7 is characterized by profuse diarrhea, abdominal cramping, and bloody stools and is most often associated with undercooked, contaminated ground beef or poultry. Salmonella contamination most often occurs with poultry, staphylococcal

infections occur with milk and salad dressings, and botulism occurs with fish and low-acid canned products.

Case Study

1. **Expected**: fatigue (due to decreased hemoglobin and hematocrit levels and malnutrition), abdominal pain (due to stomach cancer), indigestion (due to gastric reflux); **Unexpected**, gastric outlet obstruction (which is a blockage from the stomach to the duodenum impeding the emptying of stomach contents), jaundice and ascites (which indicate liver involvement from possible metastasis); **Unrelated:** peripheral neuropathy (which doesn't apply to S.E. She may develop peripheral neuropathy if she is treated with chemotherapy agents)

2. **Anemia**=decreased hemoglobin and fatigue; **Nutritionally compromised**=decreased serum albumin, weight loss and emaciated; **Impaired GI function**=nausea and vomiting

3. **1**=68; **2**=32%; **3**=smoking, *H. Pylori*, and achlorhydria; **4**=endoscopy (best diagnostic tool) **4**=PET scan (can stage the disease) **4**=laparoscopy (determines peritoneal spread); **5**= Trastuzumab

4. B, C, G, H. Unless the patient is considered terminal, the nurse shouldn't discuss hospice options. Soft-bristled toothbrush would be recommended. Patients should perform activities as tolerable and should only be on bed rest if their condition warrants. Smoked meats are contraindicated because they increase the risk of stomach cancer. Promoting fluid intake is recommended, not restricting them. Fluids are not the cause of lymphedema.

5. **1**=metoclopramide; **2**=4 mg IV every 6 hours PRN; **3**=Phenothiazine; **4**=Increases gastric motility and emptying; **5**=Anticholinergic; **6**=aprepitant; **7**=80 mg PO once daily; **8**=Blocks action of serotonin

CHAPTER 47

1. c. Antiperistaltic agents, such as loperamide (Imodium) and paregoric, should not be used in infectious diarrhea because of the potential of prolonging exposure to the infectious agent. Demulcent agents may be used to coat and protect mucous membranes in these cases. The other options are all appropriate measures to use in cases of infectious diarrhea.

2. c. Wearing gloves will avoid hand contamination. Washing hands with soap and water will remove more *Clostridium difficile* spores than alcohol-based hand cleaners and ammonia-based disinfectants. The entire room will have to be disinfected with a 10% solution of household bleach. Probiotics may help prevent diarrhea in the patient on antibiotics by replacing normal intestinal bacteria.

3. d. The first intervention to establish bowel regularity includes promoting bowel evacuation at a regular time each day, preferably by placing the patient on the bedpan, using a bedside commode, or walking the patient to the bathroom. To take advantage of the gastrocolic reflex, an appropriate time is 30 minutes after the first meal of the day or at the patient's usual individual time. Perianal pouches are used to protect the skin only when regularity cannot be established, and evacuation suppositories are also used only if other techniques are not successful.

4. d. Ignoring the urge to defecate causes the muscles and mucosa in the rectal area to become insensitive to the presence of feces and drying of the stool occurs. The urge to defecate is decreased and stool becomes more difficult to expel. Taking a bulk-forming agent with fluids or high-fiber diet with fluids prevent constipation. Hemorrhoids are the most common complication of chronic constipation, caused by straining to pass hardened stool. The straining may cause problems in patients with hypertension, but these do not cause constipation.

5. c. Of the foods listed, dried beans contain the highest amount of dietary fiber and are an excellent source of soluble fiber. (See Table 42.8.)

6. a. Enemas are fast acting and beneficial in the immediate treatment of acute constipation but should be limited in their use. Increased fluids can help decrease the incidence of constipation. Stool softeners have a prolonged action, taking up to 72 hours for an effect. Bulk-forming medication stimulates peristalsis but takes 24 hours to act.

7. a. 1; b. 5; c. 4; d. 3; e. 2. Assessment of vital signs should be the first nursing action for the patient with an acute abdomen because there may be significant fluid or blood loss into the abdomen; followed by assessment of the abdomen and the nature of the pain. Anticipate diagnostic studies to identify the cause as soon as possible. Analgesics should be used cautiously until a diagnosis can be determined so that symptoms are not masked.

8. b, c, d, f. An immediate surgical consult is needed for acute ischemic bowel, foreign body perforation, ruptured ectopic pregnancy, or ruptured abdominal aneurysm. A diagnostic laparoscopy or a laparotomy may be done to repair a ruptured abdominal aneurysm or remove the appendix. Surgery is not needed for pancreatitis or pelvic inflammatory disease, as these can be diagnosed and treated without surgery.

9. c. An adequately functioning nasogastric (NG) tube should prevent nausea and vomiting because stomach contents are continuously being removed. The first intervention in this case is to check the amount and character of the recent drainage and check the tube for patency. Decreased or absent bowel sounds are expected after a laparotomy, and the Jackson-Pratt drains only fluid from the tissue of the surgical site. Antiemetics may be given if the NG tube is patent because anesthetic agents may cause nausea.

10. a. The abdominal pain and distention that occur from the decreased motility of the bowel should be treated with increased ambulation and frequent position changes to increase peristalsis. If the pain is severe, cholinergic drugs, rectal tubes, or application of heat to the abdomen may be prescribed. Assessment of bowel sounds is not an intervention to relieve the pain, and a high Fowler's position is not indicated. Opioids may still be necessary for pain control, and motility can be increased by other means.

11. d. The patient is having symptoms of an acute abdomen and should be evaluated immediately by an HCP at a hospital able to perform surgery if needed. The patient's age, location of pain, and other symptoms are characteristic of appendicitis. Heat application and laxatives should not be used in patients with undiagnosed abdominal pain because they may cause perforation of the appendix or other inflammations. Fluids should not be taken until vomiting is controlled, nor should they be taken in the event that surgery may be performed.

12. b. Because there is no definitive treatment for irritable bowel syndrome (IBS), patients become frustrated and

discouraged with uncontrolled symptoms. It is important to develop a trusting relationship that will support the patient as different treatments are implemented and evaluated. Although IBS can be precipitated and aggravated by stress and emotions, it is not a psychogenic illness. High-fiber diets may help, but they may also increase the bloating and gas pains of IBS. Medications are available, but use is individualized because of side effects.

13. b. It is likely that the patient could be developing peritonitis, which could be life threatening, and assessment of vital signs for hypovolemic shock should be done to report to the HCP. If an IV line is not in place, it should be inserted and pain may be eased by flexing the knees.

14. b. The patient's manifestations are characteristic of appendicitis. After laboratory test and CT scan confirmation, the patient will have surgery. Laxatives are not used. The 6 hours of fluids and antibiotics preoperatively would be used if the appendix was ruptured. The NG tube is more likely to be used with abdominal trauma.

15. c. IV fluid replacement along with antibiotics, NG suction, analgesics, and potential surgery would be expected. Peritoneal lavage may be used to determine abdominal trauma. Peritoneal dialysis would not be performed. Oral fluids would be avoided with peritonitis.

16. a, c, e, f. Crohn's disease may have severe weight loss, crampy abdominal pain, and segmented distribution through the entire wall of the bowel. Rectal bleeding and toxic megacolon are more often seen with ulcerative colitis.

17. c. In the patient with ulcerative colitis, decreased serum Na^+, K^+, Mg^+, Cl^-, and HCO_3^- are a result of diarrhea and vomiting. Hypoalbuminemia may be present in severe disease. Elevated white blood cell (WBC) counts occur with toxic megacolon. Decreased hemoglobin (Hgb) and hematocrit (Hct) occur with bloody diarrhea, leading to iron-deficiency anemia.

18. d. Ulcerative colitis and Crohn's disease have many of the same extraintestinal symptoms, including erythema nodosum and osteoporosis, as well as gallstones, uveitis, and conjunctivitis. Celiac disease, peptic ulcer disease, and colonic dilation are not extraintestinal.

19. a, b, e, f. With an acute exacerbation of inflammatory bowel disease (IBD), to rest the bowel the patient will be NPO, receive IV fluids and parenteral nutrition, and have NG suction. Sedatives may be used to alleviate stress. Enteral nutrition will be used as soon as possible.

20. c. Cobalamin and iron injections will help correct malnutrition. Correcting malnutrition will also indirectly help improve quality of life and fight infections.

21. c. Antidiarrheal agents only relieve symptoms. Corticosteroids, 6-mercaptopurine, and sulfasalazine (Azulfidine) are used to treat and control inflammation with various diseases and maintain IBD remission.

22. b. The initial procedure for a total proctocolectomy with ileal pouch and anal anastomosis includes a colectomy, rectal mucosectomy, ileal reservoir construction, ileoanal anastomosis, and a temporary ileostomy. A loop ileostomy is the most common temporary ileostomy, and it may be held in place with a plastic rod for the first week. A rectal tube to suction is not indicated in any of the surgical procedures for ulcerative colitis. A colostomy is not used, and an NG tube would not be used to irrigate the pouch. A

permanent ileostomy stoma would be expected following a total proctocolectomy with a permanent ileostomy.

23. a. Initial output from a newly formed ileostomy may be as high as 1500 to 2000 mL daily, and intake and output must be accurately monitored for fluid and electrolyte imbalance. Ileostomy bags may have to be emptied every 3 to 4 hours, but the appliance should not be changed for several days unless there is leakage onto the skin. A terminal ileum stoma is permanent, and the entire colon has been removed. A return to a normal, presurgical diet is the goal for the patient with an ileostomy, with restrictions based only on the patient's individual tolerances.

24. a. Signs of malnutrition include pallor from anemia, hair loss, bleeding, cracked gingivae, and muscle weakness, which support a clinical problem that identifies impaired nutrition. Diarrhea may contribute to malnutrition but is not a defining characteristic for this patient. Anorectal excoriation and pain relate to problems with skin integrity. Hypotension relates to problems with fluid deficit.

25. b. Volvulus is an abnormal twisting of the bowel. The bowel folding in on itself is intussusception. Emboli of arterial blood supply to the bowel is vascular obstruction. Protrusion of bowel in a weak or abnormal opening is a hernia.

26. d. Intermittent crampy abdominal pain, nausea, projectile vomiting, and dehydration are characteristics of proximal small intestinal obstruction. Large bowel obstruction is characterized by constipation, low-grade abdominal pain, and abdominal distention. Esophageal sphincter blockage or achalasia feels like food is stuck in the chest. Fecal emesis is seen with distal small intestinal obstruction.

27. b. Mouth care should be done frequently for the patient with a small intestinal obstruction who has an NG tube because of vomiting, fecal taste and odor, and mouth breathing. No ice chips are allowed when a patient is NPO because of a bowel obstruction. The NG tube should be checked for patency and irrigated only as ordered. The position of the patient should be one of comfort.

28. c. Although all polyps are abnormal growths, the most common type of polyp (hyperplastic) is nonneoplastic, as are inflammatory, lipomas, and juvenile polyps. However, adenomatous polyps are characterized by neoplastic changes in the epithelium, and about 85% of colorectal cancers (CRCs) arise from these polyps. Only patients with a family history of familial adenomatous polyposis (FAP) have close to a 100% lifetime risk of developing CRC and are at greater risk for other cancers.

29. a. A diet high in red meat and low in fruit and vegetable intake is associated with development of CRC, as are alcohol intake and smoking. Family and personal history of CRC also increases the risk. Other environmental agents are not known to be related to CRC. Long-term use of nonsteroidal antiinflammatory drugs (NSAIDs) is associated with reduced CRC risk.

30. d. With an abdominal perineal-resection (APR), an abdominal incision is made, and the proximal sigmoid colon is brought through the abdominal wall and formed into a permanent colostomy. The patient is repositioned, a perineal incision is made, and the distal sigmoid colon, rectum, and anus are removed through the perineal incision, which may be closed or open and packed, and have drains.

31. d. The ileostomy drainage is extremely irritating to the skin, so the skin must be cleaned and a new solid skin barrier

and pouch applied as soon as a leak occurs to prevent skin damage. The pouch is usually worn for 4 to 7 days unless there is a leak. Because the initial drainage from the ileostomy is high, the fluid intake must be increased. The pouch must always be worn, as the liquid drainage, not formed bowel movements, is frequent.

32. b. A normal new colostomy stoma should appear rose to brick-red, have mild to moderate edema, and have a small amount of bleeding or oozing of blood when touched. A purplish stoma indicates inadequate blood supply and should be reported. Bowel sounds after extensive bowel surgery will be diminished or absent. The colostomy will not have any fecal drainage for 2 to 4 days, but there may be some earlier mucus or serosanguineous drainage.

33. d, e. The LPN can monitor and record observations related to the drainage and can measure and record the amount. The LPN could also monitor the skin around the stoma for breakdown. LPNs can irrigate a colostomy in a stable patient, but this patient is only 2 days postoperative. The other actions are responsibilities of the RN (teaching, assessing stoma, and developing a care plan).

34. d. Sexual dysfunction may result from an APR, but the nurse should discuss with the patient that different nerve pathways affect erection, ejaculation, and orgasm and that a dysfunction of one does not mean total sexual dysfunction and also that an alteration in sexual activity does not have to alter sexuality. Referral to a wound, ostomy, and continence nurse (WOCN) would also be helpful. Simple reassurance of desirability and ignoring concerns about sexual function do not help the patient regain positive feelings of sexuality.

35. d. The patient with a transverse colostomy has semiliquid to semiformed stools needing a pouch and needs to have fluid balance monitored. The ascending colostomy has semiliquid stools needing a pouch and increased fluid. The ileostomy has liquid to semiliquid stools needing a pouch and increased fluid. The sigmoid colostomy has formed stools, may or may not need a pouch but will need irrigation, and no changes in fluid needs.

36. a. Encouraging the patient to share concerns and ask questions will help the patient begin to adapt to living with the colostomy. The other options do not support the patient and do not portray the nurse's focus on helping the patient or treating the patient as an individual.

37. c. Formation of diverticuli is common when decreased bulk of stool, combined with a more narrowed lumen in the sigmoid colon, causes high intraluminal pressures that result in saccular dilation or outpouching of the mucosa through the muscle of the intestinal wall. To prevent diverticula, fecal volume and passage is increased with use of high-fiber diets and at least 2 L of fluid each day. Bulk laxatives, such as psyllium (Metamucil), may also be used. Antibiotics are used only during acute diverticulitis with infection. Colonoscopies are done to detect problems, but not yearly.

38. a. Diverticulitis can erode the bowel wall and perforate into the peritoneum. Abscesses may form to wall off the area of perforation, but complete perforation with peritonitis may occur. Systemic antibiotic therapy is often used, but medicated enemas would increase intestinal motility and increase the possibility of perforation, as would the application of heat. Surgery is only necessary to drain abscesses or to resect an obstructing inflammatory mass.

39. a, d. The ventral or incisional hernia is caused by a weakness of the abdominal wall at the site of a previous incision. It is reducible because it returns to the abdominal cavity. Inguinal hernias are at the weak area of the abdominal wall, where the spermatic cord in men or the round ligament in women emerges. A femoral hernia is a protrusion through the femoral ring into the femoral canal. Incarcerated hernias do not reduce. Strangulation occurs when the blood supply to an irreducible hernia is compromised.

40. c. A strangulated femoral hernia obstructs intestinal flow and blood supply, thus requiring emergency surgery. The other options are incorrect.

41. b. Scrotal edema is a common and painful complication after an inguinal hernia repair and can be relieved in part by elevation of the scrotum with a scrotal support and application of ice. Heat would increase the edema and the discomfort and a truss is used to keep unrepaired hernias from protruding. Coughing is discouraged postoperatively because it increases intraabdominal pressure and stress on the repair site.

42. b. The most common type of malabsorption syndrome is lactose intolerance, and it is managed by restricting the intake of milk and milk products. Antibiotics are used in cases of bacterial infections that cause malabsorption, pancreatic enzyme supplementation is used for pancreatic insufficiency, and restriction of gluten is necessary for control of adult celiac disease (celiac sprue, gluten-sensitive enteropathy).

43. c. The autoimmune process associated with celiac disease continues as long as the body is exposed to gluten, regardless of the symptoms it produces, and a lifelong gluten-free diet is necessary. The other statements regarding celiac disease are all true.

44. b. Short bowel syndrome results from extensive resection of portions of the small bowel and would occur if a patient had an extensive resection of the ileum. The other conditions primarily affect the large intestine and result in fewer and less severe symptoms.

45. b. An anorectal abscess is a collection of perianal pus. An ulcer in the anal wall is an anal fissure. Sacrococcygeal hairy tract describes a pilonidal sinus. A tunnel leading from the anus or rectum is an anorectal fistula.

46. c. Human papillomavirus (HPV) is associated with about 80% of anal cancer cases. Other risk factors include smoking, receptive anal sex, women with cervical or vulvar cancer or precancerous lesions, immunosuppression, and human immunodeficiency virus (HIV) infection. The other options are not considered risk factors for anal cancer.

47. d. Warm sitz baths provide comfort, healing, and cleansing of the area following all anorectal surgery and may be done 3 or 4 times a day for 1 to 2 weeks. Stool softeners and bulking agents help form a soft bulky stool that is easier to pass, but laxatives may cause irritation and trauma to the anorectal area and are not used postoperatively. Early passage of a bowel movement, although painful, is encouraged to prevent drying and hardening of stool, which would result in an even more painful bowel movement.

Case Study

1. **Related**: hematochezia (bloody stools), constipation (or diarrhea, any change in bowel habits), abdominal pain or discomfort, fatigue; **Unrelated**: nausea and vomiting, dyspnea on exertion, weight gain (weight loss is associated)

2. **Indicated**: ask the patient to report flatus (this indicates GI motility and the diet can be advanced), advance diet to soft food once bowel sounds are normal, apply transparent ostomy pouch over the stoma (this allows visual assessment of the stoma postoperatively); **Contraindicated**: keep the patient on bedrest (the patient should be ambulating on the same day postop; bedrest can lead to complications); tell the patient's wife the stoma is temporary (C.D.'s stoma will be permanent because the rectum was removed; telling her it is temporary will offer false hope and disappointment); **Non-essential**: report stoma drainage of 50 mL over 24 hours (this amount of drainage is expected, therefore there is no need to report it), perform daily weights (unnecessary as it doesn't provide useful information for this patient)

3. **Colostomy**: stool is semiformed, stoma may arise from the transverse colon; **Ileostomy**: stool is liquid to semiliquid, stoma arises from the ileum, dietary restrictions may be necessary to avoid obstruction; **Both**: an ostomy pouch is worn, passage of the stool cannot be regulated, may be temporary or permanent

4. **Effective**: his wife is asking questions about stoma care (shows an interest and participation in her husband's care), C.D. says he knows he will have to change his diet (to a healthier diet with less meat and more fruits and vegetables); **Ineffective**: wife is emotional (difficulty coping with the stoma), C.D. calls the stoma "Jake" and says it is "winking" (naming it and giving it a personality separates it from himself preserving his body image), attempts to use the PCA 17 times in an hour (indicates he may be anxious, fearful, lacks control, or has difficulty coping); **Unrelated**: C.D. asks for a nicotine patch (meets his need for nicotine while not being able to smoke, but isn't related to coping with the colostomy)

5. B., D., E., G. C.D. should be advised to reduce or eliminate his risk factors which includes quitting smoking. He will need to stay hydrated by drinking at least 3000 mL of fluid each day. He should refrain from heavy lifting for 6-8 weeks postoperatively. Community support groups and other resources can benefit C.D. and his wife by providing information and emotional support. Gas forming foods can quickly inflate the ostomy pouch and emit odor which can be reduced or avoided by not eating certain gas producing foods like cabbage and beans. Asparagus and garlic are odor-producing. They don't cause diarrhea. Stomas can get wet. Sexual problems do occur with this type of surgery and can be managed with giving it time and tips to hide or cover the stoma during intimacy.

CHAPTER 48

1. c. Gallstones cause obstructive or posticteric jaundice and may increase both conjugated and unconjugated bilirubin.

2. d. Hemolytic jaundice from a blood transfusion reaction is from increased breakdown of red blood cells (RBCs) producing increased unconjugated bilirubin in the blood. Hepatocellular jaundice results from damaged hepatocytes leaking bilirubin. Hemolytic jaundice occurs with malaria. Obstructive jaundice is from obstructed bile flow through the liver or biliary duct system.

3. d. Hepatitis E virus (HEV) is associated with poor sanitation and contaminated water in developing countries.

4. b. Hepatitis B virus (HBV) is a DNA virus that is transmitted via infectious blood and body products and is required for hepatitis D virus (HDV) replication, and chronic HBV along with chronic hepatitis C virus (HCV) accounts for 80% of hepatocellular cancer cases. Hepatitis A virus (HAV), HCV, HDV, and HEV are all RNA viruses.

5. c. Immunization to HBV after vaccination is identified with the hepatitis B surface antibody (anti-HBs). Anti-HBc immunoglobulin (Ig)G indicates previous or ongoing HBV infection. Surface antigen HBsAg is present in acute and chronic infection. Core antigen anti-HBc IgM indicates acute infection and does not appear after vaccination.

6. d. HBV DNA quantitation is the best indicator of viral replication and effectiveness of therapy for chronic HBV. HBsAg is present in acute or chronic infection. HBeAg shows high infectivity and can be used to determine clinical management of patients with chronic HBV. Anti-HBc IgM occurs with acute infection. Anti-HBc IgG indicates ongoing infection. Anti-HDV is present in past or current infection with HDV and therefore HBV. Anti-HBs indicate previous infection with HBV or immunization.

7. d. Anti-HAV IgM indicates acute HAV infection. Anti-HBc IgG indicates previous or ongoing infection with HBV. Anti-HBc IgM indicates acute HBV infection. Anti-HAV IgG indicates previous infection with HAV.

8. b. HCV genotyping is done to determine HCV drug choice, duration, and response to drug therapy. Anti-HCV and HCV RNA quantitation are tests completed to diagnose HCV. FibroSure (FibroTest) is used to assess the extent of hepatic fibrosis.

9. d. The systemic manifestations of rash, angioedema, arthritis, fever, and malaise in viral hepatitis are caused by the activation of the complement system by circulating immune complexes. Liver manifestations include jaundice from hepatic cell damage and cholestasis as well as anorexia. Impaired portal circulation usually does not occur in uncomplicated viral hepatitis but would be a liver manifestation.

10. b. During the incubation period, there are no symptoms, but serologic and enzyme markers of the disease are present. Earliest symptoms may include anorexia and discomfort in the upper right quadrant of the abdomen. Pruritus, dark urine, and light-colored stools occur with the onset of jaundice in the acute phase. Easy fatigability and malaise are seen in the convalescent phase as jaundice disappears.

11. d. The most common cause of acute liver failure is drugs, usually acetaminophen in combination with alcohol. HBV is the second most common cause. HAV is a less common cause.

12. d. HBV vaccine and hepatitis B immune globulin (HBIG) are used together prophylactically after a needle stick. Interferon is used to treat chronic HBV.

13. b. People who have been exposed to hepatitis A through household contact or foodborne outbreaks should be given IG within 1 to 2 weeks of exposure to prevent or modify the illness. Hepatitis A vaccine is used to provide preexposure immunity to the virus. Although hepatitis A may be spread by sexual contact, the risk is higher for transmission with the oral-fecal route.

14. c. Nucleoside and nucleotide analogs (e.g., lamivudine) and pegylated interferon are used to treat chronic hepatitis B. No specific drugs are effective in treating acute viral

hepatitis, although supportive drugs, such as antiemetics, sedatives, or antipruritics, may be used for symptom control.

15. b. The patient with acute hepatitis B is infectious for 4 to 6 months, and precautions to prevent transmission through percutaneous and sexual contact should be maintained until tests for Hbs Ag or anti-HBc IgM are negative. Close contact does not have to be avoided, but close contacts of the patient should be vaccinated. Alcohol should not be used for at least a year, and rest with increasing activity during convalescence is recommended.

16. a. Adequate nutrition is especially important in promoting regeneration of liver cells, but the anorexia of viral hepatitis is often severe, requiring creative and innovative nursing interventions. Strict bed rest is not usually required, and the patient usually has only minor discomfort with hepatitis. Diversional activities may be required to promote psychologic rest but not during periods of fatigue.

17. c. Immunosuppressive agents are indicated in hepatitis associated with immune disorders to decrease liver damage caused by autoantibodies. Autoimmune hepatitis is similar to viral hepatitis in presenting signs and symptoms and may become chronic and lead to cirrhosis.

18. c. Corneal Fleischer rings, brownish red rings in the cornea near the limbus, are the hallmark of Wilson's disease. Pruritus (not seen with Wilson's disease) is commonly seen with jaundice or primary biliary cirrhosis. Renal failure associated with hepatorenal syndrome is not seen with Wilson's disease. High serum iron levels are seen with hemochromatosis.

19. d. Most patients with primary sclerosing cholangitis (PSC) also have ulcerative colitis. The manifestations are otherwise similar to cirrhosis, and PSC may lead to cirrhosis, liver failure, and liver cancer.

20. a, c, d. The anemia of cirrhosis is related to overactivity of the enlarged spleen that removes blood cells from circulation. Vitamin B deficiencies from altered intake and metabolism of nutrients and decreased prothrombin production can increase bleeding tendencies. The other options do not contribute to anemia in the patient with cirrhosis.

21. a, b, d. There is no treatment for nonalcoholic fatty liver disease (NAFLD) except to control the other diseases that are common in these persons. These measures include weight loss for obesity, control of blood glucose for diabetes, control of hyperlipidemia, and treating hypertension if it is present. Ulcerative colitis is unrelated to NAFLD.

22. c. Esophageal varices occur when collateral channels of circulation develop inelastic fragile veins from portal hypertension. Portal hypertension is from scarring and nodular changes in the liver leading to compression of the veins and sinusoids, causing resistance of blood flow through the liver from the portal vein. It contributes to peripheral edema and ascites. Jaundice is from the inability of the liver to conjugate bilirubin. Biliary cirrhosis causes the loss of small bile ducts and ultimate cholestasis in patients with other autoimmune disorders.

23. d. Blood flow through the portal system is obstructed and causes portal hypertension that increases the BP in the portal venous system. Decreased albumin production leads to decreased serum colloidal oncotic pressure that

contributes to ascites. Hyperaldosteronism increases sodium and water retention and contributes to increased fluid retention, hypokalemia, and decreased urinary output. The retained fluid has low oncotic colloidal pressure. It escapes into the interstitial spaces, causing peripheral edema. Portal hypertension contributes to esophageal varices. Reduced renal blood flow and increased serum levels of antidiuretic hormone (ADH) contribute to impaired water excretion and ascites.

24. b. Serum bilirubin, both direct and indirect, would be expected to be increased in cirrhosis. Serum albumin and cholesterol are decreased and liver enzymes, such as aspartate aminotransferase (AST) and alanine aminotransferase (ALT), are initially increased but may be normal in end-stage liver disease.

25. a. Oral hygiene may improve the patient's taste sensation. Food preferences are important, but some foods may be restricted if the patient is on a low-sodium or low-fat diet. The patient will feel more independent with self-feeding and will be more likely to increase intake by having someone sit with the patient while the patient eats. Snacks and supplements should be available whenever the patient desires them but should not be forced on the patient.

26. b, c. With diuretic therapy, fluid and electrolyte balance must be monitored; serum levels of sodium, potassium, chloride, and bicarbonate must be monitored, especially for hypokalemia. Renal function must be monitored with blood urea nitrogen and serum creatinine. Water excess is manifested by muscle cramping, weakness, lethargy, and confusion. Gastrointestinal (GI) bleeding, body image disturbances, and bleeding tendencies seen with cirrhosis are not related to diuretic therapy.

27. d. Early signs (grade 1) of this neurologic condition include impaired computational skills, short attention span, personality change, decreased short-term memory, mild confusion, depression, and incoordination. Loss of consciousness (grade 4) is usually preceded by asterixis, abnormal reflexes, and disoriented to time (grades 2 and 3); inappropriate behavior, deficient executive function, marked confusion, loss of meaningful conversation, and incomprehensible speech. Increasing oliguria is a sign of hepatorenal syndrome.

28. c. Ammonia must be reduced to treat hepatic encephalopathy. The laxative, lactulose, decreases ammonia by trapping the ammonia and eliminating it in the feces. A β-adrenergic blocker will be used to decrease portal venous pressure and decrease variceal bleeding. The proton pump inhibitor will decrease gastric acidity but will not eliminate blood already in the GI tract. Rifaximin will decrease bacterial flora and therefore decrease ammonia formation from protein metabolism.

29. c. The patient may not be oriented or able to walk to the bathroom alone because of hyperreflexia, asterixis, or decreased motor coordination. Turning should be done every 2 hours to prevent skin breakdown. Activity is limited to decrease ammonia as a by-product of protein metabolism. Although constipation will be prevented, it will not keep the patient safe.

30. b. The patient with advanced, complicated cirrhosis requires a high-calorie, high-carbohydrate diet with moderate to low fat. Patients with cirrhosis are at risk for edema and ascites, and their sodium intake may be limited.

The tomato sandwich with salt-free butter best meets these requirements. Rough foods, such as popcorn, may irritate the esophagus and stomach and lead to bleeding. Peanut butter is high in sodium and fat, and canned chicken noodle soup is very high in sodium.

31. d. Monitoring for viral, fungal, and bacterial infection after the liver transplant is essential, as only fever may be present with an infection. Alcohol will not be any better for the patient after the transplant than it was before the transplant. HBIG is given for postexposure protection from HBV. The head of the bed is elevated to improve ventilation with severe ascites.

32. c. Bleeding esophageal varices are a medical emergency. During an episode of bleeding, management of the airway and prevention of aspiration of blood are critical factors. Portal shunting surgery may be done for esophageal varices but not during an acute hemorrhage. Occult blood as well as fresh blood from the GI tract would be expected. Vasopressin causes vasoconstriction, decreased heart rate, and decreased coronary blood flow. IV nitroglycerin may be given with the vasopressin to counter these side effects.

33. d. By shunting fluid sequestered in the portal vein into the venous system, pressure on esophageal veins is decreased and more volume is returned to the circulation, improving cardiac output and renal perfusion. However, because ammonia is diverted past the liver, hepatic encephalopathy may occur. These procedures do not prolong life or promote liver function.

34. c. Abstinence from alcohol is very important in alcoholic cirrhosis and may result in improvement if started when liver damage is limited. Although further liver damage may be reduced by rest and nutrition, most changes in the liver cannot be reversed. Exercise does not promote portal circulation, and very moderate exercise is recommended. Acetaminophen should not be used by the patient with alcoholic cirrhosis because this liver is more sensitive to the hepatotoxicity of acetaminophen.

35. c. Because the prognosis for cancer of the liver is poor and treatment is largely palliative, supportive nursing care is appropriate. The patient exhibits clinical manifestations of liver failure, as seen in any patient with advanced liver failure. Whether the cancer is primary or metastatic, there is usually a poor response to chemotherapy and surgery is indicated in the few patients that have localization of the tumor when there is no evidence of invasion of hepatic blood vessels.

36. d. Liver transplantation is indicated for patients with cirrhosis as well as for many adults and children with other irreversible liver diseases. Liver transplantation is contraindicated with severe extrahepatic disease, cancers, ongoing drug or alcohol use, and inability to comprehend or comply with the rigorous posttransplant care. Nurses should be knowledgeable about the indications for transplantation and be able to discuss the patient's questions and concerns related to transplantation. Rejection is less of a problem in liver transplants than with other organs, such as the kidney.

37. d. A pancreatic abscess, usually from an infected pseudocyst, is a collection of pus that must be drained to prevent infection of adjacent organs and sepsis. Tetany from hypocalcemia is treated with IV calcium gluconate (10%). Although pseudocysts usually resolve spontaneously, they may be treated with surgical, percutaneous catheter, or endoscopic drainage to prevent perforation. Pleural effusion is treated by treating the cause (pancreatitis) and monitoring for respiratory distress and oxygen saturation.

38. d. The predominant symptom of acute pancreatitis is severe, deep abdominal pain that is usually located in the left upper quadrant (LUQ) but may be in the midepigastrium. Bowel sounds are decreased or absent, the patient is hypotensive and may manifest symptoms of shock, and there is only a low-grade fever.

39. b. Although serum lipase levels and urinary amylase levels are increased, an increased serum amylase level is the criterion most commonly used to diagnose acute pancreatitis in the first 24 to 72 hours. Serum calcium levels are decreased and serum glucose is increased.

40. c. Pancreatic rest and suppression of secretions are promoted by preventing any gastric contents from entering the duodenum, which would stimulate pancreatic activity. Surgery is not indicated for acute pancreatitis but may be used to drain abscesses or cysts. Pancreatic enzyme supplements are necessary in chronic pancreatitis if a deficiency in secretion occurs, but not for acute pancreatitis. An endoscopic retrograde cholangiopancreatography (ERCP) pancreatic sphincterotomy may be done when pancreatitis is related to gallstones.

41. c. Positions that flex the trunk and draw the knees up to the abdomen help relieve the pain of acute pancreatitis. Positioning the patient on the side with the head elevated decreases abdominal tension. Diversional techniques are not as helpful as positioning in controlling the pain. The patient is usually NPO because food intake increases the pain and inflammation. Bed rest is indicated during the acute attack because of hypovolemia and pain.

42. c. Sodium restriction is not indicated for patients recovering from acute pancreatitis, but fat is restricted. The stools should be observed for steatorrhea, indicating that fat digestion is impaired. Alcohol is a primary cause of pancreatitis and should not be used. Glucose levels are monitored for chronic pancreatitis.

43. c. Chronic damage to the pancreas causes a deficiency of digestive enzymes and insulin resulting in malabsorption and diabetes. Abstinence from alcohol is necessary in both types of pancreatitis, as is a high-carbohydrate, high-protein, and low-fat diet. Although abdominal pain is a major manifestation of chronic pancreatitis, more commonly a constant heavy, gnawing feeling occurs.

44. a, b, c. Measures to prevent attacks of pancreatitis are those that decrease the stimulation of the pancreas. Lower fat intake and foods that are less stimulating and irritating (bland) should be encouraged. High carbohydrates are less stimulating. Avoid alcohol and nicotine, since both stimulate the pancreas. Monitor for steatorrhea to determine the effectiveness of the enzymes and because it may indicate worsening pancreatic function. Pancreatic enzymes should be taken with, not after, meals.

45. b. Major risk factors for pancreatic cancer are cigarette smoking, chronic pancreatitis, diabetes, age, family history of pancreatic cancer, high-fat diet, and exposure to benzidine. Pancreatic cancer is not directly associated with alcohol intake, as pancreatitis is.

46. a. In a Whipple procedure, the head of the pancreas, the duodenum which is next to the pancreas, distal segment of the common bile duct, the gall bladder, and the distal portion of the stomach are removed. The duodenum is responsible for the breakdown of food in the small intestine and regulates the rate of stomach emptying, which affects the patient's nutritional status.

47. a, b, c, e, f. Incidence of cholelithiasis is higher in women, multiparous women, persons over 40 years of age, and those with family history and obesity. Postmenopausal women taking estrogen replacement therapy and younger women on oral contraceptives have a higher incidence. Alcohol intake and diet do not increase the incidence of cholelithiasis.

48. a, c, d. Acalculous cholecystitis is associated with prolonged immobility, fasting, prolonged parenteral nutrition, and diabetes. Hypothyroidism, *Streptococcus pneumoniae*, and absence of bile in the intestine are unrelated to this condition.

49. b. Absence of bilirubin and bile salts in the intestine lead to clay-colored stools and steatorrhea. Soluble bilirubin in the blood excreted into the urine leads to dark urine. Contraction of the inflamed gallbladder leads to pain with fatty food intake. Obstruction of the common bile duct prevents bile drainage into the duodenum, with congestion of bile in the liver. Bilirubin absorption in the blood leads to jaundice.

50. a. Ultrasonography is accurate in detecting gallstones and is a noninvasive procedure. Magnetic resonance cholangiopancreatography (MRCP) and endoscopic ultrasound (EUS) may also be used when the patient is allergic to contrast medium. An IV cholangiogram uses radiopaque dye to outline the gallbladder and ducts. Liver function studies will be increased if liver damage has occurred but do not indicate gallbladder disease.

51. a. NPO and nasogastric (NG) suction prevent gallbladder stimulation from food or fluids moving into the duodenum. Laparoscopic cholecystectomy is used more often than incisional cholecystectomy, but both remove the gallbladder, not its stimulation. Administration of antiemetics decreases nausea and vomiting but does not decrease gallbladder stimulation. Anticholinergics counteract the smooth muscle spasms of the bile ducts to decrease pain.

52. d. The laparoscopic cholecystectomy requires 1 to 4 small abdominal incisions to visualize and remove the gallbladder, and the patient has small dressings placed over these incisions. The patient with an incisional cholecystectomy is usually hospitalized for 2 to 3 days, whereas the laparoscopic procedure allows same-day or next-day discharge with return to work within 1 week. A T-tube is placed in the common bile duct after exploration of the duct during an incisional cholecystectomy.

53. c. After removal of the gallbladder, bile drains directly from the liver into the duodenum and a low-fat diet is recommended until adjustment to this change occurs. Most patients tolerate a regular diet with moderate fat intake but should avoid excessive fat intake, as large volumes of bile previously stored in the gallbladder are not available. Steatorrhea could occur with a large fat intake.

54. a. The T-tube drains bile from the common bile duct until swelling from trauma has subsided, and bile can freely enter the duodenum. The tube is placed to gravity drainage and should be kept open and free from kinks to prevent bile from backing up into the liver. The tube is not normally clamped or irrigated.

55. c. Bile-colored drainage or pus from any incision may indicate an infection and should be reported to the HCP immediately. The bandages on the puncture sites should be removed the day after surgery, followed by showering. Referred shoulder pain is a common and expected problem following laparoscopic procedures, when carbon dioxide used to inflate the abdominal cavity is not readily absorbed by the body. Nausea and vomiting are not expected postoperatively and may indicate damage to other abdominal organs and should be reported to the HCP.

Case Study

1. **Expected**: decreased or absent bowel sounds (due to decreased GI motility; patients may have paralytic ileus), crackles in the lungs (lungs are often involved), Cullen's sign (periumbilical discoloration); **Unexpected**: palpable epigastric mass (present with a pancreatic pseudocyst), pleural effusion (indicates a systemic complication), Trousseau's sign (tetany of the arm when squeezed by BP cuff indicates hypocalcemia which is a sign of severe disease), increased abdominal girth (could indicate abdominal compartment syndrome); **Unrelated**: grade III/VI murmur (indicates cardiac regurgitation due to an incompetent heart valve)

2. **Expected**: increased serum amylase and lipase (primary diagnostic tests; occurs due to increased pancreatic enzymes being released), WBC count 20,000/μL (leukocytosis is common); **Unexpected**: calcium 7 mg/dL (hypocalcemia associated with severe disease), chest x-ray: whiteout (could be a sign of ARDS which is a complication of acute pancreatitis); **Unrelated**: echocardiogram EF 40% (is indicative of a cardiac problem), hemoglobin 10 g/dL (indicates anemia which is not associated with acute pancreatitis)

3. A., D., E., G., H. Pressures between 40-80 mm Hg are recommended when low intermittent or continuous suction is ordered. Feeding tubes are too small in diameter and should not be connected to suction or used to decompress the stomach. Salem sump NG tubes are preferred to decompress the stomach. The air vent on a Salem sump helps create adequate suction and should not be clogged or clamped. A normal adult size Salem sump NG tube is 14-Fr to 16-Fr. The HOB should be at least 30 degrees to reduce the risk of aspiration. Residuals are checked for tube feedings, not NG tubes connected to suction. Placement should be verified using pH test paper to confirm the acidity of the gastric drainage. Injecting air boluses while auscultating the epigastric area is not a reliable method to check placement as studies show that the air can be heard even though the tube is in the wrong place.

4. **Hypotension**: administer lactated Ringer's solution (to improve hydration and replace fluid loss), dopamine, if necessary (vasoactive medication that will increase SVR and treat hypotension), albumin, if necessary (a volume expander used to improve fluid status and treat hypotension); **Acute Pain**: morphine PCA (an opioid the patient can control to help with pain management), papaverine, if necessary (a calcium-channel blocker

that helps relax smooth muscle and treats spasms that may be causing pain); **Pancreatic Enzyme Production**: keep patient NPO (reduces or suppresses pancreatic enzymes that stimulate the pancreas allowing the pancreas to rest), administer pantoprazole (a PPI that reduces gastric secretion), NG tube to LIS (reduces vomiting and gastric distention and prevents acidic gastric contents from entering the duodenum which would stimulate the production of pancreatic enzymes)

5. **Effective**: SpO₂ 96% on 3 L/min nasal cannula (evidence the patient is not hypoxemic and has sufficient oxygenation), denies dizziness with position changes (no evidence of orthostatic hypotension, BP has improved), denies palpitations (evidence of a normal heart rate without dysrhythmias, patient was tachycardic); **Ineffective**: cheek twitches when tapped (Chvostek's sign indicative of hypocalcemia), flank ecchymosis (Grey Turner sign, evidence of acute pancreatitis), reports numbness around lips (evidence of hypocalcemia), reports dyspnea on exertion (indicates poor activity tolerance possibly caused by pleural effusions or pulmonary edema); **Unrelated**: pupils 4 mm equal and reactive (neurologic assessment that is unrelated to acute pancreatitis)

6. A., C., E., F., I. Using any nicotine products, including smoking, is not recommended because they stimulate the pancreas. Replacing fats with carbohydrates is recommended because fats stimulate the pancreas to produce enzymes. Because of the loss of physical and muscle strength, physical therapy may be needed. Alcohol is the main risk factor associated with acute pancreatitis; therefore, patients should abstain from drinking alcohol. Foul-smelling stools should be reported to the HCP because it indicates ongoing destruction of the pancreatic tissue and pancreatic insufficiency (chronic pancreatitis). It is better to eat small frequent meals instead of 3 large ones to decrease pancreatic stimulation. Weight loss is a sign of chronic pancreatitis and should be reported to the HCP. Acute pancreatitis can develop into chronic pancreatitis.

CHAPTER 49

1. a. Inferior vena cava; b. right adrenal gland; c. kidney; d. urethra; e. bladder; f. left ureter; g. aorta; h. diaphragm; i. fibrous capsule; j. calyx; k. renal pelvis; l. papilla; m. medulla; n. cortex; o. ureter; p. renal vein; q. renal artery; r. pyramid

2. a, 1; b, 4; c, 3; d, 6; e, 5; f, 2. Blood is filtered in the glomerulus, and the ultrafiltrate flows from the Bowman's capsule to the tubules for reabsorption of essential materials and secretion of nonessential ones. In the proximal convoluted tubule, most electrolytes, glucose, amino acids, and small proteins are reabsorbed. Water is conserved in the loop of Henle with chloride and sodium reabsorbed in the ascending loop. The distal convoluted tubules complete final water balance and acid-base balance.

3. a, c, e, f. The distal convoluted tubules regulate water and acid-base balance by reabsorption of water under antidiuretic hormone (ADH) influence, secreting H^+ and reabsorbing bicarbonate, reabsorption of Na^+ in exchange for K^+, and reabsorption of Ca^{+2} with the influence of parathormone. The reabsorption of water without ADH

occurs in the proximal convoluted tubule and descending loop of Henle. The reabsorption of glucose and amino acids occurs in the proximal convoluted tubule. Active reabsorption of Cl^- and passive reabsorption of Na^+ occurs in the ascending loop of Henle.

4. a, c. Atrial natriuretic peptide (ANP) responds to increased atrial distention by increasing sodium excretion and inhibiting renin, ADH, and angiotensin II action. Aldosterone secretion is also suppressed. ANP also causes afferent arteriole relaxation that increases the glomerular filtration rate (GFR).

5. c. GFR is primarily dependent on adequate blood flow and hydrostatic pressure. The glomerulus filters the blood. The GFR is the amount of blood filtered each minute by the glomeruli, which determines the concentration of urea in the blood. Increased permeability in the glomerulus from kidney diseases causes loss of proteins in the urine. The prostaglandins increase the GFR with increased renal blood flow.

6. a. Renin is released in response to decreased arterial BP, renal ischemia, decreased extracellular fluid (ECF), decreased serum Na^+ concentration, and increased urinary Na^+ concentration. It is the catalyst of the renin-angiotensin-aldosterone system, which raises BP when stimulated. ADH is secreted by the posterior pituitary in response to serum hyperosmolality and low blood volume. Aldosterone is secreted only after stimulation by angiotensin II. Kidney prostaglandins lower BP by causing vasodilation.

7. a. Erythropoietin is released when the oxygen tension of the renal blood supply is low and stimulates production of red blood cells in the bone marrow. Hypotension causes activation of the renin-angiotensin-aldosterone system, as well as release of ADH. Hyperkalemia stimulates the release of aldosterone from the adrenal cortex and fluid overload does not directly stimulate factors affecting the erythropoietin release by the kidney.

8. a, b, e. Testing would include urinalysis to see crystals and look for red blood cells. Abdominal ultrasound and CT scan may also be done to look for renal calculi.

9. c. When the amount of urine in the bladder has reached 1100 mL, the person would need relief and require catheterization. The bladder capacity ranges from 600 to 1000 mL. When there is 250 mL of urine in the bladder, the person will usually feel the urge to urinate, and at 400 to 600 mL the patient will be uncomfortable.

10. c. Relaxation of female urethra, bladder, vagina, and pelvic floor muscles may contribute to stress and urge incontinence and urinary tract infections. The short urethra of women allows easier ascension and colonization of bacteria in the bladder than occurs in men and the urethra does not lengthen with age. The bladder capacity of men and women is the same but decreases with aging. With aging, the urinary sphincter weakens.

11. d. Decreased renal blood flow and altered hormone levels result in a decreased ability to concentrate urine that results in an increased volume of dilute urine, which does not maintain the usual diurnal elimination pattern. A decrease in bladder capacity contributes to nocturia, but decreased bladder muscle tone results in urinary retention. Decreased renal mass decreases renal reserve, but function is generally adequate under normal circumstances.

12.

Functional Health Pattern	Risk Factor for or Response to Urinary Problem
Health perception–health management	Smoking history, occupational history, and history of exposure to carcinogenic and nephrotoxic chemicals, family history of kidney disease, geographic residence, confused older person
Nutritional-metabolic	Low fluid intake or loss of fluids, high calcium and purine intake; caffeine, alcohol, carbonated beverage, artificial sweetener, or spicy food intake; weight gain resulting from fluid retention; anorexia, nausea, or vomiting; supplements and herbal therapy
Elimination	Change in appearance and amount of urine, change in urinary patterns, necessary assistance in emptying bladder, bowel function
Activity-exercise	Change in energy level, sedentary lifestyle, urine leakage during activity
Sleep-rest	Sleep deprivation from nocturia
Cognitive-perceptual	Pain in flank, groin, or suprapubic area; dysuria; absence of pain with other urinary symptoms; cognitive impairment affecting continence; mobility, visual acuity, and dexterity
Self-perception–self-concept	Decreased self-esteem and body image because of urinary problems
Role-relationship	Problems maintaining job and social relationships
Sexuality-reproductive	Change in sexual pleasure or performance
Coping–stress tolerance	Withdrawal or ineffective coping with incontinence or urinary problem
Value-belief	Any treatment decisions that are affected by value system

13. c. To assess for kidney tenderness, the nurse strikes the fist of 1 hand over the dorsum of the other hand at the posterior costovertebral angle. The upper abdominal quadrants and costovertebral angles are auscultated for vascular bruits in the renal vessels and aorta, and an empty bladder is not palpable. The kidneys are palpated through the abdomen, with the patient supine.

14. d. Stress incontinence is involuntary urination with increased pressure when sneezing or coughing and is seen with weakness of sphincter control. Nocturia is frequent urination at night. Micturition is the evacuation of urine. Urge incontinence is involuntary urination preceded by urinary urgency.

15. a. Retention is the inability to void even though urine is in the bladder. Anuria is no urine formation. Polyuria is a large amount of urine output over time. Frequency is increased incidence of urination.

16. b. Hesitancy is difficulty starting the urine stream and is common with benign prostatic hyperplasia (BPH). Oliguria is scanty urine formation and output. Hematuria is blood in the urine. Pneumaturia is urine containing gas, as is caused by a fistula between the bowel and bladder.

17. c. Enuresis is involuntary urination at night. Ascites is excess fluid in the intraperitoneal cavity. Dysuria is painful urination. Urgency is the feeling of needing to void immediately.

18. b. Bacteria in warm urine specimens multiply rapidly and falsely elevated bacterial counts may occur with urine that has been sitting for periods of time. Glucose, specific gravity, and white blood cells (WBCs) do not change in urine specimens, but pH becomes more alkaline, red blood cells (RBCs) hemolyze, and casts disintegrate.

19. a. Cloudiness in a fresh urine specimen, RBC above 4 per high-powered field (hpf), WBC count above 5/hpf are all indicative of urinary tract infection (UTI). When the pH is elevated, it is usually because bacteria in urine split the urea into CO_2 and alkaline ammonia. Yellow urine, protein 0 to 8 mg/dL, pH 4.0 to 8.0, and bacteria $<10^3$ colony-forming units/mL indicate normal or healthy urine. Cloudy, brown urine usually indicates hematuria or the presence of bile. Colorless urine is usually very dilute, which occurs with increased glucose and ketones.

20. a. A urine specific gravity of 1.002 is low, indicating dilute urine and the excretion of excess fluid. Fluid overload, diuretics, or lack of ADH can cause dilute urine. Normal urine specific gravity is 1.003 to 1.030. A high urine specific gravity indicates concentrated urine that would be seen in dehydration.

21. d. During a renal arteriogram, a catheter is inserted, most commonly in the femoral artery. Following the procedure, the patient is positioned with the affected leg extended with a pressure dressing applied. Peripheral pulse monitoring is essential to detect the development of thrombi around the insertion site, which may occlude blood supply to the leg. Gross bleeding in the urine is a complication of a renal biopsy. Allergy to the contrast medium should be established before the procedure.

22. c. The rate at which creatinine is cleared from the blood and eliminated in the urine approximates the GFR and is the most specific test of renal function. The renal scan is useful in showing the location, size, and shape of the kidney and general blood perfusion. Serum creatinine is an end product of muscle and protein metabolism and may be elevated with body builders and decreased with older people. Blood urea nitrogen (BUN) can be altered with gastrointestinal (GI) bleeding, starvation, and hyper- or hypovolemia.

23. a. BUN is increased in patients with renal problems. It may also be increased when there is rapid or extensive tissue damage from other causes. Very low protein intake may cause a low BUN.

24.

Laboratory Finding	Impaired Kidney Function
Serum Ca^{2+}: 7.2 mg/dL (1.8 mmol/L)	Impaired conversion of inactive vitamin D to active vitamin D results in poor calcium absorption from the bowel, resulting in hypocalcemia.
Hgb: 9.6 g/dL (96 g/L)	Loss of cells that produce erythropoietin results in lack of stimulation of bone marrow to produce RBCs.
Serum creatinine: 3.2 mg/dL (283 mmol/L)	This serum creatinine level is high, indicating the loss of tubular secretion (passage of substances from the blood into the tubule) by the kidney.

25. b. Bleeding from the kidney following a biopsy is the most serious complication of the procedure and urine must be examined for both gross and microscopic blood, in addition to vital signs and hematocrit levels being monitored. Following a cystoscopy, the patient may have burning with urination, and warm sitz baths may be used. Urinary infections are a complication of any procedure requiring instrumentation of the bladder.

26. a, d, e. A clean-catch urine specimen is obtained in a sterile container after cleaning the meatus. The patient will void a small amount in the toilet, stop, and then void in the container to catch the urine midstream. The first morning specimen is best for a urinalysis. A full bladder is necessary for a urine flow study. A urinary catheter is inserted immediately after voiding to assess residual urine.

27. b. A cathartic the evening before the procedure and assessing sensitivity to iodine are important for a renal arteriogram as well as a CT scan and an intravenous pyelogram (IVP). The cystometrogram involves filling the bladder with water or saline to measure tone and stability. The kidneys, ureters, and bladder (KUB) is an x-ray that may have bowel preparation.

CHAPTER 50

1. a. An upper urinary tract infection (UTI) affects the renal parenchyma, renal pelvis, and ureters. A lower UTI is an infection of the bladder and/or urethra. A complicated UTI exists in the presence of coexisting obstruction, stones, catheters, or preexisting diseases. An uncomplicated UTI occurs in an otherwise normal urinary tract.

2. c. The usual classic manifestations of UTI are often absent in older adults, who tend to have nonlocalized abdominal discomfort and cognitive impairment characterized by confusion or decreased level of consciousness rather than dysuria and suprapubic pain.

3. c. Unless a patient has a history of recurrent UTIs or a complicated UTI, trimethoprim-sulfamethoxazole or nitrofurantoin is usually used to empirically treat an initial UTI without a culture and sensitivity or other testing. Asymptomatic bacteriuria does not justify treatment, but symptomatic UTIs should always be treated.

4. b. Fluid intake should be increased to about 2000 mL/day without caffeine, alcohol, citrus juices, and chocolate drinks, because they are potential bladder irritants. The bladder should be emptied at least every 3 to 4 hours, not waiting until an intense urge. Cleaning the urinary meatus with an antiinfective agent after voiding will irritate the meatus, but the perineal area should be wiped from front to back after urination and defecation to prevent fecal contamination of the meatus.

5. c. Ascending infections from the bladder to the kidney are prevented by the normal anatomy and physiology of the urinary tract, unless a preexisting condition, such as vesicoureteral reflux or lower urinary tract dysfunction (bladder tumors, prostatic hyperplasia, strictures, or stones), is present. Scarred and fibrotic kidney is a result of chronic pyelonephritis. Resistance to antibiotics and failure to take a full prescription of antibiotics for a UTI usually result in relapse or reinfection of the lower urinary tract.

6. a. Systemic manifestations of fever and chills with leukocytosis and nausea and vomiting are more common in pyelonephritis than in a lower UTI. Dysuria, frequency, and urgency can be present with both.

7. d. A urine specimen specifically obtained for culture and sensitivity is required to diagnose pyelonephritis because it will indicate the bacteria causing the infection and provide information on what drug the bacteria is sensitive to for treatment. The renal biopsy is used to diagnose chronic pyelonephritis or cancer. Blood cultures would be done if bacteremia is suspected. Intravenous pyelogram (IVP) would increase renal irritation, but CT urograms may be used to assess for signs of infection in the kidney and complications of pyelonephritis.

8. d. The symptoms of interstitial cystitis (IC) imitate those of an infection of the bladder, but the urine is free of infectious agents. Unlike a bladder infection, the pain with IC increases as urine collects in the bladder and is temporarily relieved by urination. Acidic urine is very irritating to the bladder in IC and the bladder is small, but urinary retention is not common.

9. d. Calcium glycerophosphate (Prelief) is an OTC dietary supplement that alkalinizes the urine and can help relieve the irritation from acidic foods. A diet low in acidic foods is recommended. If a multivitamin is used, high-potency vitamins should be avoided because these products may irritate the bladder. A voiding diary is useful in diagnosis but does not have to be kept indefinitely.

10. c. Glomerulonephritis is not an infection but rather an antibody-antigen-induced injury of the glomerulus, and complement activation causes inflammation. Prior infection by bacteria or viruses may stimulate the antibody production but is not present or active at the time of glomerular damage.

11. d. An elevated blood urea nitrogen (BUN) indicates that the kidneys are not clearing nitrogenous wastes from the blood and protein may be restricted related to the degree of proteinuria until the kidney recovers. Proteinuria indicates loss of protein from the blood and possibly a need for increased protein intake. Hypertension is treated with sodium and fluid restriction, diuretics, and antihypertensive drugs. The hematuria is not specifically treated.

12. a. Most patients recover completely from acute poststreptococcal glomerulonephritis (APSGN) with

supportive treatment. Chronic glomerulonephritis that progresses insidiously over years and rapidly progressive glomerulonephritis that results in renal failure within weeks or months occur in only a few patients with APSGN. In Goodpasture syndrome, antibodies are present against both the glomerular basement membrane (GBM) and the alveolar basement membrane of the lungs, and dysfunction of kidneys and lungs are present.

13. c. The massive proteinuria that results from increased glomerular membrane permeability in nephrotic syndrome leaves the blood without adequate proteins (hypoalbuminemia) to create an oncotic colloidal pressure to hold fluid in the vessels. Without oncotic pressure, fluid moves into the interstitium, causing severe edema. Hypercoagulability occurs in nephrotic syndrome but is not a factor in edema formation, and glomerular filtration rate (GFR) is not necessarily affected in nephrotic syndrome.

14. a. 6; b. 3; c. 1; d. 4; e. 8; f. 5; g. 2; h. 7

15. d. The manifestations of genitourinary tuberculosis are described. Urosepsis is when the UTI has spread systemically. Urethral diverticula are localized outpouching of the urethra and occur more often in women. Goodpasture syndrome manifests with flu-like symptoms with pulmonary symptoms that include cough, shortness of breath, and pulmonary insufficiency and renal manifestations that include hematuria, weakness, pallor, anemia, and renal failure.

16. c. Because crystallization of stone constituents can precipitate and unite to form a stone when in supersaturated concentrations, one of the best ways to prevent stones of any type is by drinking adequate fluids to keep the urine dilute and flowing (e.g., an output of about 2 L of urine a day). Sedentary lifestyle is a risk factor for renal stones, but exercise also causes fluid loss and a need for additional fluids. Protein foods high in purine should be restricted only for the small percentage of patients with uric acid stones. Although UTIs contribute to stone formation, prophylactic antibiotics are not indicated.

17. c. Calcium oxalate stones are most common (35% to 40%) and small enough to get trapped in the ureter. Cystine stones incidence is 1% to 2%; uric acid incidence is 5% to 8%; calcium phosphate incidence is 8% to 10%.

18. b. Struvite stones are most common in women and always occur with UTIs. They are usually large staghorn type.

19. b, e. This patient is most likely to have uric acid stones. Gout is a predisposing factor. The treatment will include allopurinol and reducing animal protein intake to reduce purine, as uric acid is a waste product from purine metabolism. Reducing oxalate and using thiazide diuretics help treat calcium oxalate stones. Giving α-penicillamine and tiopronin prevents cystine crystallization for cystine stones. Reducing intake of milk products to decrease calcium intake may be indicated for patients with calcium stones.

20. a. Calcium phosphate stones are typically mixed with struvite or oxalate stones and related to alkaline urine. Cystine stones are associated with a genetic autosomal recessive defect and defective gastrointestinal (GI) and kidney absorption of cystine. Struvite stones are 3 to 4 times more common in women than in men.

21. c. A classic sign of the passage of a stone down the ureter is intense, colicky back pain that may radiate into the testicles, labia, or groin and may be accompanied by mild shock with cool, moist skin. Many patients with renal stones do not have a history of chronic UTIs. Stones obstructing a calyx or at the ureteropelvic junction may produce dull costovertebral flank pain, and large bladder stones may cause bladder fullness and lower obstructive symptoms.

22. d. Oxalate-rich foods should be limited to reduce oxalate excretion. Foods high in oxalate include spinach, rhubarb, asparagus, cabbage, and tomatoes, chocolate, coffee, and cocoa. Encourage increased intake of calcium, fruits, and vegetables. Milk, milk products, dried beans, and dried fruits are sources of high levels of calcium. Organ meats are high in purine, which contributes to uric acid stones.

23. b. A high fluid intake maintains dilute urine, which decreases bacterial concentration in addition to washing stone fragments and expected blood through the urinary system following lithotripsy. High urine output also prevents supersaturation of minerals. Moist heat to the flank may be helpful to relieve muscle spasms during renal colic. All urine should be strained in patients with renal stones to collect and identify stone composition, but these are not related to infection. Interprofessional care usually will include antibiotics to reduce infection risk.

24. b. The patient with urethral stricture will benefit from being taught to dilate the urethra by self-catheterization every few days. Renal trauma is treated related to the severity of the injury with bed rest, fluids, and analgesia to surgery. Renal artery stenosis includes control of hypertension with possible surgical revascularization. Accelerated nephrosclerosis is associated with malignant hypertension that must be aggressively treated as well as monitoring kidney function.

25. b. Adult-onset polycystic kidney disease is an inherited autosomal dominant disorder that often manifests after the patient has had children. Therefore the children should receive genetic counseling regarding their life choices. The disease progresses slowly, eventually causing progressive renal failure. Hereditary medullary cystic disease causes poor concentration ability of the kidneys, and classic Alport syndrome is a hereditary nephritis that is associated with deafness and deformities of the optic lens.

26. d. Systemic lupus erythematosus causes connective tissue damage that affects the glomerulus. Gout deposits uric acid crystals in the kidney. Amyloidosis deposits hyaline bodies in the kidney. Diabetes causes microvascular damage affecting the kidney.

27. a. Both cancer of the kidney and cancer of the bladder are associated with smoking. A family history of renal cancer is a risk factor for kidney cancer. Cancer of the bladder has been associated with long-term indwelling catheters, recurrent renal calculi (often bladder), and chronic lower UTIs.

28. c. There are no early characteristic symptoms of cancer of the kidney, and gross hematuria, flank pain, and a palpable mass do not occur until the disease is advanced. The treatment of choice is a partial or radical nephrectomy, which can be successful in early disease. Radiation is palliative. Many kidney cancers are diagnosed as incidental imaging findings. The most common sites of metastases are the lungs, liver, and long bones.

29. d, e, f. Urge incontinence is involuntary urination preceded by urgency caused by overactivity of the detrusor muscle

when the bladder contracts by reflex, which overrides central inhibition. Treatment includes treating the underlying cause and retraining the bladder with urge suppression, anticholinergic drugs, or containment devices. The other options are characteristic of stress incontinence. Patients may have a combination of urge and stress incontinence.

30. a. Reflex incontinence occurs with no warning, equally during the day and night, and with spinal cord lesions above S2. Overflow incontinence is when the pressure of urine in the overfull bladder overcomes sphincter control and is caused by bladder or urethral outlet obstruction. Functional incontinence is loss of urine resulting from cognitive, functional, or environmental factors. Incontinence after trauma or surgery occurs when fistulas have occurred or after a prostatectomy.

31. c, d, e. α-Adrenergic blockers block the stimulation of the smooth muscle of the bladder, 5α-reductase inhibitors decrease outlet resistance, and bethanechol enhances bladder contractions. Baclofen or diazepam is used to relax the external sphincter for reflex incontinence. Anticholinergics are used to relax bladder tone and increase sphincter tone with urge incontinence.

32. c. Pelvic floor exercises (Kegel exercises) increase the tone of the urethral sphincters and should be done in sets of 10 or more contractions 4 to 5 times a day (total of 40 to 50 per day). Frequent bladder emptying is recommended for patients with urge incontinence and an increase in pressure on the bladder is recommended for patients with overflow incontinence. Absorptive perineal pads should be only a temporary measure because long-term use discourages continence and can lead to skin problems.

33. c. All urinary catheters in hospitalized patients pose a very high risk for infection, especially antibiotic-resistant, health care–associated infections, and scrupulous aseptic technique is essential in the insertion and maintenance of all catheters. Routine irrigations are not performed. Turning the patient to promote drainage is recommended only for suprapubic catheters. Cleaning the insertion site with soap and water should be performed for urethral and suprapubic catheters, but lotion or powder should be avoided. Site care for other catheters may require special interventions.

34. b. Output from ureteral catheters must be monitored every 1 to 2 hours because an obstruction will cause overdistention of the renal pelvis and renal damage. The renal pelvis has a capacity of only 3 to 5 mL, and if irrigation is ordered, no more than 5 mL of sterile saline is used. The patient with a ureteral catheter is usually kept on bed rest until specific orders for ambulation are given. Suprapubic tubes may be milked to prevent obstruction of the catheter by sediment and clots.

35. b. A nephrectomy incision is usually in the flank, just below the diaphragm or in the abdominal area. Although the patient is reluctant to breathe deeply because of incisional pain, the lungs should be clear. Decreased sounds and shallow respirations are abnormal and would require intervention.

36. a. The Kock pouch is a continent diversion created by formation of an ileal pouch with an external stoma requiring catheterization. Ileal conduit is the most common incontinent diversion using a stoma of resected ileum with implanted ureters. Orthotopic neobladder is a new bladder from a reshaped segment of intestine in the anatomic position of the bladder with urine discharged through the urethra. A cutaneous ureterostomy diverts the ureter from the bladder to the abdominal skin, but there is frequent scarring and strictures of the ureters, so ileal conduits are used more often.

37. d. Urine drains continuously from an ileal conduit and the drainage bag must be emptied every 2 to 3 hours and measured to ensure adequate urinary output. Fitting for a permanent appliance is not done until the stoma shrinks to its normal size in a few weeks. With an ileal conduit, mucus is present in the urine because it is secreted by the ileal segment as a result of the irritating effect of the urine, but the surgery causes paralytic ileus and the patient will be NPO for several days postoperatively. Self-catheterization is performed when patients have formation of a continent Kock pouch.

38. b. Because the stoma continuously drains urine, a wick formed of a rolled-up 4 × 4 gauze or a tampon is held against the stoma to absorb the urine while the skin is cleaned and a new appliance is attached. The skin is cleaned with warm water only because soap and other agents cause drying and irritation. Clean, not sterile, technique is used. The appliance should be left in place for as long as possible before it loosens and allows leakage onto the skin, perhaps up to 14 days.

39. e, f. The AP may assist the incontinent patient to void at regular intervals and provide perineal care. An RN should perform the assessments and teaching. The LPN/VN will do bladder scanning. In long-term care and rehabilitation facilities, AP may use bladder scanners after they are trained.

Case Study

1. **Expected**: microscopic or gross hematuria, urgency, frequency; **Unexpected**: severe pain in suprapubic region (bladder cancer is usually painless), bladder distention (is a sign of urinary retention, not a symptom associated with bladder cancer), dribbling (is not a symptom associated with bladder cancer), pyuria (pus in the urine is not associated with bladder cancer)

2. **Indicated**: report gross hematuria to the HCP (gross hematuria indicates active bleeding and should be investigated by the HCP), have the patient void before discharge home (it is usually a requirement that patients having urologic procedures void before being discharged to make sure they can void and eliminate urine), record hourly urine output by subtracting the amount of irrigant from the total amount emptied from the urinary bag (the difference is the urine output), insert a 3-way urinary catheter (necessary to accomplish continuous bladder irrigation); **Contraindicated**: give a B&O suppository for bladder spasms (this medication will relax the smooth muscle of the bladder which requires an indwelling urinary catheter to remain for 12 or more hours), use sterile water as the irrigation fluid (this may cause dangerous electrolyte shifts, therefore 0.9% normal saline is the preferred irrigation fluid), clamp the irrigation tubing if there are blood clots in the urinary tubing (the purpose of CBI is to flush blood and blood clots out of the bladder); **Non-essential**: strain (filter) the urine using a strainer (unnecessary), keep patient NPO (unnecessary)

3. A., C., E., G., H. Difficulty urinating should be reported to the HCP as urinary retention may necessitate catheterization. Patients should be instructed to drink lots of fluids to help flush the bladder. Since smoking is a risk factor of bladder cancer, patients should be encouraged to stop smoking. Pink urine is expected during the first 7-10 days postoperatively, but gross hematuria should be reported. Seeing brown and red flakes in the urine is expected as the bladder heals. A TURBT doesn't predispose patients to urinary incontinence. Patients need to avoid straining during bowel movements; therefore, increasing fiber or taking stool softeners is advised. Coffee and tea may irritate the bladder which may cause painful urination.

4. **1**=chemotherapy and immunotherapy; **2**=urinary catheter; **3**=1-2 hours; **4**=15 minutes; **5**=once; **6**=6-12 weeks.

5. **Effective**: "I may have flu-like symptoms after treatments." (this is a possible side effect), "I should avoid spicy foods." (spicy foods can be an irritant to the bladder), "I should drink water instead of diet soda." (most diet sodas contain aspartame which is a known bladder irritant, water is the preferred beverage); **Ineffective**: "I will expect hair loss." (this is unlikely with intravesical chemotherapy), "I can drink wine and beer as long as I stay away from hard liquor." (alcohol can be a bladder irritant); **Unrelated**: "I will not be able to swim for several months." (swimming is not contraindicated), "I will have annual PSA testing." (PSA testing is related to the prostate, not the bladder)

CHAPTER 51

1. d, e, f. Intrarenal causes of acute kidney injury (AKI) include conditions that cause direct damage to the kidney tissue, including nephrotoxic drugs, acute glomerulonephritis, and tubular obstruction by myoglobin, or prolonged ischemia. Anaphylaxis and other prerenal problems are frequently the initial cause of AKI. Renal stones and bladder cancer are among the postrenal causes of AKI.

2. c, e. Because the patient has had nothing to eat or drink for 2 days, she is probably dehydrated and hypovolemic. Decreased cardiac output (CO) is most likely because she is older and takes heart medicine, which is probably for heart failure or hypertension. Both hypovolemia and decreased CO cause prerenal AKI. Anaphylaxis is also a cause of prerenal AKI but is not likely in this situation. Nephrotoxic drugs would contribute to intrarenal causes of AKI, and renal stones would be a postrenal cause of AKI.

3. d. Acute tubular necrosis (ATN) is primarily the result of ischemia, nephrotoxins, or sepsis. Major surgery is most likely to cause severe kidney ischemia in the patient requiring a blood transfusion. A blood transfusion hemolytic reaction produces nephrotoxic injury. Diabetes, hypertension, and acetaminophen overdose will not contribute to ATN.

4. b. Injury is the stage of RIFLE classification in which urine output is <0.5 mL/kg/hr for 12 hours, the serum creatinine is increased times two, or the glomerular filtration rate (GFR) is decreased by 50%. This stage may be reversible by treating the cause or, in this patient, the dehydration by administering IV fluid and a low dose of a loop diuretic, furosemide (Lasix). Assessing the daily weight will be done to monitor fluid changes, but it is not the first treatment

the nurse should anticipate. IV administration of insulin and sodium bicarbonate would be used for hyperkalemia. Checking the urinalysis will help determine if the AKI has a prerenal, intrarenal, or postrenal cause by what is seen in the urine. With this patient's dehydration, it is thought to be prerenal to begin treatment.

5. d. In prerenal oliguria, the oliguria is caused by a decrease in circulating blood volume and there is no damage yet to the renal tissue. It can be reversed by correcting the precipitating factor, such as fluid replacement for hypovolemia. Prerenal oliguria is characterized by urine with a high specific gravity and a low sodium concentration, whereas oliguria of intrarenal failure is characterized by urine with a low specific gravity and a high sodium concentration. Malignant hypertension causes damage to renal tissue and intrarenal oliguria.

6. b. A urine specific gravity that is consistently 1.010 and a urine osmolality of about 300 mOsm/kg is the same specific gravity and osmolality as plasma. This indicates that tubules are damaged and unable to concentrate urine. Hematuria is more common with postrenal damage. Tubular damage is associated with a high sodium concentration (>40 mEq/L).

7. d. Metabolic acidosis occurs in AKI because the kidneys cannot synthesize ammonia or excrete hydrogen (H +) ions or the acid products of metabolism, resulting in an increased acid load. Sodium is lost in urine because the kidneys cannot conserve sodium. Bicarbonate is normally generated and reabsorbed by the functioning kidney to maintain acid-base balance. Impaired excretion of potassium results in hyperkalemia.

8. d. The blood urea nitrogen (BUN) and creatinine levels remain high during the oliguric and diuretic phases of AKI. The recovery phase begins when the glomerular filtration returns to a rate at which BUN and creatinine stabilize and then decrease. Urinary output of 3 to 5 L/day, decreasing sodium and potassium levels, and fluid weight loss are characteristic of the diuretic phase of AKI.

9. d. Hyperkalemia is a potentially life-threatening complication of AKI in the oliguric phase. Muscle weakness and abdominal cramping are signs of the neuromuscular impairment that occurs with hyperkalemia. In addition, hyperkalemia can cause the cardiac conduction abnormalities of peaked T wave, prolonged PR interval, prolonged QRS interval, and depressed ST segment. Urine output of 300 mL/day is expected during the oliguric phase, as is the development of peripheral edema.

10. d. Measuring daily weights with the same scale at the same time each day allows for the evaluation and detection of excessive body fluid gains or losses. Infection is the leading cause of death in AKI, so meticulous aseptic technique is critical. The fluid limitation in the oliguric phase is 600 mL plus the prior day's measured fluid loss. Dietary sodium and potassium intake are managed according to the plasma levels.

11. b. This patient has at least 3 of the 6 common indications for renal replacement therapy (RRT), including: (1) high potassium level; (2) metabolic acidosis; and (3) changed mental status. The other indications are (4) volume overload, resulting in compromised cardiac status (this patient has a history of hypertension); (5) BUN >120 mg/dL; and (6) pericarditis, pericardial effusion, or cardiac

tamponade. Although the other treatments may be used, they will not be as effective as RRT for this older patient. Loop diuretics and increased fluid are used if the patient is dehydrated. Insulin and sodium bicarbonate can be used to temporarily drive the potassium into the cells. Sodium polystyrene sulfonate (Kayexalate) is used to actually decrease the amount of potassium in the body.

12. a, b, c, d, e. High-risk patients include those exposed to nephrotoxic agents and advanced age: (a), massive trauma (b), prolonged hypovolemia or hypotension (possibly b, c, and d), obstetric complications (c), cardiac failure (d), preexisting chronic kidney disease (CKD), extensive burns, or sepsis. Patients with prostate cancer may have obstruction of the outflow tract, which increases risk of postrenal AKI (e).

13. a. Dysrhythmias may occur with an elevated potassium level and are potentially lethal. Monitor the rhythm while contacting the HCP or calling the rapid response team. Vital signs should be checked. Depending on the patient's history and cause of increased potassium, instruct the patient about dietary sources of potassium; however, this would not help at this point. The nurse may want to recheck the value, but until then the heart rhythm must be monitored.

14. b. During acidosis, potassium moves out of the cell in exchange for H^+ ions, increasing the serum potassium level. Correction of the acidosis with sodium bicarbonate will help temporarily shift the potassium back into the cells. A decrease in pH and the bicarbonate and partial pressure of carbon dioxide in arterial blood ($PaCO_2$) levels would indicate worsening acidosis.

15. b. Stages of CKD are based on the GFR. No specific markers of urinary output, mental status, or azotemia classify the seriousness of CKD.

16. a, b, d. Pruritus is common in patients receiving dialysis. It causes scratching from dry skin, sensory neuropathy, and calcium-phosphate deposition in the skin. Vascular calcifications contribute to cardiovascular disease, not to itching skin. Uremic frost rarely occurs without BUN levels >200 mg/dL, which should not occur in a patient on dialysis; urea crystallizes on the skin and also causes pruritus.

17. c. Increased ammonia in saliva, from bacterial breakdown of urea, leads to stomatitis and mucosal ulcerations. Uremic fetor, or the urine odor of the breath, is caused by high urea content in the blood. Irritation of the gastrointestinal (GI) tract from urea in CKD contributes to anorexia, nausea, and vomiting. Ingestion of iron salts and calcium-containing phosphate binders, limited fluid intake, and limited activity cause constipation.

18. c. Kussmaul respirations occur with severe metabolic acidosis when the respiratory system is attempting to compensate by removing carbon dioxide with exhalations. Uremic pleuritis would cause a pleural friction rub. Decreased pulmonary macrophage activity increases the risk of pulmonary infection. Dyspnea would occur with pulmonary edema.

19. d. As GFR decreases, BUN and serum creatinine levels increase. Although elevated BUN and creatinine indicate that waste products are accumulating, the calculated GFR is considered a more accurate indicator of kidney function than BUN or serum creatinine.

20. b. Hyperkalemia can lead to life-threatening dysrhythmias. Hypocalcemia leads to an accelerated rate of bone remodeling and potentially to tetany. Hyponatremia may lead to confusion. Elevated sodium levels lead to edema, hypertension, and heart failure. Hypermagnesemia may decrease reflexes, mental status, and BP.

21. a. 5, b. 3, c. 6, d. 1, e. 2, f. 4. Less vitamin D is converted to its active form resulting in decreased serum calcium. Hypocalcemia causes the parathyroid to secrete parathyroid hormone (PTH), which stimulates bone demineralization, releasing calcium and phosphate from the bones. Hyperphosphatemia decreases calcium levels and further reduces the kidney's ability to activate vitamin D. Low serum calcium, elevated phosphate, and decreased vitamin D further stimulate PTH secretion. Accelerated bone remodeling occurs, causing weakened bone matrix with replacement of bone tissue with fibrous tissue.

22. d. A patient with CKD may have sugars and starches (unless the patient is diabetic); hard candy is an appropriate snack and may help relieve the metallic and urine taste that is common in the mouth. Raisins are a high-potassium food. Ice cream contains protein and phosphate and counts as fluid. Pickled foods have high sodium content.

23. a. Erythropoietin is used to treat anemia, as it stimulates the bone marrow to produce red blood cells.

24. b. Both are used to treat hypertension. Nifedipine (Procardia) is a calcium channel blocker, and furosemide (Lasix) is a loop diuretic that can help decrease potassium.

25. a, b, e. Cinacalcet (Sensipar), a calcimimetic agent to control secondary hyperparathyroidism; calcium acetate, a calcium-based phosphate binder, and sevelamer carbonate (Renvela), a non–calcium-based phosphate binder, are used to treat mineral and bone disorder in CKD. IV glucose and insulin and IV 10% calcium gluconate along with sodium polystyrene sulfonate (Kayexalate) are used to treat the hyperkalemia of CKD.

26. d. In the patient with CKD, when serum calcium levels are increased, calcium-based phosphate binders are not used. The dialyzable nutrient supplemented for patients on dialysis is folic acid, although IV iron sucrose injections may be prescribed for anemia if the patient receives erythropoietin. The various body system manifestations occur with uremia, which includes azotemia. Meperidine is contraindicated in patients with CKD related to possible seizures.

27. c. The most common causes of CKD in the United States are diabetes and hypertension. The nurse should obtain information on long-term health problems that are related to kidney disease. The other disorders are not closely associated with renal disease.

28. c, e. Peritoneal dialysis (PD) is less stressful for the cardiovascular system and requires fewer dietary restrictions. PD actually contributes to more protein loss and increased hyperlipidemia. The fluid and creatinine removal are slower with PD than hemodialysis (HD).

29. c. Dextrose or icodextrin or amino acid is added to dialysate fluid to create an osmotic gradient across the membrane to remove excess fluid from the blood. Dialysate usually contains higher calcium to promote its movement into the blood. Dialysate sodium is usually less than or equal to that of blood to prevent sodium and fluid retention. The dialysate fluid has no potassium so that potassium will diffuse into the dialysate from the blood.

30. a. 3; b. 2; c. 1

31. b. Automated peritoneal dialysis (APD) is the type of dialysis in which the patient dialyzes during sleep and leaves the fluid in the abdomen during the day. Long nocturnal HD occurs while the patient is sleeping and is done up to 6 times per week. Continuous venovenous hemofiltration (CVVH) is a type of continuous RRT used to treat AKI. Continuous ambulatory peritoneal dialysis (CAPD) is dialysis that is done with exchanges of 2 to 3 L of dialysate at least 4 times daily.

32. b. Exit site infection and peritonitis are common complications of PD and may require catheter removal and termination of dialysis. Infection occurs from contamination of the dialysate or tubing or from progression of exit-site or tunnel infections, and strict sterile technique must be used by health care professionals as well as the patient to prevent contamination. Too-rapid infusion may cause shoulder pain, and pain may be caused if the catheter tip touches the bowel. Difficulty breathing, atelectasis, and pneumonia may occur from pressure of the fluid on the diaphragm, which may be prevented by elevating the head of the bed and promoting repositioning and deep breathing.

33. c. A more permanent, soft, flexible double-lumen catheter is used for long-term access when other forms of vascular access have failed. These catheters are tunneled subcutaneously and have Dacron cuffs that prevent infection from tracking along the catheter. Because the patient has chosen HD, APD would not be started. The peripheral vessels and peripherally inserted central catheter (PICC) lines are not used for HD.

34. a. While patients are undergoing HD, they can perform quiet activities that do not require the limb that has the vascular access. BP is monitored frequently, and the dialyzer monitors dialysis function, but cardiac monitoring is not usually indicated. The HD machine continuously circulates both the blood and the dialysate past the semipermeable membrane in the machine. Graft and fistula access involve the insertion of 2 needles into the site: one to remove blood from and the other to return blood to the dialyzer. A double-lumen catheter is used for temporary access.

35. b. A patent arteriovenous fistula (AVF) creates turbulent blood flow that can be assessed by listening for a bruit or palpated for a thrill as the blood passes through the graft. Assessment of neurovascular status in the extremity distal to the graft site is important to determine that the graft does not impair circulation to the extremity, but the neurovascular status does not indicate whether the graft is open.

36. c. Continuous renal replacement therapy (CRRT) is indicated for the patient with AKI as an alternative or adjunct to HD to slowly remove solutes and fluid in the hemodynamically unstable patient. It is especially useful for treatment of fluid overload, but HD is indicated for treatment of hyperkalemia, pericarditis, or other serious effects of uremia.

37. d. Extensive vascular disease is a contraindication for renal transplantation, primarily because adequate blood supply is essential for the health of the new kidney. Other contraindications include disseminated malignancies, refractory or untreated cardiac disease, chronic respiratory failure, chronic infection, or unresolved psychosocial disorders. Hepatitis B or C infection is not a contraindication. Coronary artery disease (CAD) may be treated with bypass surgery before transplantation, and transplantation can relieve hypertension.

38. a. Fluid and electrolyte balance is the priority in the transplant recipient patient, especially because diuresis often begins soon after surgery. Fluid replacement is adjusted hourly based on kidney function and urine output. Urine-tinged drainage on the abdominal dressing may indicate leakage from the ureter implanted into the bladder, and the HCP should be notified. The recipient has an abdominal incision where the kidney was placed in the iliac fossa. The urinary catheter is usually used for 2 to 3 days to monitor urine output and kidney function.

39. b. Infection is a significant cause of morbidity and mortality after transplantation because the surgery, immunosuppressive drugs, and effects of CKD all suppress the body's normal defense mechanisms, thus increasing the risk of bacterial, fungal, and viral infections. The nurse must assess the patient as well as use aseptic technique to prevent infections. Rejection may occur but for other reasons. Malignancy occurrence increases later because of immunosuppressive therapy. Cardiovascular disease is the leading cause of death after renal transplantation as it is with CKD, but this would not be expected to cause death within the first month after transplantation.

Case Study

1. **Diabetic ketoacidosis**: Glucose 404 mg/dL, HCO_3^- 18 mEq/L, RR 28 and deep; **Cardiac dysrhythmias**: K^+ 5.1 mEq/L, HCO_3^- 18 mEq/L; **Kidney failure**: Creatinine 3.0 mg/dL, BUN 70 mg/dL, K^+ 5.1 mEq/L, HCO_3^- 18 mEq/L, BP 150/90 mm Hg

2. **Indicated**: continuous infusion of insulin (treats hyperglycemia), monitor urine output hourly (monitors kidney function), administer Kayexalate PO (to treat hyperkalemia by excreting potassium in the feces), place patient on continuous cardiac monitoring (hyperkalemia can cause dysrhythmias); **Contraindicated**: administer dextrose 50% (this will worsen patient's hyperglycemia), offer juice and crackers (juice has high sugar content and is not appropriate for someone who is already hyperglycemic), transfuse 1 unit of PRBCs (there is no indication for this intervention, blood transfusion reactions pose a risk that could be harmful to this patient), eating spinach (is high in potassium which is contraindicated for someone who has cardiac dysrhythmias due to hyperkalemia); **Non-essential**: using the incentive spirometer, performing continuous SpO_2 monitoring, placing the patient on droplet precautions (all are unnecessary and won't improve this patient's current health condition)

3. **Hypertension**: furosemide (loop diuretic), nifedipine (Calcium channel blocker); **Metabolic acidosis**: sodium bicarbonate; **Renal transplant**: mycophenolate mofetil, tacrolimus, methylprednisolone, furosemide (a diuretic that promotes fluid passing through the kidneys); **Diabetes**: insulin

4. **Hemodialysis**: surgery to create a graft or fistula, dialysis at least 3 times/week, may become hypotensive; **Peritoneal dialysis**: need a catheter implanted in your abdomen, may develop peritonitis, preferred in patients with diabetes; **CRRT**: only performed in the acute care setting, filters and cleans the blood over 24 hours

5. A., B., D., E., H., I. Any signs of infection should be reported to the HCP immediately. This is because a patient on immunosuppressants is susceptible to infection which may cause her to reject the transplanted kidney. Patients on immunosuppressants should stay away from crowded spaces and those with known infection due to their susceptibility of contracting an infection. These patients are also susceptible to developing cancer. Cardiovascular disease is the leading cause of death in kidney transplant patients, plus this patient has diabetes which also increases her risk of CVD. Immunosuppressant medications are necessary to prevent the body from rejecting the organ; therefore, patients should not stop or alter these medications unless told to do so by their HCP. Corticosteroids can increase blood glucose levels, especially in patients with diabetes. Transplant recipients will need lifelong testing and monitoring to prevent or detect organ rejection.

CHAPTER 52

1. a. Pineal; b. parathyroids; c. testes (male); d. ovaries (female); e. pancreatic islets of Langerhans; f. adrenals; g. thyroid; h. pituitary; i. hypothalamus
2. a, e, f, i, j. The anterior pituitary gland secretes prolactin, growth hormone (GH), gonadotropic hormones, thyroid-stimulating hormone (TSH), and adrenocorticotropic hormone (ACTH). The pineal gland secretes melatonin. The delta cells of the islets of Langerhans secrete somatostatin. The parathyroid secretes parathormone. The posterior pituitary secretes antidiuretic hormone (ADH). The intermediate lobe produces melanocyte-stimulating hormone.
3. c. The α-cells in the islets of Langerhans in the pancreas produce and secrete the hormone glucagon. The F cells secrete pancreatic polypeptide. The β-cells produce and secrete insulin and amylin. The delta cells produce and secrete somatostatin.
4. c. Cortisol is secreted by the adrenal cortex in a diurnal pattern, creating circadian rhythm. Ovaries secrete estrogen and progesterone to maintain a woman's secondary sex

characteristic function. The thyroid secretes thyroxine (T_4) and triiodothyronine (T_3) in response to TSH, and calcitonin in response to high serum calcium levels. The adrenal medulla secretes epinephrine and norepinephrine in response to stress.

5. d. The catecholamines, epinephrine and norepinephrine, are hormones from the adrenal medulla. Androgens and cortisol are from the adrenal cortex. The thyroid and adrenal cortex are controlled by negative feedback, but the adrenal medulla's hormone production is controlled by the central nervous system.
6. a. 3, 2; b. 1, 4; c. 13, 14; d. 6, 5; e. 9, 10; f. 11, 12; g. 8, 7; h. 10, 9; i. 7, 8
7. b. ADH release is controlled by the osmolality of the blood. As the osmolality rises, ADH is released from the posterior pituitary gland and acts on the kidney to cause reabsorption of water from the kidney tubule, resulting in more dilute blood and more concentrated urine. Aldosterone, the major mineralocorticoid, causes sodium reabsorption from the kidney and potassium excretion. Calcium levels are not a factor in serum osmolality.
8. d. Atrial natriuretic peptide (ANP) is secreted in response to high blood volume and high serum sodium levels and has an inhibiting effect on ADH and the renin-angiotensin-aldosterone system, the effects of which would make the blood volume even higher. The relationship between cortisol and insulin is indirect; cortisol raises blood glucose levels, and insulin secretion is stimulated by high glucose levels. Glucagon secretion inhibits insulin secretion, but insulin does not inhibit glucagon. Testosterone and estrogen have no reciprocal action, and both are secreted by the body in response to tropic hormones.
9. d. Usually insulin and glucagon function in a reciprocal manner, except after a high-protein, carbohydrate-free meal, in which both hormones are secreted. Glucagon increases gluconeogenesis and insulin facilitates transport of amino acids across muscle membranes for protein synthesis.
10. a. Hypokalemia inhibits aldosterone release as well as insulin release. Hypokalemia does not directly affect the other options.

11.

Functional Health Pattern	Risk Factor for or Response to Endocrine Problem
Health perception–health management	Decreased energy level in relation to the past, family history of similar problems
Nutritional-metabolic	Changes in appetite and weight, difficulty swallowing. Nausea and vomiting, diarrhea. Changes in hair distribution, color, and texture. Skin changes, hot and cold intolerances
Elimination	Increased thirst with frequent urination, kidney stones, frequent defecation or constipation, change in stool consistency or pattern
Activity-exercise	Decrease in previous activity levels, fatigue, hyperactivity
Sleep-rest	Sleep disturbances, nightmares, sweating, nocturia, insomnia, excessive sleep, or snoring
Cognitive-perceptual	Memory deficits, depression, inability to concentrate. Visual disturbances or exophthalmos. Apathy, headaches
Self-perception–self-concept	Changes in body appearance and self-perception
Role-relationship	Changes in ability to maintain usual roles
Sexuality-reproductive	Menstrual irregularity and infertility, history of delivering large babies, male sexual dysfunction, changes in secondary sex characteristics, growth disorders
Coping–stress tolerance	Perception of stress in life and usefulness of previous coping mechanisms, changes in response to stress, lack of support system
Value-belief	Commitment to lifestyle changes, value of health management

12. a. Although cortisol is a glucocorticoid, it has action on mineralocorticoid receptors, which causes sodium retention and potassium excretion from the kidney, resulting in hypokalemia. Because water is reabsorbed with the sodium, serum sodium remains normal. In its effect on glucose and fat metabolism, cortisol causes an elevation in blood glucose as well as increases in free fatty acids and triglycerides.

13. b. Many symptoms of hypothyroidism, such as fatigue, mental impairment, dry skin, and constipation that would be apparent in younger persons are attributed to general aging in the older adult; as a result, hypothyroidism goes unrecognized as a treatable condition.

14. c. Assessment of the endocrine system is often difficult because hormones affect every body tissue and system, causing great diversity in the signs and symptoms of endocrine dysfunction. Weight loss, fatigue, and depression are signs that may occur with many different endocrine problems or other diseases. Goiter, exophthalmos, and the "polys" are findings of specific endocrine glands' dysfunction.

15. c. In the patient with enlarged thyroid, palpation can cause the release of thyroid hormone into circulation, increasing the patient's symptoms and potentially causing a thyroid storm. Examination should be deferred to a more experienced clinician if possible. If the thyroid is palpated correctly, the carotid arteries are not compressed. Pressure should not be so great as to damage the cricoid cartilage or laryngeal nerve.

16. b, c, e. Heat intolerance, exophthalmos, and a goiter are all related to thyroid dysfunction. Tetanic muscle spasms are related to hypofunction of the parathyroid. Hyperpigmentation is related to hypofunction of the adrenal gland. Increased hand and foot size is related to excess growth hormone secretion.

17. a. Endocrine disorders related to hormone secretion from glands that are stimulated by tropic hormones can be caused by a malsecretion of the tropic hormone or of the target gland. If the problem is in the target gland, it is known as a *primary endocrine disorder*; a problem with tropic hormone secretion is known as a *secondary endocrine disorder*. Serum levels of tropic hormones can illustrate the status of the negative feedback system in relation to target organ hormone levels. Normally, if a target organ produces low amounts of hormone, tropic hormones will be increased; if a target organ is overproducing hormones, tropic hormones will be low or undetectable.

18. c. To ensure that the level is a fasting level, a minimum of 8 hours should be allowed. Water may be taken, however, and does not affect the glucose level. Many medications may also influence results, which will have to be evaluated.

19. b, d, e. Luteinizing hormone (LH) and follicle-stimulating hormone (FSH) are used to distinguish gonad problems from pituitary insufficiency. LH and FSH are low in pituitary insufficiency and high in gonadal failure. The MRI would be used to identify tumors involving the pituitary gland or hypothalamus. Thyroglobulin is a tumor marker for thyroid cancer. Parathyroid hormone (PTH), along with calcium and phosphorus levels, are checked for parathyroid function. The ACTH suppression test assesses adrenal function, especially with hyperactivity.

20. d. The elevated cortisol of Cushing syndrome manifests in elevated BP and blood glucose. Also seen are moon face, hirsutism, decreased muscle mass from protein wasting, increased weight, and fragile skin with striae across the abdomen.

21. d. Glycosylated hemoglobin (A_1C) is used to assess blood glucose control during the previous 3 months. Water deprivation (ADH stimulation) is used to differentiate causes of diabetes insipidus. Fasting blood glucose will measure only the current blood glucose result. The oral glucose tolerance test is used to diagnose diabetes when abnormal fasting blood glucose levels do not clearly indicate diabetes.

CHAPTER 53

1. d. Insulin is an anabolic hormone that is responsible for growth, repair, and storage. It facilitates movement of amino acids into cells, synthesis of protein, storage of glucose as glycogen, and deposition of triglycerides and lipids as fat into adipose tissue. Fat is used for energy when glucose levels are depleted. Glucagon is responsible for hepatic glycogenolysis and gluconeogenesis.

2. c, e. Adipose tissue and skeletal muscle require insulin to allow the transport of glucose into the cells. Brain, liver, and blood cells require adequate glucose supply for normal function but do not depend directly on insulin for glucose transport.

3. b. The counter regulatory hormones have the opposite effect of insulin by stimulating glucose production and output by the liver and by decreasing glucose transport into the cells. The counter regulatory hormones and insulin together regulate the blood glucose level.

4. a, b, c, d, e, f. Type 2 diabetes is characterized by β-cell exhaustion, insulin resistance, genetic predisposition, altered production of adipokines, inherited defect in insulin receptors, and inappropriate glucose production by the liver. The roles of the brain, kidneys, and gut in type 2 diabetes development are being studied.

5. d. Prediabetes is defined as impaired glucose tolerance and impaired fasting glucose or both. Fasting blood glucose results between 100 mg/dL (5.56 mmol/L) and 125 mg/dL (6.9 mmol/L) indicate prediabetes. A diagnosis of impaired glucose tolerance is made if the 2-hour oral glucose tolerance test (OGTT) results are between 140 mg/dL (7.8 mmol/L) and 199 mg/dL (11.0 mmol/L).

6. a, b, e. To reduce the risk of developing diabetes, the patient with prediabetes should maintain a healthy weight, learn to monitor for symptoms of diabetes, have blood glucose and glycosylated hemoglobin (A_1C) tested regularly, exercise regularly, and eat a healthy diet.

7. b. Polydipsia is caused by fluid loss from polyuria when high glucose levels cause osmotic diuresis. Cellular starvation from lack of glucose and the use of body fat and protein for energy contribute to fatigue, weight loss, and polyphagia in type 1 diabetes.

8. c. Type 2 diabetes has a strong genetic influence (8% to 14% risk for offspring) and offspring of parents who both have type 2 diabetes have an increased chance of developing it. In contrast, type 1 diabetes is associated with a genetic susceptibility that is related to human leukocyte antigens (HLAs). Offspring of a mother with type 1

diabetes have a 1% to 4% chance of developing the disease, while offspring of a father with diabetes have 5% to 6% risk. Other risk factors for type 2 diabetes include obesity; Native American, Hispanic, or African ancestry; and age of 55 years or older. Although 50% of people with a parent with maturity-onset diabetes of the young (MODY) will develop MODY, it is autosomal dominant, and treatment depends on which genetic mutation caused it. It is not associated with obesity or hypertension and is not currently considered preventable.

9. a. Metabolic syndrome is a cluster of abnormalities that include elevated glucose levels, abdominal obesity, elevated BP, high levels of triglycerides, and low levels of high-density lipoproteins (HDLs). Overweight persons with metabolic syndrome can prevent or delay the onset of diabetes through a program of weight loss. Regular physical activity is also important, but normal weight is most important.

10. a, c. The patient has 1 prior test result of fasting plasma glucose (FPG) $\geq$ to 126 mg/dL (7.0 mmol/L) that meets criteria for a diagnosis of diabetes, and the result is confirmed on this follow-up visit. The A_1C is 7.5% and greater than diagnostic criteria of 6.5% or higher. The other diagnostic criteria include a 2-hour OGTT level $\geq$ 200 mg/dL (11.1 mmol/L), or a patient with classic symptoms of hyperglycemia (polyuria, polydipsia, polyphagia, unexplained weight loss) or hyperglycemic crisis, a random plasma glucose $\geq$ 200 mg/dL (11.0 mmol/L).

11. d. Impaired glucose tolerance exists when a 2-hour OGTT level is higher than normal but lower than the level diagnostic for diabetes (i.e., > 200 mg/dL). Impaired fasting glucose exists when fasting glucose levels are greater than the normal of 100 mg/dL but < the 126 mg/dL diagnostic of diabetes. Both abnormal values indicate prediabetes.

12. b. Patients should consistently use the same size of insulin syringe to avoid dosing errors. Errors can be made if patients switch back and forth between different sizes of syringes. Aspiration before injection of the insulin is no longer recommended, nor is the use of alcohol to clean the skin. Because the rate of peak serum concentration varies with the site selected for injection, injections should be rotated within a particular area, such as the abdomen, before changing to another area. Lipodystrophies are rare with the use of human insulin.

13. b. A split-mixed dose of insulin requires that the patient adhere to a set meal pattern to provide glucose for the peak action of the insulin, and a bedtime snack is usually required when patients take an intermediate-acting insulin late in the day to prevent nocturnal hypoglycemia. Hypoglycemia is most likely to occur with this dose late in the afternoon and during the night. When premixed formulas are used, flexible dosing based on glucose levels is not recommended.

14. d. Lispro is a rapid-acting insulin that has an onset of action of approximately 15 minutes and should be injected at the time of the meal to within 15 minutes of eating. Regular insulin is short acting with an onset of action in 30 to 60 minutes following administration and should be given 30 to 45 minutes before meals.

15. a. When mixing regular and intermediate-acting insulin, regular insulin should always be drawn into the syringe first to prevent contamination of the regular insulin vial with intermediate-acting insulin additives. Air is added to the NPH vial first. Then air is added to the regular vial and the regular insulin is withdrawn, bubbles are removed, and then the dose of NPH is withdrawn.

16. b. Checking the temperature of the bath water is part of assisting with activities of daily living (ADLs) and within the scope of care for the AP. This is important for the patient with neuropathy. Discussing complications, teaching, and assessing learning are appropriate for RNs.

17. d. Insulin glargine (Lantus), a long-acting insulin that is continuously released with no peak of action, cannot be diluted or mixed with any other insulin or solution. Mixed insulins should be stored needle-up in the refrigerator and warmed before administration. Currently used bottles of insulin may be kept at room temperature out of sunlight for 4 weeks.

18. a. Insulin pumps provide tight glycemic control by continuous subcutaneous insulin infusion based on the patient's basal profile, with bolus doses at mealtime at the patient's discretion and related to blood glucose monitoring. Errors in insulin dosing and complications of insulin therapy are still potential risks with insulin pumps.

19. c. The patient's high glucose on arising may be the result of either dawn phenomenon or Somogyi effect. The best way to determine whether the patient needs more or less insulin is by monitoring the glucose at bedtime, between 2:00 AM and 4:00 AM, and on arising. If the 2:00 AM to 4:00 AM blood glucose levels are below 60 mg/dL, the insulin dose should be reduced to prevent Somogyi effect; if it is high, the insulin should be increased to prevent dawn phenomenon.

20. b. Biguanides (e.g., metformin [Glucophage]) are most commonly used with type 2 diabetes. They reduce glucose production by the liver and increase insulin sensitivity at the tissue level that improves glucose transport into the cells. Insulin is not taken orally, as it is ineffective. Meglitinides and sulfonylureas increase insulin production from the pancreas.

21. a, d, e. Acarbose (Precose) is an α-glucosidase inhibitor that is taken with the first bite of each meal. The effectiveness is measured with 2-hour postprandial blood glucose testing, as it delays glucose absorption from the gastrointestinal (GI) tract. The other options describe rarely used thiazolidinediones.

22. d. This glucagon-like peptide-1 (GLP-1) receptor agonist stimulates GLP-1 to increase insulin synthesis and release from the pancreas, inhibit glucagon secretion, slow gastric emptying, and must be injected subcutaneously once every 7 days. The other medications are oral agents (OAs). The mechanism of action for glycemic control for the dopamine receptor agonist is unknown. Dipeptidyl peptidase-4 (DPP-4) inhibitors block the action of the DPP-4 enzyme that inactivates incretin so there is increased insulin release, decreased glucagon secretion, and decreased hepatic glucose production. Sodium-glucose co-transporter 2 (SGLT2) inhibitors block the reabsorption of glucose by the kidney and increase urinary glucose excretion.

23. b. Rapid deep respirations are symptoms of diabetic ketoacidosis (DKA), so this is the priority of care. Stage II pressure injuries and bilateral numbness are chronic complications of diabetes. The lumps and dents on the abdomen indicate the patient has lipodystrophy and may need to learn about site rotation of insulin injections.

24. a. The body needs food at regularly spaced intervals throughout the day. Omission or delay of meals can result in hypoglycemia, especially for the patient using conventional insulin therapy or OAs. Weight loss may be recommended in type 2 diabetes if the person is overweight, but many patients with type 1 diabetes are thin and do not require a decrease in caloric intake. Fewer than 7% of total calories should be from saturated fats and simple sugar should be limited, but moderate amounts can be used if counted as a part of total carbohydrate intake.

25. b. The specific goals of nutrition therapy for people with diabetes include maintaining near-normal blood glucose levels and achievement of optimal serum lipid levels and BP. Dietary modifications are believed to be important factors in preventing both short- and long-term complications of diabetes. Loss of weight, which may or may not be to ideal body weight, may improve insulin resistance. There is no longer a specific "diabetic diet," and use of dietetic foods is not necessary for glucose control. Most patients with diabetes eat 3 meals a day, and some require a bedtime snack for control of nighttime hypoglycemia. The other goals of nutrition therapy include prevention of chronic complications of diabetes, attention to individual nutritional needs, and maintenance of the pleasure of eating.

26. a. To plan for exercise, a person with diabetes must monitor blood glucose and make adjustments to insulin dose (if taken) and food intake to prevent exercise-induced hypoglycemia. Exercise is delayed if blood glucose is $\geq$ 250 mg/dL with ketones. Before exercise if blood glucose is $\leq$ 100 mg/dL a 15-g carbohydrate snack is eaten. Blood glucose levels should be monitored before, during, and after exercise to determine the effect of exercise on the levels.

27. c. Cleaning the puncture site with alcohol is not necessary and may interfere with test results and lead to drying and splitting of the fingertips. Washing the hands with warm water is adequate cleaning and promotes blood flow to the fingers. Blood flow is also increased by holding the hand down. Punctures on the side of the finger pad are less painful. Self-monitored blood glucose (SMBG) should be performed before and after exercise.

28. b. The American Diabetes Association recommends that testing for type 2 diabetes with a FPG, A_1C, or 2-hour OGTT should be considered for all persons at the age of 45 years and above and, if normal, repeated every 3 years. Testing for immune markers of type 1 diabetes is not recommended. Testing at a younger age or more frequently should be done for members of a high-risk ethnic population, including blacks, Hispanics, Native Americans, Asian Americans, and Pacific Islanders. Overweight adults with additional risk factors should be tested.

29. a. During minor illnesses, the patient with diabetes should continue drug therapy and fluid and food intake. Insulin is important because counter regulatory hormones may increase blood glucose during the stress of illness. Food or a carbohydrate liquid substitution is important because during illness the body requires extra energy to deal with the stress of the illness. Blood glucose monitoring should be done every 4 hours, and the HCP should be notified if the level is >240 mg/dL (13.9 mmol/L) or if fever, ketonuria, or nausea and vomiting occur.

30. c. When insulin is insufficient and glucose cannot be used for cellular energy, the body uses stored fats to meet energy needs. Free fatty acids from stored triglycerides are metabolized in the liver in such large quantities that ketones are formed. Ketones are acidic and alter the pH of the blood, causing acidosis. Osmotic diuresis from the elimination of both glucose and ketones in the urine causes dehydration, not ketosis. The loss of bicarbonate and skipping a meal after insulin administration do not cause ketosis.

31. a, b, c, d, e, f. In DKA, thirst occurs to replace fluid used to eliminate ketones in the urine in trying to decrease the blood glucose and ketonemia. The metabolic acidosis leads to the Kussmaul respirations trying to decrease the acid in the system. The sweet, fruity breath odor is from acetone. Thirst and dehydration are found with both DKA and hyperosmolar hyperglycemic syndrome (HHS).

32. c. The management of DKA is similar to that of HHS except that HHS requires greater fluid replacement because of the severe hyperosmolar state. Bicarbonate is not usually given in DKA to correct acidosis unless the pH is < 7.0 because administration of insulin will reverse the abnormal fat metabolism. Total body potassium deficit is possible in both conditions, requiring monitoring and possibly potassium administration, and in both conditions glucose is added to IV fluids when blood glucose levels fall to 250 mg/dL (13.9 mmol/L).

33. a, c, e, f. Manifestations of hyperglycemia include abdominal cramps, polyuria, weakness, fatigue, and headache. The headache may also be seen with hypoglycemia that is manifested by the remaining options.

34. d. If a patient with diabetes is unconscious, immediate treatment for hypoglycemia must be given to prevent brain damage, and IM or subcutaneous administration of 1 mg of glucagon should be done. If the unconsciousness has another cause, such as ketosis, the rise in glucose caused by the glucagon is not as dangerous as the low glucose level. Following administration of the glucagon, the patient should be transported to a medical facility for further treatment and evaluation. Oral carbohydrates cannot be given when patients are unconscious, and insulin is contraindicated without knowledge of the patient's glucose level.

35. a. 3; b. 2; c. 1; d. 5; e. 4; f. 6. As with all patients, first establish an airway. With a patient with diabetes and abnormal behavior, the blood glucose must then be checked to determine if the patient's symptoms are related to the diabetes. In this case, it is hyperglycemia, so an IV must be started for fluid resuscitation and insulin administration. The last food intake and times at which medications were recently taken may establish a cause for the hyperglycemia and aid in determining further treatment.

36. a. Blood glucose levels of 80 to 90 mg/dL (4.4 to 5 mmol/L) are within the normal range and are desired in the patient with diabetes, even following a recent hypoglycemic episode. Hypoglycemia is often caused by a single event, such as skipping a meal, taking too much insulin, or vigorous exercise. Once corrected, normal glucose control should be maintained.

37. b. The development of atherosclerotic vessel disease seems to be promoted by the altered lipid metabolism common in diabetes. Although tight glucose control may help delay the

process, it does not prevent it completely. Atherosclerosis in patients with diabetes does respond somewhat to a reduction in general risk factors, as it does in nondiabetics, and reduction in fat intake, control of hypertension, abstention from smoking, maintenance of normal weight, and regular exercise should be carried out by all patients.

38. b, d. Macrovascular disease causes coronary artery disease and ulceration and results in amputation of the lower extremities. However, neuropathy may contribute to not feeling ulcerations. The remaining options are related to microvascular complications of diabetes.

39. b, e, f. Autonomic neuropathy affects most body systems. Manifestations of autonomic neuropathy include erectile dysfunction in men and decreased libido, gastroparesis (nausea, vomiting, gastroesophageal reflux and feeling full), painless myocardial infarction, postural hypotension, and resting tachycardia. The remaining options would occur with sensory neuropathy.

40. d. Complete or partial loss of protective sensation of the feet is common with peripheral neuropathy of diabetes, and patients with diabetes may suffer foot injury and ulceration without ever having pain. Feet must be inspected during daily care for any cuts, blisters, swelling, or reddened areas.

41. a. Older adults have more conditions that may be treated with medications that impair insulin action. Hypoglycemic unawareness is more common, so these patients are more likely to suffer adverse consequences from blood glucose–lowering therapy. Manifestations of long-term complications of diabetes take 10 to 20 years to develop, so the goals for glycemic control are not as rigid as in the younger population. Treatment is indicated and insulin may be used if the patient does not respond to oral agents. The patient's needs rather than age determine the responsibility of others in care.

42. b. Advise the patient to seek the guidance of the HCP regarding the safety, efficacy, and specifics of using herbal therapy rather than or with the medication prescribed. Not all herbal therapy is unsafe, but dosages are not universal.

Case Study

1. **Sympathetic nervous system**: HR 120 beats/min (tachycardia due to effects of epinephrine), numbness in fingers and feels cold (due to vasoconstriction caused by epinephrine); **Hypoglycemia to the brain**: headache, slurred speech, unsteady gait, and confusion (the brain requires glucose; the lack of glucose delivery to the brain results in the patient manifesting as though they are intoxicated.)

2. **Expected**: tremors, diaphoresis, lips/mouth numbness, dizziness; **Unexpected**: flushed and warm skin, abdominal cramping (occurs with hyperglycemia), polyuria (occurs with hyperglycemia)

3. **1**=15-20 g; **2**=simple carbohydrates (quickly and easily utilized by the body); **3**=apple juice (or any fruit juice) or soft drink (regular not diet); **4**=15 minutes; **5**=70; **6**=50% dextrose; **7**=1 mg; **8**=glucagon

4. **Effective**: "carry a snack," "increase calories before exercising," "wait 60 minutes after meals before exercising"; **Ineffective**; "insulin requirements are higher with exercise," "exercise doesn't affect BG levels" (exercise increases the body's sensitivity to insulin which causes a lower insulin requirement); **Unrelated**: "I will drink lots of water during exercise" (while it is important

to remain hydrated, it doesn't prevent hypoglycemia), "I will dress lightly during strenuous exercise" (won't prevent hypoglycemia)

5. C., D., E., G. DKA can occur in both types of diabetes, but is more prevalent in patients with type 1 diabetes. DKA is caused by the lack of sufficient insulin resulting in hyperglycemia causing polyuria, polydipsia, and polyphagia. Ketones are by-products of fat metabolism in the body's attempt to increase fuel for energy. Patients with DKA need to be hospitalized to treat hyperglycemia, dehydration, and the depletion of electrolytes like potassium. The patient shouldn't restrict fluids even though they may experience nausea and vomiting. This will worsen dehydration caused by hyperglycemia.

CHAPTER 54

1. d. A normal response to growth hormone (GH) secretion is stimulation of the liver to produce insulin-like growth factor-1 (IGF-1). In acromegaly, there are increased levels of IGF-1. When both GH and IGF-1 levels are increased, overproduction of GH is confirmed. GH also causes elevation of blood glucose and normally GH levels fall during an oral glucose challenge but not in acromegaly.

2. c. The increased production of GH in acromegaly causes an increase in thickness and width of bones and enlargement of soft tissues, resulting in marked changes in facial features, feet, and head; oily and coarse skin; and speech difficulties. Infertility is not a common finding because GH is usually the only pituitary hormone involved in acromegaly. Height is not increased in adults with GH excess because the epiphyses of the bones are closed.

3. a. A transsphenoidal hypophysectomy involves entry into the sella turcica through an incision in the upper lip and gingiva into the floor of the nose and the sphenoid sinuses. Clear nasal drainage with glucose and protein content indicates cerebrospinal fluid (CSF) leakage from an open connection to the brain, putting the patient at risk for meningitis. After surgery, the patient is positioned with the head elevated to avoid pressure on the sella turcica. Although mouth care is required every 4 hours, toothbrushing should not be done because injury to the suture line may occur. Coughing and straining are avoided to prevent increased intracranial pressure and CSF leakage.

4. d. Compression of the optic chiasm can cause visual problems as well as signs of increased intracranial pressure, including headache, nausea, and vomiting. About 30% of prolactinomas will have excess prolactin secretion with manifestations of impotence in men, galactorrhea or amenorrhea in women without relationship to pregnancy, and decreased libido in both men and women. There is decreased follicle-stimulating hormone (FSH) and luteinizing hormone (LH).

5. a, b, d, e. With panhypopituitarism, lifetime hormone replacement is needed for cortisol, vasopressin, thyroid, and GH. Sex hormones will not be replaced. Her GH will be monitored closely because of the patient's history of breast cancer. Dopamine agonists will not be used because they reduce secretion of GH, which has already been achieved with the radiation.

6. b. With increased antidiuretic hormone (ADH), the permeability of the renal distal tubules is increased, so

water is reabsorbed into circulation. Decreased output of concentrated urine with increased urine osmolality and specific gravity occur. In addition, fluid retention with weight gain, serum hypoosmolality, dilutional hyponatremia, and hypochloremia occur.

7. a. The patient with syndrome of inappropriate antidiuretic hormone (SIADH) has marked dilutional hyponatremia and should be monitored for decreased neurologic function and seizures every 2 hours. Sodium intake is supplemented because of the hyponatremia and sodium loss caused by diuretics. ADH release is reduced by keeping the head of the bed flat to increase left atrial filling pressure. A reduction in BP indicates a reduction in total fluid volume and is an expected outcome of treatment.

8. b. The patient with SIADH has water retention with hyponatremia, decreased urine output, and concentrated urine with high specific gravity. Improvement in the patient's condition is reflected by increased urine output, normalization of serum sodium, and more water in the urine, thus decreasing the specific gravity.

9. d. Patients with diabetes insipidus (DI) excrete large amounts of urine with a specific gravity of <1.005. A blood glucose may be tested if acetone breath is present to diagnose diabetes, but that is not mentioned in this situation. The serum sodium level is expected to be low with DI but is not diagnostic. To diagnose central DI, a water deprivation test is needed. A CT of the head may be done to determine the cause. Nephrogenic DI is distinguished from central DI with determination of the level of ADH after an analog of ADH is given.

10. d. A patient with central DI has a deficiency of ADH with excessive loss of water from the kidney, hypovolemia, hypernatremia, and dilute urine with a low specific gravity. When desmopressin acetate (DDAVP) is administered, the symptoms are reversed, with water retention, decreased urinary output that increases urine osmolality, and an increase in BP.

11. c. Normal urine specific gravity is 1.005 to 1.030. A urine with a specific gravity of 1.002 is very dilute, indicating that there continues to be excessive loss of water and that treatment of DI is inadequate. Headache, weight gain, and oral intake greater than urinary output are signs of volume excess that occur with overmedication. Nasal irritation and nausea may also indicate overdosage.

12. b. In nephrogenic DI, the kidney is unable to respond to ADH, so vasopressin or hormone analogs are not effective. Thiazide diuretics may reduce flow to the ADH-sensitive distal nephrons and produce a decrease in urine output. Fluids are not restricted because the patient could easily become dehydrated. Low-sodium diets (< 3 g/day) are also thought to decrease urine output. An antidiabetic drug is not needed.

13. d. In Hashimoto's thyroiditis, thyroid tissue is destroyed by autoimmune antibodies. An enlarged thyroid gland is a goiter. Viral-induced hyperthyroidism is subacute granulomatous thyroiditis. Acute thyroiditis is caused by bacterial or fungal infection.

14. a. Exophthalmos or protrusion of the eyeballs may occur in Graves' disease from increased fat deposits and fluid in the orbital tissues and ocular muscles, forcing the eyeballs outward. Graves' disease is the most common form of hyperthyroidism. Increased metabolic rate and sensitivity of the sympathetic nervous system lead to the manifestations. Thyroid-stimulating hormone (TSH) level is decreased in Graves' disease.

15. d. In Graves' disease, antibodies to the TSH receptor are formed, attach to the receptors, and stimulate the thyroid gland to release triiodothyronine (T_3), thyroxine (T_4), or both, creating hyperthyroidism. The disease is not directly genetic, but persons appear to have a genetic susceptibility to develop autoimmune antibodies. Goiter formation from insufficient iodine intake is usually associated with hypothyroidism.

16. c. A thyroid storm results in marked manifestations of hyperthyroidism. Severe tachycardia, heart failure, shock, hyperthermia, agitation delirium, seizures, abdominal pain, vomiting, diarrhea, and coma occur. Although exophthalmos may be present in the patient with Graves' disease, it is not a significant factor in thyrotoxic crisis. Hoarseness and laryngeal stridor are characteristic of the tetany of hypoparathyroidism and lethargy progressing to coma is characteristic of myxedema coma, a complication of hypothyroidism.

17. c. The β-adrenergic blocker propranolol is usually used to block the sympathetic nervous system stimulation by thyroid hormones. Atenolol would be used with asthma or heart disease. Potassium iodine is used to prepare the patient for thyroidectomy or for treatment of thyrotoxic crisis to inhibit the synthesis of thyroid hormones. Propylthiouracil, an antithyroid medication, inhibits the synthesis of thyroid hormones. Radioactive iodine (RAI) therapy destroys thyroid tissue, which limits thyroid hormone secretion.

18. b, d, f. RAI causes hypothyroidism over time by damaging thyroid tissue. This decreases thyroid hormone secretion and is the treatment of choice for nonpregnant adults. Potassium iodine decreases the release of thyroid hormones and the size of the thyroid gland before surgery. Propylthiouracil blocks peripheral conversion of T_4 to T_3 and may be used with iodine to produce a euthyroid state before surgery.

19. a. To prevent strain on the suture line after surgery, the patient's head must be manually supported while turning and moving in bed. Range-of-motion exercises for the head and neck are taught preoperatively to be gradually implemented after surgery. There is no contraindication for coughing and deep breathing. These should be carried out after surgery. Tingling around the lips or fingers is a sign of hypocalcemia, which may occur if the parathyroid glands were inadvertently removed during surgery. This sign should be reported at once.

20. a. A tracheostomy tray must be in the room to use if the emergency situation of vocal cord paralysis occurs from recurrent or superior laryngeal nerve damage or for laryngeal stridor from tetany. The oxygen equipment may be useful but will not improve oxygenation with vocal cord paralysis without a tracheostomy. IV calcium salts will be used if hypocalcemia occurs from parathyroid damage. The paper and pencil for communication may be helpful, especially if a tracheostomy is done, but will not aid in emergency oxygenation of the patient.

21. d. With the decrease in thyroid hormone after surgery, calories must be reduced to prevent weight gain. When a patient has had a subtotal thyroidectomy, thyroid

replacement therapy is not given because exogenous hormone inhibits pituitary production of TSH and delays or prevents the restoration of thyroid tissue regeneration. Regular exercise stimulates the thyroid gland and is encouraged. Saltwater gargles are used for dryness and irritation of the mouth and throat after radioactive iodine therapy.

22. d. In America, atrophy from Graves' disease or Hashimoto's thyroiditis are autoimmune disorders that eventually destroy the thyroid gland, leading to primary hypothyroidism. Worldwide, iodine deficiency is the most common cause. Thyroid tumors most often result in hyperthyroidism. Secondary hypothyroidism occurs because of pituitary failure. Iatrogenic hypothyroidism results from thyroidectomy or radiation of the thyroid gland.

23. b. Cardiorespiratory response to activity is important to monitor in this patient to determine the effect of activities and plan activity increases. Monitoring changes in orientation, cognition, and behavior are interventions for impaired memory. Monitoring bowels is needed to plan care for the patient with constipation. Assisting with meal planning will help the patient lose weight if needed.

24. d. All these manifestations may occur with treatment of hypothyroidism. However, because of the effects of hypothyroidism on the cardiovascular system, when thyroid replacement therapy is started, myocardial oxygen consumption is increased, and the resultant oxygen demand may cause angina, dysrhythmias, and heart failure. So, monitoring for dysrhythmias is most important.

25. b. Because of the mental sluggishness, inattentiveness, and memory loss that occur with hypothyroidism, it is important to provide written instructions and repeat information when teaching the patient. Replacement therapy must be taken for life and alternate-day dosing is not therapeutic. Although most patients return to a normal state with treatment, cardiovascular conditions and psychoses may persist.

26. d. The patient with hyperparathyroidism may have calcium stones, skeletal pain, decreased bone density, psychomotor retardation, or dysrhythmias among other manifestations. The other endocrine problems would not be related to calcium kidney stones or decreased bone density.

27. b. A high fluid intake is indicated in hyperparathyroidism to dilute the hypercalcemia and flush the kidneys so that calcium stone formation is reduced. Seizures are not associated with hyperparathyroidism. The patient with hyperparathyroidism is at risk for pathologic fractures resulting from decreased bone density, but mobility is encouraged to promote bone calcification. Impending tetany of hypoparathyroidism after parathyroidectomy can be noted with Trousseau's and Chvostek's signs.

28. a, c, d, e, f. In hypoparathyroidism, the patient has inadequate circulating parathyroid hormone (PTH) that leads to hypocalcemia from the inability to maintain serum calcium levels. With hypocalcemia, there is muscle stiffness and spasms, which can lead to dysrhythmias and abdominal cramps. There can be personality and visual changes and dry, scaly skin.

29. b. Rebreathing in a paper bag promotes carbon dioxide retention in the blood, which lowers pH and creates an acidosis. An acidemia enhances the solubility and ionization of calcium, increasing the proportion of total body calcium available in physiologically active form and relieving the symptoms of hypocalcemia. Saline promotes calcium excretion, as does furosemide. Phosphate levels in the blood are reciprocal to calcium and an increase in phosphate promotes calcium excretion.

30. c. The hypocalcemia that results from PTH deficiency is controlled with calcium and vitamin D supplementation and possibly oral phosphate binders. Replacement with PTH is not used because of antibody formation to PTH, the need for parenteral administration, and cost. Milk products, although good sources of calcium, have high levels of phosphate, which reduce calcium absorption. Whole grains and foods containing oxalic acid impair calcium absorption.

31. a. The effects of adrenocorticotropic hormone (ACTH) excess, especially glucocorticoid excess, include weight gain from accumulation and redistribution of adipose tissue, sodium and water retention, glucose intolerance, protein wasting, loss of bone structure, loss of collagen, and capillary fragility leading to petechiae. Manifestations of adrenocortical hormone deficiency include hypotension, dehydration, weight loss, and hyperpigmentation of the skin.

32. c. Although the patient with Cushing syndrome has excess corticosteroids, removing the glands and the stress of surgery require that high doses of corticosteroids (cortisone) be given after surgery for several days before weaning the dose. The nurse should monitor the patient's vital signs to detect whether large amounts of hormones were released during surgical manipulation, obtain morning urine specimens for cortisol measurement to evaluate the effectiveness of the surgery, and provide dressing changes with aseptic technique to avoid infection as usual inflammatory responses are suppressed.

33. b. Vomiting and diarrhea are early indicators of Addisonian crisis. Fever indicates an infection, which is causing added stress for the patient. Treatment of a crisis requires immediate IV hydrocortisone replacement. Large volumes of 0.9% saline and 5% dextrose fluids are given to reverse hypotension and electrolyte imbalances until BP returns to normal. Addison's disease is a primary insufficiency of the adrenal gland and ACTH is not effective, nor would vasopressors be effective with the fluid deficiency of Addison's disease. Potassium levels are increased in Addison's disease and KCl would be contraindicated.

34. b. A weight reduction in the patient with Addison's disease may indicate a fluid loss and a dose of replacement therapy that is too low rather than too high. Because vomiting and diarrhea are early signs of crisis and because fluid and electrolytes must be replaced, patients should notify their HCP if these symptoms occur. Patients with Addison's disease are taught to take 2 to 3 times their usual dose of steroids if they become ill, have teeth extracted, or engage in rigorous physical activity and should always have injectable hydrocortisone available if oral doses cannot be taken.

35. c. Alendronate (Fosamax) is used to prevent corticosteroid-induced osteoporosis. Potassium is used to prevent the mineralocorticoid effect of hypokalemia. Furosemide (Lasix) is used to decrease sodium and fluid retention from the mineralocorticoid effect. Pantoprazole (Protonix) is used to prevent gastrointestinal (GI) irritation from an increase in secretion of pepsin and hydrochloric acid.

36. c. Taking corticosteroids on an alternate-day schedule for pharmacologic purposes is less likely to suppress ACTH production from the pituitary and prevent adrenal atrophy. This method is not used when corticosteroids are given as hormone therapy. Normal adrenal hormone balance is not maintained nor is it more effective.

37. b. Hyperaldosteronism is an excess of aldosterone, which is manifested by sodium and water retention and potassium excretion. Furosemide is a potassium-wasting diuretic that would increase the potassium deficiency. Ketoconazole decreases adrenal corticosteroid secretion. Eplerenone and spironolactone are potassium-sparing diuretics.

38. b. Pheochromocytoma is a catecholamine-producing tumor of the adrenal medulla, which may cause severe, episodic hypertension and severe, pounding headache; tachycardia; and profuse sweating. Monitoring for a dangerously high BP before and after surgery is critical, as is monitoring for BP fluctuations during medical and surgical treatment.

Case Study

1. **Glucocorticoids**: truncal obesity, weakness, purple striae, peripheral edema, insomnia, hyperglycemia, acne, hypertension; **Mineralocorticoids**: peripheral edema, hypokalemia, hypertension; **Androgens**: weakness, acne (Refer to Table 54.16)

2. **Indicated**: MRI (or CT scan) of the head, 24-hour urine cortisol, dexamethasone suppression test, salivary cortisol; **Unrelated**: ultrasound of the adrenal glands (MRI or CT scans are preferred), creatinine clearance (measures glomerular filtration rate {GFR}), d-dimer (measures fibrin split products in blood clotting disorders)

3. Answers are listed in order of their appearance: cortisol; ketoconazole and mitotane; prednisone or hydrocortisone; mifepristone.

4. **Hypophysectomy**: "moustache" dressing (to absorb nasal drainage), report severe headaches (could indicate increased intracranial pressure {ICP} caused by bleeding or tissue swelling), elevate HOB ≥ 30° (to decrease swelling and ICP and promote drainage), assess peripheral vision (changes indicate a possible hematoma or pressure on the optic nerve or optic chiasma); **Adrenalectomy**: splint abdominal incision (during coughing, moving, sneezing to promote comfort and reduce risk wound dehiscence), report BP fluctuations (BP is increased after an adrenalectomy due to a surge of hormones released during the procedure), perform sterile dressing changes (not applicable to hypophysectomy, but having an adrenalectomy may suppress the body's response to infection), monitor electrolytes (fluctuations can occur after an adrenalectomy due to large amounts of hormones released during surgery); **Both**: administer hydrocortisone (both require steroid replacement), monitor blood glucose (to monitor for hyperglycemia while on steroid medications)

5. C., D., E., H., I. The patient is not to brush their teeth for 10 days due to the suture line in the upper gum. Clear drainage could indicate a CSF leak which should have resolved in the first 72 hours after surgery. Saline irrigation may be recommended to clean the nasal passages. Any vision changes should be reported to the HCP as this could indicate swelling or a hematoma pressing on the optic nerve or chiasma. The patient will need to take lifelong thyroid hormones, glucocorticoids, and sex hormones after the pituitary gland is removed. It is not normal to have frequent urination which could indicate diabetes insipidus. Patients should sneeze and cough with their mouth open to avoid increasing intracranial and nasal pressure. Patients can gently blow their nose usually 48 hours after surgery unless instructed otherwise. A stiff neck should be reported to the HCP as it could indicate meningitis.

CHAPTER 55

1. a. Seminal vesicle; b. ejaculatory duct; c. prostate gland; d. rectum; e. Cowper's gland; f. anus; g. epididymis; h. testis; i. scrotum; j. glans; k. penis; l. urethra; m. ductus deferens; n. bladder; o. ureter; p. fallopian tube; q. ovary; r. body of uterus; s. fundus of uterus; t. bladder; u. vagina; v. vaginal introitus; w. anus; x. rectum; y. urethra; z. cervix; aa. ureter

2. a. Prepuce; b. clitoris; c. labia minora; d. urethral meatus; e. vestibule; f. Bartholin's gland; g. perineum; h. hymen; i. vaginal introitus; j. labia majora; k. mons pubis; l. pectoralis major; m. alveoli; n. areola; o. nipple

3. a. 3; b. 8; c. 2; d. 6; e. 1; f. 7; g. 4; h. 5

4. a. Ducts carry milk from the alveoli to the lactiferous sinuses. The areola is the pigmented center of the breast, the nipple is the erectile tissue that contains pores, and adipose tissue makes up the majority of the nonlactating breast tissue.

5. c. Montgomery's tubercles are similar to sebaceous glands and lubricate the nipple. Milk is stored in the lactiferous sinuses and secreted from the alveoli during lactation. The nipple has erectile tissue and contains pores for milk delivery.

6. c. Menopause is identified after 1 year of amenorrhea. The ovum is fertilized by the sperm in the fallopian tube. A Papanicolaou (Pap) test includes cells from both the endocervix and the ectocervix. The reabsorption of oocytes by the body is called *atresia*. Follicle-stimulating hormone (FSH) stimulates the initial stage of follicular maturation, while luteinizing hormone (LH) must be present for complete maturation and ovulation to occur.

7. b, c, f. LH completes follicle maturation in women and stimulates testosterone production. LH is called *interstitial cell-stimulating hormone* (ICSH) in men. Progesterone maintains an implanted egg. Estrogen develops and maintains secondary sex characteristics of women, the proliferative phase of the menstrual cycle after menstruation, and uterine changes essential to pregnancy. Prolactin stimulates the growth of the mammary glands.

8. b, c, f. FSH is increased at menopause. In men, it is responsible for spermatogenesis. FSH stimulates growth and maturity of ovarian follicles. Testosterone is made by the testes and produces male sex characteristics. Gonadotropin-releasing hormone (GnRH) is stimulated by increased estrogen levels and decreased testosterone levels.

9. b. Age-related changes in sexual function in men include a need for increased stimulation for an erection and a possible decreased response to sexual stimuli. There may be a decreased ability to attain an erection, but it is not related to prostatic changes. A negative social attitude toward sexuality in older adults may affect the sexual activity of people in this age-group.

10.

Factor	Problem Identified During Assessment
Rubella	Potential congenital anomalies if rubella occurs during the first trimester of pregnancy
Mumps	Increased sterility in young men with mumps because of testicular atrophy resulting from orchitis
Diabetes	Erectile dysfunction and retrograde ejaculation in men in addition to erectile problems from neuropathies. In women, sexual performance and health of mother and fetus may be affected if diabetes is uncontrolled
Antihypertensive agents	Many may cause erectile dysfunction in men

11. b. A slow and difficult-to-start urinary stream indicates a need for further examination for benign prostatic hyperplasia (BPH). A mass could indicate cancer or other scrotal problems. A single, painless, small blister could indicate lymphogranuloma venereum or cancer. Palpating a bulging inguinal ring while the patient bears down is indicative of an inguinal hernia.

12. a. A decrease in the size of the penis is a normal finding in the older man. Loss of pubic hair is not normal, nor is the enlargement of 1 breast. The normally darker color of the scrotum does not change with aging.

13. c. Vaginal dryness occurs with decreased estrogen and increased androgens circulating in the aging female. This also leads to breast and genital atrophy, reduction in bone mass, and increased atherosclerosis. A rectocele may occur and cause sexual or fecal elimination problems for the patient that will need treatment, but this is not a normal finding. Severe osteoporosis is not a normal change of aging.

14.

Functional Health Pattern	Risk Factor for or Patient Response to Reproductive Problem
Health perception–health management	Lack of Pap testing, clinical breast prostate or testicular examinations. Smoking, alcohol, and illicit drug use. Family history of breast, ovarian, uterine, or prostate cancer. Allergies
Nutritional-metabolic	History of anemia, anorexia nervosa, obesity, decreased calcium intake
Elimination	Urge and stress incontinence. Difficulty urinating in male patients. Vaginal and bladder infections
Activity-exercise	Fatigue and activity intolerance related to menorrhagia
Sleep-rest	Sleep interruption related to hot flashes and sweating. Insomnia, nocturia
Cognitive-perceptual	Pelvic pain, dyspareunia
Self-perception–self-concept	Changes in self-concept related to sexuality and changes of aging
Role-relationship	Occupational hazards related to sexual functioning and reproductive capacity. Dysfunctional or changing roles and relationships with others
Sexuality-reproductive	Obstetric history, contraceptive methods, recent changes in sexual practices, dissatisfaction with sexual expression, reproductive problems that affect sexual satisfaction, changes in menstrual patterns, multiple sexual partners, no protection against/history of sexually transmitted infections (STIs)
Coping–stress tolerance	Effect of STI on sex partners, stress of sexual problems or changes, infertility, coping methods
Value-belief	Conflict between value system and treatment, abortion issues, infertility issues

15. b. Candidiasis is a white, thick, or curd-like discharge and causes itching and inflammation. Cancer would be more likely to produce a bloody discharge. Trichomonas vaginalis produces a malodorous frothy green or yellow discharge. Bacterial vaginosis infection produces copious amounts of thin gray or white drainage with a fishy odor.

16. d. The vulva should be the color of the skin or slightly pink. Redness indicates inflammation and possible genital herpes. A small amount of clear vaginal discharge is normal in females, as are episiotomy scars in women who have had children. Skene's glands should not be palpable.

17. b, d. Gram stain smears, nucleic acid amplification test (NAAT), and cultures can screen for *Chlamydia* from vaginal, endocervical, urinary, and urethral samples. The NAAT can also be used to detect gonorrhea. A Pap test detects potentially cancerous cells. The rapid plasma reagin (RPR), the Venereal Disease Research Laboratory (VDRL), and fluorescent treponemal antibody absorption (FTA-Abs) tests all screen for syphilis.

18. c. Serum estradiol measures ovarian function to assess estrogen-secreting tumors and precocious female puberty or to confirm perimenopausal status in women. It may be indicative of testicular tumors in men. Pregnancy is detected with urinary or serum human chorionic gonadotropin (hCG). Prostate cancer is detected with prostate-specific antigen (PSA). Gonadal failure caused by pituitary dysfunction is identified with urine or serum FSH studies.

19. b. The risk for bleeding is increased following a dilation and curettage (D&C) because the endometrial lining is scraped and injury to the uterus can occur. The nurse should closely assess the amount of bleeding with frequent pad checks for the first 24 hours. Infection following D&C is uncommon, and the urinary system is not affected. Infection could occur after a biopsy. Urinary retention occurs with BPH.

20. a, b, c, e. A D&C and laparoscopy are operative procedures requiring surgical anesthesia. A culdoscopy involves insertion of an endoscope through an incision made through the posterior fornix of the cul-de-sac and requires sedation, as does the removal of cervical tissue during a conization. Colposcopy and endometrial biopsies do not require surgical anesthesia.

21. b. A semen analysis requires a couple to have no sexual intercourse 2 to 3 days before an examination of semen for the volume, viscosity, number, mobility, and structure of sperm. Urinary LH is an OTC test to identify midcycle LH surge that precedes ovulation by 1 to 2 days. An endometrial biopsy provides a sample of endometrium to evaluate its changes under the influence of progesterone. A hysterosalpingogram is a contrast x-ray of the uterine cavity and fallopian tubes. Intercourse does not affect these other 3 test results.

CHAPTER 56

1. c. The value of breast self-examination (BSE) in reducing mortality rates from breast cancer in women is currently controversial and under review. However, it is still a useful tool in helping women become self-aware of how their breasts normally look and feel. None of the other options has been confirmed at this time.

2. Screening recommendations:
   a. Women ages 40 to 44 years should have the choice to start annual breast cancer screening with mammograms if they wish to do so.
   b. Women aged 45 to 54 years should get mammograms every year.
   c. Women 55 years and older should transition to biennial screening or have the opportunity to continue screening annually.
   d. Screening should continue as long as a woman is in good health and is expected to live 10 more years or longer.
   In women with increased risk, decisions for additional and more frequent testing should be determined with the HCP.

3. a. One of the major reasons why women do not examine their breasts regularly is because of a lack of confidence in BSE skill. A teaching program should include allowing time for women to ask questions and perform a return demonstration of the examination on themselves. Fear and denial often interfere with BSE even when women know that the perceived risk for cancer is high, know the statistics, and know that they should seek medical care if an abnormality is detected. Examinations in premenopausal women should be done right after the menstrual period and specific dates are set for postmenopausal women or those who have had hysterectomies.

4. d. A histologic examination of biopsied tissue is the only means of making a definitive diagnosis of breast cancer. A core (core needle) biopsy is as reliable as an excisional biopsy and has the advantages of decreased length of time for the procedure and recovery and reduced cost. A limitation of fine-needle aspiration is that if negative results are found, more definitive biopsy procedures are needed.

5. c. Oncotype DX is the most commonly used early stage breast cancer genomic assay test to assess risk of recurrence and the likely benefit of chemotherapy. CA 27-29 is a cancer marker produced by the *MUC1* gene. TNM is not a genomic assay but a system for staging cancer using tumor size, nodal involvement, and the presence of metastasis. Direct to consumer genetic testing enables consumers to supply their own samples but does not include genetic counseling and only tests single nucleotide variants, not representative of diseases.

6. d. Most breast lesions are benign. Many mobile cystic lesions change in response to the menstrual cycle, while most cancer tumors do not. Caffeine has been associated with fibrocystic changes in some women, but research has not proven caffeine as a cause of breast pain or cysts. Questions about a patient's last mammogram or family history are not closely related to the nurse's findings.

7. c. Fibrocystic changes make breasts difficult to examine because of fibrotic changes and multiple lumps. A woman with this condition should be familiar with the characteristic changes in her breasts and monitor them closely for new lumps that do not respond in a cyclic manner over 1 to 2 weeks. Estrogen antagonizes the condition and fibrocystic changes are not precancerous.

8. c, e, f. Intraductal papilloma is more common in women 30- to 50-years-old, is associated with increased cancer risk, and is a wartlike growth in mammary ducts beneath the areola. Fat necrosis is associated with breast trauma. Fibroadenoma generally occurs in women in their teens and twenties and has well-delineated, very mobile tumors. Multicolored, sticky nipple discharge is seen in ductal ectasia.

9. a. Mastitis occurs during lactation and is usually caused by *Staphylococcus aureus*. Ductal ectasia involves subareolar area ducts and has multicolored sticky nipple discharge and inflammatory signs. It is not associated with malignancy. Fibroadenoma is the most common cause of benign breast lumps in women under 25 years of age and may be caused by increased estrogen sensitivity. A biopsy must be done to exclude malignancy. Senescent gynecomastia occurs in older men, probably from increased conversion of androgens to estrogens in peripheral circulation. It generally regresses in 6 to 12 months.

10. d. After the age of 60 years, the incidence of breast cancer increases dramatically, and advanced age is the highest risk factor for females. Ninety-nine percent of breast cancer cases occur in women. A first-degree relative with breast cancer is a contributing factor for breast cancer. Genetic mutations in *BRCA1, BRCA2, p53, ATM,* and *CHEK2* genes may increase the risk of breast cancer. Obesity and lack of physical activity are other contributing factors. Fibrocystic breast changes are neither a precursor of breast cancer nor a known risk factor for cancer.

11. b. On palpation, malignant lesions are characteristically hard, irregularly shaped, poorly delineated, nontender, and nonmobile and the most common site is the upper outer quadrant of the breast. Fibrocystic lesions are usually large, tender, moveable masses found throughout the breast tissue. A fibroadenoma is firm, defined, and mobile. A painful, immobile mass under a reddened area of skin is most typical of a local abscess.

12. a. Axillary lymph node status is one of the most important prognostic factors in primary breast cancer; the more nodes involved, the higher the risk for relapse or metastasis. Aneuploid DNA tumor content shows that cells have abnormally high or low DNA content compared with normal cells and is associated with tumor aggressiveness. Cells in S-phase have a higher risk for recurrence and can produce earlier cancer death. Hormone receptor–negative tumors are usually poorly differentiated histologically, often recur, and are usually unresponsive to hormonal therapy.

13. b. Either treatment choice is indicated for women with early stage breast cancer because the 10-year survival rate with lumpectomy with radiation is about the same as that with modified radical mastectomy. Each procedure has advantages and disadvantages that the patient must consider in making an informed choice and the nurse should make that information available to the patient to aid in decision making.

14. d. Sentinel lymph node dissection (SLND) has become the standard of care, with axillary lymph node dissection reserved for patients with clinical indications of disease in the axilla. SLND provides prognostic information and helps determine further treatment. A lumpectomy, or breast-conservation surgery, is followed by radiation therapy to the entire breast and the use of chemotherapy or hormone therapy depends on the characteristics of the tumor and evidence of metastases.

15. d. In a sentinel lymph node biopsy (SLNB) radioisotopes or dye identify lymph nodes that drain from the tumor site, and they are removed. Those nodes are examined for malignant cells. If any of the nodes have malignant cells, the next step is a complete axillary lymph node dissection (ALND). If the sentinel nodes are negative, no other lymph nodes are removed.

16. a, c. High-dose brachytherapy may be completed in 5 days and is an alternative to traditional, longer-term radiation for early stage breast cancer. External radiation is a primary treatment after mastectomy for breast cancer. Radiation as an adjuvant to surgery is used to treat possible residual cancer cells postmastectomy. Palliative radiation is used to reduce tumor size and relieve pain.

17. a. Tamoxifen is an antiestrogen agent that blocks the estrogen-receptor sites of malignant cells and is the usual first choice of treatment in women with hormone receptor–positive tumors, with or without nodal involvement. Tamoxifen reduces the risk for recurrent breast cancer and new primary tumors. The side effects of the drug are minimal and are those associated with decreased estrogen.

18. c. As early as in the recovery room following a modified radical mastectomy, the patient should start flexing and extending the fingers and wrist of the affected arm with daily increases in activity. Postoperative mastectomy exercises, such as wall climbing with the fingers, shoulder rotation and extension, and hair care, are instituted gradually to prevent disruption of the wound.

19. b. Removal of the axillary lymph nodes impairs lymph drainage from the affected arm and predisposes the patient to infection of the arm. The arm must be protected from even minor trauma. BP, venipunctures, and injections should not be done on the arm. The arm should never be dependent, even during sleep, and should be elevated to promote lymph drainage.

20. c. The Reach-to-Recovery program consists of volunteers, all women, who have had breast cancer and can answer questions about what to expect at home, how to tell people about the surgery, and what prosthetic devices are available. It is a valuable resource for patients who have breast cancer and should be used if available in the community. If a volunteer is not available, the nurse is responsible for assisting the patient in the same manner. Although the nurse can discuss wearing a prosthesis, a permanent prosthesis cannot be used until healing is complete and inflammation is resolved.

21. b. It is most important for the patient planning a mammoplasty that she has a realistic idea about what the surgery can accomplish and about possible complications. Currently, surgery cannot restore nipple sensation or erectility, and the breast will not fully resemble its premastectomy appearance, but the outcome is usually more acceptable than the mastectomy scar. The woman's motives for breast reconstruction should not be questioned. There have been allegations of immune-related diseases associated with the use of silicone gel implants but after further evaluation the U.S. Food and Drug Administration (FDA) has approved these implants for use.

22. a. When an expander is used to stretch the skin and muscle at the mastectomy site, the expander is gradually increased in size by weekly to monthly injections of sterile saline until the site is large enough for an implant to be inserted or stays in place to become the implant. Placement of the expander can be at the time of mastectomy or at a later date. An autologous tissue flap procedure is a type of reconstruction using the patient's own tissue. The nipple of the affected breast is removed at mastectomy, and a new nipple can be reconstructed after breast reconstruction from various normal tissues.

Case Study

1. **Recommended**: monthly self-breast exams (to detect changes early), annual clinical breast exam, annual mammograms starting at age 45; **Not Recommended**: genetic testing (unless there is a familial predisposition involving first-degree relatives), mammogram every 5 years starting at age 25 (younger people have a lower risk of breast cancer and mammograms in younger women are less sensitive because of greater density breast tissue), annual Pap smear testing for HPV (unrelated to breast cancer, but is important to detect cervical cancer), annual MRIs (only recommended for high risk patients, like first-degree relatives with BRCA mutation)

2. **Risk Factor**: age (advancing age is a risk factor), uses estrogen therapy to treat hot flashes (increases the risk), weight (obesity increases the risk), used contraceptives (increases risk when used within past 10 years); **Clinical Manifestation**: clear nipple discharge (may be normal or abnormal, but since she has a palpable tumor it is considered related); **Unrelated**: fibrocystic changes (are benign changes), round breasts (normal finding), menopausal (unrelated unless hormonal therapy is being used to treat symptoms during menopause), no family history (first-degree relatives with BRCA mutation increases the risk of breast cancer)

3. **1**= ductal carcinoma in situ; **2**=20%; **3**= lobular carcinoma in situ; **4**= invasive ductal carcinoma; **5**=80%; **6**= invasive lobular carcinoma; **7**=10%-15%; **8**=inflammatory breast cancer; **9**=1%-3%

4. B., C., D., F., G., H. HER-2 positive, not HER-2 negative, tumors tend to be more aggressive and have a poorer prognosis. Triple-negative tumors do not respond to hormone therapy and tend to be more aggressive and have a poorer prognosis. Surgery is the main treatment followed by chemotherapy or radiation as necessary. BRCA1 and BRCA2 mutations increase the risk of breast cancer in both breasts, therefore a double mastectomy is recommended. Estrogen receptor-negative and progesterone receptor-

negative tumors, not positive, have a greater chance of recurrence and are poorly differentiated. Tamoxifen is a chemotherapeutic drug used to treat estrogen receptor-positive tumors, but a side effect is it increases the risk of developing endometrial cancer.

5. **Effective**: phantom breast pain may occur after a mastectomy, patients should not raise the arm on the affected side greater than 90 degrees due to the stretch on the incision, blood pressures shouldn't be measured on the right arm for the remainder of her life, she is a candidate for breast implants which is why they put in tissue expanders; **Ineffective**: blood draws should not occur on the right arm for the remainder of her life because of lymph node removal, lymphedema is less common after a SLND but there is still a risk, ice shouldn't be placed on the breast tissue because it impedes circulation but it can be used on the axillary incision.

CHAPTER 57

1. c. Although many factors relate to the current sexually transmitted infections (STI) rates, a major factor is the widespread use of oral contraceptives instead of condoms (both male and female). Condoms are the only contraceptive device that protects against STIs.
2. c. *Chlamydia trachomatis* can cause nongonococcal urethritis in men and cervicitis in women. Herpes simplex virus (HSV) causes genital herpes. *Treponema pallidum* causes syphilis. *Neisseria gonorrhoeae* causes gonorrhea.
3. a. A positive fluorescent treponemal antibody (FTA) test indicates syphilis infection caused by *T. pallidum*. Gonorrhea is caused by *N. gonorrhoeae*. Genital warts are caused by human papillomavirus (HPV). Genital herpes are caused by HSV.
4. d. Gonorrhea has become very resistant to most antibiotics, so it is treated with dual therapy of a single dose of IM ceftriaxone and oral azithromycin (Zithromax). Acyclovir would be used for HSV. Penicillin G is used to treat syphilis. Nucleic acid amplification testing (NAAT) is used to confirm the diagnosis in women. Because of a short incubation period and high rates of infectivity, treatment for gonorrhea is often given without waiting for positive test results.
5. a. Upward extension of gonorrhea or chlamydia commonly causes pelvic inflammatory disease (PID), which can cause adhesions and fibrous scarring, leading to tubal pregnancies and infertility. Disseminated gonococcal infection is rare, and endocarditis and aneurysms are associated with syphilis. Polyarthritis and adenopathy are not seen in gonorrhea or chlamydia.
6. d. All sexual contacts of patients with gonorrhea must be notified, evaluated, and treated for STIs to prevent reinfection and further transmission. The other information may be helpful in diagnosis and treatment, but the nurse must try to identify the patient's sexual partners.
7. a, b, c, d, f. In the tertiary (or late) stage of syphilis, there can be cardiovascular problems (heart failure, aneurysms, valve insufficiency), gummas (chronic destructive lesions), and neurosyphilis manifestations (mental deterioration, tabes dorsalis, and speech disturbances). Generalized cutaneous rash occurs in the secondary stage of syphilis, a few weeks after the chancre appears.

8. a. Lack of manifestations but a positive treponemal antibody test with normal cerebrospinal fluid (CSF) occurs in the latent stage. The primary stage is characterized by a chancre, regional lymphadenopathy, and genital ulcers. The secondary stage has flu-like symptoms and cutaneous lesions. The late or tertiary stage is characterized by gummas, cardiovascular changes, and neurosyphilis.
9. c. Many other diseases or conditions may cause false-positive test results on nontreponemal Venereal Disease Research Laboratory (VDRL) or rapid plasma reagent (RPR) tests and additional testing is needed before a diagnosis is confirmed or treatment is administered. The diagnosis is confirmed by specific treponemal tests, such as the fluorescent antibody absorption (FTA-Abs) test or the Treponema pallidum particle agglutination (TP-PA) test. Analysis of CSF is used to diagnose asymptomatic neurosyphilis.
10. d. The risk factors of drug use and sexual activity with multiple partners, men who have sex with men, or those who have unprotected sex are found in patients with both syphilis and human immunodeficiency virus (HIV) infection. Persons at highest risk for acquiring syphilis are at high risk for acquiring HIV. Syphilitic lesions on the genitals enhance HIV transmission. HIV-infected patients with syphilis appear to be at greatest risk for central nervous system (CNS) involvement and may need more intensive treatment with penicillin to prevent this complication of HIV.
11. b. Notification and treatment of sexual partners are necessary to prevent recurrence and the "ping-pong" effect of passing STIs between partners. Doxycycline is prescribed twice a day for 7 days, and although alcohol may cause more urinary irritation in the patient with chlamydia, it will not interfere with treatment. Avoiding sexual intercourse for 7 days after the medication is to prevent transmission.
12. b. The NAAT is more sensitive than other diagnostic tests, can be done with a urine sample, and has results within 24 hours. A cell culture can be used to detect chlamydia organisms, but it requires specific handling and is not as easy or as fast to perform as the NAAT. Gonorrhea and chlamydia have very similar symptoms in men and frequently occur together. Gram stain smears and cultures for *N. gonorrhoeae* do not definitively diagnose *Chlamydia*. Manifestations of epididymitis or proctitis may be present, as with other STIs, but are not diagnostic.
13. c, e. Sexual activity and stress may precipitate the recurrence of genital herpes symptoms of painful vesicular lesions that rupture and ulcerate. Acyclovir only decreases recurrences of genital herpes. Herpes simplex virus type 2 (HSV-2) may cause oral or genital lesions. Prevention of the spread of genital herpes is best done with avoidance of sexual activity when lesions are present.
14. d. HPV is responsible for causing genital warts, which manifest as discrete single or multiple white to gray warts that may coalesce to form large cauliflower-like masses on the vulva, vagina, cervix, and perianal area. Purulent vaginal discharge is associated with gonorrhea or chlamydia. Painful perineal vesicles and ulcerations are characteristic of genital herpes and a chancre of syphilis is a painless indurated lesion on the vulva, vagina, lips, or mouth.

15. a. Some types of genital warts are associated with cancer of the cervix, vagina, vulva, and throat or pharynx. Cancer of the penis, rectum, throat, or pharynx may occur in men. Regular Papanicolaou (Pap) tests in women are critical in detecting early malignancies of the cervix. Oral acyclovir is used to treat HSV-2, but topical use has no value in treating viral STIs. Sexual partners of patients with HPV should be examined and treated, but because treatment does not destroy the virus, condoms should always be used during sexual activity. Genital warts often grow more rapidly during pregnancy, but pregnancy is not contraindicated.

16. d. Women with an active HSV genital lesion at the time of delivery have the highest risk of transmitting genital herpes to the neonate, so delivery will be done with a cesarean section (C-section). Syphilis is spread to the fetus in utero and has a high risk of stillbirth, but C-sections are not required. Treatment with parenteral penicillin will cure both the mother and fetus. Prevention of the spread of gonorrhea to the neonate's eyes is done with erythromycin ophthalmic ointment or silver nitrate aqueous solution. *Chlamydia* spread to the fetus can be prevented by treating the pregnant woman, so a C-section is not required.

17. c. A vaccine is available for 9 types of HPV and protects against genital warts and cervical cancer. Although sexual abstinence is the most certain method of avoiding all STIs, it is not usually a feasible alternative. Undamaged condoms also protect against infection. Conscientious hand washing and voiding after intercourse are positive hygienic measures that will help prevent secondary infections but will not prevent STIs.

18. a. STIs, such as syphilis, that can be treated with a single dose or short course of antibiotic therapy often lead to a casual attitude about the outcome of the disease, which leads to nonadherence with instructions and delays in treatment. This is particularly true of diseases that initially show few distressing or uncomfortable symptoms, such as syphilis.

Case Study

1. **Indicated** (a symptom of gonorrhea): vaginal discharge, bleeding after intercourse, urinary frequency; **Unrelated**: breast tenderness, fever (present with a complication like PID), shortness of breath, dysmenorrhea (present with complications of the disease)

2. **Indicated for C.J.:** history of symptoms (men are usually symptomatic so with the history of an infected sexual partner along with symptoms a predictive diagnosis can be made), urethral swab; **Indicated for Ms. A.:** endocervical swab; **Indicated for Both:** oropharyngeal swab, gram-staining swab specimens, NAAT (nucleic acid amplification test), HIV testing; **Unrelated to Both:** treponemal serologic test (diagnostic test for syphilis), PCR testing (diagnostic test for genital herpes)

3. B., C., E., F. His fiancé needs to be informed and tested. Females tend to be asymptomatic more often than males with gonorrhea infection. In some states, the PHD will be notified and perform contact tracing and notification, while others depend on the infected person to perform these notifications. You can be infected and then reinfected with gonorrhea. If his fiancé develops complications from gonorrhea, infertility can occur. It is recommended that patients with a gonorrhea infection abstain from sexual

contact for at least 7 days after beginning treatment. Repeat testing is recommended in 3 months. Any type of sexual contact, including oral sex, can transmit this infection.

4. **Epididymitis**: swelling of external genitalia (testis and epididymis become indistinguishable), scrotal pain; **Pelvic inflammatory disease**: increased abdominal pain with walking (due to tenderness involving cervix, uterus, and adnexa), painful urination (dysuria), chills (and fever); **Disseminated Gonococcal Infection**: chest pain, skin lesions, joint pain (arthralgia and arthritis)

5. Answers are in order they appear in the sentences: Ceftriaxone; Syphilis; Doxycycline; Acyclovir or Valacyclovir; Azithromycin.

CHAPTER 58

1. a. The initial visit of a couple seeking assistance with infertility includes a history and physical for both partners, psychosocial functioning, testing for medical problems and sexually transmitted infections (STIs), a cervical Papanicolaou (Pap) test, possible semen analysis, and at-home ovulation testing. A discussion of possible future testing options and cost is also done. If the couple decides to continue with treatment, further visits will include more intensive evaluation, including postcoital testing, a hysterosalpingogram, pelvic ultrasound, and midluteal progesterone and prolactin levels.

2. c. Drug therapy will be used before more invasive treatments. Drugs may include selective estrogen receptor modulators, menotropin (human menopausal gonadotropin), follicle-stimulating hormone agonists, gonadotropin-releasing hormone (GnRH) antagonists, GnRH agonists, or human chorionic gonadotropin (hCG). If the husband's reproductive system is functioning, intrauterine insemination with his sperm may later be done. The assisted reproductive technologies may be used if this is not successful. Surgery for endometriosis could be done if this was diagnosed, but that is not included in this question.

3. b. In the presence of a confirmed pregnancy, uterine cramping with vaginal bleeding is the most important sign of spontaneous abortion. Other conditions causing vaginal bleeding, such as an incompetent cervix, do not usually cause cramping. There is no evidence that any medical treatment improves the outcome for spontaneous abortion. Some patients with significant blood loss may need a blood transfusion. Dilation and curettage (D&C) (if needed) is done after the abortion to minimize blood loss and reduce the chance of infection.

4. d. There is physical and emotional pain and grieving after an abortion that puts the patient in need of support. D&C is needed only if the products of conception do not pass completely or bleeding becomes excessive. The time it takes for the products of conception to pass depends on the type of abortion being done. It is immediate with surgical abortion and slower with medical abortion.

5. d. Premenstrual syndrome (PMS) is diagnosed when other possible causes for symptoms have been eliminated. A diagnosis is based on: (1) consistency of the syndrome complex, (2) occurrence of symptoms in the luteal phase and resolution after menses begins, (3) documented ovulatory cycles, and (4) symptoms that disrupt the

woman's life. Oral contraceptives may be used to control the symptoms of PMS by suppressing ovulation. Although progesterone may relieve the symptoms of PMS, its effectiveness is not associated with PMS. There are no laboratory findings that account for the premenstrual symptoms.

6. c. Vitamin B$_6$, calcium, and magnesium are recommended, as well as foods high in tryptophan, which may promote serotonin production, to improve mood changes. Limiting refined sugar and caffeine in the diet may decrease the PMS symptoms of abdominal bloating, increased appetite, and irritability. Estrogen is not used during the luteal phase, but progesterone may be tried. Exercise is encouraged because it increases the release of endorphins, which elevate the mood, and has a tranquilizing effect on muscle tension.

7. c. The release of excess prostaglandins from the endometrium at the time of menstruation or increased sensitivity to the prostaglandins is responsible for symptoms of primary dysmenorrhea. Drugs that inhibit prostaglandin production and release, such as nonsteroidal antiinflammatory drugs (NSAIDs), are effective in many patients with primary dysmenorrhea. Oral contraceptives may be used for primary dysmenorrhea by reducing endometrial hyperplasia.

8. c. Young female athletes may have amenorrhea related to excessive exercise, low body weight, stress, or severe dieting. If she had increased sexual activity, she would be assessed for pregnancy, but decreased sexual activity will not affect her menses. Excess prostaglandin production leads to dysmenorrhea. Intermenstrual bleeding is associated with endometrial cancer or uterine fibroids.

9. c. When ovulation does not occur, estrogen continues to be unopposed by progesterone and excessive buildup of the endometrium occurs. To prevent the risk of endometrial cancer by the buildup of the endometrium or to prevent heavy menstrual bleeding from an unstable endometrium, progesterone or combined oral contraceptives are prescribed to ensure regular shedding of the endometrial lining. Balloon therapy to treat heavy menstrual bleeding is contraindicated in women who desire future fertility and does not apply to amenorrhea.

10. d. Heavy menstrual bleeding is increased duration or amount of bleeding with menses. Pain with menses is called *dysmenorrhea*. Chronic abnormal uterine bleeding is classified as uterine bleeding that is abnormal in volume, timing, or regularity and has been present for most of the past 6 months. Intermenstrual bleeding is bleeding between regular menstrual cycles.

11. b. Ectopic pregnancy is a life-threatening condition. If the fallopian tube ruptures, profuse bleeding can lead to hypovolemic shock. While all the interventions are indicated, the priority is monitoring the vital signs and pain for evidence of bleeding.

12. a, c. The lack of estrogen in menopause contributes to many of the signs of aging, including cessation of menses, vasomotor instability (hot flashes), atrophic changes of vaginal and external genitalia and breast tissue, increased risks for osteoporosis and coronary artery disease, redistribution of fat, muscle and joint pain, loss of skin elasticity, and atrophic lower urinary tract changes.

13. b. Taking combination hormone replacement therapy (HRT) increases bone marrow density and decreases fractures.

Both progesterone and estrogen are recommended for a menopausal woman with a uterus. Progesterone alone is not as effective as estrogen. The risk for breast cancer is increased and the risk for endometrial cancer is decreased with combination HRT. Evidence does not support using HRT to prevent cardiovascular disease.

14. c. Bacterial vaginosis is characterized by watery vaginal discharge with a fishy odor. Cervicitis displays mucopurulent discharge and postcoital spotting. Trichomoniasis has frothy greenish or gray discharge. Vulvovaginal candidiasis has thick, white, curdy discharge.

15. a, d. "Yeast infection" or vulvovaginal candidiasis has intense itching and dysuria from urine coming in contact with fissures or irritated areas in the vulva. The discharge is thick, white, and cottage cheese-like. Hemorrhagic cervix and vagina occur with trichomoniasis and produce a pruritic, frothy greenish or gray discharge. Mucopurulent discharge and postcoital spotting from cervical inflammation are seen with cervicitis.

16. a. *Gardnerella vaginalis* infection is a bacterial vaginosis that may be sexually transmitted, and both partners may be infected. Treatment of the condition includes vaginal treatment with metronidazole (Flagyl) or clindamycin (Cleocin) or treatment via the oral route. Sexual activity is avoided until both partners are infection free. Pads may be used to contain vaginal secretions but do not prevent reinfection. Vaginal suppositories and creams are used at bedtime so that the medication stays in the vagina for a long time.

17. b. Sexual activity with multiple partners increases the risk for pelvic inflammatory disease (PID). There is often a history of an acute infection of the lower genital tract caused by gonococcal or chlamydia microorganisms. The only significant contraceptive issue related to PID is that condom use will help prevent STIs that may lead to PID.

18. a. Resting in semi-Fowler's position promotes drainage of the pelvic cavity by gravity and may prevent the development of abscesses high in the abdomen. Coitus, douching, and tampon use should be avoided to prevent spreading infection upward from the vagina. Frequent perineal care should be done to remove infectious drainage.

19. b. The risk for infertility following PID is high. The nurse should allow time for the patient to express her feelings, clarify her concerns, and begin problem solving with regard to the outcomes of the disease. Responses that do not allow for discussion of feelings and concerns and that tell the patient how she should feel or what she should worry about are not therapeutic.

20. c. The treatment of endometriosis and leiomyomas is surgical when the patient does not tolerate the symptoms. The type of surgery for endometriosis depends on the desire for pregnancy. Endometriosis and leiomyomas subside with the onset of menopause. Therefore the medications to treat them create a pseudomenopause. The ectopic uterine tissue is endometriosis, while leiomyomas are fibrous smooth muscle tumors.

21. c. Left untreated, polycystic ovary syndrome (PCOS) may lead to cardiovascular disease and abnormal insulin resistance with type 2 diabetes. Hirsutism may be treated with spironolactone. Leuprolide is used to treat hyperandrogenism, but PCOS cannot be cured. Severity of symptoms is associated with obesity, but the hormone

abnormalities will be treated along with the obesity to prevent complications. If other treatment is not successful, a hysterectomy with bilateral salpingectomy and oophorectomy may be done.

22. c. A stage 0 cervical cancer indicates cancer in situ that is confined to the epithelial layer of the cervix and requires treatment. Stage 0 is the least invasive. Stage I is confined to the cervix. Stage II has spread beyond the cervix to the upper two-thirds of the vagina but not the tissues around the uterus. Stage III involves the pelvic wall, lower third of the vagina, and/or kidney problems. Stage IV indicates spread to distant organs.

23. c. Conization (an excision of a cone-shaped section of the cervix) and laser treatment both are effective to locally remove or destroy malignant cells of the cervix and preserve fertility. Radiation treatments often impair ovarian and uterine function and lead to sterility. A subtotal hysterectomy would be contraindicated in the treatment of cervical cancer because the cervix would be left intact in this procedure.

24. a. Postmenopausal vaginal bleeding is an early sign of endometrial cancer. When it occurs, a sample of endometrial tissue must be taken to exclude cancer. An endometrial biopsy can be done as an office procedure and is indicated in this case. Abdominal x-rays and Pap tests are not reliable tests for endometrial cancer. Laser treatment of the cervix is indicated only for cervical dysplasia.

25. b. Treatment of ovarian cancer is determined by staging from the results of laparotomy with multiple biopsies of the ovaries and other tissue throughout the pelvis and lower abdomen. The patient's desire for fertility is not a consideration because of the high mortality rate associated with ovarian cancer. Although diagnosis of ovarian tumors may be made by transvaginal ultrasound or CT scan, the treatment of ovarian cancer depends on the staging of the tumor.

26. a. Vaginal cancer is usually related to metastases of other cancers or intrauterine exposure to diethylstilbestrol (DES). Cervical, endometrial, and ovarian cancer have other or unknown causes.

27. a, b, e, f. Endometrial cancer is at higher risk in obese patients because adipose cells store estrogen, which is the major risk factor, especially unopposed estrogen. Smoking is a risk factor for endometrial and cervical cancers. Early menarche and late menopause are risk factors for endometrial cancer. Early sexual activity is a risk factor for cervical cancer. Family history is a risk factor for ovarian cancer.

28. a. Early signs of cancer of the vulva include pruritus, or burning, soreness of the vulva, and discharge or bleeding of the vulva, with edema of the vulva and lymphadenopathy occurring as the disease progresses. Labial lesions and excoriation more commonly occur with infections, and nodules are more often cysts or lipomas.

29. c. A total hysterectomy involves the removal of the uterus and cervix, with the fallopian tubes and ovaries left intact. Although menstruation is terminated, normal ovarian production of estrogen continues. When the uterus, tubes, and ovaries are removed, it is called a *total hysterectomy and bilateral salpingo-oophorectomy (TAH-BSO)*.

30. c. A pelvic exenteration is the most radical gynecologic surgery and results in removal of the uterus, ovaries, fallopian tubes, vagina, bladder, urethra, and pelvic lymph nodes and, in some situations, the descending colon, rectum, and anal canal. There are urinary and fecal diversions on the abdominal wall, the absence of a vagina, and the onset of menopausal symptoms, all of which result in severe altered body structure and changes in body image. The patient and family will need much understanding and support during the long recovery period, including verbalization of feelings.

31. d. To prevent displacement of the intrauterine implant, the patient is maintained on absolute bed rest with turning from side to side. Bowel elimination is discouraged during the treatment by cleaning the colon before implantation and urinary elimination is maintained by an indwelling catheter. Because the patient is radioactive, the principles of ALARA (as low as reasonably achievable) are used so that caregivers limit time and distance and use shielding for protection.

32. a. The muscles that should be exercised are those affected by trying to stop an expulsion of gas from the rectum or stop urine midflow. Kegel exercises help strengthen muscular support of the perineum, pelvic floor, and bladder and are beneficial for problems with pelvic support and stress incontinence.

33. c. A uterine prolapse occurs when the uterus is displaced through the vagina, causing the feeling of something coming down her vagina, a backache, dyspareunia, or a heavy feeling in the pelvis.

34. d. The primary goal of care is to prevent wound infection and pressure on the vaginal incision, which requires perineal cleansing at least twice daily and after each urination and defecation. While an ice pack and stool softener will be used, they are not the priority. The enema would have been done preoperatively.

35. a. An anterior colporrhaphy involves repair of a cystocele and an indwelling urinary catheter is left in place for several days postoperatively while healing occurs. Bowel function should not be altered and is maintained with a low-residue diet and a stool softener if necessary, to avoid straining and pressure on the incision.

36. b. Sexual assault is an act of violence and the first priority of care for the patient should be assessment and treatment of serious injuries involving extragenital areas, such as fractures, subdural hematomas, cerebral concussions, and intraabdominal injuries. While all the other options as well as preserving forensic evidence are appropriate treatments, treatment for shock and urgent medical injuries is the first priority.

37. a. Specific informed consent must be obtained from the rape victim before any examination can be made or rape data collected. Following consent, the patient is advised not to wash, eat, drink, or urinate before the examination so that evidence can be collected for medicolegal use. Prophylaxis for STIs, hepatitis B, and tetanus is administered following examination and follow-up testing for pregnancy and human immunodeficiency virus (HIV) is done in several weeks.

Case Study

1. **Gynecological Cancer:** purulent vaginal discharge (all GYN cancers except vulvar cancer), abdominal pain (ovarian cancer), increased pain during vaginal exam

(ovarian and uterine cancers), young age (cervical cancer); **Vaginitis:** purulent vaginal discharge, young age (due to increased sexual activity and multiple partners); **PID:** purulent vaginal discharge, fever, malaise, abdominal pain (with walking), increased pain during vaginal examination, young age (due to increased sexual activity and multiple partners)

2. **Indicated:** Pap test (will test for STIs and assess cervical cells for dysplasia), HIV testing (this patient has PID which occurs due to STIs, therefore other STIs, like HIV, should be tested for), pregnancy test (to rule-out ectopic pregnancy), STI testing (primary cause of PID); **Non-essential:** chest x-ray, genetic testing (pertinent to evaluate risk of certain types of cancers), abdominal CT (unless cancer or other cause is suspected)

3. A., C., D., E., H. HPV is the most common sexually transmitted infection in the U.S. and is the leading cause of cervical, not ovarian, cancer. It can also increase the risk of vaginal and vulvar cancers. It is usually asymptomatic. It isn't treatable and resolves on its own, but there is a vaccine to help prevent HPV. HPV can be transmitted through oral sex, causing oropharyngeal problems including cancers. Annual Pap tests are recommended for sexually active women.

4. **Indicated:** high-dose ceftriaxone and doxycycline (are recommended to treat co-infection causing PID {chlamydia and gonorrhea}), assess and document vaginal discharge (to note color, amount, odor and report any changes if necessary), ask about her recent sexual partners (they should be tested for STIs because of her known infection); **Contraindicated:** high-dose cephalosporin (is not the recommended antibiotic to treat PID caused by chlamydia and gonorrhea), fluid restriction (the patient should be receiving hydration especially with a fever); **Non-essential:** contact precautions (this isn't transmissible through casual contact), palpate abdomen for deep pain (is unnecessary and will cause the patient to have pain)

5. A., C., D., F., G., H. Gardasil is the vaccine to prevent HPV and is safe to receive during a HPV infection; however, this vaccine won't treat the current HPV infection. Antibiotics should be taken as directed until gone. It is recommended that patient's with STIs abstain from sexual intercourse until fully treated to avoid transmitting the infection. Condoms are barriers that can drastically decrease the risk of transmitting and being infected with STIs. Birth control pills only prevent pregnancy, not STIs. Complications of PID can lead to infertility, especially if the infection goes untreated. Abdominal pain should resolve as the PID resolves, so persistent pain should be reported to the HCP. Douching can cause PID and should be avoided.

CHAPTER 59

1. d. Hyperplasia is an increase in the number of cells and in benign prostatic hyperplasia (BPH). It is thought that the enlargement caused by the increase in new cells results from hormonal changes associated with aging. The hyperplasia is not considered a tumor, nor has BPH been proven to predispose to cancer of the prostate. Hypertrophy refers to an increase in the size of existing cells.

2. c. Classic symptoms of uncomplicated BPH are those associated with irritative symptoms, including nocturia, frequency, urgency, dysuria, bladder pain, and incontinence associated with inflammation or infection. Obstructive symptoms caused by prostate enlargement include diminished caliber and force of the urinary stream, hesitancy or difficulty initiating voiding, intermittent urination, dribbling at the end of urination, and a feeling of incomplete bladder emptying because of urinary retention. Bladder spasms, hematuria, perineal pain, and cloudy urine do not occur with BPH.

3. a. Uroflowmetry is used to measure the volume of urine expelled from the bladder to determine the extent of urethral blockage. Cystourethroscopy may also evaluate the degree of obstruction, but a cystometrogram measures bladder tone. A transrectal ultrasound may determine the size and configuration of the prostate gland. Postvoiding catheterization measures residual urine.

4. a. Finasteride results in suppression of dihydrotestosterone (DHT) formation, which reduces the size of the prostate gland. Drugs affecting bladder tone are not indicated. α-Adrenergic receptor blockers are used to cause smooth muscle relaxation in the prostate, which improves urine flow.

5. c. Because of edema, urinary retetion, and delayed sloughing of tissue that occurs with a laser prostatectomy, the patient will have a postprocedure urinary catheter for up to 7 days. The procedure is done under local anesthetic, and incontinence or urinary retention is not usually a problem with laser prostatectomy.

6. d. The prostate gland can be easily palpated by rectal examination, and enlargement of the gland is detected early if yearly examinations are performed. If symptoms of prostatic hyperplasia are present, further diagnostic testing, including prostate-specific antigen (PSA), a urinalysis, and cystoscopy may be indicated.

7. b. The transurethral needle ablation (TUNA) uses low-wave radiofrequency to heat the prostate, causing necrosis. Laser prostatectomy uses a laser beam. Transurethral microwave thermotherapy (TUMT) uses microwave radiating heat to produce coagulative necrosis of the prostate and is not used for men with rectal problems. Transurethral electrovaporization of prostate (TUVP) uses electrosurgical vaporization and desiccation to destroy prostate tissue.

8. e, f. The transurethral resection of the prostate (TURP) is the most common surgical procedure to treat BPH and uses a resectoscopic excision and cauterization of prostate tissue. Photovaporization of the prostate (PVP) or a simple open prostatectomy may be used for a very large prostate and has an external incision. TUMT is not approved for men with rectal problems. Transurethral incision into the prostate to expand the urethra for a small to moderate-sized prostate is done with a transurethral incision of the prostate (TUIP).

9. b, c, d, e. PVP, TUNA, TUIP, and TUMT can be done on an outpatient basis or in a HCP's office.

10. d. An indwelling urinary catheter is placed to provide hemostasis and facilitate urinary drainage. This procedure does not have an external incision and is done using a resectoscope inserted into the urethra. Urinary infections are not increased and this procedure is not done under local anesthesia.

11. d. Bleeding and blood clots from the bladder are expected after a TURP. Continuous irrigation is used to keep

clots from obstructing the urinary tract. The rate of the irrigation may be titrated to keep the clots from forming, if ordered, but the nurse should check the vital signs because hemorrhage is the most common complication of prostatectomy. The traction on the catheter applies pressure to the operative site to control bleeding and should be relieved on schedule. The catheter will be manually irrigated only to release a blockage. Clamping the drainage tube is contraindicated because it would distend the bladder.

12. b. The nurse should first check for the presence of clots obstructing the catheter or tubing and remove them by irrigation. Pain management interventions should be implemented as indicated and ordered. The flow rate of the irrigation fluid may be decreased if orders permit because fast-flowing, cold fluid may also contribute to spasms. The patient should not try to void around the catheter because this will increase the spasms.

13. b. Activities that increase intraabdominal pressure should be avoided until the HCP approves these activities at a follow-up visit. Stool softeners and high-fiber diets may be used to promote bowel elimination. Enemas should not be used because they increase intraabdominal pressure and may start bleeding. Because TURP does not remove the entire prostate gland, the patient needs annual prostatic examinations to screen for cancer of the prostate. Fluid intake should be high, but caffeine and alcohol should not be used because they have a diuretic effect and increase bladder distention.

14. c. Most prostate cancers (about 75%) are considered sporadic. About the only modifiable risk factor for prostate cancer is its association with a diet high in red and processed meat and high-fat dairy products along with a low intake of vegetables and fruits. Age, ethnicity, and family history are risk factors for prostate cancer but are not modifiable. Environment may also play a role. Simple enlargement or hyperplasia of the prostate is not a risk factor for prostate cancer. There is no evidence that saw palmetto is more effective than a placebo.

15. c. A prostatectomy performed with a perineal approach has a high risk for infection because of the proximity of the wound to the anus, so wound care is the priority. Chemotherapy is usually not the first choice of drug therapy after surgery, nor is sildenafil. The catheter size would not be changed but the catheter would be removed. Urinary incontinence is a bigger problem than retention.

16. a, c, f. Typically, prostate cancer is asymptomatic, but lumbosacral pain radiating to the hips or legs and a hard, asymmetric, enlarged prostate may be present. Annual prostate examination is recommended starting at a younger age for black men because of increased diagnosis and mortality from prostate cancer in this ethnic group. An orchiectomy may be done with prostatectomy or for metastatic stages of prostate cancer. Hormonal treatment includes androgen deprivation therapy, luteinizing hormone–releasing hormone agonists, and androgen receptor blockers. Early detection of prostate cancer is best detected with annual rectal examinations and serum PSA. High prostatic acid phosphatase (PAP) will be seen with metastasis, not a new diagnosis.

17. d. Chronic bacterial prostatitis commonly causes urinary tract infections (UTIs) in adult men and recurs frequently.

The other options are true of both chronic and acute prostatitis, although not as severe with chronic.

18. c. Hypospadias is the urethral meatus located on the ventral surface of the penis. Scrotal lymphedema is called a *hydrocele*. An undescended testicle is cryptorchidism. Inflammation of the prepuce or foreskin is called *phimosis*.

19. d. Paraphimosis is tightness of the foreskin and the inability to pull it forward from a retracted position to return it over the glans. It is usually associated with leaving the foreskin pulled back during a bath, use of a urinary catheter, or intercourse. Painful, prolonged erection is priapism. Epididymitis is inflammation of the epididymis. A painful downward curvature of an erect penis is chordee.

20. d. The cremasteric reflex is elicited by light stroking of the inner aspect of the thigh in a downward direction with a tongue blade. In testicular torsion, or a twisted spermatic cord that supplies blood to the testes and epididymis, this reflex is absent on the swollen side. Hydrocele is scrotal lymphedema from interference with lymphatic drainage of the scrotum. Varicocele is dilation of the veins that drain the testes. Spermatocele is a sperm-containing cyst of the epididymis.

21. b. α-Fetoprotein (AFP) and human chorionic gonadotropin (hCG) are glycoproteins that may be high in testicular cancer. If they are high before surgical treatment, the levels are noted, and if response to therapy is positive, the levels will decrease. Lactate dehydrogenase (LDH) may be increased. Tumor necrosis factor (TNF) is a normal cytokine responsible for tumor surveillance and destruction. C-reactive protein (CRP) is found in inflammatory conditions and widespread malignancies. PSA and PAP are used for screening of prostatic cancer. Carcinoembryonic antigen (CEA) is a tumor marker for cancers of the gastrointestinal (GI) system. Antinuclear antibody (ANA) is found most frequently in autoimmune disorders. HER-2 is used as a marker in breast cancer.

22. d. Until sperm distal to the anastomotic site is ejaculated or absorbed by the body, the semen will contain sperm and alternative contraceptive methods must be used. When a postoperative semen examination reveals no sperm, the patient is considered sterile. After vasectomy, there is rarely noticeable difference in the amount of ejaculate because ejaculate is primarily seminal and prostatic fluid. Vasectomy does not cause erectile dysfunction (ED), nor does it affect testicular production of sperm or hormones.

23. a. Before treatment for ED is initiated, reversibility must be determined so that appropriate treatment can be planned. The actual cause may be determined, but this is more expensive. Only a small percentage of ED is caused by psychologic factors. In the case of the 80% to 90% of ED that is of physiologic causes, interventions are directed at correcting or eliminating the cause or restoring function by medical means. Patients with systemic diseases can be treated medically if the cause cannot be eliminated. New invasive or experimental treatments are not widely used and should be limited to research centers.

24. d. Intraurethral devices include the use of vasoactive drugs administered as a topical gel or medication pellet (alprostadil) inserted into the urethra (intraurethral) using a medicated urethral system for erection (MUSE) device, or an injection into the penis (intracavernosal self-injection). The vasoactive drugs enhance blood flow into the penile

arteries for erection. Erectogenic drugs (e.g., tadalafil [Cialis]) cause smooth muscle relaxation and increase blood flow to promote an erection. Blood drawn into corporeal bodies and held with a ring is achieved with a vacuum constriction device (VCD). Devices implanted into corporeal bodies to firm the penis are penile implants. Androgen or testosterone replacement therapy may also be used for erectile dysfunction.

25. a. The gel may spread the testosterone to others if it is not washed off of his hands after application. If his wife applies the gel, she should wear gloves to prevent absorption of the testosterone and its effects on her body. Clothing over the area until it has dried is recommended. The gel is only topical; a buccal testosterone tablet is called *Striant*.

26. d. Varicocele is the most common testicular cause of infertility. Surgical ligation of the spermatic vein is done to correct the problem. Antibiotics are used if there is an infection, but this is not as common as a varicocele. Semen analysis is the first study done when investigating male infertility, but it is not a treatment. Avoidance of scrotal heat is a lifestyle change that may be used with idiopathic infertility.

Case Study

1. B., C., E., H. Testicular cancer is rare. It accounts for less than 1% of all cancers found in males. However, it is the most common cancer in young men between 15 and 34 years of age. Risk factors include family predisposition, orchitis, having had undescended testes (cryptorchidism), HIV infection, maternal exposure to exogenous estrogen, and testicular cancer in other testis. Not all forms of testicular cancers are aggressive. Seminoma germ cell cancers are the most common but are the least aggressive. Nonseminoma testicular germ cell tumors are rare but very aggressive. Acute pain is the first symptom in about 10% of patients. Most testicular cancers develop from 2 types of embryonic germ cells.

2. **Indicated**: palpation of scrotal contents (1st step in diagnosing), α-fetoprotein (AFP) marker (serum tumor marker), hCG level (serum tumor marker), CT scans of the abdomen and pelvis (to stage and assess for metastases), liver functions tests (may be increased in metastatic disease); **Unrelated**: PSA level (assesses for prostate cancer), LDL level (measures a type of cholesterol; LDH is a serum tumor marker)

3. **Effective**: storing semen in a sperm bank is recommended as the treatments for testicular cancer may cause infertility, C.E.'s tumor type (seminoma germ cell tumor) is sensitive to radiation therapy, ejaculatory dysfunction may occur from the lymph node dissection, lung damage from chemotherapy treatment, especially bleomycin, can occur; **Ineffective**: testicular cancer has a 95% survival rate, an orchiectomy will most likely be necessary; **Unrelated**: therapies to treat testicular cancer will not cause gynecomastia (male breast enlargement)

4. **Indicated**: SCDs while on bedrest (to prevent VTE), wearing a scrotal support like a jock strap, applying ice to the scrotum (to reduce swelling and decrease pain); **Contraindicated**: applying oxygen (patients having had bleomycin may have lung damage, therefore oxygen is contraindicated even if the patient is mildly hypoxemic), the patient should be ambulating the same day

postoperatively; **Non-essential**: coagulation studies and 12-lead ECG (are unnecessary unless there are indications for these diagnostics)

5. A., B., C., G., H. The patient should avoid bicycle riding and other strenuous activities until approved by their HCP. Bicycle seats will put pressure on the incision. Any SOB or other unexpected symptoms should be reported to the HCP. Scrotal support is recommended for at least the first 48 hours, but the patient may continue if he finds it more comfortable. Ice is recommended for the first 48-72 hours to decrease swelling and pain, but heat is not recommended as it may promote bleeding. Taking showers after 48 hours may be acceptable, but soaking in water like bathtubs, swimming pools, hot tubs, etc. will not be recommended until the incision has healed, usually 2 weeks postoperatively at the earliest. There are driving restrictions if taking opioids for pain, but not Tylenol or ibuprofen. Ibuprofen should be taken with food to decrease the risk of gastritis or GI ulcers. Any foul smelling drainage should be reported to the HCP as it may be a sign of infection.

CHAPTER 60

1. a. Mitochondrion; b. nucleolus; c. nucleus; d. axon; e. Schwann cell; f. myelin sheath; g. collateral axon; h. node of Ranvier; i. telodendria; j. synaptic knobs; k. neuron cell body; l. dendrites

2. a. Superior temporal gyrus; b. Broca's motor speech; c. frontal lobe; d. precentral gyrus; e. postcentral gyrus; f. parietal lobe; g. Wernicke's receptive speech; h. occipital lobe; i. temporal lobe; j. cerebellum; k. medulla

3. d. The cerebrospinal fluid (CSF) protects the central nervous system (CNS). The synaptic cleft is the space where neurotransmitters cross from neuron to neuron. The limbic system is the area of the brain concerned with emotion, aggression, feeding behavior, and sexual response. Myelin sheath is the insulator for the conduction of impulses in the CNS and peripheral nervous system (PNS).

4. c. Schwann cells are the macroglial cells that myelinate peripheral nerve fibers. Neurons are not glial cells. Astrocytes provide structural support to neurons and form the blood-brain barrier with the endothelium of blood vessels. Ependymal cells line the brain ventricles and aid in secretion of CSF.

5. c. The presynaptic terminal submits neurotransmitter impulses through the synaptic cleft to the receptor site on the postsynaptic cell (another neuron or a gland or muscles). If there are enough presynaptic cells releasing excitatory neurotransmitters on a single neuron, the sum of their input is enough to generate an action potential. The synapse is not a physical connection between neurons, as there is a space between them where the neurotransmitter goes from 1 neuron to another.

6. b. The dendrite carries impulses to the nerve cell body. The gap in the peripheral nerve axons (node of Ranvier) allows an action potential to travel faster by jumping from node to node without traversing the insulated membrane segment. The axon carries impulses from the nerve cell body. Regeneration may occur with damage to peripheral axons.

7. b. The fasciculus gracilis and fasciculus cuneatus tracts carry information and transmit impulses concerned with touch, deep pressure, vibration, position sense,

and kinesthesia. Spinothalamic tracts carry pain and temperature sensations. The spinocerebellar tracts carry subconscious information about muscle tension and body position. Descending corticobulbar tracts carry impulses responsible for voluntary impulses from the cortex to the cranial and peripheral nerves.

8. a. The cell bodies of lower motor neurons that send impulses to skeletal muscles in the arms, trunk, and legs are located in the anterior horn of the spinal cord. Lesions generally cause weakness or paralysis, decreased muscle tone, hyporeflexia, and flaccidity. Upper motor neurons include the brainstem and cerebral cortex motor neurons that influence skeletal muscle movement. Lesions at this point cause weakness and paralysis with hyperreflexia and spasticity.

9. a. The medulla contains the vital centers concerned with respiratory, vasomotor, and cardiac function. The cerebellum maintains trunk stability and equilibrium but is not related to respiratory or cardiac function. The parietal lobe interprets spatial information and controls the sensory cortex. Wernicke's area is responsible for language comprehension.

10. b. The occipital lobe is responsible for visual perception. This patient may experience inability to identify colors, hallucinations, vision loss, or total blindness. Heat is sensed with the sensory part of the brain. The olfactory nerve is responsible for identifying smells. Broca's area regulates verbal expression.

11. c. The hypothalamus regulates functions of the endocrine system and autonomic nervous system (ANS). The basal ganglia function includes initiation, execution, and completion of voluntary movements, learning, emotional response, and automatic movements associated with skeletal muscle activity. The temporal lobe integrates somatic, visual, and auditory data; it also contains Wernicke's area. The reticular activating system regulates arousal and sleep-wake transitions with communication among the brainstem, reticular formation in the brainstem, and the cerebral cortex.

12. c. The thalamus relays sensory and motor input to and from the cerebrum and basal ganglia. Auditory input is registered by the superior temporal gyrus. Past experiences are integrated by the anterior temporal lobe. The basal ganglia controls and facilitates learned and automatic movements associated with skeletal muscle activity.

13. d. All spinal nerves have both afferent sensory and efferent motor fibers. Some cranial nerves (CNs) are only efferent (e.g., III, IV, VI, VII, XI, XII), some are only afferent (e.g., I, II, VIII), and some have both motor and sensory functions (e.g., V, IX, X). Both cranial and spinal nerves occur in pairs. Most CNs affect the head, neck, and shoulder area, but CN X affects the thorax and abdomen as well. Cranial cell bodies are located in specific areas of the brainstem, except CN I and II are located in the brain.

14. b. The falx cerebri is a fold of the dura that separates the cerebral hemispheres and slows expansion of brain tissue. The ventricles are filled with and produce CSF. The arachnoid layer is a delicate membrane that lies next to the dura mater with the subarachnoid space between the arachnoid and pia mater. The tentorium cerebella is a fold of dura that separates the cerebral hemispheres from the posterior fossa that contains the brainstem and cerebellum.

15. b. The blood-brain barrier physiologically protects the brain from harmful agents in the blood. The skull protects the brain from external trauma. The vertebral column allows flexibility while protecting the spinal cord. The dura mater is the outer protective membrane.

16. c. A decrease in sensory receptors caused by degenerative changes leads to a diminished sense of touch, temperature, and pain in the older adult. Reflexes are decreased but not normally absent. Intelligence does not decrease, although there may be some loss of memory. Hypothalamic modifications lead to increased frequency of spontaneous awakening with interrupted sleep and insomnia.

17. a, c, e. When taking the history of a patient with a neurologic problem, avoid suggesting symptoms or asking leading questions. The mode of onset and course of the illness are especially important. Validate the history if the patient's mental status causes question as to the reliability of the history. The other options are part of the physical assessment and will depend on the patient's history and manifestations.

18.

Functional Health Pattern	Risk Factor for or Patient Response to Neurologic Problem
Health perception–health management	Uncontrolled hypertension, lack of appropriate helmet or seat belt use, family history of neurologic problems, substance abuse, smoking, malnutrition, mental or physical changes noticed by others
Nutritional-metabolic	Difficulty chewing and swallowing, deficiency of B vitamins
Elimination	Bowel or bladder incontinence, constipation. Frequency of episodes, sensations, and measures to control
Activity-exercise	Problems in mobility, strength, and coordination. History of falling, activities of daily living (ADL) performance
Sleep-rest	Sleep disturbances from pain or immobility. Insomnia, frequent awakening, hallucinations
Cognitive-perceptual	Pain, sensory changes, dizziness, cognitive changes, language difficulties
Self-perception–self-concept	Decreased self-worth and body image. Unkempt physical appearance and hygiene
Role-relationship	Changes in roles at work or in family from neurologic problems
Sexuality-reproductive	Decreased sexual desire, hypersexuality
Coping–stress tolerance	Sense of being overwhelmed, inadequate coping patterns. Support system available
Value-belief	Life-changing effects. Religious or cultural beliefs that interfere or assist with planned treatment

19. b, d, e. The trochlear (CN IV), abducens (CN VI), and oculomotor (CN III) nerves cause oblique eye movement. The optic nerve (CN II) is for vision. The trigeminal nerve (CN V) provides sensation from the face and the motor function of mastication.

20. c. The trigeminal (CN V) and facial (CN VII) nerves respond to the corneal reflex test. The optic (CN II) nerve is tested by confrontation or field of vision. The vagus (CN X) nerve provides the gag reflex with the glossopharyngeal (CN IX) nerve. The spinal accessory (CN XI) nerve is tested with the resistive shoulder shrug.

21. c, e, f. The facial (CN VII) nerve is assessed with the corneal (blink) reflex test; smile, frown, and close eyes; and salt and sugar discrimination. Gag reflex is used to evaluate the glossopharyngeal (CN IX) and vagus (CN X) nerves. Visual field testing is used to assess the optic (CN II) nerve. Light touch to the face and the corneal (blink) reflex test are used to evaluate the trigeminal (CN V) nerve.

22. c. The hypoglossal (CN XII) nerve is tested with tongue protrusion. The vagus (CN X) and glossopharyngeal (CN IX) nerves are tested with the gag reflex. The olfactory (CN I) nerve is tested with odor identification.

23. d. The cochlear branch of the acoustic (CN VIII) nerve should enable the patient to hear. The patient may be distracted or hard of hearing, but the damage to this nerve is the most likely neurologic problem causing the inability to hear the ticking watch. The nurse should ensure that there are no distractions or extraneous noise when performing this test. The vagus (CN X) nerve is unrelated to hearing.

24. c. This nursing neurologic assessment of the motor system shows a potential for falls, which the nurse should help protect the patient from. Cerebellar dysfunction is present, but a diagnosis cannot be established only with this information. Assisting the patient to cope or planning a rehabilitation program will also not occur with only this part of the assessment.

25. b. The heel-to-shin test assesses coordination and cerebellar function. Muscle tone is assessed by passively moving limbs through their range of motion and feeling slight resistance. Extensor plantar response is tested with plantar stimulation and may indicate an upper motor neuron lesion. Loss of proprioception (or position sense) is assessed by placing the thumb and forefinger on either side of the patient's forefinger or great toe and gently moving it up and down, then asking the patient to indicate the direction in which the digit was moved.

26. d. Extinction is assessed by simultaneously touching both sides of the body; it is abnormal if the patient extinguishes 1 stimulus and perceives the stimulus only on 1 side. The cotton wisp assesses light touch. Pain sensation is assessed by touching the sharp and dull end of a pin to each of the patient's limbs with the patient responding "sharp" or "dull" each time. A tuning fork to bony prominences assesses vibration sense.

27. c. A positive Romberg test is demonstrated when the patient is unable to maintain balance with the feet together and then closing the eyes. Pronator drift is observed when the patient holds both arms fully extended at shoulder level in front of him with the palms upward and eyes closed; the downward drift and palm pronation indicates a problem in the opposite motor cortex. Absent patellar reflex is when there is no response to striking the patellar tendon just below the patella. Absence of 2-point discrimination is seen when the 2 points of a calibrated compass are on the tips of the fingers and are not recognized as 2 distinct points.

28. b. The normal response of the triceps reflex is extension of the arm or visible contraction of the triceps. The normal response of the biceps reflex is flexion of the arm at the elbow. Flexion and supination at the elbow are seen with the presence of the brachioradialis reflex.

29. b. This grade is 2/5 as it is a normal patellar reflex response. Deep-tendon grading is as follows: 0/5 = absent; 1/5 = weak response; 2/5 = normal response; 3/5 = brisk response; 4/5 = hyperreflexia with nonsustained clonus; 5/5 hyperreflexia with sustained clonus.

30. d. To facilitate insertion of the spinal needle between the third and fourth lumbar vertebrae, the patient should round the spine by flexing the knees, hips, and neck while in a lateral recumbent position, although a seated position may also be used. Sedation is used for more invasive tests, such as myelograms and angiography. Stimulants are withheld for 8 hours before an electroencephalogram (EEG). Assessing for stroke symptoms is not needed before a lumbar puncture but is done before cerebral angiography.

31. a. A spinal headache, which may be caused by loss of CSF at the puncture site, is common following a lumbar puncture or a myelogram, and nuchal rigidity may also occur as a result of meningeal irritation. The patient is not in danger of paralysis with a lumbar puncture, nor does hemorrhage from the site occur. Contrast media are not used with a lumbar puncture.

32. b. Following a myelogram (and a lumbar puncture), the patient is positioned flat in bed for several hours to avoid a spinal headache. Fluids are encouraged to help in the excretion of the contrast medium. Pain at the insertion site is rare and the most common complaint after a myelogram is a headache.

33. b. Cerebral angiography involves the injection of contrast media through a catheter inserted into the femoral or brachial artery and passed into the base of a carotid or vertebral artery and is performed when vascular lesions or tumors are suspected. Allergic reactions to the contrast medium may occur, and vascular spasms or dislodgement of plaques is possible. Neurologic status and vital signs must be monitored every 15 to 30 minutes for 2 hours, every hour for the next 6 hours, and then every 2 hours for 24 hours following the test. Electromyelography, EEG and transcranial Doppler sonography are not invasive studies.

34. c. Normal glucose levels in CSF are 40 to 70 mg/dL. All types of organisms consume glucose, and a decreased glucose level reflects bacterial activity. Increased levels are associated with diabetes. The other results are all normal.

CHAPTER 61

1. a, c, e. Blood adapts with increased venous outflow, decreased cerebral blood flow (CBF), and collapse of veins and dural sinuses. Brain tissue adapts with distention of the dura, slight compression of tissue, or herniation. Cerebrospinal fluid (CSF) adapts with increased absorption, decreased production, and displacement into the spinal canal. Skull bone and scalp tissue do not adapt to changes in intracranial pressure (ICP).

2. 56 mm Hg

   Mean arterial pressure(MAP) = diastolic blood

   pressure $(DBP) + \frac{1}{3}($systolic blood pressure

   $[SBP] - DBP) = 52 + 18 = 70$

   Cerebral perfusion pressure(CPP) = MAP − ICP

   $= 70 - 14 = 56$

3. 45 mm Hg

   $MAP = DBP + \frac{1}{3}(SBP - DBP) = 64 + 15 = 79$

   $CPP = MAP - ICP = 79 - 34 = 45$

4. a, c, e. Cerebral blood flow is decreased when the MAP and the partial pressure of carbon dioxide in arterial blood ($PaCO_2$) are decreased and ICP is increased. The other options increase cerebral blood flow.

5. b, e. A variety of insults, such as brain tumors, abscesses, and ingested toxins, lead to vasogenic cerebral edema. It is the most common type of cerebral edema and characterized by leakage of macromolecules from the capillaries into the surrounding extracellular space. This results in an osmotic gradient that favors the flow of fluid from the intravascular to the extravascular space. Hydrocephalus causes interstitial cerebral edema. Destructive lesions or trauma destroy cell membranes and cause cytotoxic cerebral edema.

6. a, b, d. Increased ICP is caused by vasodilation and edema from an initial brain insult or necrotic tissue. Blood vessel compression and brainstem compression and herniation occur because of increased ICP.

7. c. One of the most sensitive signs of increased ICP is a decreasing level of consciousness (LOC). A decrease in LOC will occur before changes in vital signs, ocular signs, or projectile vomiting occur.

8. c. Cushing's triad consists of 3 vital sign measures that reflect increased ICP and its effect on the medulla, hypothalamus, pons, and thalamus. Because these structures are very deep, Cushing's triad is usually a late sign of increased ICP. The signs include an increasing SBP with a widening pulse pressure, a bradycardia with a full and bounding pulse, and irregular respirations.

9. c. The dural structures that separate the 2 hemispheres and the cerebral hemispheres from the cerebellum influence the patterns of cerebral herniation. A cingulate herniation occurs where there is lateral displacement of brain tissue beneath the falx cerebri. Uncal herniation occurs when there is lateral and downward herniation. Tentorial herniation occurs when the brain herniates down through the opening created by the brainstem. The temporal lobe can be involved in central herniation.

10. a. An intraventricular catheter is a fluid-coupled system that can provide direct access for microorganisms to enter the ventricles of the brain and aseptic technique is a very high nursing priority to decrease the risk for infection. Constant monitoring of ICP waveforms is not usually necessary and removal of CSF for sampling or to maintain normal ICP is done only when specifically ordered.

11. b. An inaccurate ICP reading can be caused by CSF leaks around the monitor device, obstruction of the intraventricular catheter, kinks or bubbles in the tubing, and incorrect height of the transducer or drainage system relative to the patient's reference point, the tragus of the ear (cartilage projection anterior to the opening of the ear). The P2 wave being higher than the P1 wave shows poor ventricular compliance. The drain of the CSF drainage device should be closed for 6 minutes preceding the reading.

12. b. The normal pressure of oxygen in brain tissue ($PbtO_2$) is 20 to 40 mm Hg. The normal jugular venous oxygen saturation ($SjvO_2$) is 60% to 75% and indicates total venous brain tissue extraction of oxygen; this is used for short-term monitoring. The MAP of 70 to 150 mm Hg is needed for effective autoregulation of CBF. The normal range for partial pressure of oxygen in arterial blood (PaO_2) is 80 to 100 mm Hg.

13. d. Mannitol (Osmitrol) (25%) is an osmotic diuretic that expands plasma and causes fluid to move from tissues into the blood vessels. Hypertonic saline reduces brain swelling by moving water out of brain tissue. The corticosteroid dexamethasone is used to treat vasogenic edema to stabilize cell membranes and improve neuronal function by improving CBF and restoring autoregulation. Oxygen administration is done to maintain brain function. Pentobarbital (Nembutal) and other barbiturates are used to reduce cerebral metabolism.

14. d. A patient with increased ICP is in a hypermetabolic and hypercatabolic state and needs adequate glucose to maintain fuel for the brain and other nutrients to meet metabolic needs. Malnutrition promotes cerebral edema and if a patient cannot take oral nutrition, other means of providing nutrition should be used, such as tube feedings or parenteral nutrition. Glucose alone is not adequate to meet nutritional requirements, and 5% dextrose solutions may increase cerebral edema by lowering serum osmolarity. Patients should remain in a normovolemic fluid state with close monitoring of clinical factors, such as urine output, fluid intake, serum and urine osmolality, serum electrolytes, and insensible losses.

15. a. The Glasgow Coma Scale (GCS) is used to quickly assess the LOC with a standardized system. The 3 areas assessed are the patient's ability to open eyes, speak, and obey commands to verbal or painful stimulus. Although best motor response is an indicator, it is not used to assess coordination.

16. b. No opening of eyes = 1; incomprehensible words = 2; flexion withdrawal = 4. Total = 7

17. d. Of the body functions that should be assessed in an unconscious patient, cardiopulmonary status is the most vital function and gives priorities to the ABCs (airway, breathing, and circulation).

18. c. One of the functions of cranial nerve (CN) III, the oculomotor nerve, is pupillary constriction. Testing for pupillary constriction is important to identify patients at risk for brainstem herniation caused by increased ICP. Nystagmus is often associated with specific lesions or chemical toxicities and not a definitive sign of ICP. The corneal reflex is used to assess the functions of CN V and VII and the oculocephalic reflex tests all cranial nerves involved with eye movement.

19. a. Nursing care activities that increase ICP include hip and neck flexion, suctioning, clustering care activities, and noxious stimuli. They should be avoided or done as little as possible in the patient with increased ICP. Lowering the

PaCO$_2$ below 20 mm Hg can cause ischemia and worsening of ICP.

20. c. A PaO$_2$ of 70 mm Hg reflects hypoxemia that may lead to further decreased cerebral perfusion. The goal is to keep PaO$_2$ at ≥ 100 mm Hg. The pH and arterial oxygen saturation (SaO$_2$) are within normal range and a PaCO$_2$ of 35 mm Hg reflects a normal value.

21. a, b, d, e. The first sign of increased ICP is a change in LOC. Other manifestations are dilated ipsilateral pupil, changes in motor response, such as posturing, and fever, which may indicate pressure on the hypothalamus. Changes in vital signs would be an increased SBP with widened pulse pressure and bradycardia.

22. b. If reflex posturing occurs during range of motion (ROM) or positioning of the patient, these activities should be done less often until the patient's condition stabilizes because posturing can cause increases in ICP and may indicate herniation. Neither restraints nor central nervous system (CNS) depressants would be indicated.

23. d. A cerebral concussion may include a brief disruption in LOC, retrograde amnesia, and a headache, all of short duration. A parietal fracture may have deafness, loss of taste, and CSF otorrhea. A basilar skull fracture may have a dural tear with CSF or brain otorrhea, rhinorrhea, hearing difficulty, vertigo, and Battle's sign. A temporal fracture would have a boggy temporal muscle because of extravasation of blood, Battle's sign, or CSF otorrhea.

24. c. The posterior fossa fracture causes occipital bruising resulting in cortical blindness or visual field defects. A cerebral contusion is bruising of brain tissue within a focal area. An orbital skull fracture would cause periorbital ecchymosis (raccoon eyes) and possible optic nerve injury. A frontal lobe skull fracture would expose the brain to contaminants through the frontal air sinus and the patient would have CSF rhinorrhea or pneumocranium.

25. c. The compound skull fracture is a depressed skull fracture and scalp lacerations with communicating pathway(s) to the intracranial cavity. A linear skull fracture is a straight break in the bone without alteration in the fragments. A depressed skull fracture is an inward indentation of the skull that may cause pressure on the brain. A comminuted skull fracture has multiple linear fractures with bone fragmented into many pieces.

26. b. Testing clear drainage for CSF in nasal or ear drainage may be done with a Dextrostix or Tes-Tape strip, but if blood is present, the glucose in the blood will produce an unreliable result. To test bloody drainage, the nurse should test the fluid for a "halo" or "ring" that occurs when a yellowish ring encircles blood dripped onto a white pad or towel within a few minutes.

27. d. An arterial epidural hematoma is the most acute neurologic emergency, and typical symptoms include unconsciousness at the scene with a brief lucid interval followed by a decrease in LOC. An acute subdural hematoma manifests signs within 48 hours of an injury. A chronic subdural hematoma develops over weeks or months.

28. d. When there is a depressed fracture or a fracture with loose fragments, a craniotomy is indicated to elevate the depressed bone and remove free fragments. A craniotomy is also indicated in cases of acute subdural and epidural hematomas to remove the blood and control the bleeding.

Burr holes may be used in an extreme emergency for rapid decompression or to aid in removing a bone flap but with a depressed fracture, surgery would be the treatment of choice.

29. a. 1, b. 6, c. 2, d. 5, e. 4, f. 3.

30. a. Residual mental and emotional changes of brain trauma with personality changes are often the most incapacitating problems following head injury and are common in patients who have been comatose for longer than 6 hours. Families must be prepared for changes in the patient's behavior to avoid family-patient friction and maintain family functioning, and professional assistance may be required. There is no indication the patient will be dependent on others for care, but he likely will not return to pretrauma status.

31. d. The positron emission tomography (PET) scan or MRI is used to detect very small tumors. The CT and brain scans are used to identify the location of a lesion. Angiography could be used to determine blood flow to the tumor and further localize it. Electroencephalography (EEG) would be used to rule out seizures.

32. b. Frontal lobe tumors often lead to loss of emotional control, confusion, memory loss, disorientation, seizures, and personality and judgment changes that are very disturbing and frightening to the family. Physical symptoms, such as blindness, speech disturbances, or disturbances in sensation and perception that occur with other tumors, are more likely to be understood and accepted by the family.

33. d. A craniectomy is excision of cranial bone without replacement, so the patient will need to protect the brain from trauma in this surgical area. Burr holes are opened into the cranium with a drill to remove blood and fluid. A craniotomy is opening the cranium with removal of a bone flap to open the dura. The replaced bone flap is wired or sutured after surgery. A cranioplasty replaces part of the cranium with an artificial plate.

34. b. A stereotactic radiosurgery technique uses precisely focused radiation to destroy tumor cells. The radiation is computer and imagery guided. Brachytherapy uses radioactive seeds to deliver radiation. Ventricular shunts are used to redirect CSF from 1 area to another. A craniotomy is done by first making burr holes and then opening the cranium by connecting the holes to remove a flap of bone to expose the dura mater.

35. a. To prevent undue concern and anxiety about hair loss and postoperative self-esteem disturbances, a patient undergoing cranial surgery should be informed preoperatively that the head is usually shaved in surgery while the patient is anesthetized and that a turban, scarf, or cap may be used after the dressings are removed postoperatively, and a wig also may be used after the incision has healed to disguise the hair loss. In the immediate postoperative period the patient is very ill and the focus is on maintaining neurologic function. Before surgery, the nurse should anticipate the patient's postoperative need for self-esteem and maintenance of appearance.

36. d. The primary goal after cranial surgery is prevention of increased ICP, and interventions to prevent ICP and infection postoperatively are nursing priorities. The residual deficits, rehabilitation potential, and ultimate

function of the patient depend on the reason for surgery, the postoperative course, and the patient's general state of health.

37. c. The symptoms of brain abscess closely resemble those of meningitis and encephalitis, including fever, headache, nausea, vomiting, and increased ICP, except that the patient also may have some focal symptoms that reflect the local area of the abscess.

38. c, d, e. Encephalitis is usually caused by a virus that inflames the brain and can be transmitted by ticks and mosquitoes. The other options are characteristics of meningitis.

39. d. Meningitis is often a result of an upper respiratory infection or a penetrating wound of the skull, where organisms gain entry to the CNS. Ticks and mosquitoes transmit epidemic encephalitis. Nonepidemic encephalitis may occur as a complication of measles, chickenpox, or mumps. Encephalitis caused by the herpes simplex virus has a high fatality rate.

40. b. High fever, severe headache, nuchal rigidity, nausea, and vomiting are key signs of meningitis. Other symptoms, such as papilledema, generalized seizures, hemiparesis, and decreased LOC, and cranial nerve dysfunction may occur as complications of increased ICP in meningitis.

41. b. LOC must be monitored because it will decrease with the increased brain metabolism that the fever causes. Analgesics will not aid in lowering the body temperature, although acetaminophen will be used as an antipyretic. Rapid cooling may lead to shivering that increases metabolism. Monitoring cerebral edema will be done. Peripheral edema is unrelated and there will not be a rapid fluid infusion for the fever. Fluid replacement will be calculated with 800 mL/day for respiratory losses and 100 mL for each degree of temperature above 100.4°F (38°C).

Case Study

1. **Indicated**: mannitol (osmotic diuretic to reduce ICP), assess pupils (may indicate increased ICP), use EVD to drain CSF (to reduce ICP); **Contraindicated**: HOB flat (HOB should be 30-45° to reduce ICP), beta-blocker (HR is elevated due to the fever, administering this medication may cause a decrease in BP which will affect CPP); **Non-essential**: auscultate bowel sounds (irrelevant to the neurologic problems), applying antibiotic ointment on cranial staples (doesn't address the main problems)

2. Information to highlight that is evidence of DI: HR 120 beats/min (tachycardia is a result of the SNS trying to compensate for dehydration), BP 95/55 (loss of fluid will cause hypotension), urine output that is clear (without any yellow color is evidence), output of 400 mL/hr (indicates diuresis), specific gravity 1.0 (which is < 1.005), Hct 50% (higher than normal which could indicate dehydration causing more viscous blood), sodium 155 mg/dL (hypernatremia occurs with fluid loss), urine osmolality 50 mOsm/kg (normal is > 100 mOsm/kg)

3. **Risk for Injury:** pad the side rails and administer antiseizure medications, like phenytoin (patient is at increased risk for seizures), lock all bed controls when EVD is open to drain (to prevent too much CSF draining off, which could collapse the ventricles and cause brain herniation); **Increased Intracranial Pressure:** keep HOB 30-45° (reduces ICP by using gravity to reduce cerebral edema), drain 10 mL/hr from EVD (drains CSF to reduce ICP), 3% saline (a hypertonic solution that has an osmotic effect); **Altered Temperature:** administer antibiotics (to treat infection causing fever), obtain CSF culture (to identify microorganisms causing infection), aseptic technique (for all dressing changes and invasive lines)

4. A., C., D., F., G., I. A key sign of meningitis is nuchal rigidity (neck stiffness). Seizures occur in 1/3rd of these patients. Meningitis contributes to increase in ICP and is likely a contributing factor to the change in GCS for J.K. Unequal pupils can occur due to the compression of the optic nerve which indicates increased ICP, but this is a complication not an expected finding. J.K. may have headaches for months due to the irritation and inflammation of the meninges. Photophobia can occur with meningitis; therefore, patients should be kept in quiet dark rooms or their eyes should be covered. Bacterial meningitis is very contagious; therefore, respiratory isolation is necessary. If fevers are not responsive to acetaminophen or aspirin, a cooling blanket can be used to reduce the patient's body temperature.

5. **Effective**: urine specific gravity 1.025 (is normal which means the patient doesn't have DI), BP 125/75 (92) (is higher than it was which improves this patient's CPP), temperature 38°C (has decreased from the initial assessment which decreases the metabolic demand by the brain and indicates therapies are working), patient withdraws to painful stimulus (the patient is becoming more responsive than he was before and is no longer posturing); **Ineffective**: ICP 22 mm Hg (is still above the goal of < 20 mm Hg), pupils are unequal (indicates increased ICP compressing the optic nerve which is an abnormal finding); **Unrelated**: HR 100 beats/min (is decreased from the initial assessment, but it doesn't prove treatment has been effective for this patient's neurologic problems), peripheral pulses assess peripheral circulation and isn't related to this patient's neurologic problems)

CHAPTER 62

1. c. The highest risk factors for the most common stroke, thrombotic stroke, are hypertension and diabetes. Blacks have a higher risk for stroke than do white persons, probably because they have a greater incidence of hypertension, diabetes, and obesity. Factors, such as diet high in saturated fats and cholesterol, cigarette smoking, metabolic syndrome, sedentary lifestyle, and excessive alcohol use are also risk factors but carry less risk than hypertension.

2. c. The communication between the anterior and posterior cerebral circulation in the circle of Willis provides a collateral circulation, which may maintain circulation to an area of the brain if its original blood supply is obstructed. Atherosclerotic plaques are not readily reversed, and all areas of the brain require constant blood supply. Neurologic deficits can result from ischemia caused by many factors.

3. d. A transient ischemic attack (TIA) is a temporary focal loss of neurologic function caused by ischemia of an area of the brain, usually lasting an hour or less. TIAs may be caused by microemboli that temporarily block blood flow and are a warning of progressive cerebrovascular disease. Evaluation is necessary to determine the cause of the

neurologic deficit and provide prophylactic treatment if possible.

4. a, b, c, e. Strokes from intracerebral hemorrhage have a poor prognosis, are caused by the rupture of a blood vessel, are associated with hypertension, and may create a mass that compresses the brain. Hypertension is also related to thrombotic strokes that often occur during sleep or after sleep.

5. a. Embolic strokes are associated with endocardial disorders, such as atrial fibrillation, have a rapid onset, and are likely to occur during activity. Hemorrhage also commonly occurs during activity but is unrelated to cardiac disorders.

6. c. Clinical manifestations of altered neurologic function differ, depending primarily on the specific cerebral artery involved and the area of the brain that is perfused by the artery. The prognosis is related to the amount of brain tissue area involved. The degree of impairment depends on rapidity of onset, the size of the lesion, and the presence of collateral circulation.

7. a. L; b. R; c. R; d. L; e. R; f. R; g. L

8. c. Receptive aphasia is the lack of comprehension of both verbal and written language. Dysarthria is disturbance in muscular control of speech. In fluent dysphasia, speech is present but contains little meaningful communication. Expressive aphasia is the loss of the production of language.

9. c. MRI could be used to rapidly distinguish between ischemic and hemorrhagic stroke and determine the size and location of the lesion. A noncontrast CT scan could also be used. Lumbar punctures are not performed routinely because of the chance of increased intracranial pressure causing herniation. Cerebral arteriograms are invasive and may dislodge an embolism or cause further hemorrhage. They are performed only when no other test can provide the needed information.

10. d. A carotid endarterectomy is the removal of an atherosclerotic plaque in the carotid arteries that may impair circulation enough to cause a stroke. The other procedures described may also be used to prevent strokes. An extracranial-intracranial bypass involves cranial surgery to bypass a sclerotic intracranial artery. Stenting may improve circulation in the brain. A percutaneous transluminal angioplasty uses a balloon to compress stenotic areas in the carotid and vertebrobasilar arteries and often includes inserting a stent to hold the artery open.

11. d. Administering antiplatelet agents, such as aspirin, ticlopidine, clopidogrel (Plavix), dipyridamole (Persantine), and combined dipyridamole and aspirin (Aggrenox), reduces the incidence of stroke in those at risk. Anticoagulants are used for prevention of embolic strokes but increase the risk for hemorrhage. The calcium channel blocker, nimodipine, is used in patients with subarachnoid hemorrhage to decrease the effects of vasospasm and minimize tissue damage. Diuretics are not used for stroke prevention other than for their role in controlling BP. Warfarin, although it is an anticoagulant, is used for patients with atrial fibrillation, not TIA.

12. d. The first priority in acute management of the patient with a stroke is preservation of life. Because the patient with a stroke may be unconscious or have a reduced gag reflex, it is most important to maintain a patent airway for the patient

and provide oxygen if respiratory effort is impaired. IV fluid replacement, treatment with osmotic diuretics, and avoiding hyperthermia may be used for further treatment depending on the patient's manifestations.

13. b. Surgical management with clipping of an aneurysm to decrease rebleeding and vasospasm is an option for a stroke caused by rupture of a cerebral aneurysm. Placement of coils provides immediate protection against hemorrhage by reducing the blood pulsations within the aneurysm, then a thrombus forms and the aneurysm is sealed off from the parent vessel. Hyperventilation therapy would increase vasodilation and the potential for hemorrhage. Osmotic diuretics may leak into tissue, pulling fluid out of the vessel and increasing edema. Thrombolytic therapy would be absolutely contraindicated.

14. a. The body responds to the vasospasm and decreased circulation to the brain that occurs with a stroke by increasing the BP, frequently resulting in hypertension. The other options are important cardiovascular factors to assess, but they do not result from impaired cerebral blood flow.

15. a, b, c, d, f. The secondary assessment and ongoing neurologic monitoring include the gaze, sensation, facial palsy, proprioception, distal motor function, cognition, motor abilities, cerebellar function, and deep tendon reflexes. Current medications and history of hypertension are part of the primary assessment.

16. d. Active range of motion (ROM) should be started on the unaffected side as soon as possible. Passive ROM of the affected side should be started on the first day. Having the patient actively exercise the unaffected side provides the patient with active and passive ROM as needed. Use of footboards is controversial because they stimulate plantar flexion. The unaffected arm should be supported, but immobilization may precipitate a painful shoulder-hand syndrome. The patient should be positioned with each joint higher than the joint proximal to it to prevent dependent edema.

17. a. The presence of homonymous hemianopia in a patient with right hemisphere brain damage causes a loss of vision in the left field bilaterally. Early in the care of the patient, objects should be placed on the right side of the patient in the field of vision, and the nurse should approach the patient from the right side. Later in treatment, patients should be taught to turn the head and scan the environment and should be approached from the affected side to encourage head turning. Eye patches are used if patients have diplopia (double vision).

18. a. Usually the speech therapist will have completed a swallowing study before a diet is ordered. The first step in providing oral feedings for a patient with a stroke is ensuring that the patient has an intact gag reflex because oral feedings will not be provided if the gag reflex is impaired. After placing the patient in an upright position, the nurse may then evaluate the patient's ability to swallow ice chips or ice water.

19. c. Soft foods that provide enough texture, flavor, and bulk to stimulate swallowing should be used for the patient with dysphagia. Thin liquids are difficult to swallow, and patients may not be able to control them in the mouth. Pureed foods are often too bland and too smooth, and milk products should be avoided because they tend to increase the viscosity of mucus and increase salivation.

20. d. Recombinant tissue plasminogen activator (tPA) dissolves clots and increases the risk for bleeding. It is not used with hemorrhagic strokes. If the patient had a thrombotic or embolic stroke, the timeframe of 3 to 4.5 hours after onset of clinical signs of the stroke would be important as well as a history of surgery. The nurse should answer the question as accurately as possible and then encourage the wife to talk with the HCP if she has further questions.

21. c, d, f. The patient's rehabilitation potential, physical status of all body systems, and the expectations of the patient and caregiver related to the rehabilitation program will have a big impact on planning and carrying out the rehabilitation plan. The other things the rehabilitation nurse will assess are the presence of complications caused by the stroke or other chronic conditions, the patient's cognitive status, and the family (including the patient and caregiver) resources and support.

22. a. During rehabilitation, the patient with aphasia needs time to process and complete thoughts for verbal response. Conversation by the nurse and family should include meaningful verbal stimulation that is relevant to the patient. Gestures, pictures, and simple statements are more appropriate in the acute phase, when patients may be overwhelmed by verbal stimuli. Not responding verbally does not promote communication. Flashcards are often perceived by the patient as childish and meaningless.

23. c. Unilateral neglect, or neglect syndrome, occurs when the patient with a stroke is unaware of the affected side of the body, which puts the patient at risk for injury. During the acute phase, the affected side is cared for by the nurse with positioning and support, but during rehabilitation the patient is taught to care consciously for and attend to the affected side of the body to protect it from injury. Patients may be positioned on the affected side for up to 30 minutes.

24. c. Patients with left-brain damage from stroke often experience emotional lability, inappropriate emotional responses, mood swings, and uncontrolled tears or laughter disproportionate to or out of context with the situation. The behavior is upsetting and embarrassing to both the patient and family, and the patient should be distracted to minimize its presence. Maintaining a calm environment and avoiding shaming or scolding the patient are important. Patients with right-brain damage often have impulsive, rapid behavior that requires supervision and direction.

25. d. The patient and family need accurate and complete information about the effects of the stroke to problem solve and make plans for chronic care of the patient. The patient's specific needs for care must be identified and rehabilitation efforts should be continued at home. It is uncommon for patients with major strokes to return completely to prestroke function, behaviors, and role. Both the patient and family will mourn these losses. Family therapy and support groups may be helpful for some patients and families.

26. c. Medication administration is within the scope of practice for an LPN. Assessment and teaching are within the scope of practice for the RN.

Case Study

1.

Category	Orders (Rationale)
Imaging	□ PET scan (This identifies chemical activity in the brain) □ Echocardiogram (This would be helpful if cardiac involvement was suspected, i.e., atrial fibrillation) ■ **CT scan** (This is a rapid diagnostic to identify hemorrhage) □ Chest x-ray (This isn't helpful when identifying causes for neurological changes)
Monitoring	□ Continuous EEG monitoring (An EEG is a diagnostic to measure brain wave activity and isn't routinely done continuously) ■ **Neurologic assessment every hour** (The nurse should be performing this assessment frequently to quickly identify any changes) ■ **Continuous pulse oximetry** (It is important to supply a sufficient amount of oxygen to the brain. This would be important to monitor to quickly identify hypoxemia and/or issues with an obstructed airway) ■ **Intracranial pressure (ICP) monitoring** (This should be monitored and treated as necessary to decrease the risk of more brain injury)
Medications	■ **Nimodipine** (SAH often cause cerebral vasospasms, calcium channel blockers decrease the occurrence of these vasospasms as well as decrease BP) □ Aspirin (Contraindicated in patients with cerebral hemorrhage because aspirin potentiates bleeding) □ Atropine (The patient's HR is bradycardic, but it is asymptomatic as indicated by the elevated BP; therefore this medication is not currently indicated) □ Metoprolol (This medication may help decrease BP, but will also decrease HR. This patient's HR is already < 60 causing the administration of this medication to be contraindicated.) ■ **Mannitol** (This is an osmotic diuretic that is used to decrease intracranial pressure by decreasing cerebral edema.)

2. **Indicated**: Raise the HOB to 30 degrees (to help decrease ICP); Orient the patient to place and time (An unconscious patient can still hear; therefore, they should be treated as though they are conscious.); Prepare the patient for surgery (The patient will need surgery to stop the bleeding and evacuate the hematoma.); **Contraindicated**: Use the Trendelenburg position to treat hypotension (Trendelenburg will increase ICP which is contraindicated for a patient who already has increased ICP); Prepare to administer t-PA (This patient had a subarachnoid hemorrhage. This medication will increase the risk of bleeding.); **Non-essential**: Perform a 12-lead ECG (not applicable to this situation); Insert an oropharyngeal airway (There isn't any

evidence the patient cannot protect her airway or that there is an airway obstruction; therefore, it is unnecessary.)

3. The following data needs follow-up by the nurse: GCS of 3; HR 48 beats/min; BP 160/70 mm Hg; RR 10 and irregular; saturation 95% on 100% NRB; pupils sluggish to light; doesn't have an indwelling urinary catheter; bladder scan shows 650 mL. **Rationale**: The GCS was 5 and is now 3 which indicates a deterioration. This patient is showing signs of Cushing's triad as evidenced by the decrease in HR from 56 to 48 beats/min, the SBP increasing from 150 to 160 mm Hg, and a widening pulse pressure when compared to the ED admission. Oxygen saturation of 95% on 100% non-rebreather mask isn't ideal for this patient, which could indicate the patient needs to be intubated and placed on mechanical ventilation to maintain airway patency as well as improve oxygenation. Pupils are equal but sluggish, which may be a sign of increased intracranial pressure. The bladder scan indicates urinary retention which necessitates an indwelling urinary catheter especially since this patient is unconscious.

4. A, B, F, G, H. SAH may be genetic; therefore, people who have at least 2 first-degree relatives with a history of SAH should be screened. Smoking, taking oral contraceptives and baby aspirin are risk factors for intracranial hemorrhage, including SAH. SAH can be caused by aneurysms in the Circle of Willis which can manifest as a headache if they are leaking. Alcohol may increase the risk if this patient drank more than one drink/day. Sedentary lifestyles increase the risk, but this patient exercised 3x/week. Sleep or lack of sleep is not a risk factor.

5. **Indicated**: Use a specialized air mattress (This patient is immobile so a specialized mattress can aid in preventing pressure ulcer development.); Apply SCDs to BLE (Immobility can increase the risk of VTE [DVT]. SCDs will help prevent DVT formation.); Turn the patient every 2 hours (This is indicated for immobile patients to reduce the risk of pressure ulcer injury as well as promote oxygenation.); Administer enteral nutrition through a feeding tube (Nutrition is essential. If a patient cannot ingest food orally, a feeding tube inserted into the stomach to allow for enteral feeding is preferred over parenteral feeding.); **Contraindicated**: Massage calves twice a day (This is contraindicated in immobile patients as it may cause a PE if a DVT is dislodged by massaging the calves.); Suction the endotracheal tube every 2 hours (The ETT should only be suctioned when there is evidence of secretions as suctioning will increase ICP.); Perform mouth care once daily (Mouth care should be performed multiple times per day to reduce the risk of ventilator-associated pneumonia.); **Non-essential**: Place the patient on Contact Precautions (There isn't any indication for these precautions.); Start an additional IV for extra access (This isn't essential as there isn't any indication of necessity.); Place the patient on fall precautions (The patient is currently unconscious which doesn't pose an immediate risk for falls. If the patient becomes conscious, then this would be indicated.)

CHAPTER 63

1. b. Migraine headaches are frequently unilateral and usually throbbing. They may be preceded by a premonitory symptom or aura, and there is often a family history.

Cluster headaches are also unilateral with severe bone-crushing pain, but there is no premonitory symptom or family history. Frontal-type headache is not a functional type of headache but does describe the area of discomfort. Tension-type headaches are bilateral with constant, squeezing tightness without premonitory symptoms or family history.

2. b, c, d, f. Cluster headaches have only alcohol as a dietary trigger and have an abrupt onset of severe, sharp, penetrating pain lasting 5 minutes to 3 hours. Cluster headaches may be accompanied by unilateral ptosis, lacrimation, rhinitis, facial flushing, or pallor. They commonly recur several times each day for several weeks, with months or years between clustered attacks. Family history and nausea, vomiting, or irritability may be seen with migraine headaches. Bilateral pressure occurring between migraine headaches and intermittent occurrence over long periods of time are characteristics of tension-type headaches.

3. d. The primary way to diagnose and differentiate between headaches is with a careful history, requiring assessment of specific details related to the headache. Electromyelography (EMG) may reveal contraction of the neck, scalp, or facial muscles in tension-type headaches, but this is not seen in all patients. CT scans and cerebral angiography are used to rule out organic causes of the headaches.

4. d. Triptans (e.g., sumatriptan [Imitrex]) affect selected serotonin receptors that decrease neurogenic inflammation of the cerebral blood vessels and produce vasoconstriction. Because both migraine headaches and cluster headaches appear to be related to vasodilation of cranial vessels, drugs that cause vasoconstriction are useful in their treatment. Tricyclic antidepressants and β-adrenergic blockers are used prophylactically for migraine headaches but are not effective for cluster headaches. Nonsteroidal antiinflammatory drugs (NSAIDs) may be used for treatment of migraine headaches, but do not change the pathophysiologic process of migraine or cluster headaches.

5. a. When anxiety is related to a lack of knowledge about the etiology and treatment of a headache, helping the patient identify stressful lifestyle patterns and other precipitating factors and ways of avoiding them are appropriate nursing interventions. Interventions that teach alternative therapies to supplement drug therapy also give the patient some control over pain and are appropriate teaching regarding treatment of the headache. The other interventions may help reduce anxiety, but they do not address the cause of the anxiety.

6. c. The AP is able to obtain equipment from the supply cabinet or department. The RN may need to provide a list of necessary equipment and should set up the equipment and ensure proper functioning. The RN is responsible for the initial history and assessment as well as assessing and documenting seizure events. Padded tongue blades are no longer used, and no effort should be made to place anything in the patient's mouth during a seizure.

7. d. Generalized seizures are the result of bilateral synchronous epileptic discharge affecting the entire brain at onset of the seizure. Focal seizures begin in 1 side of the brain but may spread to involve the entire brain. Loss of consciousness is characteristic of generalized seizures but complex focal seizures also include an altered

consciousness. Focal seizures that start with a local focus and spread to the entire brain, causing a secondary generalized seizure, are associated with a transient residual neurologic deficit postictally known as *Todd's paralysis*.

8. b. In typical absence seizures, the child has staring spells that last for a few seconds. Atonic seizures occur when the patient falls from loss of muscle tone. Focal impaired awareness seizures have focal motor, sensory, or autonomic symptoms related to the area of the brain involved without loss of consciousness. Staring spells in atypical absence seizures last longer than those in typical absence seizures and are accompanied by peculiar behavior during the seizure or confusion after the seizure.

9. c, d, f. Focal impaired awareness seizures are psychomotor seizures with automatisms, such as lip smacking. They cause altered consciousness or loss of consciousness producing a dreamlike state and may involve behavioral, emotional, or cognitive experiences without memory of what was done during the seizure. Generalized tonic-clonic seizures, (previously known as *grand mal seizures*) are characterized by loss of consciousness and stiffening of the body with subsequent jerking of extremities. Incontinence or tongue or cheek biting may also occur.

10. a. Status epilepticus is most dangerous because the continuous seizing can cause potentially fatal respiratory insufficiency, hypoxemia, dysrhythmia, hyperthermia, and systemic acidosis. Myoclonic seizures may occur in clusters with a sudden, excessive jerk of the body that may hurl the person to the ground. Subclinical seizures may occur in a patient who is sedated, so there is no physical movement. Psychogenic seizures are psychiatric in origin and diagnosed with video-electroencephalography (EEG) monitoring. They occur in patients with a history of emotional abuse or a specific traumatic episode.

11. c. A seizure is a paroxysmal, uncontrolled discharge of neurons in the brain that interrupts normal function; however, the cause of the abnormal firing is not clear. Many factors may precipitate seizures. Although scar tissue may make the brain neurons more likely to fire, it is not the usual cause of seizures. Epilepsy is established only by a pattern of spontaneous, recurring seizures.

12. b. Most patients with seizure disorders maintain seizure control with medications. If surgery is considered, 3 requirements must be met: the diagnosis of epilepsy must be confirmed, there must have been an adequate trial with drug therapy without satisfactory results, and a there must be a defined electroclinical syndrome. The focal point must be localized, but the presence of scar tissue is not required.

13. c. Serum levels of antiseizure drugs are monitored regularly to maintain therapeutic amounts of the drug (above which patients are likely to have toxic effects, below which seizures are likely to occur). Many newer drugs do not require drug level monitoring because of large therapeutic ranges. A daily seizure log and urine testing for drug levels will not assess compliance or monitor toxicity. EEGs have limited value in diagnosis of seizures and even less value in monitoring seizure control.

14. c. Abruptly discontinuing antiseizure drugs can precipitate seizures. Missed doses should be made up if the omission is remembered within 24 hours. Patients should not adjust medications without professional guidance because this can increase seizure frequency and cause status epilepticus.

Antiseizure drugs have many interactions with other drugs, and the HCP should evaluate the use of other medications. If side effects occur, the HCP should be notified, and drug regimens evaluated.

15. a, b, c. The focus is on maintaining a patent airway and preventing patient injury. The nurse should not place objects in the patient's mouth or restrain the patient.

16. b. In the postictal phase of a generalized tonic-clonic seizure, the patient is usually very tired and may sleep for several hours. The nurse should allow the patient to sleep as long as necessary. Suctioning is performed only if needed. Decreased level of consciousness is not a problem postictally unless a head injury has occurred during the seizure.

17. b. One of the most common complications of seizure disorder is the effect on the patient's lifestyle. For example, the social stigma attached to seizures may cause the patient to hide the diagnosis and to prefer not to be identified as having epilepsy. Medication regimens usually require only once- or twice-daily dosing. Major lifestyle restrictions usually involve driving and high-risk environments. Job discrimination against the handicapped is prevented by federal and state laws. Patients only need to identify their disease in case of medical emergencies.

18. c. Restless legs syndrome that is unrelated to other pathologic processes (e.g., diabetes or rheumatic disorders) may be caused by a dysfunction in the basal ganglia circuits that use the neurotransmitter dopamine, which controls movements. Dopamine precursors and dopamine agonists, such as those used for parkinsonism, are effective in managing sensory and motor symptoms. Polysomnography studies during sleep are the only tests that have diagnostic value. Although exercise should be encouraged, excessive leg exercise does not have an effect on the symptoms.

19. c. Huntington's disease (HD) involves deficiency of acetylcholine and γ-aminobutyric acid (GABA) in the basal ganglia and extrapyramidal system that causes the opposite symptoms of parkinsonism. Myasthenia gravis involves autoimmune antibody destruction of cholinergic receptors at the neuromuscular junction. Amyotrophic lateral sclerosis (ALS) involves degeneration of motor neurons in the brainstem and spinal cord.

20. a. Most patients with multiple sclerosis (MS) have remissions and exacerbations of neurologic dysfunction or a relapsing-remitting initial course followed by progression with or without occasional relapses, minor remissions, and plateaus that progressively cause loss of motor, sensory, and cerebellar functions. Intellectual function generally is intact, but patients may have anger, depression, or euphoria. A few people have chronic progressive deterioration, while some may have only occasional and mild symptoms for several years after onset.

21. c. Specific neurologic dysfunction of MS is caused by destruction of myelin and replacement with glial scar tissue at specific areas in the nervous system. Motor, sensory, cerebellar, and emotional dysfunctions, including paresthesia, patchy blindness, blurred vision, pain radiating along the dermatome of the nerve, ataxia, and severe fatigue, are the most common manifestations of MS. Constipation and bladder dysfunction, short-term memory loss, sexual dysfunction, anger, and depression or euphoria may occur. Excess involuntary movements and tremors are not seen in MS.

22. d. There is no specific diagnostic test for MS. A diagnosis is made primarily by history and clinical manifestations. Certain diagnostic tests may be used to help establish a diagnosis of MS. Positive findings on MRI include evidence of at least 2 inflammatory demyelinating lesions in at least 2 different locations within the central nervous system (CNS). Cerebrospinal fluid (CSF) may have increased immunoglobulin G and the presence of oligoclonal banding. Evoked potential responses are often delayed in persons with MS.

23. b. Ocrelizumab is an immunosuppressant given IV when the patient has inadequate responses to other drugs. It increases the risk of infection and breast cancer.

24. c. The main goals in care of the patient with MS is to keep the patient active and maximally functional, and promote self-care as much as possible to maintain independence. Assistive devices encourage independence while preserving the patient's energy. No care activity should be done by others if the patient can do it for himself or herself. Family involvement in the patient's care and maintaining social interactions are important but not the priority.

25. b. Corticosteroids used in treating acute exacerbations of MS should not be abruptly stopped by the patient because adrenal insufficiency may result; tapering doses should be prescribed and followed. Infection may worsen symptoms and should be avoided. High-fiber diets with vitamin supplements are recommended. Long-term planning for increasing disability is also important.

26. d. The degeneration of dopamine-producing neurons in the substantia nigra of midbrain and basal ganglia lead to these signs. Muscle soreness, pain, and slowness of movement are consequences of patient function related to rigidity. Shuffling gait, absent arm swing while walking, absent blinking, masked facial expression, saliva drooling, and difficulty initiating movement are all related to akinesia. Impaired handwriting and hand activities are related to the tremor of Parkinson's disease (PD). Being unable to stop the self from going forward or backward results from postural instability.

27. b. Although clinical manifestations are characteristic in PD, no laboratory or diagnostic tests are specific for the condition. A diagnosis is made when the presence of tremor, rigidity, akinesia, and postural instability occur with asymmetric onset. It is confirmed with a positive response to antiparkinsonian drugs. Research about the role of genetic testing and MRI to diagnose PD is ongoing. Essential tremors increase during voluntary movement, while the tremors of PD are more prominent at rest.

28. c. The akinesia of PD prevents automatic movements. Activities, such as beginning to walk, rising from a chair, or even swallowing saliva, cannot be executed unless they are consciously willed. Handwriting is affected by the tremor and results in the writing trailing off at the end of words. Specific limb weakness and muscle spasms are not characteristic of PD.

29. c. Peripheral dopamine does not cross the blood-brain barrier. However, its precursor levodopa is able to enter the brain, where it is converted to dopamine, increasing the supply that is deficient in PD. Bromocriptine is used to treat PD to stimulate dopamine receptors in the basal ganglia. Amantadine stimulates dopamine release and blocks the reuptake of dopamine into presynaptic neurons. Carbidopa and entacapone are usually given with levodopa to prevent the levodopa from being metabolized in peripheral tissues before it can reach the brain.

30. d. The shuffling gait of PD causes the patient to be off balance and at risk for falling. A more balanced gait can be promoted by teaching the patient to use a wide stance with the feet apart, to consciously think about stepping over an imaginary object when walking, and to look ahead. Use of an elevated toilet seat will enable a patient to initiate movement but not prevent falls. Using a wheelchair will not maintain independence or optimize psychosocial well-being. Canes and walkers are hard for the patient with PD to maneuver and may increase the risk for injury.

31. b. Serum acetylcholine receptor antibodies will confirm a diagnosis of myasthenia gravis (MG). The history and physical revealing weakness is part of the diagnosis, but not the confirmation. Impaired respiratory function is a sign of MG, but not a confirmation of the diagnosis. The EMG will show muscle fatigue with a decreased response.

32. c. The patient in myasthenic crisis has severe weakness and fatigue of all skeletal muscles, affecting the patient's ability to breathe, swallow, talk, and move. However, the priority of nursing care is monitoring and maintaining adequate respiratory function.

33. b. Gradual degeneration of motor neurons occurs in ALS, with extreme muscle wasting from lack of stimulation and use. However, cognitive function is not impaired and the patient feels trapped in a dying body. Chorea manifested by writhing, involuntary movements is characteristic of HD. As an autosomal dominant genetic disease, HD has a 50% chance of being passed to each offspring.

34. c. The nurse can try to help patients maximize neurologic function and self-care abilities, alleviate physical symptoms, and prevent complications for as long as possible. Many chronic neurologic diseases involve progressive deterioration in physical or mental capabilities and have no cure, with devastating results for patients and families.

Case Study

1. **Expected**: 32 years of age (most are diagnosed between 20-40 years of age), European descent (most prevalent in people of Northern European descent), born and raised in Minneapolis (more prevalent further away from the equator), vitamin D deficiency (some evidence of causing a greater risk), viral neuritis 2 years ago (viruses are thought to be a trigger of this autoimmune disease); **Unrelated**: smoking cigarettes, drinking alcohol and having hypercholesterolemia (are unrelated)

2. 1=central nervous system; 2=50; 3=autoimmune; 4=T cells; 5=glial; 6=white, grey and axonal

3. **Diagnostic**: Liver function tests (due to effects of medications used to treat MS), Lumbar puncture (CSF analysis may show an increase in immunoglobulin G and the presence of oligoclonal banding), CT scan (may show changes in the brain caused by MS); **Nursing Care**: vision assessment (due to visual changes patients with MS experience), out of bed with assistance (due to weakness and paresthesias), bladder ultrasound if unable to void (patients can experience urinary retention); **Ancillary Care**: speech therapy (MS patients can have speech problems), physical therapy (assist with ADLs

and optimizing mobility); **Medications**: cladribine (suppresses lymphocytes), alemtuzumab (helps slow the inflammation of the central nervous system caused by MS), hydrocortisone (a corticosteroid that reduces inflammation and suppresses the immune system)

4. **1**=may cause suicidal ideation; **2**=teriflunomide; **3**=slows attack on myelin by lymphocytes; **4**=susceptible to fatal brain infection; **5**=prednisone

5. B., C., D., F. MS patients should not get live virus vaccines because they are immunosuppressed. Patients should rest when tired and avoid extreme heat because becoming over-heated can exacerbate MS symptoms. Annual eye exams will be important to identify and possibly correct changes in vision caused by MS. Medications may improve symptoms and may slow the progression, but will not prevent MS from getting worse. MS is a progressive disease without a cure. It is recommended to limit caffeine intake. Urinary incontinence should be reported to the HCP because there are medications that may help. Acute exacerbations will occur and may interfere with ADLs, including causing immobility.

CHAPTER 64

1. a, d, e. Manifestations of delirium include cognitive impairment with reduced awareness, reversed sleep/wake cycle, and distorted thinking and perception. The other options are characteristic of dementia.

2. d. The diagnosis of vascular dementia can be aided by neuroimaging studies showing vascular brain lesions along with exclusion of other causes of dementia. Overproduction of β-amyloid protein contributes to Alzheimer's disease (AD). Vascular dementia can be prevented or slowed by treating underlying diseases (e.g., diabetes, cardiovascular disease). Dementia caused by hepatic or renal encephalopathy can potentially be reversed.

3. a. Depression is often associated with AD, especially early in the disease when the patient has awareness of the diagnosis and progression of the disease. When dementia and depression occur together, intellectual deterioration may be more extreme. Depression is treatable. Use of antidepressants often improves cognitive function.

4. c. The Mini-Mental State Examination is a tool to document the degree of cognitive impairment. It can be used to determine a baseline from which changes over time can be evaluated. It does not evaluate mood or thought processes but can detect dementia and delirium and distinguish these from psychiatric mental illness. It cannot help determine the cause.

5. c. Hypothyroidism can cause dementia, but it is a treatable condition if it has not been long standing. The other conditions are causes of irreversible dementia.

6. d. In mild cognitive impairment, people often forget people's names and begin to forget important events. Delirium changes usually occur abruptly. In AD, the patient may not remember knowing a person and loses the sense of time and which day it is. Normal forgetfulness includes momentarily forgetting names and occasionally forgetting to run an errand.

7. b. The only definitive diagnosis of AD can be made on examination of brain tissue during an autopsy, but a clinical diagnosis is made when all other possible causes of dementia have been eliminated. Patients with AD may have β-amyloid proteins in the blood, brain atrophy, or isoprostanes in the urine, but these findings are not exclusive to those with AD.

8. c. In the moderate stage of AD, the patient may need help with getting dressed. In the severe stage, patients will be unable to dress or feed themselves and are usually incontinent.

9. b. Because there is no cure for AD, collaborative management is aimed at controlling the decline in cognition, controlling the undesirable manifestations that the patient may have and providing support for the family caregiver. Cholinesterase inhibitors help to increase acetylcholine (ACh) in the brain, but a variety of other drugs are also used to control behavior. Memory-enhancing techniques have little or no effect in patients with AD, especially as the disease progresses. Patients with AD have limited ability to communicate health symptoms and problems, leading to a lack of professional attention for acute and other chronic illnesses.

10. c. Lorazepam (Ativan) is a benzodiazepine used to manage behavior with AD. Sertraline (Zoloft) is a selective serotonin reuptake inhibitor used to treat depression. Donepezil (Aricept) is a cholinesterase inhibitor used for decreased memory and cognition. Risperidone (Risperdal) is an antipsychotic used for behavior management.

11. d. Memantine (Namenda) is the N-methyl-D-aspartate (NMDA) receptor antagonist often used for AD patients with decreased memory and cognition. Zolpidem (Ambien) is a sedative to help with sleep problems. Olanzapine (Zyprexa) is an antipsychotic medication used for behavior management. Rivastigmine (Exelon) is a cholinesterase inhibitor used for decreased memory and cognition.

12. b. Patients with moderate to severe AD often become agitated, but because their short-term memory loss is so pronounced, distraction is a very good way to calm them. "Why" questions are upsetting to them because they do not know the answer and cannot respond to normal relaxation techniques.

13. a, b, f. Avoiding trauma to the brain, treating depression early, and exercising regularly can maintain cognitive function. Staying socially active, avoiding intake of harmful substances, getting enough sleep, a healthy diet, and challenging the brain to keep its connections active and create new ones also help keep the brain healthy.

14. a. The risk is higher for the children of parents with early onset AD. Women do get AD more often than men, but that is more likely related to women living longer than men than to the type of AD. Gene testing for *ApoE-4* allele of the 19th chromosome is used for research with late-onset AD but does not predict who will develop the disease. Late-onset AD is more genetically complex than early-onset AD and is more common in those over age 60 years.

15. b. Adhering to a regular, consistent daily schedule helps the patient avoid confusion and anxiety and is important both during hospitalization and at home. Clocks and calendars may be useful in early AD, but they have little meaning to a patient as the disease progresses. Questioning the patient about activities and events they cannot remember is threatening and may cause severe anxiety. Maintaining a safe environment for the patient is important but does not change the disturbed thought processes.

16. b. Family caregiver role strain is characterized by such symptoms of stress as the inability to sleep, make decisions, or concentrate. It is often seen in family members who are responsible for the care of the patient with AD. Assessment of the caregiver may reveal a need for assistance to increase coping skills, effectively use community resources, or maintain social relationships. Eventually the demands on a caregiver exceed the resources, and the person with AD may be placed in an institutional setting.

17. a. Adult day care is an option to provide respite for caregivers and a protective environment for the patient during the early and middle stages of AD. There are also in-home respite care providers. The respite from the demands of care allows the caregiver to maintain social contacts, perform normal tasks of living, and be more responsive to the patient's needs. Visits by home health nurses involve the caregiver and cannot provide adequate respite. Institutional placement is not always an acceptable option at earlier stages of AD, nor is hospitalization available for respite care.

18. b, e. Dementia with Lewy bodies (DLB) is diagnosed with dementia with the following symptoms: (1) extrapyramidal signs, such as bradykinesia, rigidity, and postural instability but not always a tremor; (2) fluctuating cognitive ability; and (3) hallucinations. The extrapyramidal signs plus tremors would more likely indicate Parkinson's disease. Disturbed behavior, sleep, personality, and eventually memory are characteristics of frontotemporal lobe degeneration (FTLD).

19. a, b, d. All caregivers are responsible for the patient's safety. Basic care activities, such as those associated with personal hygiene and activities of daily living (ADLs) can be delegated to the AP. The RN will perform ongoing assessments and develop and revise the plan of care as needed. The RN will assess the patient's safety risk factors, provide education, and make referrals. The LPN could check the patient's environment for potential safety hazards.

20. a. Age; b. infection (pneumonia); c. hypoxemia (lung disease); d. ICU hospitalization (change in environment, sensory overload); e. preexisting dementia; f. dehydration. Hyperthermia and potentially medications to treat chronic obstructive pulmonary disease (COPD) and pneumonia.

21. d. Delirium is an acute problem that usually has a rapid onset in response to a precipitating event, especially when the patient has underlying health problems, such as heart disease and sensory limitations. In the absence of prior cognitive impairment, a sudden onset of confusion, disorientation, and agitation is usually delirium. Delirium may manifest with both hypoactive and hyperactive symptoms.

22. c. Care of the patient with delirium is focused on identifying and eliminating precipitating factors if possible. Treating underlying medical conditions, changing environmental conditions, and stopping medications that induce delirium are important. Drug therapy is reserved for those patients with severe agitation because the drugs themselves may worsen delirium.

23. d. In the severe stage of AD, the patient is at a developmental level of 15 months or less. Therefore appropriate distractions would be infant toys. Watching TV and playing games are more appropriate in the mild to moderate stage. Books to read should be at developmentally appropriate levels to be used as a diversion.

24. b. The patient's history and symptoms most likely indicate delirium associated with sleep deprivation and sensory overload related to the ICU environment. Informing the receiving nurse and transferring the patient is appropriate. Postponing the transfer is likely to prolong the delirium. Benzodiazepines and restraints contribute to delirium and agitation.

Case Study

1. Answers are in the order they appear in the statements: CT scan; atrophy; PET scan; amyloid; B-complex.

2. **Mini-Cog**: repeat 3 words previously stated before the other 2 tasks and then have the patient repeat them as the last step of the examination, draw a clock and put the clock hands on 11:10; **MMSE**: ask the patient to name an object (like a pen or pencil), read an instruction and do what it says (i.e., clap hands, close eyes); ask "What is today's date?"

3. **Mild**: occasionally misplaces eyeglasses, has trouble finding the right word; **Moderate**: wanders, has trouble recognizing children (or other family members and friends), becomes easily agitated; **Severe**: difficulty with speech, places objects in the wrong place (i.e., keys in the refrigerator or TV remote in the dryer)

4. 1=trazodone; 2=clonazepam; 3=SSRI; 4=cholinesterase inhibitor; 5=forgetfulness; 6=insomnia; 7=depression; 8=disinhibition

5. A., B., C., F., G. Advance directive, living wills, durable powers of attorney for healthcare and finances should be completed before progression of the disease, while G.D. still has the capacity to make these decisions. Distraction and diversion is recommended to cope with behavior issues. Correcting or chastising the behavior will cause anger and frustration and may illicit a violent reaction from the person with AD. G.D. should wear a MedicAlert bracelet to identify his disease to others who may find him wandering. Interactions with family and friends is encouraged. G.D. should stop driving even in the mild stage of AD as his judgment and driving skills may be impaired putting him and others at risk. Community support groups can help caregivers the most, sharing their experiences and learning about experiences of others. Safety in the home is important and can be accomplished by labeling the faucets hot and cold, removing throw rugs (tripping hazard), having good lighting, and installing hand rails in the bathroom/shower. It is not recommended to correct mistakes made by a person with AD as it may cause embarrassment, anger, frustration, or behavior problems.

CHAPTER 65

1. d. Young adult men ages 16 to 30 years, who may be impulsive or risk takers in daily living, have the greatest risk for spinal cord injury (SCI). Other risk factors include alcohol and drug use, taking part in sports, and occupational exposure to trauma or violence.

2. b. At the C7 level, spinal shock is manifested by tetraplegia and sensory loss. The neurologic loss may be temporary or permanent. Paraplegia with flaccid paralysis would

occur at the level of T1 or below. Hemiplegia occurs with central (brain) lesions affecting motor neurons and spastic tetraplegia occurs when spinal shock resolves.

3. a. In central cord syndrome, motor weakness and sensory loss are present in upper extremities; lower extremities are not usually affected.

4. b. Brown-Séquard syndrome is characterized by ipsilateral loss of motor function and position and vibratory sense, and contralateral loss of pain and temperature sensation below the level of the injury. Damage to the most distal cord and nerve roots with flaccid paralysis of the lower limbs and areflexic bowel and bladder is seen with cauda equina syndrome or conus medullaris syndrome. Posterior cord syndrome is rare; cord damage results in loss of proprioception below the lesion level but retention of motor control and temperature and pain sensation. Anterior cord syndrome is often caused by flexion injury, with acute compression of the cord resulting in complete motor paralysis and loss of pain and temperature sensation below the level of injury; touch, position, vibration, and motion remain intact.

5. c. The primary SCI rarely affects the entire cord, but the pathophysiology of secondary injury may result in damage that is the same as mechanical severance of the cord. Complete cord dissolution occurs through autodestruction of the cord by hemorrhage, ischemia, edema, and the presence of metabolites, which lead to cell death and permanent neurologic deficit.

6. c. Spinal shock occurs in many people with acute SCI. In spinal shock, the entire cord below the level of the lesion fails to function, resulting in flaccid paralysis and hypomotility of most processes without any reflex activity. Return of reflex activity, although spastic, signals the end of spinal shock. Rehabilitation activities are not contraindicated during spinal shock and should be started if the patient's cardiopulmonary status is stable. Neurogenic shock results from loss of vascular tone from the injury. It is manifested by hypotension, peripheral vasodilation, and decreased cardiac output (CO). Sympathetic function is impaired below the level of the injury because sympathetic nerves leave the spinal cord at the thoracic and lumbar areas. Cranial parasympathetic nerves predominate in control over respirations, heart, and all vessels and organs below the injury, which includes autonomic functions.

7. b. Until edema and necrosis at the site of the injury are resolved, it is not possible to determine how much cord damage is present from the initial injury, how much secondary injury occurred, or how much the cord was damaged by edema that extended above and below the level of the original injury. The return of reflexes signals the end of spinal shock. Reflexes may be inappropriate and excessive, causing spasms that complicate rehabilitation.

8. a. SCI below C4 will result in diaphragmatic breathing and usually hypoventilation from decreased vital capacity and tidal volume from intercostal muscle impairment. The nurse's priority actions will be to monitor rate, rhythm, depth, and effort of breathing to observe for changes from the baseline and identify the need for ventilation assistance. Loss of all respiratory muscle function occurs above C4, and the patient needs mechanical ventilation to survive. Although the decreased sympathetic nervous system response (from injuries above T6) and gastrointestinal (GI)

hypomotility (paralytic ileus and gastric distention) will occur (with injuries above T5), they are not the patient's initial priority needs.

9. b. Neurogenic shock associated with SCI above the level of T6 greatly decreases the effect of the sympathetic nervous system, leading to bradycardia and hypotension. A heart rate of 42 bpm is not adequate to meet the oxygen needs of the body. While low, the BP is not at a critical point. The oxygen saturation is satisfactory and the motor and sensory losses are expected.

10. c. With the injury at T4, the highest-level realistic goal for this patient is to be independent in self-care and wheelchair use because arm function will not be affected. Indoor mobility in a manual wheelchair will be achievable, but it is not the highest-level goal. Ambulating with crutches and leg braces can be achieved only by patients with injuries in T6-12 area. Independent ambulation with short leg braces and canes could occur for a patient with an L3-4 injury. (See Table 60.2.)

11. d. Although surgical treatment of SCI often depends on the preference of the HCP, surgery is usually indicated when there is continued compression of the cord by extrinsic forces or there is evidence of cord compression. Other indications may include progressive neurologic deficit, compound fracture of the vertebra, bony fragments, and penetrating wounds of the cord.

12. a. The need for a patent airway is the first priority for any injured patient. A high cervical injury may decrease the gag reflex and the ability to maintain an airway as well as the ability to breathe. Maintaining cervical stability is then a consideration, along with assessing neurologic status and for the presence of other injuries.

13. c. The development of better surgical stabilization has made surgery the more frequent treatment of cervical injuries. However, when surgery cannot be done, skeletal traction with the use of Crutchfield, Gardner-Wells, or other types of skull tongs is required to immobilize the cervical vertebrae, even if a fracture has not occurred. Special turning or kinetic beds may be used to turn and mobilize patients who are in cervical traction. Hard cervical collars or a sternal-occipital-mandibular immobilizer brace may be used for stabilization during emergency transport of the patient, after cervical stabilization surgery, or for minor injuries.

14. d. Norepinephrine is a vasopressor that is used to maintain BP during states of hypotension that occur during neurogenic shock associated with SCI. Atropine would be used to treat bradycardia. The temperature reflects some degree of poikilothermism, but this is not treated with medications.

15. c. Because pneumonia and atelectasis are potential problems related to ineffective coughing and the loss of intercostal and abdominal muscle function, the nurse should assess the patient's breath sounds and respiratory function to determine if secretions are being retained or respiratory impairment is progressing. If the patient cannot count to 10 aloud without taking a breath, immediate attention is needed. Suctioning is not indicated unless lung sounds indicate retained secretions. Position changes will help mobilize secretions. Intubation and mechanical ventilation are used if the patient becomes exhausted from labored breathing or if arterial blood gases (ABGs) deteriorate.

16. d. During the first 2 to 3 days after SCI, paralytic ileus may occur. Nasogastric suction must be used to remove secretions and gas from the GI tract until peristalsis resumes. IV fluids are used to maintain fluid balance but do not specifically relate to paralytic ileus. Tube feedings would be used only for patients who have difficulty swallowing, but not until peristalsis returns. Parenteral nutrition would be used only if the paralytic ileus was unusually prolonged.

17. a. The bladder is atonic during the acute phase of SCI, causing urinary retention with the risk for reflux into the kidney or rupture of the bladder. An indwelling catheter is used to keep the bladder empty and monitor urinary output. Intermittent catheterization or other urinary drainage methods may be used in long-term bladder management. Use of incontinent pads is inappropriate because they do not help the bladder empty.

18. b. When spinal shock ends, reflex movement and spasms will occur that may be mistaken for return of function. However, with the resolution of edema, some normal function may also occur. When movement occurs, it is important to determine if the movement is voluntary and can be consciously controlled because this would indicate some return of function. If movement is not voluntary, reflex return will be explained.

19. a. 5; b. 2; c. 6; d. 3; e. 1; f. 4. The patient has autonomic dysreflexia. The first response by the nurse should be to elevate the head of bed (HOB) to decrease BP and then to remove noxious stimulation. Often the trigger is bladder distention, which can be addressed quickly by catheterization or ensuring drainage. The HCP must be notified as soon as possible. Meanwhile, the nurse should stay with the patient. If bladder distention was not the cause, a digital rectal examination with anesthetic ointment may be done. Loosen restrictive clothing. The HCP may order an antihypertensive. Documentation of the entire episode should be accurate and thorough.

20. b. Intermittent self-catheterization 4 to 6 times a day is the recommended method of bladder management for the patient with SCI and reflex neurogenic bladder because it more closely mimics normal emptying and has less potential for infection. The patient and family should be taught the procedure using clean technique at home. If the patient has use of the arms, self-catheterization should be performed. Indwelling catheterization is used during the acute phase to prevent overdistention of the bladder. Surgical urinary diversions are used if urinary complications occur.

21. b. If S2-S4 nerve pathways are intact, the patient with a complete lower motor neuron lesion is able to have reflex erections and use drugs to maintain erection for sexual satisfaction. The patient with complete upper motor neuron lesions usually has only reflex sexual function with rare ejaculation. The patient with incomplete lower motor neuron lesions has the highest possibility of successful psychogenic erections with ejaculation. The patient with incomplete upper motor neuron lesions may have reflex erections with ejaculation.

22. a. Working through grief is a lifelong process. It is triggered by new experiences, such as marriage, child rearing, employment, or illness, to which the patient must adjust throughout life within the context of their disability. The goal of recovery is related to adjustment rather than complete acceptance, and many patients do not experience all components of the grief process. During the anger phase, the patient should be allowed outbursts. The nurse may use humor to displace some of the patient's anger.

23. b. Most metastatic or secondary tumors are extradural lesions in which treatment, including surgery, is palliative. Primary spinal tumors may be removed with the goal of cure. Most spinal cord tumor are slow-growing and do not cause autodestruction. If removal is possible, complete function may be restored. Radiation is used to treat metastatic tumors that are sensitive to radiation and that have caused only minor neurologic deficits in the patient. Radiation is used as adjuvant therapy to surgery for intramedullary tumors.

24. a. The pain of trigeminal neuralgia is excruciating and may occur in clusters that continue for hours. The condition is considered benign with no major effects except the pain. Corneal exposure is a problem in Bell's palsy or it may occur after surgery for the treatment of trigeminal neuralgia. Maintaining optimal nutrition is important but not urgent. Chewing may trigger trigeminal neuralgia and the patient then avoids eating. Except during an attack, there is no change in facial appearance in a patient with trigeminal neuralgia. Body image is more disturbed in response to the paralysis typical of Bell's palsy.

25. a. Glycerol rhizotomy causes less sensory loss and fewer sensory aberrations with comparable pain relief and less danger than microvascular decompression and percutaneous radiofrequency rhizotomy, although these provide greater pain relief. Gamma knife radiosurgery provides precise high doses of radiation useful for persistent pain after other surgery.

26. c. Because attacks of trigeminal neuralgia may be precipitated by hot or cold air movement on the face, jarring movements, or talking, the environment should be of moderate temperature and free of drafts. The patient should not be expected to converse during the acute period. Patients often prefer to carry out their own oral care because they are afraid someone else may inadvertently injure them or precipitate an attack. The nurse should stress that oral hygiene be done because patients often avoid it. Residual food in the mouth after eating occurs more often with Bell's palsy.

27. a, d, e, f. Bell's palsy affects the motor branches of the facial nerve. Herpes simplex virus 1 or herpes zoster virus may be a precipitating factor. Moist heat, gentle massage, electrical nerve stimulation, and exercises are prescribed. Care must be taken to protect the eye with sunglasses and artificial tears or gel. Taping the eyelid closed at night may be helpful. Bell's palsy is treated with corticosteroids (usually prednisone), not antiseizure drugs. Oral hygiene is important. Avoiding hot foods is not needed.

28. a. The most serious complication of Guillain-Barré syndrome is respiratory failure. It is essential that respiratory rate and depth, ABGs, and vital capacity are monitored to detect involvement of autonomic nerves that affect respiration. Corticosteroids do not appear to have an effect on the prognosis or duration of the disease. Rather, plasmapheresis or high-dose immunoglobulin result in shortening recovery time. The involvement of peripheral nerves of the sympathetic and parasympathetic nervous systems in the disease may cause orthostatic hypotension,

hypertension, and abnormal vagal responses affecting the heart. Guillain-Barré syndrome may affect the lower brainstem and cranial nerves (CNs) VII, VI, III, XII, V, and X, affecting facial, eye, and swallowing functions.

29. c. As nerve involvement ascends, it is very frightening for the patient. While 80% of patients with Guillain-Barré syndrome recover completely with care, 65% may have a residual weakness. Patients have a poor prognosis but recover if ventilatory support is provided during respiratory failure. Guillain-Barré syndrome affects only peripheral nerves and does not affect the brain.

30. b. The patient with chronic inflammatory demyelinating polyneuropathy (CIDP) will respond to corticosteroids, and the patient with Guillain-Barré syndrome will not. Both patients will benefit from rehabilitation, plasmapheresis, and IV immunoglobulin.

31. a. Tetanus is transmitted through wound contamination, causes painful tonic spasms or seizures, and can be prevented with immunization.

Case Study

1. **Indicated**: maintain MAP > 85 mm Hg (to maintain adequate spinal cord perfusion), maintain SpO_2 > 92% (cervical level SCIs are associated with respiratory impairment), monitor $EtCO_2$ (can help indicate the need for intubation), administer a PPI (or H2 antagonist to prevent GI stress ulcer); **Contraindicated**: raise HOB to 45°(patients with SCI of T5 and above are predisposed to being hemodynamically unstable due to neurogenic shock); turn patient every 2 hours (patients with spinal cord injuries should be logrolled when necessary, but the nurse should place SCI patients on kinetic beds to reduce the chance of causing further injury by turning the patient every 2 hours); **Non-essential**: encourage use of incentive spirometer and performing ROM exercises (are not priorities during the acute phase of care as the focus of care are *ABCs* and to make sure the patient's SCI is stabilized and secondary injuries from tissue swelling are being treated)

2. **1**=famotidine; **2**=methylprednisolone; **3**=anticoagulant; **4**=anticholinergic; **5**=prevent VTE; **6**=treat hypotension (resulting from neurogenic shock); **7**=treat bradycardia (resulting from neurogenic shock); **8**=extravasation (can occur when not using a central line for administration); **9**=hyperglycemia

3. A., C., E., F. It is important for the nurse to assess for urinary retention or a kinked urinary catheter, if applicable. If urinary retention occurs, the nurse should straight catheterize the patient to eliminate the stimulus causing autonomic dysreflexia (AD). Since rectal stimulation, including fecal impaction or constipation, can also cause AD, stool elimination should be promoted using stool softeners and laxatives. Neck alignment is important to treat a cervical SCI, but isn't relevant to AD. If the patient experiences symptoms of AD, such as high blood pressure, throbbing headache, flushing above the injury level, the nurse should raise the HOB to decrease BP. Visual changes can be a sign of AD. Logrolling isn't relevant to preventing or treating AD, but it is important to not cause further injury. Acetaminophen won't treat AD which is causing the headache. The underlying cause needs to be eliminated.

4. **Therapeutic**: "Tell me how you are feeling." (Opens up communication and allows patients to express themselves),

"You may experience depression, but there is professional help if you need it." (Grieving the loss of function and an old way of living is expected and depression may result. This response is truthful while offering support.), "Rehabilitation can help you function at your highest potential." (This is the goal of rehab); **Nontherapeutic**: "You only have an incomplete spinal cord injury, so you have a good chance for a full recovery." (This diminishes the patient's injury and is misleading as the patient may not fully recover, which may mean to her that she will resume her life the same as it was before the injury), "You shouldn't be angry, unfortunately these accidents happen." (The patient should be allowed to be angry and express these feelings openly, it is also dismissive), "I understand how you feel." (The focus should be on the patient and by using *I* you are now the focus. No one can fully understand how they feel especially if never experiencing this type of life-altering injury.), "You must eventually accept what has happened to you." (The goal will be to make adjustments to her life, not necessarily accept what has happened. Patients shouldn't be told how to feel.)

5. **Effective**: wearing a T-shirt under the vest (for comfort and to absorb perspiration is acceptable), pin site care with hydrogen peroxide (can use chlorhexidine, water, or possibly antibiotic ointment), reporting fevers (may be a sign of infection related to the pin sites); **Ineffective**: wearing high heels (wearing flats are recommended, high-heels may cause patients to lose their balance and fall), sheepskin pad cannot be washed (this is not true), severe headaches mean the pins are too tight (headaches are more likely a sign of autonomic dysreflexia); **Unrelated**: avoid wearing tight clothing (this is unrelated to wearing a halo vest, but could cause autonomic dysreflexia to occur)

CHAPTER 66

1. a. Epiphysis; b. diaphysis; c. articular cartilage; d. spongy bone; e. epiphyseal line; f. red marrow cavities; g. compact bone; h. medullary cavity; i. yellow marrow; j. periosteum

2. a. Periosteum; b. canaliculi; c. blood vessels; d. osteon

3. a. Joint cavity with synovial fluid; b. bursa; c. tendon sheath; d. articular cartilage; e. bone; f. periosteum; g. joint capsule; h. nerve; i. blood vessel; j. synovial membrane; k. bone

4. c. Osteoblasts form bone. Osteocytes are mature bone cells. Osteoclasts are responsible for the resorption of bone. A sarcomere is the contractile unit of myofibrils.

5. b. *Atrophy* describes a decrease in muscle size. Hyaline is the most common type of cartilage tissue. *Isometric* describes a muscle contraction that produces hypertrophy. *Hypertrophy* refers to the increase in the size of cells, causing an increase in the organ.

6. d. A loss of elasticity in ligaments and tendons increases stiffness in the neck, shoulders, back, hips, and knees of older patients. Actin (thin) filaments and myosin (thick) filaments make up the contractile unit of the myofibrils, which decrease in strength with lack of use. Fascia is connective tissue that can withstand limited stretching.

7. d. Periosteum is the fibrous connective tissue covering bone. Synovium is the lining of a joint capsule. *Striated* refers to a characteristic of skeletal muscle. Hyaline is the most common type of cartilage.

8. a. The function of the tendon is to attach muscle to bone. The ligament attaches bone to bone at the joint. Fascia

encloses individual muscles but does not connect cartilage to muscle in joints. The bursae are lined with synovial membrane; they are located in joints to relieve pressure and decrease friction between moving parts.

9. a, c, e, f. *Abduction* is moving the part away from the midline of the body, and *adduction* is moving the part toward the midline of the body. These movements can be done with the hip, wrist, thumb, and shoulder. The knee and elbow move with flexion and extension.

10. d. Loss of water from discs between vertebrae, vertebral disc compression, and narrowing of intervertebral spaces all contribute to a loss of height in the older adult. Although bone density decreases and cartilage is lost from joints, these do not affect the long bones or the height of the person.

11. d. Exercise will decrease the older adult's risk of falls. Loss of muscle mass and strength, decreased motor neurons, limited movement because of joint changes, cartilage

deterioration, and less flexible tendons and ligaments are changes that contribute to this risk. Although rest and nutrients are important, fatigue and a high risk for impaired skin integrity are not directly related to changes associated with aging in the musculoskeletal system. Being overweight will increase stress on joints. Providing all care only contributes to weakening of muscles and decreased independence.

12. a. Corticosteroids affect both bone and muscle function by causing avascular necrosis with tiny breaks in bone tissue; protein catabolism with skeletal muscle wasting; and increased osteoclast activity with loss of bone mass, which can have a marked detrimental effect on mobility and activity. Potassium-depleting diuretics may cause hypokalemia, which is associated with muscle weakness and cramps. Oral hypoglycemic drugs and nonsteroidal antiinflammatory drugs (NSAIDs) are not known to affect the musculoskeletal system.

13.

Functional Health Pattern	Risk Factor for or Response to Musculoskeletal Problem
Health perception–health management	History of musculoskeletal injuries, poor use of body mechanics or excessive muscular or joint stress, family history of joint and bone disease. Mechanism and circumstances of injury, methods of treatment, current status, need for assistive devices, interference with activities of daily living, safety practices, tetanus and polio immunizations
Nutritional-metabolic	Presence of obesity; inadequate calcium, vitamin D or C, or protein intake
Elimination	Inability to physically access toilet, constipation
Activity-exercise	Limitation or clumsiness of movement. Pain, weakness, crepitus. Extremes of occupational activity and recreational activities—sedentary or heavy use of body
Sleep-rest	Pain interfering with sleep, frequent position changes, bedtime routine
Cognitive-perceptual	Musculoskeletal pain and intensity, pain management measures
Self-perception–self-concept	Loss of body image or self-worth caused by musculoskeletal deformity
Role-relationship	Change in work and family roles and responsibilities caused by immobility or pain. Available assistance
Sexuality-reproductive	Decreased sexual activity and satisfaction because of pain, movement, and positioning
Coping–stress tolerance	Decreased coping ability related to effect of musculoskeletal problems
Value-belief	Cultural or religious beliefs that influence the patient's acceptance of treatment related to diet, exercise, medication, or lifestyle modifications

14. 4. Muscle strength is graded on a scale of 0 to 5, with 0 = no detection of muscle contraction and 5 = active movement against full resistance without evident fatigue (normal). Active movement against gravity and some resistance = 4. (See Table 61.4.)

15. b. Because a short-leg gait is noticed, the length of both legs should be measured between the anterosuperior iliac crest and the bottom of the medial malleolus; both sides should be compared. Palpating for crepitus will identify friction between bones, usually at joints. Joint movement and muscle mass size may affect gait in various ways, but differences in limb length will always affect gait.

16. c. A goniometer is a protractor device that measures the angle of joints and can be used to determine specific degrees of joint range of motion (ROM). It is used when a specific musculoskeletal problem that affects ROM has been identified. An ergometer measures the amount of work done by a muscle. A myometer measures the extent of muscle contraction. A peak flow meter measures peak expiratory flow for asthma patients.

17. b. Scoliosis is a lateral "S" curve of the thoracic and lumbar spine. Lordosis is an exaggerated lumbar curvature or swayback. *Ankylosis* refers to fixation of a joint. Kyphosis is an exaggerated forward thoracic curvature.

18. c. A contracture is shortening of a muscle or ligament that causes resistance of movement. A fluid-filled cyst is a ganglion cyst. Generalized muscle pain is myalgia. Crepitation is a grating sensation between bones with movement.

19. d. With torticollis, the neck twisted in an unusual position to 1 side; the nurse should provide enough pillows to support the patient's head comfortably. An immobilizer to hold bones in place may be used with dislocation or for a joint with subluxation. Exercises to increase or maintain muscle strength and maintain ROM are appropriate for most patients. Pillows to support the knees while sleeping may be done for valgum or varum deformities or for any patient's comfort.

20. c. Plantar fasciitis presents as burning sharp pain at the sole of the foot that is worse in the morning. Pes planus

is abnormal flatness of the sole and arch of the foot. Tenosynovitis involves inflammation and swelling of a tendon, with pain along a tendon sheath. Muscle atrophy presents as flabby-appearing muscle with decreased function and tone.

21. d. Steppage gait uses increased hip and knee flexion to clear the foot from the floor, and then the foot slaps down on the walking surface. Ataxic gait is a staggering, uncoordinated gait, often with a sway. Spastic gait has short steps with dragging of the foot in a jerky cross-knee movement. Antalgic gait has a shortened stride with as little weight bearing as possible on the painful side.

22. c. A standard x-ray evaluates structural or functional changes of bones and joints and can help in determination of bone density. Myelogram is a sensitive test for nerve impingement and can detect very subtle lesions and injuries. Arthroscopy involves visualizing the inside of joint; it is used to diagnose, or repair joint problems. MRI is used to view soft tissue.

23. d. Dual energy x-ray absorptiometry (DEXA) measures bone mass of spine, femur, forearm, and total body. It is used to diagnose osteoporosis and monitor changes in bone density with treatment. Bone scan is done with the injection of a radioisotope that is taken up by the bone to identify osteomyelitis and primary and metastatic malignant lesions. A diskogram is an x-ray with contrast media to evaluate intervertebral disc abnormalities. Quantitative ultrasound (QUS) evaluates density, elasticity, and strength of bone, and is commonly performed at the calcaneus (heel).

24. c, d, e, f. Increases in rheumatoid factor (RF), antinuclear antibody (ANA), and anticyclic citrullinated peptide (anti-CCP) may occur in rheumatoid arthritis. Increased C-reactive protein (CRP) and presence of human leukocyte antigen (HLA)-B27 may be found. Uric acid may be elevated in gout. Anti-DNA antibody is the most specific test for systemic lupus erythematosus.

CHAPTER 67

1. d. Almost all older adults have some degree of decreased muscle strength, joint stiffness, and pain with motion. Warming up before and strengthening exercises help decrease aches and pains. Musculoskeletal problems in the older adult can be prevented with appropriate strategies, especially exercise. Walkers and canes should be used as necessary to decrease stress on joints so activity can be maintained. Stair walking can create enough stress on fragile bones to cause a hip fracture.

2. b. An avulsion fracture occurs when a ligament pulls a bone fragment loose. The pain is similar to a sprain. A fracture with 2 or more fragments is a comminuted fracture. A spiral fracture is twisted around a bone shaft. A transverse fracture occurs when the line of fracture is at right angles to the longitudinal axis.

3. c. A pathologic fracture is a spontaneous fracture at the site of bone disease, such as osteoporosis. An open fracture occurs when there is communication with the external environment. The oblique fracture has a slanted fracture line. A greenstick fracture is splintered on the convex side, and the other side is in intact with a concave bend.

4. d. Carpal tunnel syndrome would be expected related to continuous wrist movements. Injuries of the meniscus

(fibrocartilage in the knee) are common with athletes. Radial-ulnar fractures are seen with great force, such as a fall or a car accident. Rotator cuff injuries occur with sudden adduction forces applied to the cuff while the arm is held in abduction. They are often seen with repetitive overhead motions.

5. c. Bursitis is inflammation of the synovial membrane sac at friction sites. Tearing of a ligament is a sprain. Stretching of muscle and fascia sheath is a strain. Incomplete separation of articular surfaces of joints caused by ligament injury is subluxation.

6. b. Rest, ice, compression, and elevation (RICE) are indicated to decrease edema resulting from sprains and some strains. Muscle spasms are usually treated with heat application and massage. Repetitive strain injuries require cessation of the precipitating activity and physical therapy. Dislocations or subluxations require immediate reduction and immobilization to prevent vascular impairment and bone cell death.

7. a, b, c, e. Consider the principle of RICE. *R*est: movement should be restricted. *I*ce: cold should be used to promote vasoconstriction and reduce edema. *C*ompression: helps decrease swelling. *E*levate: the extremity above the level of the heart. Mild nonsteroidal antiinflammatory drugs (NSAIDs) may be needed to manage pain. Warm, moist compresses may be used after 48 hours for 20 to 30 minutes at a time to reduce swelling and provide comfort.

8. a. Ossification is the stage of fracture healing when there is clinical union and enough strength to prevent movement at the fracture site. Remodeling is the return to preinjury structural strength and shape. Consolidation is when the distance between bone fragments eventually closes and radiologic union first occurs. The callus formation stage appears by the end of the second week of injury, when minerals and new bone matrix are deposited in the osteoid produced in the granulation tissue stage.

9. a, b, c, e. When the remodeling stage of healing occurs, radiologic union is present. Excess bone tissue is resorbed in the final stage of healing and union is complete. The bone gradually returns to its preinjury structure strength and shape. The osteoblasts and osteoclasts function normally in response to physical loading stress. The fracture hematoma stage occurs when the hematoma at the ends of the fragments becomes a semisolid blood clot. There is an unorganized network of bone composed of cartilage, osteoblasts, calcium, and phosphorus woven around fracture parts in the callus formation stage.

10. b. Deformity is the cardinal sign of fracture but may not be apparent in all fractures. Other supporting signs include edema and swelling, localized pain and tenderness, muscle spasm, ecchymosis, loss of function, crepitation, and an inability to bear weight.

11. a. A malunion occurs when the bone heals in the expected time but in an unsatisfactory position, possibly resulting in deformity or dysfunction. Nonunion occurs when the fracture fails to heal completely despite treatment. Delayed union is healing of the fracture at a slower rate than expected. In posttraumatic osteoporosis, the loss of bone substances occurs as a result of immobilization.

12. a. Open reduction involves use of a surgical incision to visualize the fracture and correct bone alignment. The main disadvantage is the risk of infection. Anesthesia

complications are also possible. Preexisting medical conditions may have impact on surgical success. Skin irritation and nerve impairment are most likely with skin traction. Prolonged immobility is possible with skeletal traction.

13. d. Abdominal pain or pressure, nausea, and vomiting are signs of cast syndrome that occur when hip spica casts or body jacket braces cause compression of the superior mesenteric artery against the duodenum because of swelling or tight application. The cast may have to be split or removed, and the HCP should be notified. Elevation is not indicated for a spica cast. The patient with a spica cast should not be placed in the prone position during the initial drying stage because the cast may break because it is so large and heavy. A cast should never be covered with a blanket because heat builds up in the cast and may cause tissue damage.

14. b. Tetanus prevention is always indicated if the patient has not been immunized or does not have a current booster. Infection is the greatest risk with an open fracture, and all open fractures are considered contaminated. Although prophylactic antibiotics are used in management of open fractures, neither recent antibiotic therapy nor previous injury to the site is relevant. Dirt or gravel contamination will be evident on physical assessment.

15. d. Sensation, motor function, and pain distal to the injury should be checked before and after splinting to assess for nerve damage. Document results to avoid doubts about whether a problem discovered later was missed during the original examination or was caused by the treatment. Peripheral vascular assessment is needed and the HCP is notified. Elevation of the limb and application of ice should be instituted after the extremity is splinted.

16. c. Neurologic assessment includes evaluation of sensation, motor function, and pain in the upper extremity. Ask the patient to abduct the fingers (ulnar nerve), oppose the thumb and small fingers (median nerve), and flex and extend the wrist (or fingers if in a cast) (radial nerve). The nurse will assess pain and sensory function in the fingers. Evaluation of the feet would occur in lower extremity injuries. Assessment of color, temperature, capillary refill, peripheral pulses, and edema evaluates vascular condition.

17. b. A patient with any type of cast should exercise the joints above and below the cast frequently. Moving the fingers will improve circulation and help prevent edema. Unlike plaster casts, thermoplastic resin or fiberglass casts are relatively waterproof. If they become wet, they can be dried with a hair dryer on low setting. Tape petals are used on plaster casts to protect the edges from breaking and crumbling but are not needed for synthetic casts. After the cast is applied, the extremity should be elevated at the level of the heart to promote venous return. Ice may be used to prevent edema.

18. c. Pain that is distal to the injury and unrelieved by opioid analgesics is the earliest sign of compartment syndrome; paresthesia is also an early sign. Paralysis and absence of peripheral pulses will eventually occur if there is no treatment, but these are late signs that often appear after permanent damage has occurred. The overlying skin may appear normal because the surface vessels are not occluded.

19. a. Soft tissue edema in the area of the injury may cause increased pressure within the closed tissue compartments formed by the nonelastic fascia, causing compartment syndrome. If symptoms occur, surgical incision of fascia may be needed (*fasciotomy*). Amputation is usually needed only if the limb becomes septic because of untreated compartment syndrome.

20. c. A fractured humerus may cause radial nerve and brachial artery damage. It may be reduced nonsurgically with a hanging arm cast. A fractured tibia and femur are in the leg. The Colles' fracture is in the wrist and manifests with pronounced swelling and obvious deformity of the wrist. It is treated with closed manipulation and immobilization.

21. c. A Colles' fracture most often occurs in patients over 50 years of age with osteoporosis, frequently when the patient attempts to break a fall with an outstretched arm and hand. Dislocation is the complete separation of articular surfaces of the joint caused by a ligament injury. Open fracture occurs when there is communication with the external environment. A fracture is incomplete if only part of the bone shaft is fractured and the bone is still in 1 piece.

22. a, c. Airway patency and cervical spinal cord injury are the emergency considerations with facial fractures. Oral examination and cranial nerve assessment will be done after the patient is stabilized. Immobilization of the jaw is done surgically for a mandibular fracture.

23. b. The spine should be kept straight by turning the shoulders and hips together (logrolling). This keeps the spine in good alignment until union has been accomplished. Bed rest may be required for a short time but not until the pain is gone. Bone cement is used by the surgeon to stabilize vertebral compression fractures. Analgesics should be taken only as ordered. If they do not manage the pain, the HCP should be notified.

24. a. Initial manifestations of fat embolism usually occur 24 to 48 hours after injury. They are associated with fractures of long bones and multiple fractures related to pelvic injuries, including fractures of the femur, tibia, ribs, and pelvis. Venous thromboemboli (VTEs) tend to form later after injury of the extremities and pelvis.

25. c. Patients with fractures are at risk for both fat embolism and pulmonary embolism from VTE, but there is a difference in the time of occurrence. Fat embolism occurs shortly after the injury and thrombotic embolism occurring several days after immobilization. They both may cause pulmonary symptoms of chest pain, tachypnea, dyspnea, apprehension, tachycardia, and cyanosis. However, only fat embolism may cause petechiae found around the neck, anterior chest wall, axilla, buccal membrane of the mouth, and conjunctiva of the eye.

26. a. A hip prosthesis is usually used for intracapsular fractures. The other options are all for extracapsular fractures.

27. d. The classic signs of a hip fracture are external rotation and shortening of the leg accompanied by severe pain at the fracture site. Additional injury could be caused by weight bearing on the extremity. The patient may not be able to move the hip or the knee, but movement in the ankle and toes is not affected.

28. c. Although surgical repair is the preferred method of managing intracapsular and extracapsular hip fractures, patients may be treated initially with skin traction (e.g., Buck's traction) to relieve the painful muscle spasms before surgery is performed. Prolonged traction would be required

to reduce the fracture or immobilize it for healing, creating a very high risk for complications of immobility.

29. a. Because the fracture site is internally fixed with pins or plates, the fracture site is stable and the patient is moved from the bed to the chair on the first postoperative day. Ambulation begins on the first or second postoperative day without weight bearing on the affected leg. Weight bearing on the affected extremity is usually restricted for 6 to 12 weeks until adequate healing is evident on x-ray. Abductor pillows are used for patients who have total hip replacements by the posterior surgical approach. The patient may be positioned on the operative side following internal fixation as prescribed by the HCP.

30. d. Having someone else put the patient's socks and shoes on for patients with hip prostheses with a posterior approach will protect the patient from extreme flexion, adduction, or internal rotation for at least 6 weeks to prevent dislocation of the prosthesis. Gradual weight bearing on the limb is allowed and ambulation should be encouraged. The leg should be not be internally rotated but kept in a neutral position.

31. c. The low-bulk, high-carbohydrate liquid diet and intake of air through a straw after mandibular fixation often lead to constipation and flatus, which may be relieved with bulk-forming laxatives, prune juice, and ambulation. Hard candy should not be held in the mouth. Wires or rubber bands should be cut only in the case of cardiac or respiratory arrest, and the patient should be taught to clear the mouth of vomitus or secretions. The mouth should be thoroughly cleaned with water, saline, or alkaline mouthwashes or using a Water Pik as necessary to remove food debris.

32. c. The compression dressing or bandage supports the soft tissues, reduces edema, hastens healing, minimizes pain, and promotes residual limb shrinkage. If the dressing is left off, edema will form quickly and may delay rehabilitation. Elevation and ice will not be as effective at preventing the edema that will form. Dressing the incision with dry gauze will not provide the benefits of a compression dressing.

33. b. Phantom limb sensation or pain may occur after amputation, especially if pain was present in the affected limb preoperatively, and is a real sensation to the patient. It will first be treated with analgesics and other pain interventions (i.e., tricyclic antidepressants, antiseizure drugs, transcutaneous electrical nerve stimulation [TENS], mirror therapy, acupuncture). As recovery and ambulation progress, phantom limb sensation usually subsides.

34. a. Because the device covers the residual limb, the surgical site cannot be directly seen, and postoperative hemorrhage is not apparent on dressings. This requires vigilant assessment of vital signs for signs of bleeding. Elevation of the residual limb with an immediate prosthetic fitting is not necessary because the device itself prevents edema formation. Leg exercises are not done in the immediate postoperative period to avoid disruption of ligatures and the suture line.

35. a. Flexion contractures, especially of the hip, may be debilitating and delay rehabilitation for the patient with a leg amputation. To prevent hip flexion, the patient should avoid sitting in a chair with the hips flexed or having pillows under the surgical extremity for prolonged periods. The patient should lie on the abdomen for 30 minutes 3 to 4 times a day to extend the hip.

36. a. Skin breakdown on the residual limb can delay the use of a prosthesis, so the limb should be inspected every day for signs of irritation or pressure areas. A residual limb shrinker is an elastic stocking that is used to mold the limb in preparation for prosthesis use. A cotton residual limb sock is worn with the prosthesis. Range-of-motion (ROM) exercises are not necessary when the patient is using a prosthesis. No substances except water and mild soap should be used on the residual limb.

37. c. Debridement removes devitalized tissue from joints. Osteotomy corrects bone deformity by removal of a wedge or slice of bone. Arthrodesis surgically fuses a joint to relieve pain. Synovectomy removes tissue involved in joint destruction from rheumatoid arthritis (RA).

38. c. An arthroplasty is reconstruction or replacement of a joint to relieve pain and correct deformity, especially with osteoarthritis, RA, avascular necrosis, congenital deformity, or dislocation. Arthrodesis is the surgical fusion of a joint to relieve pain. An osteotomy removes a wedge of bone to correct a bone deformity. Synovectomy is used in RA to remove the tissue involved in joint destruction.

39. d. Physical therapy is initiated on the first postoperative day with ambulation using a walker and limited weight bearing for a patient with a cemented prosthesis and non–weight-bearing on the operative side for an uncemented prosthesis. In addition, the patient sits in the chair at least twice a day and is turned to the back and unaffected side with the operative leg supported. Crutches would be difficult to use the first postoperative day.

40. b. During hospitalization, after a total hip arthroplasty with a posterior approach, an abduction pillow is placed between the legs to maintain abduction and the leg is extended. Extremes of internal rotation, adduction, and 90-degree flexion of the hip must be avoided for 4 to 6 weeks postoperatively to prevent dislocation of the prosthesis.

41. b. Continuous passive motion (CPM) machines may be used after knee surgery to promote early joint mobility. Because joint dislocation is not a problem with knee replacements, early ambulation to prevent deep vein thrombosis (DVT) and improve circulation, exercise with straight leg raises, and gentle ROM maybe encouraged postoperatively.

42. b. Neurovascular checks following surgery are essential to detect compromised neurologic and vascular function caused by trauma or edema. Postoperatively, the hands are elevated with a bulky dressing in place. When the dressing is removed, a guided splinting program is started. After discharge, exercises are done 3 to 4 times each day. Before surgery, the patient is taught that the goal of the surgery is to restore function related to grasp, pinch, stability, and strength and the hands, not cosmetic appearance.

43. d. The patient with a tight cast may be at risk for neurovascular compromise (impaired circulation and peripheral nerve damage) and should be assessed first. The other patients should be seen as soon as possible. Providing analgesia for the patient with phantom pain would be the next priority. The patient in skeletal traction needs explanation of the purpose and functioning of the traction. She may need analgesia or muscle relaxants to help tolerate the traction. Checking on the patient being transferred would include reassurance and paperwork completion.

Case Study

1. **Expected**: 2+ dorsalis pedis pulse, RLE edema (due to injury), able to move toes and ankle on RLE; **Unexpected**: RLE feels like pins and needles, RLE is pale and cool, and significant amount of tightness in the RLE (all of these findings could indicate compartment syndrome or compromised circulation); **Unrelated**: burning with urination (not applicable to this injury)

2. **Indicated**: apply ice to RLE (part of RICE, ice reduces swelling), no weight bearing on RLE (bone is unstable, applying weight could displace the fracture and lead to complications), immobilize RLE (part of RICE, stabilizes the fracture), obtain a CBC (assesses bleeding by evaluating the hematocrit and hemoglobin values); **Contraindicated**: SCD to RLE (may impair circulation or dislodge fat embolus or blood clot that developed from the tibial injury), perform ROM exercises with RLE (the extremity needs to be immobilized, performing ROM exercises could worsen the injury and cause complications); **Non-essential**: perform a 12-lead ECG (doesn't apply to this patient unless he complains of chest pain or has a dysrhythmia), administer 1 liter of normal saline solution (no indication for this intervention which would be applicable if the patient was hypotensive or hemorrhaging)

3. **Delegated**: elevate the casted extremity on 2 pillows (the fracture is stabilized with a cast which means it is safe to move the extremity), offer a urinal, measuring vital signs, transporting to x-ray; **Cannot be Delegated**: assessing, teaching and documenting are functions of the RN as is administering an opioid drug.

4. A., C., D., F., G. Patients should not put anything down the cast due to the increased risk of tissue injury. The cast should not get wet. Weight bearing will be decided by the HCP, but until the fracture is healed weight bearing is discouraged. Elevating the extremity above the level of the heart can help reduce swelling thereby reducing pain. It is contraindicated to drive while taking opioids as they can impair judgment, cause drowsiness, and is considered driving under the influence or while intoxicated. Opioids can cause constipation; therefore, increasing fluids, dietary fiber, or taking a stool softener is recommended. Discoloration of the toes should be reported as this may indicate impaired tissue perfusion. Foul odor is not expected and should be reported as this may indicate an infection.

5. 1=Contractures; 2=atrophy; 3=isometric exercises; 4=high-top tennis shoes; 5=Achilles tendon; 6=thermotherapy; 7=muscle spasms

CHAPTER 68

1. b. Chronic infection of the bone leads to formation of scar tissue from granulation tissue. This avascular scar tissue provides an ideal site for continued microorganism growth and is impenetrable to antibiotics. Surgical debridement is often necessary to remove the poorly vascularized tissue and dead bone, and to instill antibiotics directly to the area. Bone and skin grafting may be needed after surgical removal of infection if destruction is extensive. Involucrum is new bone laid down at the infection site, which seals off areas of dead bone (sequestra) that may hold microorganisms that spread to other sites. Antibiotics can be effective during acute osteomyelitis. Prevention of chronic osteomyelitis requires early antibiotic treatment.

2. b. The patient with osteomyelitis is at risk for pathologic fractures at the infection site because of weakened, devitalized bone so careful handling of the extremity is needed. Careful handling of dressings is needed to prevent the spread of infection to others but is not related to preventing injury to this patient. Splints may be used to immobilize the limb. Edema is not a common finding in osteomyelitis. Range-of-motion (ROM) exercises will be limited because of the possibility of spreading infection.

3. c. Because large doses of appropriate antibiotics are needed in the treatment of acute osteomyelitis, it is important to identify the causative microorganism. The definitive way to determine the causative agent is by bone biopsy or biopsy of the soft tissue surrounding the site. The other tests may help establish the diagnosis but do not identify the causative agent.

4. d. Activities, such as exercises that increase circulation and serve as stimuli for the spread of infection, should be avoided by patients with acute osteomyelitis. Oral or IV antibiotic therapy is continued at home for 4 to 6 weeks. The HCP should be notified if increased pain occurs. Weight bearing is contraindicated to prevent pathologic fractures. Monitoring for side effects and complications of antibiotic therapy must be done.

5. b. One of the most common adverse effects of prolonged and high-dose antibiotic therapy is overgrowth of *Candida albicans* in the oral cavity and genitourinary tract. These infections are marked by whitish-yellow, curdlike lesions of the mucosa. A dry, cracked, furrowed tongue is characteristic of severe dehydration and vesicles are characteristic of herpes simplex infections. Mouth and lip ulcers are characteristic of aphthous stomatitis (canker sores).

6. d. Osteochondroma is a benign overgrowth of bone and cartilage near the end of the bone at the growth plate, especially in long bones, pelvis, or scapula. It may transform to a malignant form. Enchondroma is a benign intramedullary cartilage tumor found in a cavity of a single hand or foot bone. Osteoclastoma is a benign bone tumor with a high rate of recurrence but does not become malignant. Ewing's sarcoma develops in the medullary cavity of long bones, especially the femur, humerus, pelvis, and tibia.

7. b. Osteosarcoma, the most common primary bone cancer, occurs in the metaphyseal region of long bones of the arms, legs, or pelvis. It is extremely malignant, metastasizes rapidly, and is often brought to attention by injury. A high rate of local recurrence occurs with osteoclastoma that arises in the cancellous ends of long bones. Ewing's sarcoma develops in the medullary cavity of long bones.

8. b. Promoting muscle activity is important in any patient with muscular dystrophy. However, when the disease has progressed to cardiomyopathy or respiratory failure, activity must be balanced with oxygen supply. At this stage of the disease, care should be taken to prevent skin or respiratory complications. The patient should be encouraged to perform as much self-care and exercise as energy allows, but this will be limited.

9. d. Lumbar disc herniation is generally indicated by radicular pain radiating down the buttock, below the knee,

and along the distribution of the sciatic nerve. Cervical disc disease has pain radiating into the arms and hands. Acute lumbosacral strain causes acute low back pain. Degenerative disc disease is a structural degeneration of discs that often occurs with aging and results in intervertebral discs losing their elasticity, flexibility, and shock-absorbing capabilities.

10. a. Proper daily stretching and strengthening exercises are an important part of the prevention of back injury, with the goal of maintaining mobility and strength in the back. Patients should sit with the knees level with the hips and should sleep in a side-lying position, with knees and hips bent, or on the back, with a device to flex the hips and knees. Good body mechanics with proper transfer and turning techniques are necessary in all jobs and activities.

11. b. Urinary incontinence after spinal surgery may indicate nerve damage and should be reported to the HCP. Paralytic ileus is not unexpected after this type of surgery. Pain at the graft site, usually the iliac crest or the fibula, is more often severe than pain at the fused area. Although movement and sensation of the arms and legs should not be more impaired than before surgery, deficits are not often relieved immediately after surgery.

12. c. After spinal surgery, patients are logrolled to maintain straight alignment of the spine. This involves turning the patient with a pillow between the legs and moving the body as a unit. The head of the bed is usually kept flat and the legs are extended.

13. a. A plantar wart is a painful papillomatous growth on the sole of the foot. Thickened skin on the weight-bearing part of the foot is a callus. Local thickening of skin caused by pressure on bony prominences is a corn. A tumor on nerve tissue between the third and fourth metatarsal heads is a Morton's neuroma.

14. c. This patient has a hallux valgus (bunion) that will be treated surgically by removing the bursal sac and bony enlargement and correcting the lateral angle of great toe. Metatarsal arch support is conservative treatment for hammer toe. A corn is trimmed with a scalpel after softening. Intraarticular corticosteroids and passive manual stretching are conservative treatment for hallux rigidus from osteoarthritis.

15. c. Poorly fitted shoes selected for fashion rather than comfort are the primary factor in the development of foot problems. A few congenital problems predispose to foot problems. Poor hygiene in patients with peripheral vascular disease may lead to foot infections but these factors are in the minority compared with the effect of ill-fitting shoes.

16. c, f. Paget's disease involves abnormal remodeling and resorption of bone with replacement of normal marrow with vascular connective tissue. Osteoporosis is loss of total bone mass and substance with abnormal remodeling and resorption of bone; it is most common in bones of the spine, hips, and wrists. Osteomalacia results from vitamin D deficiency and causes generalized bone decalcification with bone deformity.

17. b, d, e. Risk factors for osteoporosis include age >65 years, white or Asian ethnicity, cigarette smoking, low body weight, inactive lifestyle, and estrogen deficiency (either postmenopausal, or from premature or surgical menopause). Other factors include family history; diet low in calcium; vitamin D deficiency; excessive alcohol use;

and long-term use of medications, such as corticosteroids, thyroid replacement, heparin, long-acting sedatives, or antiseizure drugs.

18. b, c. Increased calcium and vitamin D intake and weight-bearing exercises (i.e., walking) are the best methods to prevent osteoporosis in postmenopausal women. Beef is not high in calcium or vitamin D. Although 20 minutes in the sun each day provides vitamin D for most women, postmenopausal women should take supplemental vitamin D doses of 800 to 1000 IU per day. Although estrogen replacement may protect the woman against bone loss and fractures, it is no longer given specifically to prevent osteoporosis because of increased risk of heart disease and breast or uterine cancer.

19. a. The bisphosphonates, such as alendronate, must be taken with a full glass of water at least 30 minutes before food or other medications to promote their absorption. Because they are very irritating to the stomach and esophagus, the patient must remain upright for at least 30 minutes after taking these medications to prevent reflux into the esophagus. Although these drugs will prevent further bone loss and increase bone density, calcium and vitamin D supplementation is still needed for bone formation.

Case Study

1. **Risk factors**: weight (patient is obese), occupation (sits for long periods of time), smokes cigarettes (impairs circulation to intervertebral discs contributing to low back pain); **Unrelated**: height, BP, history of femur fracture, age (he is 38-years-old, which is considered young; older adults > 50 are at greater risk)

2. **Indicated**: MRI, leg raise test (an increased pain response indicates nerve root irritation or muscle strain), epidural venogram (may be necessary if other tests are not conclusive); **Unrelated**: ABG (arterial blood gas evaluates ventilation and oxygenation), PET scan (evaluates diseases in the body, such as cancer), CBC (isn't indicated for an orthopedic injury that isn't associated with blood loss), lumbar puncture (obtains CSF for analysis)

3. The following should be highlighted as signs of cauda equina syndrome: urge to urinate but is unable and has a bladder scan of 650 mL (urinary retention), right inner thigh and buttocks are numb (Saddle anesthesia), weakness (3/5 dorsiplantar flexion) in RLE, increased pain with leg raise test. **Not chosen**: 5 out of 10 pain is moderate not severe; tingling in the toes is expected with low back pain or injury and is unrelated to cauda equina syndrome; the remaining descriptions are expected findings or are unrelated to this syndrome.

4. **Indicated**: assess dressing (for any signs of active bleeding and prevent contamination of the incision), report complaints of a headache to the HCP (could indicate a CSF leak), encourage the use of an incentive spirometer (to prevent atelectasis and promote oxygenation), place pillows under knees and thighs (supports lower back and reduces pain and strain at the incision site); **Contraindicated**: have the patient turn independently (patient should be logrolled which requires several people to assist; he shouldn't be twisting to turn), raise HOB if patient reports a headache (patients should be supine if a CSF leak is suspected); **Non-essential**: keep the HOB supine at all times (is unnecessary unless patient has a CSF leak),

collaborate with occupational therapy (physical therapy should be consulted), report lower extremity weakness that was present preoperatively (this is considered a baseline finding, meaning it was present before surgery; only new changes from baseline should be reported to the HCP)

5. B., C., E., F., G. Patients with back pain or who are status-post back surgery shouldn't be lifting anything heavier than 5-10 pounds. Physical therapy will teach appropriate exercises and ergonomics. Standing or sitting for long periods of time should be avoided. Patients should sleep on a firm mattress, supine with legs and thighs supported by pillows. Any motor or sensation deficits that weren't present preoperatively should be reported to the patient's HCP. This patient's occupation as a truck driver, which requires sitting for long periods, will prevent him from going back to work in 2 weeks. Patients should avoid twisting and stretching, unless advised by PT, and may be required to wear a brace or orthotics.

CHAPTER 69

1. d. Cartilage destruction in the joints affects most adults by the age of 40 years. When the destruction becomes symptomatic, osteoarthritis (OA) is said to be present. Degenerative changes cause symptoms after age 50 or 60 years. More than half of adults over age 65 years have x-ray evidence of OA. Joint pain and functional disability are not to be considered a normal finding in aging persons. OA is not a systemic disease but may be caused by a known event or condition that directly damages cartilage or causes joint instability (e.g., menopause, obesity).

2. a. 3; b. 5; c. 6; d. 1; e. 4; f. 2

3. d. The pain in later OA is caused by bone surfaces rubbing together after the articular cartilage has deteriorated. Crepitation occurs earlier in the disease with loose particles of cartilage in the joint cavity. Bouchard's nodes and Heberden's nodes are tender; they occur as joint space decreases and appear as early as 40 years of age.

4. b. Principles of joint protection and energy conservation are critical in being able to maintain functional mobility in the patient with OA. Help patients find ways to perform activities and tasks with less stress. ROM, isotonic, and isometric exercises of the affected joints should be balanced with joint rest and protection. During an acute flare of joint inflammation, the joints should be rested. If a joint is painful, it should be used only to the point of pain and masking the pain with analgesics may lead to greater joint injury.

5. a. Results from studies on the use of glucosamine and chondroitin have been mixed. The American College of Rheumatology and American Academy of Orthopaedic Surgeons do not recommend their use. The nurse should encourage the patient to discuss all herbs and supplements with the HCP before taking them.

6. a. Common side effects of nonsteroidal antiinflammatory drugs (NSAIDs) include gastrointestinal (GI) irritation and bleeding, dizziness, rash, headache, and tinnitus. Misoprostol is used to prevent NSAID-induced gastric ulcers. Gastritis and would increase the patient's tolerance of any of the NSAIDs. Naproxen could cause the same gastric effects as ibuprofen. It is generally recommended that the daily dose of acetaminophen should not exceed 3

g/day to prevent liver damage. Antacids interfere with the absorption of NSAIDs.

7. a. OA is not systemic or symmetric. In OA, morning joint stiffness resolves in about 30 minutes. Rheumatoid arthritis (RA) is often rheumatoid factor (RF) positive, occurs more in women than men, is systemic, and affects small joints symmetrically. In RA, morning joint stiffness lasts 60 minutes to all day.

8. d. Pain and immobility of OA may be aggravated by falling barometric pressure. OA primarily first affects weight-bearing joints of knees and hips. Stiffness occurs on arising but usually resolves after 30 minutes. Pain during the day is relieved with rest. Fatigue, anorexia, and weight loss are nonspecific manifestations of the onset of RA.

9. c. In early disease, the fingers of the patient with moderate RA may become spindle shaped from synovial hypertrophy and thickening of the joint capsule. The patient may not have joint deformities but may have limited joint mobility, adjacent muscle atrophy, and inflammation. Splenomegaly may be found with Felty syndrome in those with severe nodule-forming RA. Heberden's nodes and crepitus on movement are associated with OA.

10. d. The antibody to citrullinated peptide (anti-CCP) is more specific than RF for RA and may allow earlier and more accurate diagnosis. Other tests include C-reactive protein (CRP) that is elevated from inflammation of RA, a finding that is useful in monitoring the response to therapy. Anemia, rather than polycythemia, is common. Immunoglobulin G (IgG) levels are normal. The white blood cell (WBC) count may be increased in response to inflammation and is also elevated in synovial fluid.

11. b. Rheumatoid nodules develop in about half of patients with RA. Felty syndrome is most common in patients with long-standing RA. It is characterized by splenomegaly and leukopenia. Sjögren's syndrome occurs as a disease by itself or with other arthritic disorders. Lyme disease is a spirochetal infection transmitted by an infected deer tick bite. Spondyloarthropathies are interrelated multisystem inflammatory disorders that affect the spine, peripheral joints, and periarticular structures; they do not have serum antibodies.

12. b. Etanercept binds to tumor necrosis factor (TNF) and blocks its interaction with the TNF cell surface receptors, thus decreasing the inflammatory response. Anakinra is an interleukin-1 receptor antagonist that also decreases the inflammatory response. Leflunomide is an antiinflammatory that blocks immune cell overproduction. Azathioprine is a rarely used immunosuppressant that inhibits DNA, RNA, and protein synthesis.

13. b. Certolizumab is a monoclonal antibody that is a TNF inhibitor. It stays in the system longer and may cause a rapid reduction in RA symptoms. Parenteral gold alters immune responses that may suppress synovitis of active RA, but it takes 3 to 6 months to be effective. Tocilizumab blocks the action of the proinflammatory cytokine interleukin-6 (IL-6). Hydroxychloroquine is a slow-acting antimalaria drug used initially for mild RA. Periodic eye examinations are needed with hydroxychloroquine therapy to assess for retinal damage.

14. c. The use of multidrug therapy in RA is particularly problematic in older adults because of the increased likelihood of adverse drug interactions and toxicity.

Rheumatic disorders affect younger and older adults. Older adults are not less compliant with drug treatment but may need help with complex regimens. Interpretation of laboratory values in diagnosing RA in older adults is more difficult because of age-related serologic changes, but the disease can be diagnosed.

15. b. Most patients with RA have morning stiffness. Morning activities should be scheduled later in the day after the stiffness subsides. Taking a warm shower in the morning and allowing time to become more mobile before activity are advised. Ice for 10 minutes or splinting are helpful during increased disease activity. Management of RA includes daily exercises for the affected joints and protection of joints with devices and movements that prevent joint stress.

16. b. Pacing activities and alternating rest with activity are important in maintaining self-care and independence of the patient with RA. These strategies also prevent deconditioning and improve patient attitude. The nurse should not complete activities for the patient but instead should support and assist the patient as necessary. A warm shower or sitting in a tub with warm water and towels over the shoulders may help relieve some stiffness.

17. d. Cold therapy is indicated to relieve pain during an acute inflammation. It can be applied for 10 to 15 minutes at a time with packages of frozen vegetables. Heat in the form of heating pads, moist warm packs, paraffin baths, or warm baths or showers is indicated to relieve stiffness and muscle spasm. Heat should not be applied for more than 20 minutes at a time.

18. c. The best aerobic exercise is aquatic exercise in warm water. This allows easier joint movement because of the buoyancy of the water. Water produces more resistance and can strengthen the muscles. Tai Chi is a gentle, stretching exercise that would be appropriate. Dancing and walking impact the joints of the feet and even low-impact aerobics could be damaging. Exercises for the patient with RA should be gentle.

19. d. The definitive diagnosis of gout is established by finding needle-like monosodium urate crystals in the synovial fluid of an inflamed joint or tophus. Although there is a familial predisposition to hyperuricemia, environmental and genetic factors contribute to gout. Hyperuricemia and elevated urine uric acid are not diagnostic for gout because they may be related to a variety of drugs or may exist as a totally asymptomatic abnormality in the general population.

20. b. Colchicine has an antiinflammatory action specific for gout. It is the treatment of choice during an acute attack, often producing dramatic pain relief when given within 12 to 24 hours. Probenecid is a uricosuric drug used to control hyperuricemia by increasing the renal excretion of uric acid. Aspirin inactivates the effect of uricosuric drugs and should not be used when the patient is taking probenecid or other uricosuric drugs. Allopurinol, a xanthine oxidase inhibitor, is used to control hyperuricemia by blocking uric acid production.

21. b. During therapy with probenecid or allopurinol, the patient must have periodic determination of serum uric acid to evaluate therapy effectiveness and to ensure uric acid is kept low enough to prevent future gout attacks. With the use of medications, strict dietary restrictions on alcohol and high-purine foods are usually not necessary.

When the patient is taking probenecid, urine output should be maintained at 2 to 3 L per day to prevent urate from precipitating in the urinary tract and causing kidney stones. The patient should not change the dose of medication without direction of the HCP. Drugs used for control of gout are not useful in the treatment of an acute attack. Joint immobilization is used for an acute attack of gout.

22. d. An unusually high frequency of human leukocyte antigen (HLA)–B27 is found in patients with ankylosing spondylitis, psoriatic arthritis, and reactive arthritis. These diseases have a predilection for involvement of the peripheral joints (especially lower extremities), sacroiliitis, uveitis, intestinal inflammation, and skin lesions. They are marked by the absence of RF.

23. d. Kyphosis and involvement of costovertebral joints in ankylosing spondylitis lead to a bent-over posture and a decrease in chest expansion. These manifestations are managed with chest expansion and deep-breathing exercises. Postural training emphasizes avoiding forward flexion during any activities. The patient should sleep on the back without using pillows.

24. b, f. Reactive arthritis is self-limiting and follows genitourinary or GI tract infection. Symptoms include urethritis and conjunctivitis. Methotrexate is the first treatment of choice for psoriatic arthritis. Hypersensitive tender points diagnose fibromyalgia. There is increased risk of septic arthritis in the person with decreased host resistance. Joint infection may be caused by the hematogenous route.

25. a. In systemic lupus erythematosus (SLE), autoantibodies are made against nucleic acids, erythrocytes, coagulation proteins, lymphocytes, platelets, and many other self-proteins. This is a hypersensitivity response, not an immunodeficiency. Overproduction of collagen is characteristic of systemic sclerosis. Abnormal IgG reactions with autoantibodies are characteristic of RA.

26. c. All body systems are affected by SLE. Fibrosis of the atrioventricular and sinus nodes and occurrence of dysrhythmias are ominous. Although lupus nephritis can occur and lead to chronic kidney disease, treatment is available. Anemia, mild leukopenia, and thrombocytopenia are often present. Disordered thought processes, disorientation, memory deficits, and depression may occur.

27. b. The patient with SLE often finds that one of the most difficult facets of the disease is its extreme variability in severity and progression. There is no characteristic pattern of progressive organ involvement. SLE is not predictable in terms of which systems may become affected. SLE is now associated with a normal life span, but the patient must be helped to adjust to the unknown course of the disease.

28. a. Efficacy of treatment with corticosteroids or immunosuppressive drugs is best monitored by serial anti-DNA titers and serum complement levels, both of which will decrease as the drugs have an effect. The patient with SLE often has a chronic anemia that is not affected by drug therapy. A reduction in erythrocyte sedimentation rate (ESR) is not as specific.

29. a. Acute exacerbations of SLE may be precipitated by overexposure to ultraviolet light, physical and emotional stress, fatigue, and infection or surgery. Dietary recommendations include small, frequent meals and adequate iron intake. Although SLE has an identified

genetic association with HLA-DR2 and HLA-DR3, genetic counseling is not a usual recommendation. The major concern in planning a pregnancy is the increased risks for the mother and fetus during pregnancy. Exacerbations are common following delivery. Although nonpharmacologic methods of pain management are encouraged, the use of NSAIDs is often needed to help with inflammation and pain.

30. a. Scleroderma is a disorder of connective tissue that causes skin thickening and tightening, resulting in symmetric, painless swelling or thickening of the skin of the fingers and hands, expressionless facial features, puckering of the mouth, and a small oral orifice. It does not cause the swan neck or ulnar drift deformities seen in RA. Low back pain and spinal stiffness are associated with ankylosing spondylitis.

31. d. One of the most common and early manifestations of CREST syndrome (calcinosis, Raynaud's phenomenon, esophageal dysfunction, sclerodactyly, and telangiectasia) is Raynaud's phenomenon. This causes paroxysmal vasospasms of the digits with decreased blood flow to the fingers and toes on exposure to cold or stress, followed by cyanosis and then erythema on rewarming. The hands and feet must be protected from cold exposure and possible burns or cuts that may heal slowly. Smoking is contraindicated. Fluid intake and sensitivity to ultraviolet light are not factors in scleroderma. Cardiovascular involvement may occur but does not require daily monitoring.

32. b. Dermatomyositis produces symmetric weakness of striated muscle. Weak neck and pharyngeal muscles may cause dysphagia. Weakened pharyngeal muscles lead to a poor cough, difficulty swallowing, and increased aspiration risk. Joint involvement, muscle tenderness, and pain are uncommon. During an acute attack the patient is so weak that bed rest and passive ROM are needed.

33. b. The patient with fibromyalgia typically has nonrestorative sleep, morning stiffness, irritable bowel syndrome, and anxiety in addition to the widespread, nonarticular musculoskeletal pain and fatigue. Fibromyalgia is nondegenerative, nonprogressive, and noninflammatory. Neither muscle weakness nor muscle spasms are associated with the disease, although there may be tics in the muscle at the tender points.

34. c. The American College of Rheumatology identifies 2 criteria for the diagnosis of fibromyalgia: (1) pain is experienced in 11 of the 18 tender points on palpation, and (2) a history of widespread pain for at least 3 months. The other findings may be present but are not diagnostic for fibromyalgia.

35. d. The pain and related symptoms of fibromyalgia cause significant stress, and anxiety is a common finding. Stress management is an important part of the treatment and may include any of the commonly used relaxation strategies as well as psychologic counseling.

36. a, c, d, g. The diagnostic criteria for SEID include: (1) profound fatigue interfering with occupational, educational, social or personal activities lasting at least 6 months; (2) postexertional malaise (total exhaustion after even minor physical or mental exertion that patients sometimes describe as a "crash"); and (3) unrefreshing sleep with at least 1 of the following manifestations: (a) cognitive impairment ("brain fog"), or (b) worsening of symptoms upon standing (orthostatic intolerance).

Case Study

1. **Rheumatoid arthritis**: age (RA affects young to middle age persons mostly women, such as N.M. who is 36-years-old, while osteoarthritis usually affects those older than 40), fatigue and fever (are not present in osteoarthritis), mild ulnar drift (is a deformity associated with RA); **Osteoarthritis**: overweight (RA is associated with normal to lower body mass while OA is associated with obesity causing stress on joints); **Both**: painful stiff hands and feet (OA is usually localized while RA is more systemic, both involve painful stiff hands and feet in the morning and with activity), puffy hands (OA is an inflammatory disease affecting usually one or more joints on one side of the body, RA is systemic affecting multiple areas of the body)

2. **Indicated**: rheumatoid factor (present in about 80% of patients), C-reactive protein (indicates inflammation), antinuclear antibody (ANA) titer (likely increased in RA), bone scans (are more useful than x-rays to identify joint changes); **Unrelated**: joint ultrasound (ultrasounds are not helpful), electrolyte panel (unnecessary as it doesn't help diagnose RA), V/Q scan (unnecessary as it evaluates ventilation and perfusion in the lungs)

3. **Indicated**: physical therapy (to assist with mobility and appropriate joint exercises), assess for evidence of leukocytosis (an increased WBC is likely to occur in RA due to systemic inflammation), assist with ROM exercises (to improve joint function), use assistive devices as necessary (promotes safety and independence); **Contraindicated**: administer antibiotics (isn't indicated unless patient has a concurrent bacterial infection, antibiotics shouldn't be used unless there is an indication), administer calcium channel blockers (not a therapy to treat RA, will decrease HR and BP which may cause harm); **Non-essential**: restrict purines in her diet (this is applicable to gout to decrease uric acid levels), check urine for hematuria (blood in the urine is not associated with RA)

4. **1**=methotrexate; **2**=report vision changes; **3**=diclofenac; **4**=monoclonal antibody; **5**=may cause orange-yellow urine or skin; **6**=adalimumab; **7**=taper dose to withdrawal from drug; **8**=depletes substance P

5. A., C., D., E., G. Methotrexate is the first drug of choice to treat RA. It is a chemotherapeutic agent but is prescribed in lower doses for RA so patients will not lose their hair. It has a lower risk for toxicity than other drugs. Rare side effects include bone marrow suppression, which increases the risk for infection, and liver toxicity, not kidney failure. Therapeutic effects should occur within 4-6 weeks, but not everyone gets adequate relief from methotrexate alone; therefore, additional drugs may be prescribed. Methotrexate is teratogenic which means pregnancy must be excluded before starting this drug. Women should wait at least 3 months before becoming pregnant after the drug is stopped.